LA volume > 100 cc / m^2
is enlarged

Heart Failure

Heart Failure

A Case-Based Approach

Editor

Peter S. Rahko, MD, FACC, FASE
Professor of Medicine
Division of Cardiovascular Medicine
Department of Medicine
University of Wisconsin School of Medicine and Public Health
Madison, Wisconsin

demosMEDICAL
New York

Visit our website at www.demosmedpub.com

ISBN: 978-1-936287-51-2
e-book ISBN: 978-1-61705-094-7

Acquisitions Editor: Rich Winters
Compositor: Newgen

Library of Congress Cataloging-in-Publication Data
Heart failure (Rahko)
Heart failure : a case-based approach / [edited by] Peter S. Rahko.
p. ; cm.
Includes bibliographical references and index.
ISBN 978-1-936287-51-2 — ISBN 978-1-61705-094-7 (e-book)
I. Rahko, Peter S., editor of compilation. II. Title.
[DNLM: 1. Heart Failure—Case Reports. WG 370]
RC685.C53
616.1'29—dc23

2013024824

Printed in the United States of America by Bradford and Bigelow.

13 14 15 16 17 / 5 4 3 2 1

Contents

Contributors

William T. Abraham, MD, FACP, FACC, FAHA, FESC
Professor of Internal Medicine, Physiology and Cell Biology
Chair of Excellence in Cardiovascular Medicine
Director, Division of Cardiovascular Medicine
Deputy Director, Davis Heart and Lung Research Institute
The Wexner Medical Center at The Ohio State University
Columbus, Ohio

Salman Allana, MD
Fellow in Cardiovascular Medicine
Division of Cardiovascular Medicine
Department of Medicine
University of Wisconsin School of Medicine and Public Health
Madison, Wisconsin

Manrique Alvarez, MD
Fellow in Cardiovascular Diseases
Department of Medicine, Section of Cardiology
Wake Forest University School of Medicine
Winston-Salem, North Carolina

Ebere Chuckwu, MD
Assistant Professor
Department of Medicine, Section of Cardiology
Wake Forest University School of Medicine
Winston-Salem, North Carolina

William G. Cotts, MD, FACP, FACC, FAHA
Clinical Director, Heart Transplantation and Mechanical Assistance
Advocate Christ Medical Center
Oak Lawn, Illinois

Todd F. Dardas, MD, MS
Assistant Professor of Medicine
Division of Cardiology
University of Washington
Seattle, Washington

Brandon Drafts, MD
Fellow in Cardiovascular Diseases
Department of Medicine, Section of Cardiology
Wake Forest University School of Medicine
Winston-Salem, North Carolina

Steven M. Ewer, MD
Assistant Professor of Medicine
Division of Cardiovascular Medicine
Department of Medicine
University of Wisconsin School of Medicine and Public Health
Madison, Wisconsin

Ray E. Hershberger, MD
Professor of Medicine and Director
Division of Human Genetics
The Wexner Medical Center at The Ohio State University
Columbus, Ohio

Mariell Jessup, MD
Professor of Medicine
University of Pennsylvania Perelman School of Medicine
Philadelphia, Pennsylvania

Roy M. John, MD, PhD
Associate Director
Cardiac Electrophysiology Laboratory
Brigham and Women's Hospital;
Assistant Professor of Medicine
Harvard Medical School
Boston, Massachusetts

Maryl R. Johnson, MD
Professor of Medicine
Medical Director, Heart Failure and Transplantation
University of Wisconsin School of Medicine and Public Health
Madison, Wisconsin

Walter Kao, MD
Associate Professor of Medicine
Division of Cardiovascular Medicine
Heart Failure and Transplant Cardiology
University of Wisconsin School of Medicine and Public Health
Madison, Wisconsin

Eric S. Ketchum, MD
Division of Cardiology
Yale University School of Medicine
New Haven, Connecticut

Ryan Kipp, MD
Fellow in Cardiovascular Medicine
Division of Cardiovascular Medicine
Department of Medicine
University of Wisconsin School of Medicine and Public Health
Madison, Wisconsin

Wayne C. Levy, MD
Professor of Medicine
Division of Cardiology
University of Washington
Seattle, Washington

Ana Morales, MS
Certified Genetic Counselor, Assistant Professor
Division of Human Genetics
The Wexner Medical Center at The Ohio State University
Columbus, Ohio

David Murray, MD
Associate Professor of Medicine
University of Wisconsin School of Medicine and Public Health;
Medical Director, Heart Failure and Transplantation
Chief, Section of Cardiology
William S. Middleton Memorial Veteran's Hospital
Madison, Wisconsin

Catherine M. Otto, MD
Professor of Medicine and Cardiology
University of Washington
Seattle, Washington

Adam P. Pleister, MD
Fellow, Advanced Heart Failure and Cardiac Transplant
Division of Cardiovascular Medicine
Department of Internal Medicine
The Wexner Medical Center at The Ohio State University
Columbus, Ohio

Peter S. Rahko MD, FACC, FASE
Professor of Medicine
Division of Cardiovascular Medicine
Department of Medicine
University of Wisconsin School of Medicine and Public Health
Madison, Wisconsin

Scott W. Sharkey, MD
Senior Consulting Cardiologist
Minneapolis Heart Institute Foundation
Minneapolis, Minnesota

Paul Sorajja, MD
Professor of Medicine
Division of Cardiovascular Diseases and Internal Medicine
Mayo Clinic
Rochester, Minnesota

Rachel Steckelberg, MD
Division of Cardiovascular Diseases and Internal Medicine
Mayo Clinic
Rochester, Minnesota

William G. Stevenson, MD
Director
Clinical Cardiac Electrophysiology
Brigham and Women's Hospital;
Professor of Medicine
Harvard Medical School
Boston, Massachusetts

William J. Stewart, MD, FACC, FASE
Staff Cardiologist
Heart and Vascular Institute
Department of Cardiovascular Medicine
Section of Cardiovascular Imaging
Cleveland Clinic Foundation;
Professor of Medicine
Director of Cardiovascular Disease Curriculum
Cleveland Clinic Lerner College of Medicine
Cleveland, Ohio

Nancy K. Sweitzer, MD, PhD
Associate Professor of Medicine
Department of Medicine
University of Wisconsin School of Medicine and Public Health
Madison, Wisconsin

Vinay Thohan, MD, FACC, FASE
Professor of Medicine
Director, Advanced Cardiac Care, Heart Transplant, Mechanical Assist Device Program
Department of Medicine, Section of Cardiology
Wake Forest University School of Medicine
Winston-Salem, North Carolina

Anjali Vaidya, MD
Co-Director, Pulmonary Hypertension Program
Advanced Heart Failure & Cardiac Transplant
Department of Medicine
University of Pennsylvania Perelman School of Medicine
Philadelphia, Pennsylvania

Mauricio Velez, MD
Senior Staff Physician
Henry Ford Hospital
Detroit, Michigan

Amanda R. Vest, MBBS, MRCP
Fellow in Cardiovascular Medicine
Cleveland Clinic, Heart and Vascular Institute
Cleveland, Ohio

Jane E. Wilcox, MD
Cardiology and AHA Postdoctoral Fellow
Division of Cardiology
Department of Preventive Medicine
Northwestern University Feinberg School of Medicine
Chicago, Illinois

Elaine Winkel, MD
Associate Professor of Medicine
Heart Failure and Transplant Program
Division of Cardiovascular Medicine
Department of Medicine
University of Wisconsin School of Medicine and Public Health
Madison, Wisconsin

Kari B. Wisinski, MD
Assistant Professor of Medicine
Division of Hematology and Oncology
Department of Medicine
University of Wisconsin School of Medicine and Public Health
Carbone Cancer Center
Madison, Wisconsin

Preface

This is a book about heart failure—a common and expanding problem in our society. In many respects, heart failure is a product of our success, as we learn how to better keep people alive after catastrophic events or as they develop chronic, progressive diseases. Heart failure can be a manifestation of almost any underlying cardiovascular disease and thus can touch the lives of a wide array of clinicians.

All of us learn case by case as we move through our careers. Less frequently, however, do we write about cases. This book attempts to take on heart failure by using cases to illustrate important points about the management of heart failure. Each expert author has been asked to write on a topic related to various manifestations of heart failure. Each chapter revolves around a case, or sometimes multiple cases, chosen to illustrate important points about care of the wide variety of patients who can develop heart failure.

The book is divided into five major parts. The first part talks about cases that manifest common ways that heart failure is newly diagnosed. Included are examples of newly diagnosed non-ischemic dilated cardiomyopathy, post-myocardial infarction heart failure, tako-tsubo cardiomyopathy, atrial fibrillation as a cause of heart failure, and manifestations of diastolic dysfunction causing heart failure. The second section discusses optimizing therapy for patients with known heart failure. What are the next steps when the initially stabilized patient begins to decline and presents with an acute exacerbation? What are the next therapies, and how do we treat patients with devices such as defibrillators, resynchronization pacemaker systems, and the combinations thereof? Finally, what can be done when despite all our best medication and device efforts our patient is still symptomatic or gradually deteriorating? Hemodynamic optimization and advanced therapy for end-stage failure are discussed by example.

The third part discusses heart failure associated with other cardiac diseases, in particular heart failure that occurs as a consequence of aortic stenosis and heart failure associated with mitral valve insufficiency. Hypertrophic cardiomyopathy, with all its potential manifestations, is also discussed in this section.

The next part talks about heart failure in patients with other significant systemic diseases. These patients are frequently difficult to deal with because they have at least two major manifestations of problems, with heart failure frequently being a substantial complicating issue. Discussed here are patients who have heart failure and chronic pulmonary disease, heart failure as a complication of cancer therapy, heart failure associated with amyloidosis, and heart failure complicated by significant renal failure.

The final two chapters are special chapters. One deals with the rapidly expanding field of familial-based cardiomyopathies. The final chapter discusses what is always a difficult problem—determining prognosis.

I hope you enjoy this book as much as I have enjoyed reading and editing all the chapters from this wonderful set of authors. A profound set of thanks are in order to all of the contributors who did an outstanding job presenting best practices in heart failure care. I also wish to thank Deb Pittz, my program assistant, who has been invaluable in the editing process to help make all of these chapters consistently formatted. Finally, I thank Rich Winters from Demos Medical Publishing, who originally came to me with the idea and has been patient and highly supportive during this entire process.

Peter S. Rahko, MD, FACC, FASE

Video Captions

Chapter 3: Tako-Tsubo (Stress) Cardiomyopathy

Video 3-1 *(referred to on page 51)*

Left ventriculogram shows "apical ballooning" with hyper-contractile basal segments, typical of tako-tsubo cardiomyopathy.

To view the video, please visit the following link: http://www.demosmedpub.com/video/?vid=829

Video 3-2A *(referred to on page 51)*

Two-dimensional echocardiogram (apical 4 chamber) demonstrates systolic anterior mitral leaflet motion resulting in left ventricular outflow tract obstruction. Left ventricular contraction is abnormal with typical "apical ballooning" and hyper-contractile basal segments.

To view the video, please visit the following link: http://www.demosmedpub.com/video/?vid=830

Video 3-2B *(referred to on page 51)*

Cine cardiac MRI demonstrates systolic anterior mitral leaflet motion resulting in left ventricular outflow tract obstruction. Left ventricular contraction is abnormal with typical "apical ballooning" and hyper-contractile basal segments.

To view the video, please visit the following link: http://www.demosmedpub.com/video/?vid=831

Video 3-3 *(referred to on page 53)*

Cine MRI (4 chamber) of patient with tako-tsubo cardiomyopathy demonstrates left ventricular "apical ballooning" pattern and normal right ventricular contraction.

To view the video, please visit the following link: http://www.demosmedpub.com/video/?vid=832

Video 3-4 *(referred to on page 53)*

Cine MRI (4 chamber) of patient with tako-tsubo cardiomyopathy demonstrates left ventricular "mid-ventricular ballooning" pattern and normal right ventricular contraction.

To view the video, please visit the following link: http://www.demosmedpub.com/video/?vid=833

Video 3-5 *(referred to on page 53)*

Cine MRI (4 chamber) of patient with tako-tsubo cardiomyopathy demonstrates left ventricular "inverted ballooning" pattern and normal right ventricular contraction.

To view the video, please visit the following link: http://www.demosmedpub.com/video/?vid=834

Video 3-6 *(referred to on page 53)*

Cine MRI (4 chamber) of patient with tako-tsubo cardiomyopathy demonstrates right ventricular ballooning and left ventricular "apical ballooning" pattern.

To view the video, please visit the following link: http://www.demosmedpub.com/video/?vid=835

Chapter 7: Optimizing Heart Failure Management in Idiopathic Non-Ischemic Dilated Cardiomyopathy Complicated by Ventricular Arrhythmia

Video 7-1A and B *(referred to on page 105)*

Four chamber view of two dimensional echocardiography in end-systole. The left panel shows images at presentation with heart failure symptoms. There is LV dilatation with LV endsystolic diameter of 43 mm. LV ejection fraction was 35% due to global hypokinesis with dyssychrony of septal and lateral wall motions. The right panel demonstrates reverse remodeling of the LV with reduction in LV end systolic diameter to 32 mm. LV ejection fraction had improved to 45%.

Note: LV = left ventricle.

To view the videos, please visit the following links: http://www.demosmedpub.com/video/?vid=836 and http://www.demosmedpub.com/video/?vid=837

Chapter 12: Left Ventricular Dysfunction With Mitral Regurgitation

Video 12-1 *(referred to on page 163)*

Parasternal long axis view of the mitral valve on two-dimensional echocardiogram.

To view the video, please visit the following link: http://www.demosmedpub.com/video/?vid=820

Video 12-2 *(referred to on page 163)*

Parasternal short axis view of the mitral valve on two-dimensional echocardiogram.

To view the video, please visit the following link: http://www.demosmedpub.com/video/?vid=821

Video 12-3 *(referred to on page 163)*

Apical four-chamber view on two-dimensional echocardiogram with Doppler color flow across the mitral valve.

To view the video, please visit the following link: http://www.demosmedpub.com/video/?vid=822

Video 12-4 *(referred to on page 163)*

Zoomed in apical-four chamber view of the mitral valve on two-dimensional echocardiogram with Doppler color flow on the right panel.

To view the video, please visit the following link: http://www.demosmedpub.com/video/?vid=823

Video 12-5 *(referred to on page 163)*

Zoomed in apical-four chamber view of the left ventricle on two-dimensional echocardiogram.

To view the video, please visit the following link: http://www.demosmedpub.com/video/?vid=824

Video 12-6 *(referred to on page 163)*

Coronary angiogram of the left anterior descending and left circumflex arteries.

To view the video, please visit the following link: http://www.demosmedpub.com/video/?vid=825

Video 12-7 *(referred to on page 163)*

Coronary angiogram of the right coronary artery.

To view the video, please visit the following link: http://www.demosmedpub.com/video/?vid=826

Chapter 16: Cardiac Amyloidosis

Video 16-1A *(referred to on page 214)*

Parasternal long axis view of the left ventricle with thickening of the inter-ventricular septum and posterior left ventricular wall indicating infiltration. The granular appearance of the thickened myocardium is characteristic of amyloid infiltration. The mitral valve leaflets are also thickened, which can be seen with amyloidosis.

To view the video, please visit the following link: http://www.demosmedpub.com/video/?vid=827

Video 16-1B *(referred to on page 214)*

Parasternal short axis view of the left ventricle, at the level of the mitral valve, demonstrates hypertrophy of the left ventricle with granular appearance of the myocardium, characteristic of amyloid infiltration.

To view the video, please visit the following link: http://www.demosmedpub.com/video/?vid=828

I

Newly Diagnosed Heart Failure

1

Initial Presentation of Heart Failure: The Non-Ischemic Dilated Cardiomyopathy

PETER S. RAHKO

CASE PRESENTATION

The patient is a 61-year-old man who works as an information systems consultant. He had come to the city 8 months before to work on a project. For the first several months he felt well, but approximately 3 months before admission, he began to notice increasing fatigue and mild shortness of breath with exertion. Typically, he would work full days, go home, and ride his bike for a few miles, without any limitation, and feel well rested. He would regularly walk up four flights of stairs at work without difficulty. The symptoms gradually worsened to the point that approximately 3 weeks before admission, he could only walk up one flight of stairs before becoming short of breath. After work, he felt increasingly fatigued, stopped riding his bike, and started going to bed early. He started waking up at night with episodes of dyspnea requiring him to sit up. He noted a modest weight gain of 5 pounds, and started feeling mildly bloated in his abdomen and swollen in his feet. Two days before admission, he found it impossible to lie down in bed and started sleeping in a chair. He thought he might be getting pneumonia because he was so short of breath even though he had no fevers, chills, sweats, or pain. These symptoms brought him to the emergency department.

His past medical history was benign. He had hypertension that was treated several years in the past, but he had stopped treatment at least 5 years before and stopped seeing a primary care physician. He denied diabetes, had not had any lipids checked recently, and had a remote 5-pack-year history of smoking. His only previous surgery was an appendectomy and a tonsillectomy, and his only medications were a multivitamin, occasional nonsteroidal anti-inflammatory, and one capsule of omega-3 fatty acid fish oil. His alcohol history was minimal and he denied use of any other drugs.

His father had coronary artery disease and heart failure but died at the age of 89. His mother also had heart failure but died of cancer at the age of 83. No other siblings had known heart disease.

Physical exam revealed blood pressure 143/98, a heart rate of 117, a respiration rate of 23, and no fever. His extremities were warm and well perfused. Peripheral pulses were intact. Central venous pressure by neck vein exam was at least 14 cm of H_2O. Carotids were intact bilaterally. His lung exam was clear in the upper fields but rales were present in the lower one third of both lung fields. His cardiac exam revealed a soft first heart sound, a persistently split second heart sound, a summation gallop, and a soft 2/6 mitral insufficiency murmur at the apex. The apical impulse was lateralized, downward, and quite diffuse. His abdomen did not appear to be significantly distended nor was there any apparent hepatomegaly. His liver was nontender and no bruits were heard. His lower extremities revealed mild edema bilaterally, and he was fully oriented with no focal neurologic signs.

SYMPTOMS AND SIGNS OF HEART FAILURE

What aspects of the history and physical are most reliable for making the diagnosis of heart failure? This is a difficult question, since most symptoms of heart failure are relatively general and nonspecific. Frequently, it is the combination of several symptoms and the time course of presentation, as in our patient, that help turn a sequence of symptoms into a diagnosis of heart failure. In the modern era, there have been several studies evaluating signs and symptoms of heart failure. Most of these are a byproduct of studies evaluating the performance of and pro–B-type natriuretic peptide (BNP) assays for detecting heart failure. These studies have recently been systematically reviewed (1). In **Table 1-1**, the most commonly recognized symptoms and signs of heart failure are listed and, if available, sensitivity and specificity from the systematic review are noted. Major and minor criteria from the Framingham Study are also noted, as this remains one of the most frequently cited set of criteria used to diagnose heart failure (2). Note that some findings such as paroxysmal nocturnal dyspnea, the presence of a third heart sound, a pulsatile liver, and a displaced apical impulse are very specific, but lack sensitivity. The opposite is true for exertional dyspnea. Most other signs and symptoms fall in the middle.

In a more focused evaluation of severely limited New York Heart Association (NYHA) Class IV heart failure patients, all of whom had a right heart catheterization, signs and symptoms were evaluated to determine their efficacy for detecting a pulmonary

Table 1-1
Diagnosis of Heart Failure: Common Symptoms and Signs

IMPORTANT SYMPTOMS	SENSITIVITY	SPECIFICITY
Disorders of Breathing		
Exertional dyspnea++	87%	51%
Orthopnea	44%	89%
Paroxysmal nocturnal dyspnea+	29%–47%	78%–98%*
Cough++	—	—
Disorders of Fluid Overload		
Edema++	53%	72%
Nocturia	—	—
Abdominal bloating/anorexia	—	—
Disorders of Functional Capacity		
Fatigue	—	—
Weakness	—	—
Decreased mental acuity/depression/anxiety	—	—
Disorders of Cardiac Performance		
Angina/atypical chest pain	—	—
Orthostatic hypotension	—	—
Palpitations	—	—
IMPORTANT PHYSICAL EXAM FINDINGS		
Cardiovascular		
Elevated central venous pressure/hepatojugular reflux+	52%	70%**
Displaced and diffuse apical impulse (cardiomegaly)+	27%	85%
Third heart sound+	11%	99%
Valvular insufficiency murmurs	—	—
Edema++	53%	72%
Pulmonary		
Rales/rhonchi/wheezing+	51%	81%
Dullness to percussion	—	—
Increased respiratory rate/work of breathing	—	—
Abdominal		
Ascites	—	—
Hepatomegaly/pulsatile liver++	17%	97%
General Systemic		
Reduced mentation/alertness	—	—
Cachexia	—	—
Tachycardia/hypotension++	—	—

* No summary data available, results taken from three studies and shown as a range (72–74)
** The level of central venous pressure is not uniformly designated in these studies
\+ Major criterion for heart failure as defined in the Framingham Study (2)
\++ Minor criterion for heart failure as defined in the Framingham Study

Source: Sensitivity and specificity adapted from reference 1.

capillary wedge pressure greater than 22 mmHg. The presence of jugular venous distention (greater than 12 mmHg) on exam and the symptom of orthopnea were most effective (3).

Most important in our patient was not only the combination of several symptoms but also the progressive nature of the disease. Exercise limitation progressed from mild to severe and physical findings occurred late in the progression. This is a common course of events and frequently patients with only a complaint of dyspnea may first be treated for respiratory disease, feel partially improved, only to be diagnosed with heart failure after further progression of disease.

CASE PRESENTATION

A 12-lead electrocardiogram (ECG) was obtained. It showed a left bundle branch block with a very wide QRS complex, with secondary ST and T-wave changes (**Figure 1-1**). His chest x-ray showed significant cardiomegaly with cephalization and evidence of increased congestion. Initial laboratories: sodium 137 mEq/L, potassium 4.6 mEq/L, chloride 104 mmol/L, bicarbonate 22 mEq/L, BUN 24 mg/dL, creatinine 1.2 mg/dL, glucose 113 mg/dL, calcium 8.5 mg/dL, B-type natriuretic peptide 1247 pg/mL, troponin 0.05 ng/mL, hemoglobin 15.2 g/dL, hematocrit 48%, WBC count 9,500 × 10^6/L, platelet count 135,000 × 10^6/L.

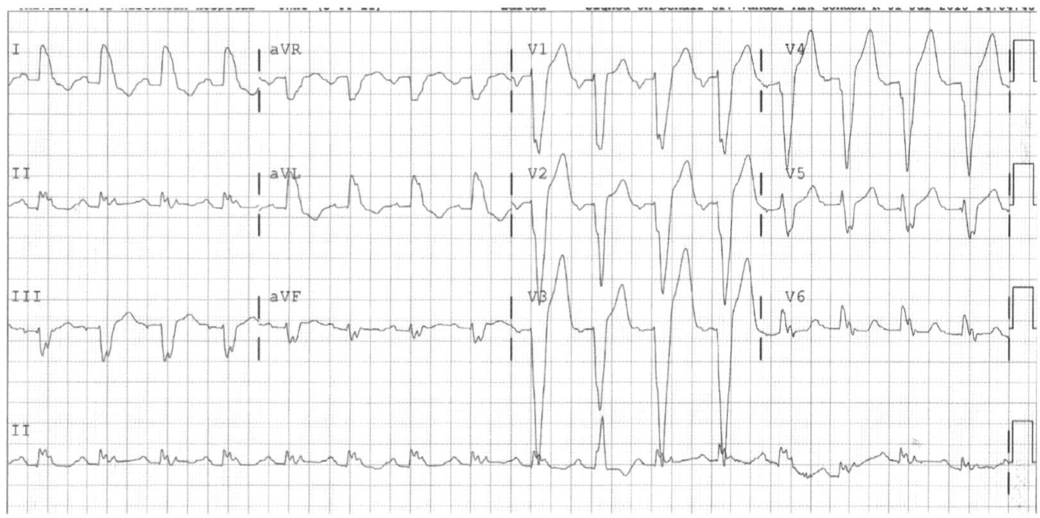

(A)

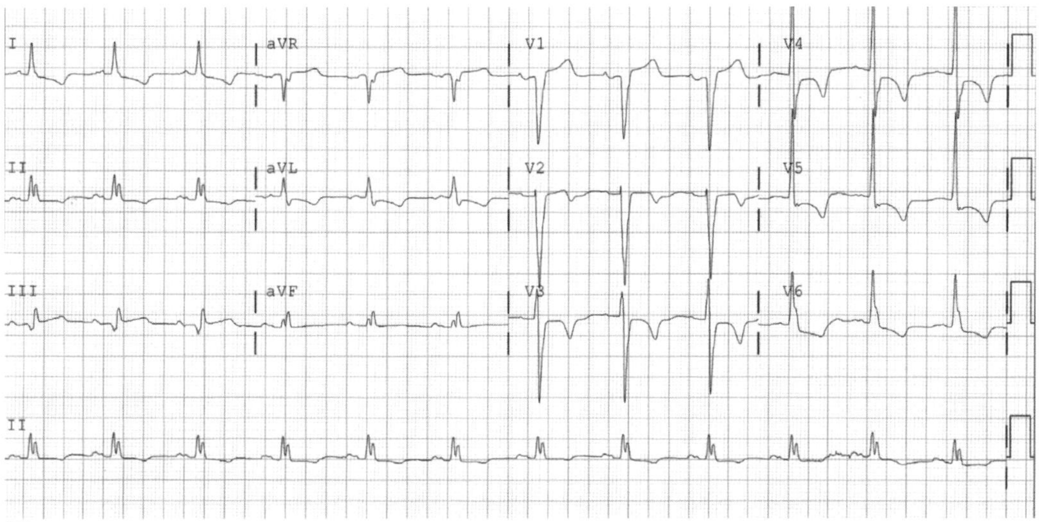

(B)

Figure 1-1
Four examples of common electrocardiograms (ECG) seen in patients presenting with heart failure. (A) Wide complex left bundle branch block. This is the ECG of the index patient discussed in the text. Typical of very large left ventricles, the QRS complex is very wide. (B) A patient with a narrow complex QRS showing classic signs of left ventricular hypertrophy with markedly increased voltage and secondary ST-T wave changes typical of left ventricular strain. Patients with very large dilated ventricles can have marked findings of left ventricular hypertrophy. *(Continued)*

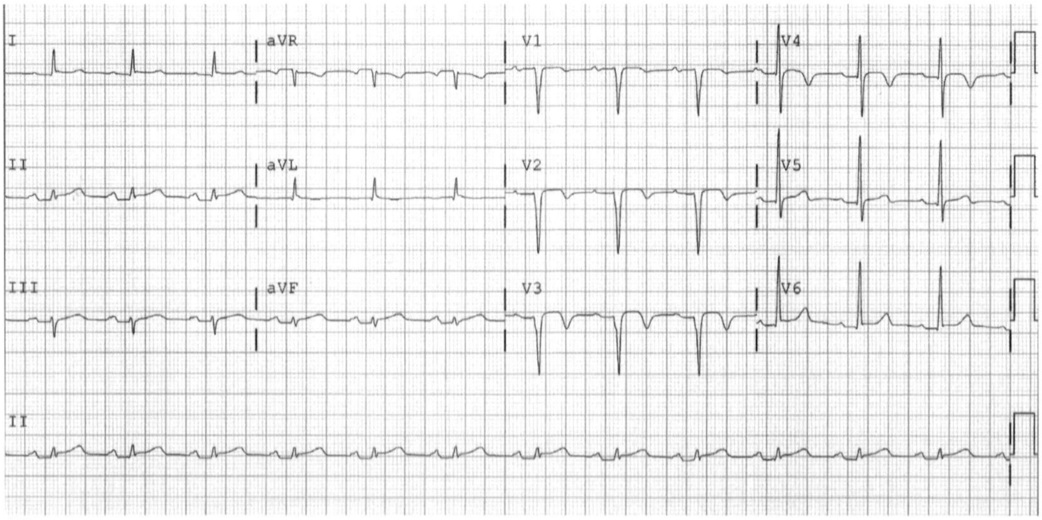

(C)

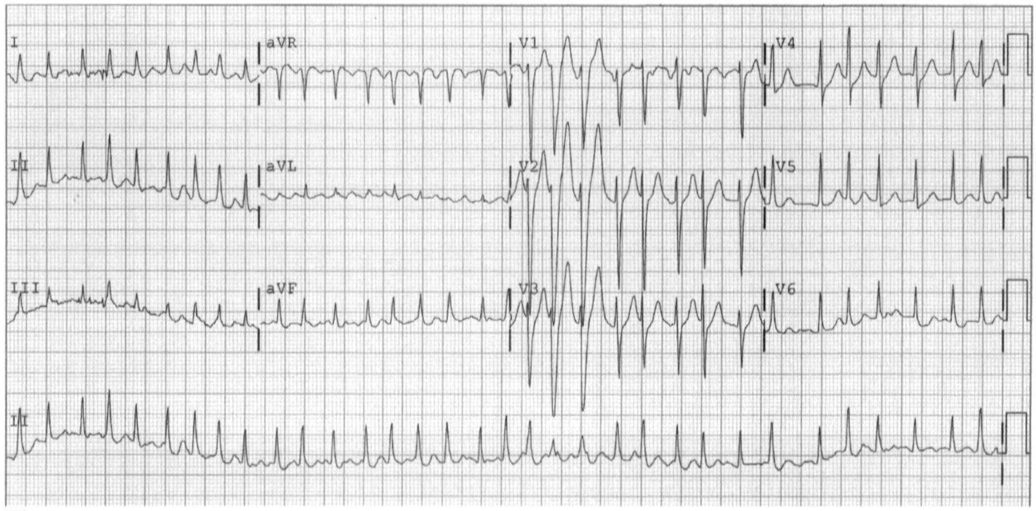

(D)

Figure 1-1 *(Continued)*
(C) Anterior wall myocardial infarction. This is an ECG of a patient who recently had a large anterior wall myocardial infarction. Note the very poor R wave progression and secondary ST and T wave changes in the precordial leads. Some patients present with no history of symptomatic infarct, their first presentation being symptoms of heart failure. (D) Atrial fibrillation with a rapid ventricular response coupled with some evidence of aberrancy, particularly seen in leads V1, V2, and V3. This manifestation can result in relatively rapid onset symptoms of heart failure and sometimes is fully or considerably reversible.

ECG, CHEST X-RAY, LABORATORY EXAM

Common ECG findings in heart failure are shown in **Table 1-2** and four examples of these findings are shown in **Figure 1-1**. The ECG should be the initial diagnostic test when a patient initially presents with symptoms of suspected heart failure. In the acute setting, a rapid assessment for acute ischemia or infarction, tachyarrhythmias, or bradyarrhythmias helps rapidly triage initial acute care. In the more stable office setting, comparison to prior ECGs for changes and examination of the ECG for additional changes such as findings of ventricular hypertrophy, P wave changes or conduction delays, particularly left bundle branch block as seen in our patient, may provide valuable data confirming the presence of organic heart disease (4). Low amplitude of the QRS complex deserves special mention. It may be a finding associated with infiltration cardiomyopathy, particularly amyloid heart disease (5). It may also be associated with decompensation with significant volume overload. As fluid overload resolves, ECG amplitude may increase

Table 1-2
Twelve-Lead Electrocardiogram Findings That May Be Associated With Heart Failure

ECG CHANGE	CLINICAL IMPLICATION
Sinus tachycardia	Reduced stroke volume and reduced cardiac output or high output demand state
Q waves, infarct pattern	Prior myocardial infarction suggesting coronary artery disease
Persistent ST elevation after myocardial infarction	Left ventricular aneurysm
Left ventricular hypertrophy with or without strain pattern	Left ventricular enlargement Cardiomyopathy Hypertensive heart disease
Atrial fibrillation	Atrial chamber enlargement Secondary finding in multiple etiologies of heart failure Primary cause of tachycardia related LV dysfunction
Left bundle branch block, interventricular conduction delay	Dilated cardiomyopathy, ischemic or non-ischemic
Prolonged P wave and biphasic with accentuated negative component V_1	Left atrial enlargement/hypertrophy
Sinus bradycardia, heart block	Reduced cardiac output

(4,6). In cases where low voltage persists, long-term prognosis has been shown to be worse (5).

In the context of heart failure, the chest x-ray is the next logical imaging procedure. Findings on chest x-ray that may help confirm the presence of heart failure are cardiomegaly, signs of pulmonary congestion, and the presence of pleural effusions, most commonly bilateral. In a systematic review of five studies of the use of the chest x-ray in the diagnosis of heart failure, the presence of any one finding consistent with heart failure had a 63% sensitivity and 83% specificity (1). Taken alone, these findings are nonspecific, but in the context of symptoms of dyspnea, of great value. The chest x-ray is also of great value for detection of noncardiac causes of dyspnea, particularly pneumonia and other infiltrates or findings suggesting chronic obstructive pulmonary disease.

A final aspect of the initial evaluation of our patient is to obtain a comprehensive set of routine laboratory tests (**Table 1-3**). The completeness of the evaluation should be guided by available data on the patient. For a brand new patient, all basic laboratory studies should be obtained for a comprehensive baseline. Several alternative causes of heart failure symptoms can be rapidly excluded such as severe anemia, renal failure, hepatic failure, hyperthyroidism, diabetes, and iron overload. Other studies noted in **Table 1-3** may be indicated depending on history and further findings as the evaluation progresses (7,8).

NATRIURETIC PEPTIDE BIOMARKERS

BNP and aminoterminal proB-type natriuretic peptide (NT-proBNP) are two related biomarkers strongly associated with heart failure. These natriuretic peptide biomarkers (NPBs) are produced in response to activation of myocardial stretch receptors, which typically are responsive to increased filling pressures (the "wet" NPB response). In addition, there is a "dry" NPB elevation associated with chronic dysfunction such as fibrosis, infiltration, hypertrophy, and ischemic disease (9). Acute heart failure symptoms are most closely related to elevated filling pressures. In this setting, NPBs are valuable for excluding the fact that filling pressures are high, particularly when the clinical presentation of dyspnea is of uncertain etiology. A BNP of less than 100 pg/ml has an 89% negative predictive value and a proBNP less than 300 pg/ml has a 99% negative predictive value (10,11). When it is clinically obvious that the cause of the symptoms is fluid overload, NPBs are of less immediate value. To date, NPBs have not been adequately tested to guide acute heart failure therapy, but several trials have demonstrated a strong association of NPB levels with long-term prognosis at the time of hospital discharge (12,13).

In ambulatory patients, NPB levels have been shown to be of prognostic value. While a single-point measurement is of value, change over time from multiple measurements is considerably more powerful

Table 1-3
Routine Laboratory Testing at the Time of Initial Presentation of Heart Failure

LABORATORY TEST	COMMENT
Complete blood count	Anemia could be a primary cause of chronic high output demand state or secondary to chronic disease
Electrolytes, calcium, magnesium	Baseline, important for several types of medical therapy
Renal function	Potential cause of symptoms of HF Implications for choice of medical therapy
Hepatic function	Potential cause of systems of HF Changes also can be secondary to HF
Troponin	Particularly important when an acute coronary syndrome or myocarditis is suspected. May be mildly abnormal in other circumstances.
Glucose, $HgbA_1C$	Screening for diabetes
Lipid profile	Risk factor assessment if not done in recent past, treatment of ischemic based HF
Thyroid function tests	Both hyper- and hypothyroidism may cause HF
Fasting transferring	Screening for hemochromatosis
HIV screening	Controversial
Viral titers	Only in select patients with recent onset HF. Implications of positive results not certain
Chagas antibody titers	Only for those from endemic areas of the world
Cardiac biopsy	Not routine, highly selected cases where management may be affected: giant cell myocarditis, sarcoid heart disease, cardiac involvement in amyloidosis, hemochromatosis, Loeffler's syndrome

Note: HF = heart failure

for predicting outcomes (9). These observations have led to the conclusion that NPB levels might help guide long-term heart failure therapy, allowing optimization of treatment. It would appear obvious that diuretic therapy should lower NPB levels, and that actually all major classes of heart failure drugs, devices, and exercise have been shown to have a beneficial effect (9). Several trials have tested the hypothesis of NPB guided ambulatory treatment of heart failure. Results have been variable as has trial design. A meta-analysis of six trials demonstrated positive benefit (14) and more recent trials have also shown benefit (15). It appears that NPBs are most valuable when an aggressive goal is chosen (BNP less than 125 pg/ml or proBNP less than 1,000 pg/ml). Patients achieving these goals through long-term comprehensive treatment adjustments (not just diuretics) appear to benefit the most (15).

CASE PRESENTATION

The patient was started on oxygen supplementation. His room air saturation was 90%. He was given 40 mg of furosemide intravenously. He was started on 6.25 mg three times daily of captopril and admitted to the cardiovascular medicine service. He began producing urine rapidly and his shortness of breath began to abate. Within 24 hours he had a net diuresis of 2.8 liters with stable renal function and potassium. The patient was feeling symptomatically improved. The blood pressure had come down and he was tolerating captopril now at 12.5 mg three times daily.

An echocardiogram was obtained the afternoon of admission. It showed evidence of a severe dilated cardiomyopathy with marked enlargement of his left ventricle, which had a markedly spheroid shape. Ejection fraction was reduced at 10% with severe, diffuse hypokinesis noted. His mitral inflow pattern was consistent with restrictive physiology, indicating severe diastolic dysfunction and high left atrial pressures. His right ventricle was mildly dilated and moderately and diffusely reduced in systolic function. Substantial pulmonary hypertension was noted with an estimated pulmonary artery pressure of 73 mmHg. Both atrial chambers were moderately enlarged. The mitral valve annulus was significantly stretched and leaflet excursion reduced typical of papillary muscle dysfunction. Moderate valvular insufficiency was present due to malcoaptation of otherwise normal leaflets. His other valves were unremarkable. The inferior vena cava was moderately dilated and blunted in its response to respiration, consistent with significantly elevated central venous pressure.

ECHOCARDIOGRAPHY

The comprehensive two-dimensional Doppler echocardiogram is the next logical diagnostic procedure and the single most useful test for evaluating a case of suspected heart failure (8). The first issue to be addressed is whether or not actual structural heart disease exists. In some cases the study will be normal, which will lead the clinician toward assessment for alternate causes of the symptoms. One caveat: it is important to differentiate a true normal study from normal systolic function with associated diastolic abnormalities. The entire study is important, not just the ejection fraction.

The second important issue is determining the presence of structural heart disease other than disease of the myocardium. Here the echocardiogram excels and can rapidly tell the clinician if there is: (a) primary heart valve disease (mitral stenosis and aortic insufficiency being the lesions least likely to cause an easily audible murmur); (b) pericardial disease such as chronic constriction or less likely, tamponade; (c) evidence of a prior silent myocardial infarction that has developed a mechanical complication such as a ventricular septal defect, mitral regurgitation from papillary muscle disease, or a ventricular aneurysm; (d) unknown congenital heart disease that has evolved into ventricular dysfunction (congenitally corrected transposition of the great arteries or a large ventricular septal defect or atrial septal defect that never caused a murmur); (e) right heart disease such as isolated right-sided valve disease, primary pulmonary hypertension, or a silent pulmonary embolism, all of which should manifest with marked right ventricular dysfunction; or (f) evidence of a chronic high-output state.

Once the above structural changes have been eliminated from consideration, the study can focus on myocardial disease. If there is a cardiomyopathy present, what type is it? Again the echocardiogram may lead us toward a specific diagnosis such as restrictive cardiomyopathy (Chapter 16), hypertrophic cardiomyopathy (Chapter 13), or less commonly suspicion for arrhythmogenic right ventricular dysplasia. All three of these cardiomyopathies have distinct findings differentiating them from the most common forms of ventricular dysfunction (16–19).

Having eliminated the less common causes of heart failure, the next major consideration is to determine if the cause of our patient's symptoms are due to predominantly systolic or diastolic dysfunction. It is not possible by either symptoms or physical examination to differentiate between a systolic or diastolic cause of heart failure. Imaging information is necessary to make this determination. In the current case, the findings clearly indicate the presence of marked systolic dysfunction. However, to add another layer of complexity, it is important to remember that patients with marked systolic dysfunction virtually all have evidence of associated diastolic dysfunction. This has led some to recommend differentiating the two most common causes of heart failure as patients with a preserved ejection fraction (greater than or equal to 45%) or patients without a preserved ejection fraction (8). The relative frequency of a systolic versus diastolic cause varies by study. Diastolic dysfunction may be the predominant cause in 20% to up to 60% of cases, with the higher frequency being observed in elderly patients (8).

Let us now consider what information the echocardiogram should supply in our patient (**Table 1-4**).

Table 1-4
Echocardiographic Information Valuable for the Evaluation of a Dilated Cardiomyopathy

CHAMBER SIZE AND FUNCTION
Left Ventricle
Ejection fraction
End diastolic and end systolic dimensions/wall thickness
End diastolic and end systolic volumes
Shape changes/aneurysm/effects of remodeling
Ventricular thrombi
Right Ventricle
Size
Function
Systolic pressure
Atrial Chambers
Left atrial volume
Left atrial dimension
Estimated right atrial size
MITRAL VALVE AND TRICUSPID VALVE
Annular enlargement
Leaflet tethering and malcoaptation
Severity of regurgitation
NONINVASIVE HEMODYNAMICS
Estimated central venous pressure
Vena cava size
Vena cava response to respiration
Right ventricular and pulmonary artery pressure
Tricuspid regurgitation gradient added to estimated central venous pressure
Stroke volume
(Doppler flow velocity integral in left ventricular outflow tract) x (area of outflow tract)
Left atrial pressure
Algorithm using multiple sources of data:
Left atrial volume
Mitral inflow pattern analysis
Mitral annular tissue Doppler
Pulmonary venous inflow pattern

The first important data is that related to left ventricular function. The report should characterize the ejection fraction; this is of prognostic importance in that mortality is inversely related to ejection fraction (20). Most laboratories still use visual analysis for reporting the number; in experienced labs, this is more reliable than dimension-based calculations or 2-D–based quantification. There is gradually more availability of 3-D quantification (**Figure 1-2**), which still is not routine for clinical use. It is hoped that this technique will eventually become commonly

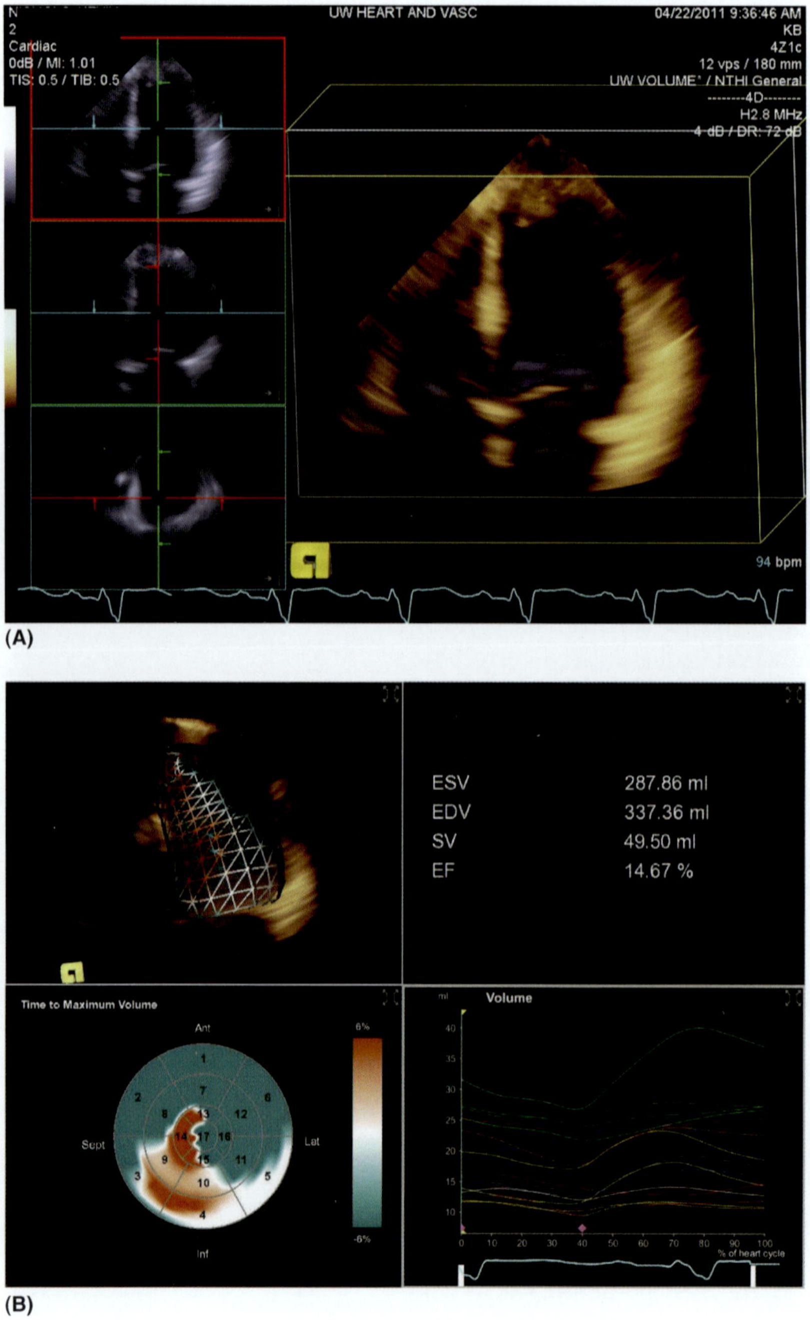

Figure 1-2
(A) Sample of a three-dimensional acquisition of the left and right ventricular volumes in a heart failure patient. Using cropping, multiple portions of the ventricle can be examined in multiple planes for further enhancement of evaluation. (B) Examples of some of the semi-automated calculations possible. In the upper left-hand corner there is an example of the volumetric model calculated by frame-by-frame analysis. The results of the calculation are shown in the upper right panel for volumes and ejection fraction. Other possible analytic information is shown in the bottom panels, one being the time to maximal volume displacement on the left side and the right side showing individual segmental time volume curves for each of the traditional 17 segments of the heart. It may be possible to get information about synchrony, and also regional function, from this type of analysis. Current three-dimensional analyses show great promise but still suffer from time and spatial resolution problems.

available and reliable (21,22). Alternate forms of assessment such as strain imaging are under evaluation but not yet adequately validated (**Figure 1-3**; 23).

The second important data is left ventricular size. In this case, 2-D–based dimension measurements (**Figure 1-4**) are simple, well known, and remain the most reproducible data for characterization of size (22). A measurement of longitudinal function of the right ventricular free wall: tricuspid annular plane systolic excursion (TAPSE) has been used extensively

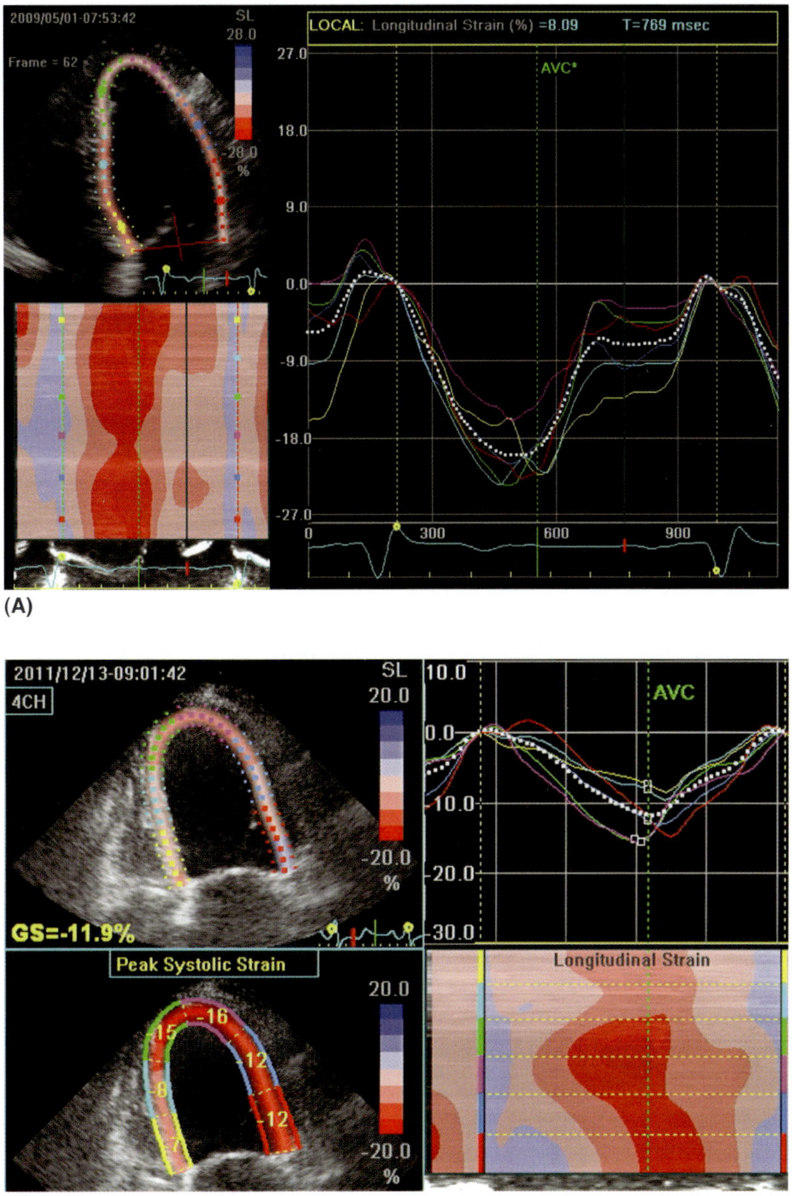

Figure 1-3

Examples of the use of longitudinal strain from apical views. Strain has been investigated by a large number of laboratories and shows promise as an alternative method of calculating ventricular function. Several examples are shown. In (A) a normal patient, strain is calculated in six different segments of the apical four-chamber view. These segments are demonstrated in the upper left-hand corner and are color coded, and also demonstrated in an M-mode format in which the walls of the ventricle are rolled out from base to apex, back to base again, with time being the variable on the X-axis. In this patient at end-systole (the green dotted line, AVC = aortic valve closure) maximum strain is achieved in most of the segments. This is also shown by the color coded change in the lower left, with maximum strain being shown as the deepest red color. Expansion of a segment would display in blue, and this is demonstrated by the light blue at end-diastole. Typical strain values for segments are about 20% and a typical average value for the view is shown as the dotted line, which is a compilation of all six segments. In (B) is an example of a patient with moderate systolic dysfunction from a dilated cardiomyopathy. Notice that the strain remains relatively synchronous in appearance but the average strain value for all six segments has now dropped to about 11.9%, consistent with definite ventricular dysfunction. *(Continued)*

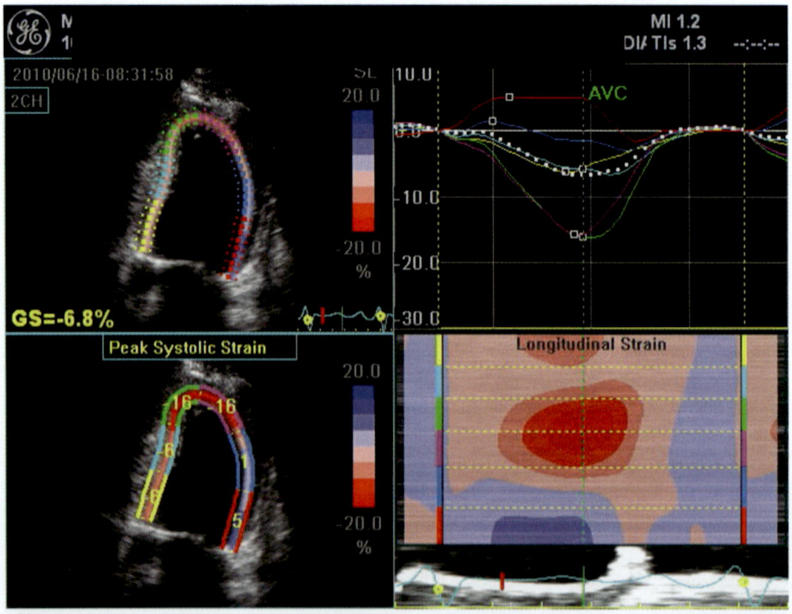

(C)

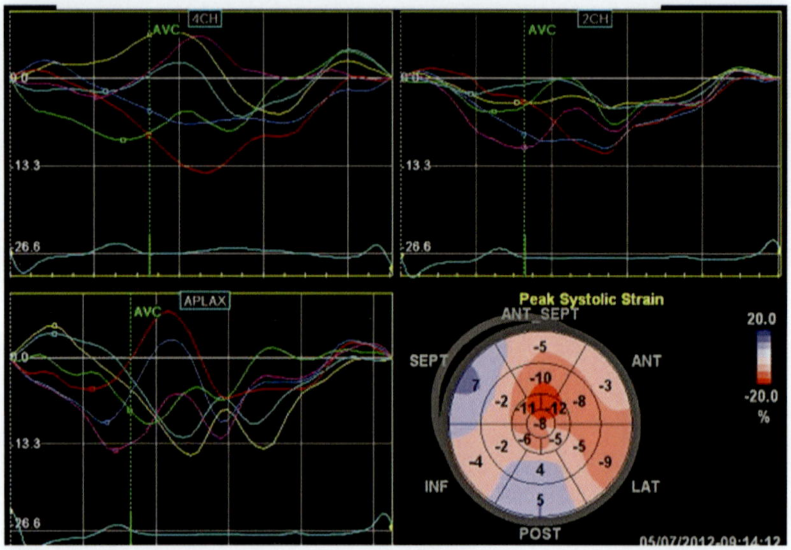

(D)

Figure 1-3 *(Continued)*
In (C) is an example of a patient with more severe reduction in function. In this case the global strain has now fallen to 6.8%. Notice, however, there is great heterogeneity in strain. As ventricles become more dysfunctional, one sees wide varieties of strain segment by segment. In this case two of the segments show essentially no compression and only elongation throughout the cardiac cycle, whereas two of the segments show relatively good compression, and the other two segments show relatively poor but still synchronous compression. The implication of these findings are still being evaluated. In (D) is an example of the six strain curves from the traditional three apical views from a two-dimensional echo. Notice that there is a marked reduction in effectiveness of contractility as demonstrated by strain, with some segments predominantly elongating, and others compressing but only to a much lower than normal value. The summation of this is shown in the bulls-eye pattern of all 18 segments. The areas in blue show segments that only elongated as one reached peak systole, whereas the segments in red show some inward motion. A global value averaging all 18 segments can be easily calculated, and this value actually shows promise in that it has a narrower range than the individual segments and also has been shown in preliminary data to have some prognostic information over and above traditional measurements of ejection fraction.

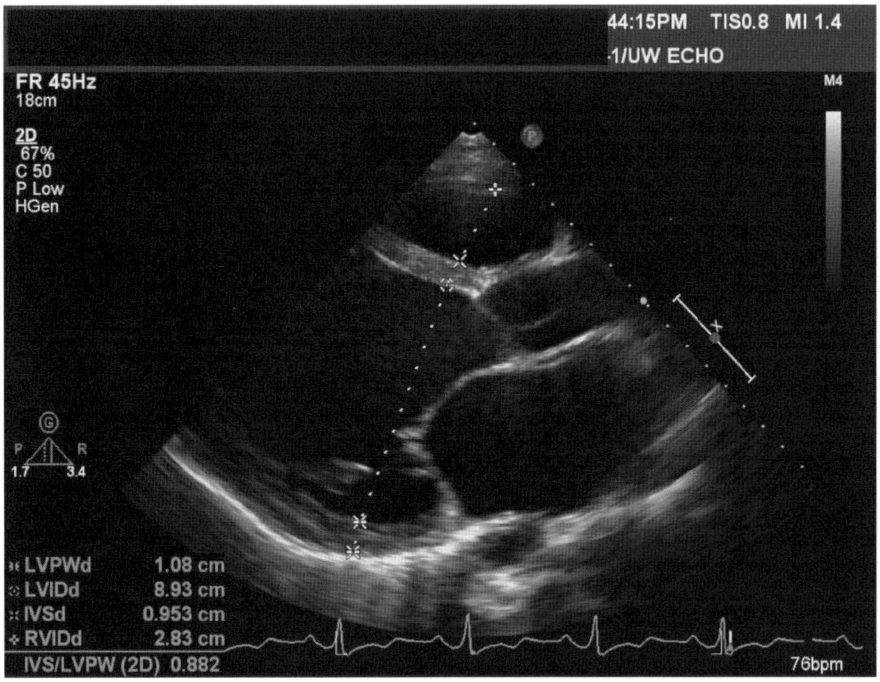

(A)

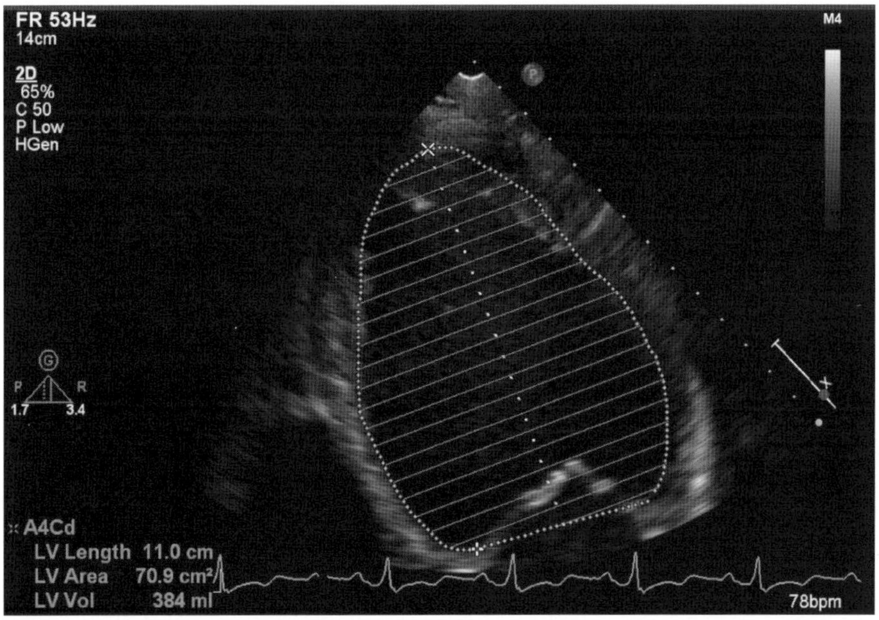

(B)

Figure 1-4

(A) Example of standardized two-dimensional measurements of ventricular size and wall thickness. These segmental diameters remain the most standardized measurements of left ventricular size and in most laboratories are now calculated directly off the two-dimensional image. In (B) and (C) are shown standardized volumetric measurements of the left ventricle calculated typically in two planes orthogonal to each other at end-systole and end-diastole. In this case there is severe enlargement at both end-systole and end-diastole. *(Continued)*

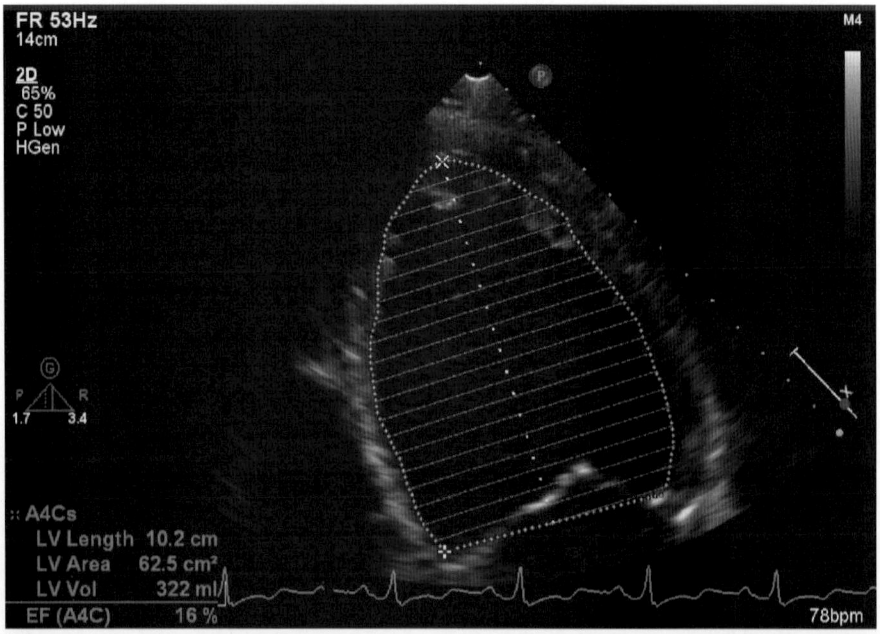

(C)

Figure 1-4 *(Continued)*

to evaluate function in multiple circumstances including dilated cardiomyopathy. It appears to offer additional functional and prognostic data in some studies, but its role is unclear (24,25). As with ejection fraction, it is hoped that 3-D volume-based data may eventually supplement dimension measurements (21). Comments on shape and structural changes from remodeling may also help further characterize disease chronicity. As remodeling progresses, the left ventricular shape tends to change to a more globular configuration that is associated with relatively thinner walls. These large, more remodeled ventricles are relatively less likely to show significant reversal with medical therapy (26).

The third important data relates to right ventricular size and function (**Figure 1-5**). Most laboratories, given the difficulty of routine quantification, characterize right ventricular size and also function as normal, mild, moderate, or severely abnormal. In heart failure, the severity of right ventricular involvement is highly variable, ranging from normal to severe. Patients with good residual right ventricular function tend to have less need for diuretics because central venous pressure may still be normal, have better preservation of exercise capacity, have a better prognosis, and a greater predominance of symptoms of dyspnea (24). The status of the right ventricle can indicate long-term prognosis. Those with right ventricular dysfunction and enlargement equal in severity to the left ventricle have a much worse prognosis. Similarly, those showing the combination of reduced right ventricular systolic function and pulmonary hypertension have much greater long-term mortality risk (27,28).

The fourth piece of data relates to the atria (**Figure 1-6**). If the patient remains in sinus rhythm, atrial size may reflect both the severity of the cardiomyopathy and the chronic status of filling pressures. Increased left atrial volume has been associated with reduced prognosis (29). Most labs have converted to reporting left atrial volumes, which much more realistically depict atrial size. The critical value defining severe enlargement is 100 ml/m^2 (29). Volume, corrected for body surface area, is most useful and superior to M-mode dimensions or raw 2-D volumes. Right atrial size is still mainly semi-quantitative in characterization.

All four valves should be carefully evaluated for primary valve disease. In most cases, this will not be present. There may, however, be significant functional disease of the mitral and tricuspid valves (see also Chapter 12). Changes in performance of these valves are generally caused by changes in ventricular size, atrial size, and ventricular function. The amount of regurgitation of these valves may vary from virtually none to severe. Valve coaptation is related to the amount of overlap of the leaflets. Enlargement of the valve annulus stretches the leaflets away from each other. Enlargement of the ventricle tethers the leaflets toward the apex, further restricting motion,

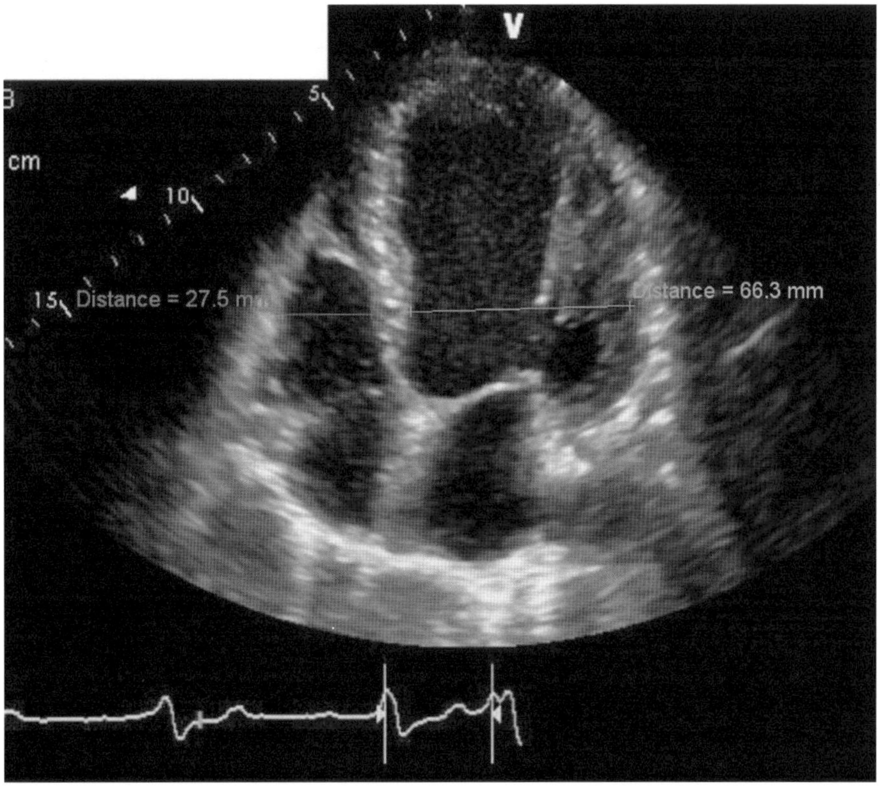

(A)

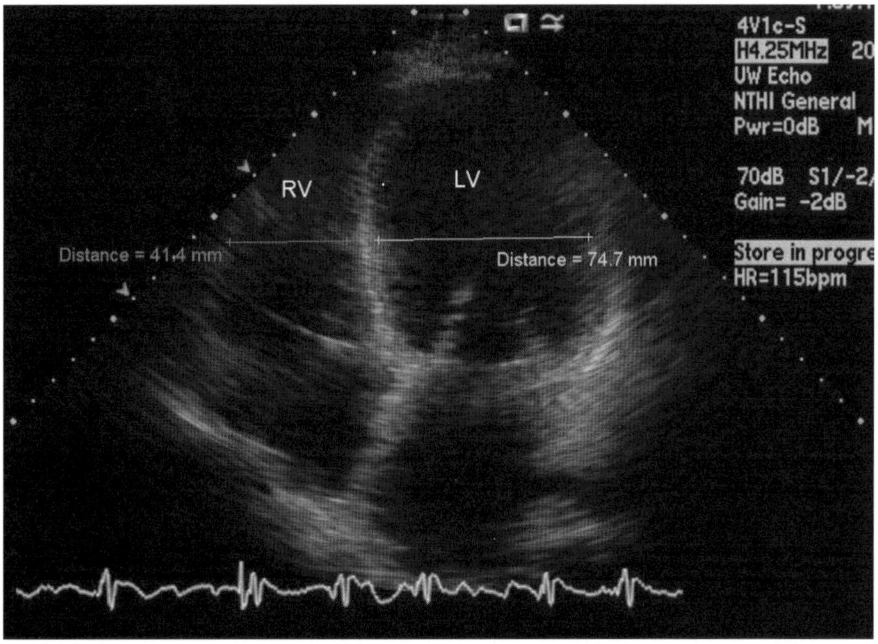

(B)

Figure 1-5

(A) This is an example of a patient with a dilated cardiomyopathy with an ejection fraction of 30% but a totally normal right ventricle. This patient remains almost entirely asymptomatic. Some patients present with relatively normal right ventricular size and function, and the relative diameter of these two chambers is shown in the example. In (B) is an example of a patient with much more severe ventricular dysfunction. Both chambers are significantly increased, but the relative size of the right ventricle as opposed to the patient in (A) is much larger. Typically, these patients are more symptomatic, with reduced exercise capacity, and overall prognosis is less favorable.

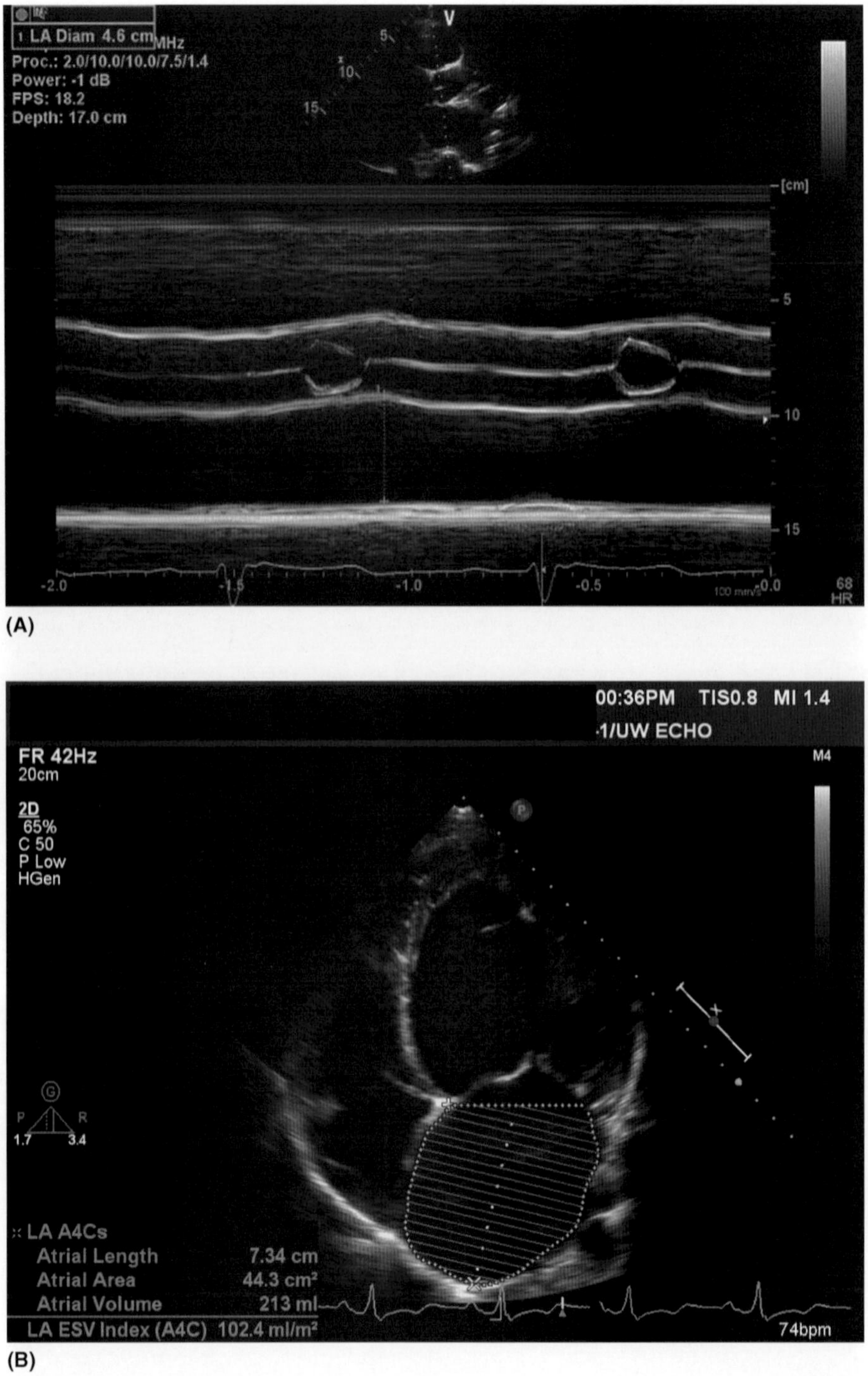

Figure 1-6

(A) The most traditional measurement of left atrial size, the M-mode measurement of the short axis. This measurement, while still commonly used, has several limitations. Many laboratories have converted to biplane volumetric calculations (B) of the left atrium, similar to what is used for the left ventricle. These measurement techniques have been found to be very successful and reproducible and should be considered the current gold standard for evaluating left atrial size.

particularly the ability to close. Remodeling of the ventricle malpositions the papillary muscles. Reduced contractility prohibits longitudinal shortening of the papillary muscles (which may also be displaced outward), further affecting closure. Dyssynchrony of contraction may further reduce the effectiveness of closure of the leaflets. All of these factors can combine to cause valvular regurgitation (**Figure 1-7**). The severity of the regurgitation may have a profound effect on symptoms and prognosis. Response to medical therapy, resynchronization therapy, and preload reduction from diuresis can have marked effects on

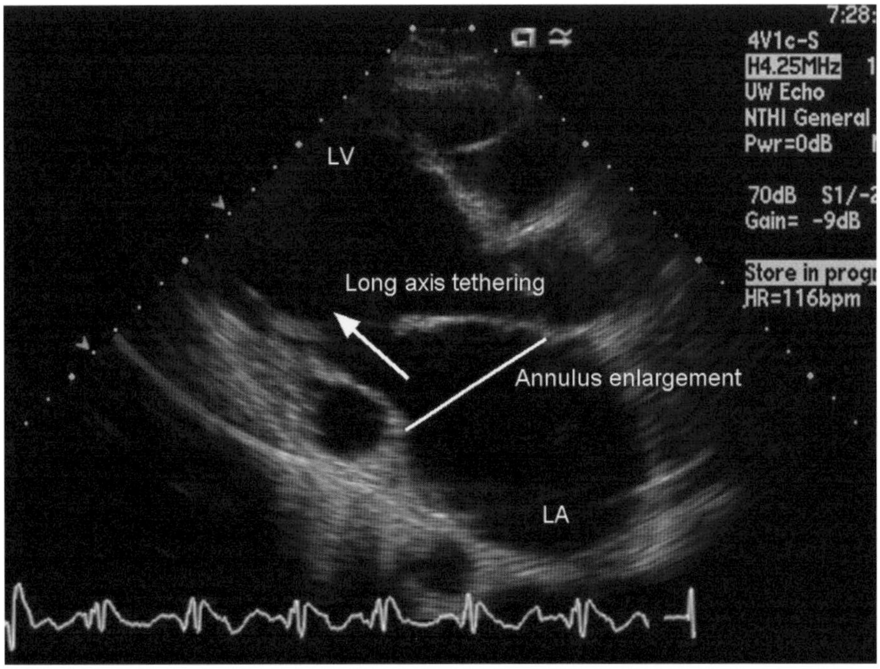

(A)

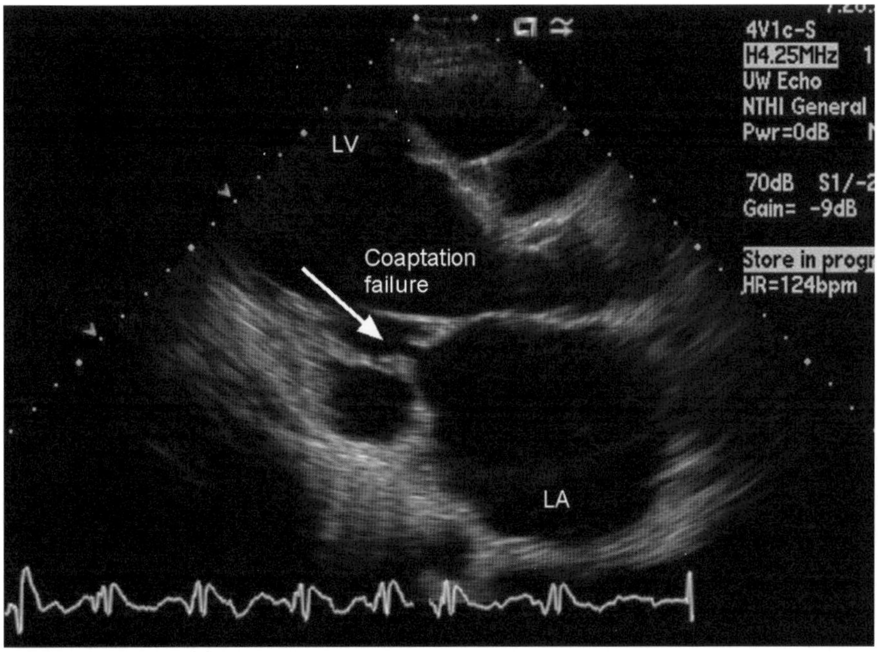

(B)

Figure 1-7

(A) This is an example of papillary muscle dysfunction. In this case the patient has a markedly enlarged left ventricle and also a markedly enlarged left atrium (LA). The consequence of chamber enlargement is typically marked enlargement of the mitral annulus, as demonstrated by the horizontal line. This pulls the base of the mitral valve apart and expands the overall orifice size. In addition, there is considerable tethering of the tips of the leaflets (arrow). As the left ventricle enlarges, the leaflets are pulled further and further toward the apex of the left ventricle and the ability of excursion back toward the annular plane becomes further and further reduced. This is further enhanced by reduced contractility of the papillary muscles and malpositioning of the papillary muscles as the chamber enlarges and becomes more globular. The consequence of papillary muscle dysfunction is demonstrated in (B). *(Continued)*

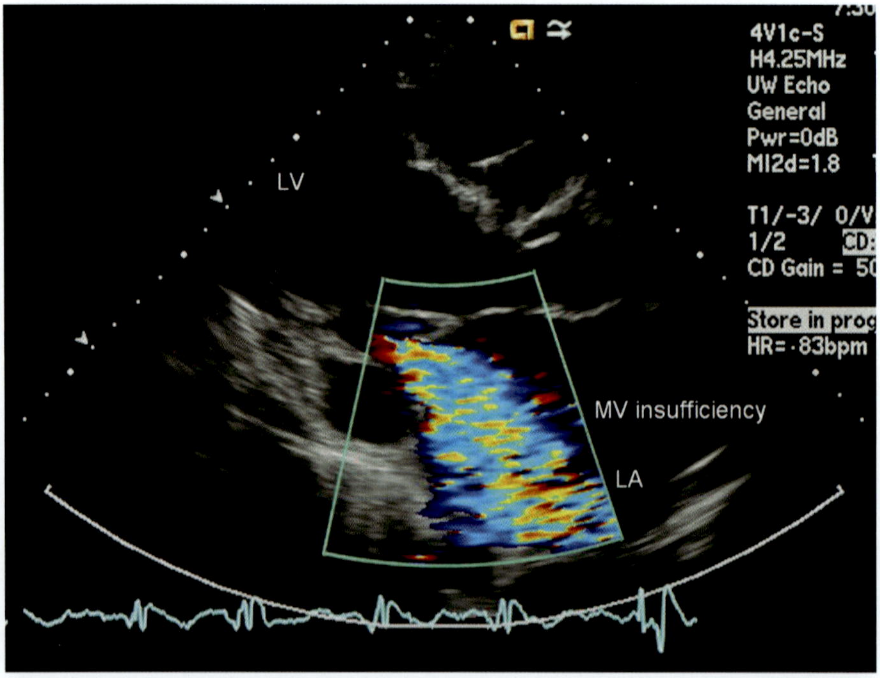

(C)

Figure 1-7 *(Continued)*
A severe case, in which there is visible coaptation failure of the two leaflets. Excursion, as is seen here, is markedly reduced and the coaptation point is markedly moved apically from the annular plane of the valve. Color Doppler positively demonstrates the consequence of this malcoaptation in (C), where there is severe mitral insufficiency present.

the severity of valve regurgitation (30–36). In many cases, regurgitation may gradually decline over time. When it does not, mitral repair surgery may be considered (37).

Hemodynamics can be estimated noninvasively. The presence of tricuspid valve regurgitation allows calculation of the right ventricular–right atria pressure gradient, which has been shown in correlation studies to be close to hemodynamics measured during right heart catheterization (37,38). This gradient is added to an estimate of central venous pressure (**Figure 1-8**). Physical examination tends to underestimate central venous pressure. Echocardiography, using assessment of the inferior vena cava diameter and response to respiration is better but still not perfect. Nevertheless, this value gives a good estimate of central venous pressure and right ventricular systolic pressure, and if the pulmonic valve is not stenotic, pulmonary artery systolic pressure (39). Cardiac output may be estimated using a combination of Doppler and dimension measurements, best done in the left ventricular outflow tract to obtain stroke volume, which can then be multiplied by heart rate (37).

Evaluation of left ventricular filling and filling pressure is complex and highly variable. Virtually all patients have some degree of diastolic dysfunction; the issue is not if it is present but how severe it is. A detailed grading system for severity has evolved and been summarized in algorithms. Multiple components of the examination are used to arrive at a conclusion: mitral valve Doppler inflow, particularly the E/A ratio and early diastolic deceleration time, tissue Doppler evaluation of the motion of the mitral annulus in diastole, pulmonary vein Doppler inflow patterns, left atrial volume, estimated pulmonary artery pressure, and other derived ratios. These are summarized in **Figure 1-9**. From this information, two algorithms may be used—one to estimate the severity of diastolic dysfunction and the other to estimate whether filling pressure is normal or elevated. These are beyond the scope of this chapter and are discussed in detail in the American Society of Echocardiography Guidelines (40). The classification system of diastolic dysfunction is summarized in **Table 1-5**. It should be noted that there also is the question of reversibility. During the echo, a Valsalva maneuver should be done to determine if the mitral flow pattern changes. This helps further classify and characterize the severity of diastolic dysfunction. Over time, with treatment, the severity of diastolic dysfunction may also change. This may be due to acute reductions in preload from diuresis that lower filling pressure. In many cases, the classification of diastolic dysfunction may change. This may also be due to chronic improvement in systolic function due to reverse remodeling over time. In both situations,

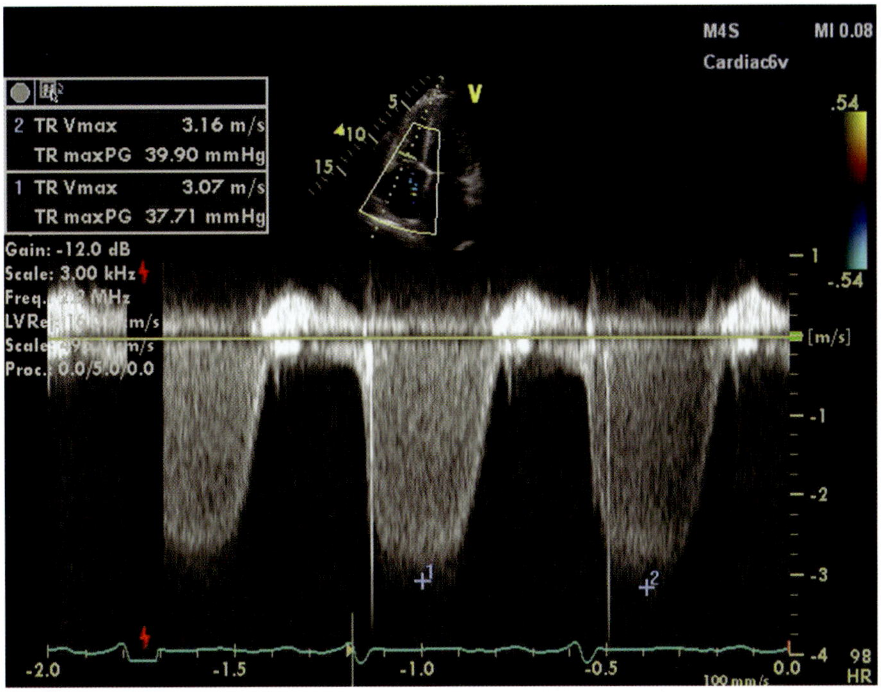

(A)

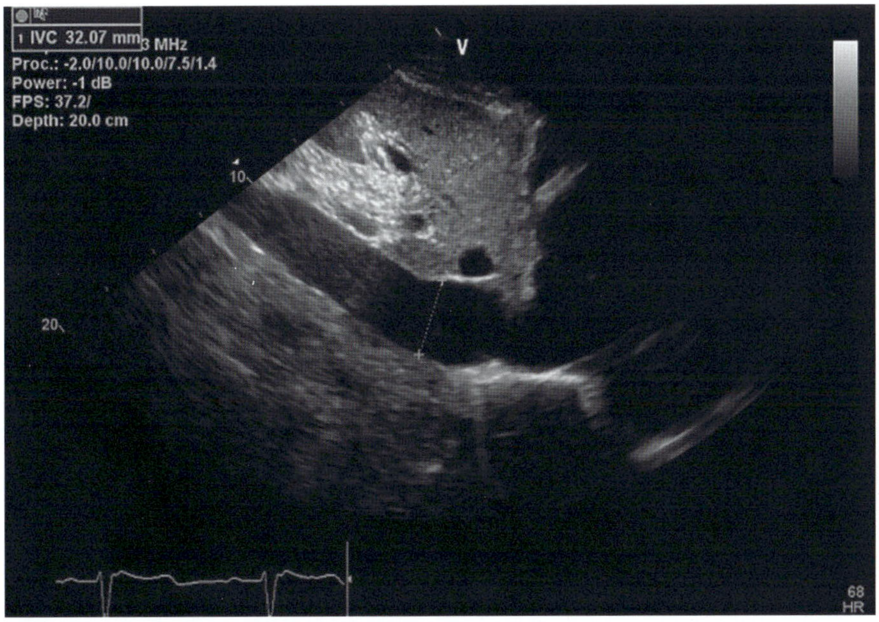

(B)

Figure 1-8
This figure demonstrates the rudiments of calculation of right ventricular systolic pressure. Tricuspid valve regurgitant velocity is calculated by continuous wave Doppler as shown in (A). In this case, the gradient is approximately 39 mmHg. To calculate central venous pressure, the inferior vena cava is utilized, as shown in (B). Overall dimension of the inferior vena cava, and also its response to respiration, are combined together to estimate central venous pressure. In this particular example, there is severe enlargement of the inferior vena cava, resulting in an estimate of central venous pressure of 25 mmHg. Thus, in this case, the patient would have an estimated right ventricular systolic pressure of 64 mmHg.

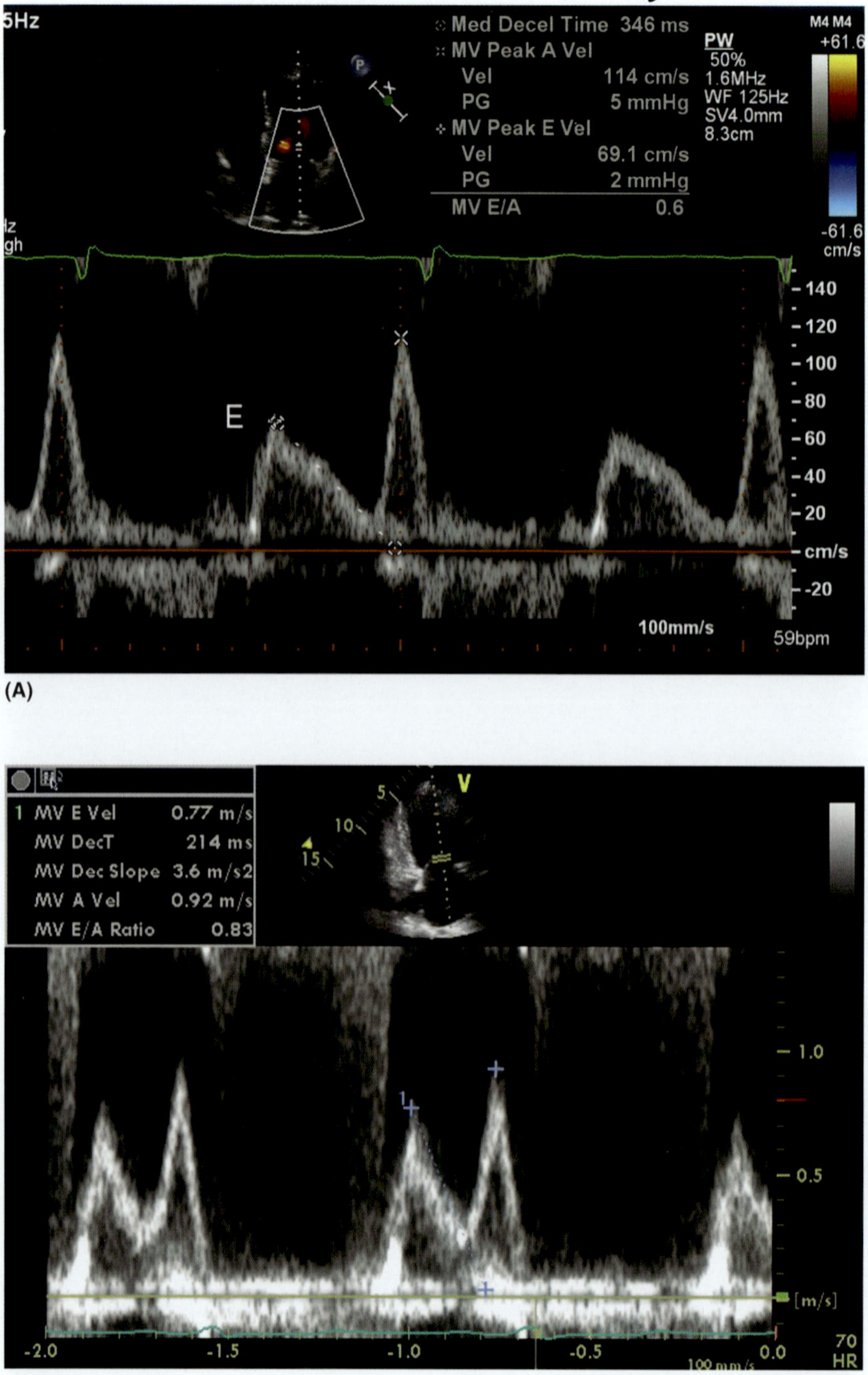

Figure 1-9

A series of figures showing the building blocks utilized by echocardiography to estimate the severity of diastolic dysfunction (see **Table 1-5**). Measurements of mitral forward flow, tissue Doppler analysis of annular motion, and pulmonary venous inflow are demonstrated. In (A) is shown a typical example of Type 1 diastolic dysfunction, where early relaxation slowing is the predominant abnormality. The E velocity of early diastole is reduced in comparison to the A velocity from atrial contraction. The deceleration time between E and A is also prolonged in this case. This finding is typical of Type 1 diastolic dysfunction and is usually associated with low filling pressures at rest. As filling pressures start to rise, the mitral flow pattern may begin to look like that seen in (B). *(Continued)*

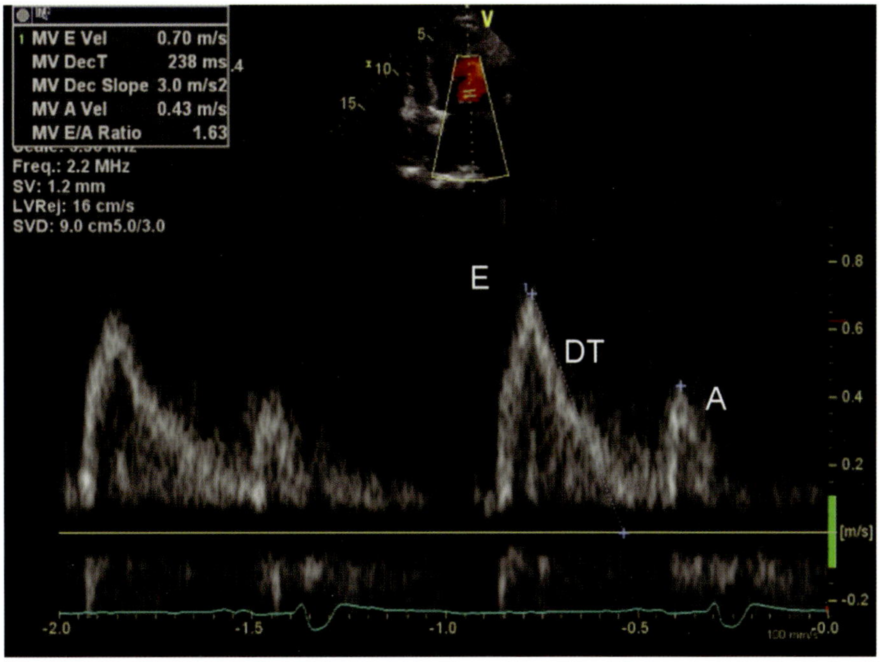

(C)

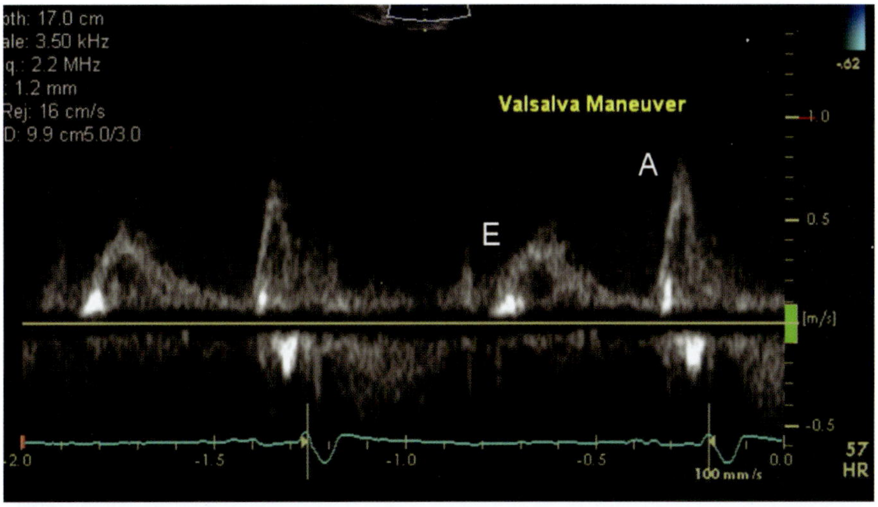

(D)

Figure 1-9 *(Continued)*
In this case the E velocity is now increased but is still less than the A velocity, and the deceleration time has come back into the normal range. As velocity of the E wave rises above 50 cm/sec (in this case it is up to 77), there is evidence that filling pressures are starting to rise. This pattern would be consistent with Type 1B diastolic dysfunction, still predominantly caused by early relaxation slowing, but now there is preload elevation also. In (C), a normal pattern of mitral inflow is shown. In heart failure patients the question becomes, is this truly normal or pseudonormal? Further elevations in filling pressures caused by high preload can "normalize" the mitral flow pattern. Diastolic relaxation is still significantly slowed and abnormal, but the high pressures in the left atrium tend to accelerate early flow velocities into the left ventricle. This remains the most difficult pattern to analyze and decide between normal or pseudonormal. One maneuver during the echocardiographic study which can help considerably in sorting out the pattern is shown in (D). *(Continued)*

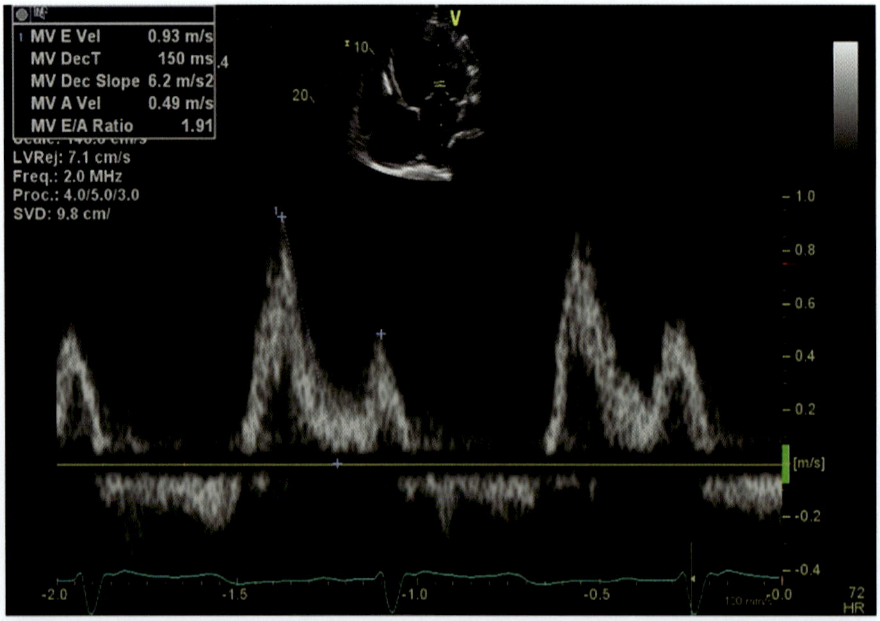

(E)

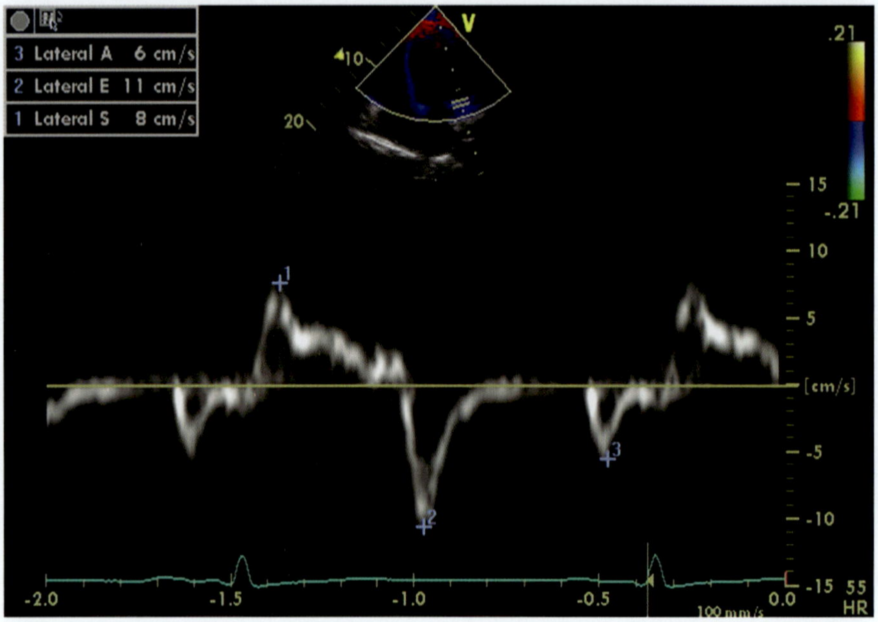

(F)

Figure 1-9 *(Continued)*
In this case a patient has performed a Valsalva maneuver and caused a marked reduction in the filling pattern, back to a Type 1 pattern. In this situation, a reduction in preload has markedly changed the filling pattern. This is a typical finding in a truly pseudonormalized Type 2 diastolic dysfunction abnormality. In (E) is shown a pattern of flow that is more severely abnormal, with now even higher E velocities and lower A velocities. This pattern is approaching the Types 3 and 4 restrictive patterns of filling of the ventricle, where filling pressures are very high but diastolic performance is markedly abnormal. Deceleration time becomes shorter and shorter as filling pressures become even higher. This finding in a dilated cardiomyopathy carries the worst prognosis with regard to diastolic function. (F) is an example of tissue Doppler obtained at the mitral annulus. In this case the pattern is still normal with normal velocities. *(Continued)*

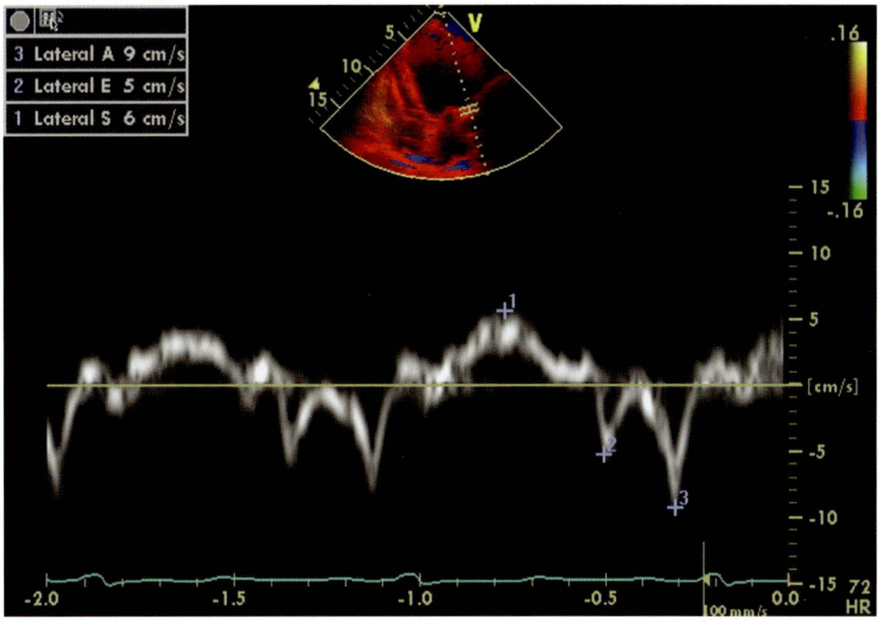

(G)

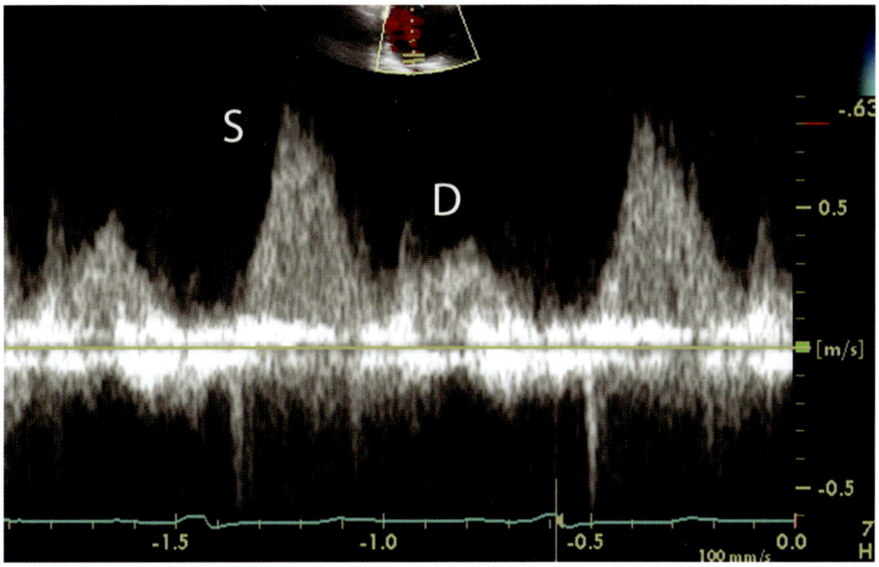

(H)

Figure 1-9 *(Continued)*
In (G) is shown the change that typically occurs as diastolic performance deteriorates in dilated cardiomyopathies. There is a shift in velocity so that the E velocity, now markedly reduced to 5 cm/sec, becomes less than the A velocity. Absolute values of less than 8 cm/sec are considered findings typical of diastolic dysfunction. The greater the severity of the diastolic dysfunction, typically the lower the velocity of E is found. Pulmonary venous inflow is shown in (H). In this pattern there is still considerable inflow in systole (S), the higher wave, and a reduction of flow in diastole (D), the smaller wave. In this particular example, filling pressures are still low, allowing a considerable amount of inflow during ventricular systole into the left atrium. However, since relaxation is slow, the amount of filling occurring during diastole is markedly attenuated. *(Continued)*

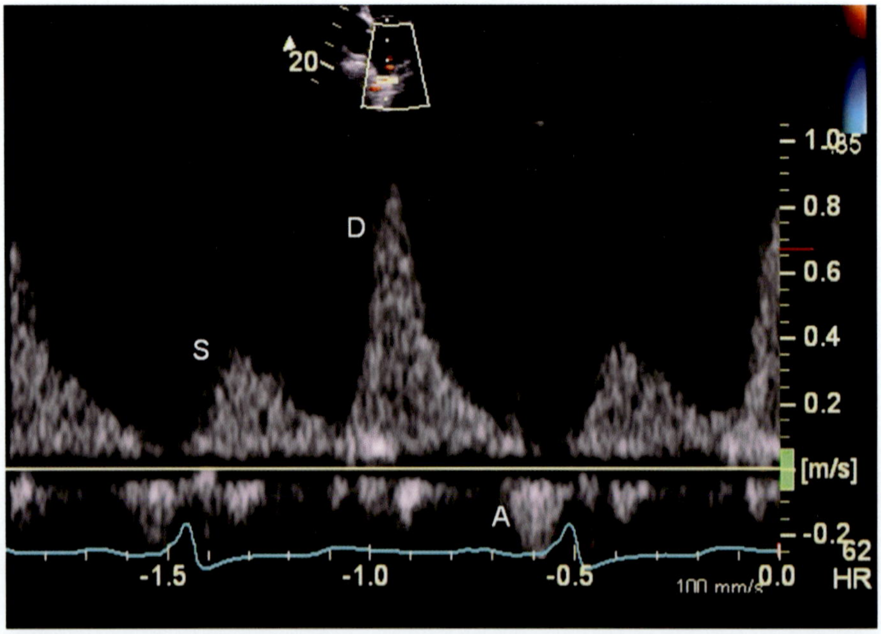

(I)

Figure 1-9 *(Continued)*
This pulmonary venous inflow pattern would corroborate a finding of a Type 1 abnormality of diastolic function. As filling pressures and preload rise, the pattern of pulmonary venous inflow changes to that seen in (I). In this case the systolic inflow wave (S) is markedly attenuated in relationship to D, the diastolic inflow wave. This pulmonary venous finding is typical of that seen in patients with Type 2, 3, or 4 diastolic dysfunction and persistently elevated left atrial pressures. (I). In this case the systolic inflow wave (S) is markedly attenuated in relationship to D, the diastolic inflow wave. This pulmonary venous finding is typical of that seen in patients with Type 2, 3, or 4 diastolic dysfunction and persistently elevated left atrial pressures.

Table 1-5
Classification of Diastolic Dysfunction in Dilated Cardiomyopathy

DIASTOLIC GRADE	ESTIMATED FILLING PRESSURE	DIASTOLIC FUNCTION
Type I	Low	Predominant early relaxation slowing
Type IB	Elevated	Predominant early relaxation slowing with some preload elevation
Type II "pseudonormal"	Elevated but drops with Valsalva	Early relaxation slowing more severe Reduced LV compliance now significant
Type III and IV severe	Elevated and may (III) or may not (IV) reverse with Valsalva	Marked reduction in relaxation rate Marked reduction in compliance Both rate and extent of relaxation limited

improvement is associated with a better long-term prognosis (40). It should also be noted that there is a poor correlation of symptomatic limitation from heart failure with diastolic filling patterns, similar to the poor correlation noted with ejection fraction (8).

CASE PRESENTATION

Based on the patient's presentation and echocardiographic and EKG findings, cardiac catheterization was planned for the next day. In addition, serial troponins had revealed a further small rise to a peak of 0.17 ng/mL.

Cardiac catheterization revealed large coronary arteries, all of which had only minimal luminal irregularities. Right heart catheterization was performed. This revealed a mean right atrial pressure of 7 mmHg, a mean pulmonary capillary wedge pressure of 18 mmHg, a pulmonary artery pressure of 41/18 with a mean of 26, a central aortic pressure of 123/88, a cardiac output of 3.9 L/min, and a cardiac index of 1.74 L/min. Pulmonary vascular resistance was 165, pulmonary artery oxygen saturation 61%, and SVR was 1,949 dynes/sec/cm^5.

EVALUATION FOR CORONARY ARTERY DISEASE

Definitive evaluation for the presence of coronary artery disease is important because it is the underlying cause of heart failure in about two out of every three patients with a low ejection fraction (EF) (8). The first consideration is how best to make the diagnosis of coronary artery disease. While a multitude of noninvasive evaluations are possible, all have limitations compared to coronary angiography. Thus, it would appear that coronary angiography remains the test of choice for most patients presenting with new heart failure with no known etiology. It can be argued that angiography may not be of much value in the very young if the pretest probability is very low and in the elderly where coronary interventions may not affect prognosis. If no significant coronary artery disease is present, ongoing medical therapy should be optimized. If coronary artery disease is discovered, the second important consideration is what should be the optimal treatment. Current data remains controversial. Older trials of intervention with coronary artery bypass surgery in patients with angina and left ventricular dysfunction showed evidence of improved symptoms and survival (41). For patients without symptomatic angina, several trials have used imaging to search for myocardial viability, the hypothesis being that those with evidence of hibernating and presumably viable myocardium will show reverse remodeling and improvement in prognosis. One meta-analysis done of 24 studies in the 1990s showed that for patients with evidence of hibernating myocardium, there was a marked reduction in mortality of 80% when patients were revascularized versus treated medically. However, those with no evidence of hibernation did not benefit from revascularization (42). More modern evaluations showed similar findings of hibernation presence being associated with improvement in EF (43), and improvement in EF being associated with better prognosis (44). The best method of defining hibernation also remains controversial, making evaluation of the efficacy of revascularization more difficult (45). These problems are exemplified by the recently published Surgical Treatment for Ischemic Heart Failure (STICH) trial, which was a randomized trial of 1,212 patients with severe ischemic cardiomyopathy (EF less than 35%), who were assigned to best medical therapy versus best medical therapy plus coronary artery bypass surgery. There was no significant mortality benefit but these results have been disputed. A recent long-term observational "real world" trial using STICH entry criteria followed patients treated with bypass surgery versus a propensity-matched medical therapy group over 10 years and found bypass surgery was associated with a survival benefit (46). Thus, more long-term data are needed. Even less information exists for percutaneous-based revascularization strategies, none randomized (47,48).

CASE PRESENTATION

On the third hospital day, the patient was started on carvedilol 3.125 mg twice daily and upward titration of his ACE inhibitor was continued. He was switched to a long-acting ACE inhibitor, lisinopril, at 10 mg per day and his diuretics were reduced to 40 mg orally once per day. The patient was introduced to nursing personnel and a clinical nutritionist from the Heart Failure Clinic and set up for long-term follow-up. He was discharged on the fourth hospital day after a total diuresis of 3.6 L. He was ambulating in the halls without significant shortness of breath for short distances and had no further orthopnea or nocturnal dyspea, denied lightheadedness or orthostasis, but still felt fatigued. Over the course of the next 2 months, he was seen approximately every 2 weeks in the Heart Failure Clinic. Medications were titrated further and the patient was able to return to work. Initially at work, he felt fatigued easily. He did not feel mentally sharp in the later part of the morning. After adjustment of timing of his medications, these symptoms gradually improved, and ultimately the patient was titrated up to 40 mg per day of lisinopril, 25 mg twice daily of carvedilol, and 40 mg once daily of furosemide.

MEDICAL TREATMENT OF HEART FAILURE

Optimal treatment of a new heart failure patient starts with patient education. The clinician must take time to educate the patient about the findings of diagnostic testing, the severity of the disease, the expected chronicity of the disease, and the plan for long-term therapy. Rarely do patients revert to normal; instead they are entering into a lifelong odyssey of chronic disease. How well he or she does will be critically dependent on compliance with treatment, vigilance for change in status, and close communication with providers.

Treatment is best performed using a team approach—a disease management system approach—with multiple providers (49): nutritionists for dietary instruction, social workers to help manage life consequences of heart failure, nurse clinicians to educate and provide close communication and frequent follow-up, nurse practitioners or physician assistants for drug titration and urgent follow-up visits, and physicians for direct patient management and overall supervision of the care plan. Several basic initial case and education issues are summarized in **Table 1-6**.

The cornerstone of treatment for the non-ischemic cardiomyopathy patient is medical therapy. The most commonly used pharmaceuticals are summarized in **Table 1-6**. Initial therapy starts with diuretics to relieve signs and symptoms of acute congestion. Typically, IV forms of diuretics are needed in substantial and

Table 1-6
Ambulatory Medical Therapy for Dilated Cardiomyopathy

PATIENT EDUCATION AND LIFESTYLE CHANGES

Sodium intake restriction to 2–3 gm
Fluid intake restriction as needed
Understanding of sodium content of food
Weight loss in obese patients (BMI > 30)
Smoking cessation
Education in the natural history of heart failure for the individual being treated based on conclusions of the initial evaluation
Limited alcohol consumption
Initiation of daily blood pressure and weight monitoring
Education as to when to call for help in management
Recommendations for exercise
Education to understand the purpose of each component of medical therapy

MEDICAL THERAPY

Diuretics
Purpose: Eliminate excessive sodium and water retention
Reduce symptoms of congestion
Achieve a "euvolemic state"

Typical drugs used:	*Initial Dose*
Furosemide	40 mg
Bumetanide	1 mg
Torsemide	10 mg

Angiotensin Converting Enzyme Inhibitors
Purpose: Reduce symptoms, reduce hospitalizations, reduce mortality

Typical drugs used:	*Initial Dose*	*Target Dose*
Captopril	6.25 mg 3 times daily	50 mg 3 times daily
Enalapril	2.5 mg 2 times daily	10 mg 2 times daily
Lisinopril	2.5–5 mg once daily	20–40 mg once daily

Angiotensin Receptor Blockers
Purpose: Reduce symptoms, reduce hospitalizations, reduce mortality
Reduce left ventricular remodeling

Typical drugs used:	*Initial Dose*	*Target Dose*
Candesartan	4–8 mg daily	32 mg daily
Losartan	12.5–25 mg twice daily	50–75 mg twice daily
Valsartan	40 mg twice daily	160 mg twice daily

Beta Blocker
Purpose: Reduce mortality, reduce hospitalizations, reduce symptoms
Reduce left ventricular remodeling, improve systolic function

Typical drugs used:	*Initial Dose*	*Initial Dose Target*
Bisoprolol	1.25 mg daily	10 mg daily
Carvedilol	3.125 mg twice daily	25–50 mg twice daily
Metoprolol succinate CR/XL	12.5–25 mg daily	200 mg daily

Aldosterone Antagonists
Purpose: Reduce mortality

Typical drugs used:	*Initial Dose*	*Target Dose*
Spironolactone	12.5–25 mg daily	25 mg daily
Eplerenone	25 mg daily	50 mg daily

Digoxin
Purpose: Reduce severity of persistent symptoms
Control ventricular rate in atrial fibrillation

Adjust digoxin to trough blood level 0.5–0.9 ng/ml
Typical starting dose 0.125 mg daily

(Continued)

Table 1-6 *(Continued)*
Ambulatory Medical Therapy for Dilated Cardiomyopathy

Hydralazine/Nitrates
Purpose: Alternative for patients not tolerant of renin-angiotensin inhibiting agents
Treatment of African Americans with heart failure
Reduce symptoms, reduce mortality, reduce LV remodeling

Typical drugs used:	*Initial Dose*	*Target Dose*
Isosorbide Dinitrate	10 mg 4 times daily	40 mg 4 times daily
Hydralazine	10 mg 4 times daily	75 mg 4 times daily
Fixed dose combination (BiDi1)	37.5 mg/20 mg 3 times daily	75 mg/40 mg 3 times daily

Source: Adapted from references 8 and 52.

frequent doses at the time of acute presentation to rapidly control symptoms. These diuretics have a rapid onset (within 30 minutes) and reach a peak effect with 2 hours. This allows the clinician to rapidly determine the effectiveness of initial therapy and decide on continuation or escalation of therapy. Diuretic naive patients with good renal function can be started at 40 mg of IV furosemide, those on chronic diuretics now presenting with an exacerbation of volume overload should be switched to IV therapy at least at the same dose of chronic oral therapy or higher (50). Once the patient is decongested, the diuretics should be switched to an oral dose. Simultaneously, establish a diet with appropriate sodium and fluid restriction. Diuretics are much more effective when combined with a low sodium diet. Expect the dose will need adjustment after the patient is discharged. Careful monitoring of blood pressure, weight, and symptoms are important as are frequent follow-up clinic visits within a week. The chronic diuretic dose is adjusted to maintain "dry weight" once that is established. Compliant patients, particularly those who show ventricular function improvement over time, may be able to reduce or sometimes eliminate the use of diuretics. Careful monitoring of electrolytes and renal function is necessary, as the most frequent side effects of diuretics are hypokalemia and renal dysfunction.

The next group of drugs to initiate is angiotensin converting enzyme inhibitors. These agents have acute hemodynamic effects of balanced preload and afterload reduction, which may help symptoms and improve cardiac performance. They are beneficial for all levels of severity of heart failure. Long-term benefits are related to reduced mortality, reduced repeat hospitalization, improved symptoms, and an antiremodeling effect on the left ventricle that slows and sometimes reverses structural deterioration of the heart (51). The medication should be started at a low dose to prevent hypotension and gradually uptitrated over several weeks. In general, one should titrate to goal doses (**Table 1-6**); however, pushing the dose to maximal levels has been questioned. Some studies have suggested benefit, others have not and it has been difficult in randomized trials to prove definite benefit of higher doses (52–54). There has also been concern about worsening renal function after initiation of ACE-inhibitors. In most circumstances, it may be due to lowering of efferent arteriolar tone in the glomerular apparatus. This can be particularly troublesome when bilateral renal artery stenosis is present or if the patient becomes intravascularly volume depleted. In the latter case, reduction in diuretic dose may restore homeostasis. Small changes in renal function are generally well tolerated and are not a reason to discontinue therapy (55).

Perhaps the most troubling side effect of ACE-inhibitors is cough. It occurs in about 10% of patients, usually within weeks to months of treatment initiation and persists, going away within 1 to 4 weeks after discontinuation of the drug, coming back on rechallenge. It should not be confused with bronchospasm or nocturnal cough from congestion (56). If real, switching to angiotensin receptor blockers (ARBs) usually eliminates the problem. The ARBs have been extensively investigated in heart failure and appear to have substantially equal efficacy as ACE-inhibitors (57). Initiation of ARBs require the same methods and precautions as with ACE-inhibitors. Typical initial and goal doses are listed in **Table 1-6**. Achieving target dose of Losartan (100 mg–150 mg/day) appears to be important to achieve maximum efficacy (58). Combined use of ACE-inhibitors and ARBs is not recommended (59).

Maximizing inhibition of the rennin-angiotensin system is best done by adding aldosterone antagonists to existing therapy with ACE-inhibitors or ARBs. Both spironolactone and eplerenone have shown benefit in small fixed doses (**Table 1-6**; 60–62) for reduction in mortality, now across the spectrum of patients from post large myocardial infarction to Class II to Class IV heart failure. It is important to take precautions of careful monitoring of electrolytes and renal function as hyperkalemia can be lethal (63). Patients should be started with spironolactone; if gynecomastia develops in men, most will benefit from a change to eplerenone.

Inhibition of the adrenergic receptors in heart failure patients leads to symptomatic improvement, reduced hospitalization, reduced mortality, and an antiremodeling effect on the left ventricle. Substantial numbers of patients show significant improvement in left ventricular ejection fraction, and the magnitude of improvement appears to be positively related to prognosis (64). All of the major trials have been performed with patients on ACE-inhibitors, so the considerable benefit seen is additive to conventional therapy. Therefore, it is of vital importance for inhibition of the renin-angiotensin system and beta blockade to go forward at once after the diagnosis is made. It is safe to initiate beta blockade at low doses in the hospital after initial stabilization of the patient (65,66). Three beta blockers are recommended for use based on clinical trial evidence (Table 1-6). They should all be started at low doses and gradually uptitrated over several weeks to goal doses. Patients should be warned that they may temporarily feel worse every time the dose is increased and be careful to monitor themselves for fluid retention that may necessitate adjustment of other therapy. Bradycardia, heart block, hypotension, or bronchospasm may also limit use.

The use of digoxin has declined in the last decade and is now recommended for use in two situations: persistence of symptoms after all of the above discussed therapy has been maximized and for rate control for heart failure patients in chronic atrial fibrillation (8,59). More recent reanalysis of an older trial has pointed to the importance of appropriate blood levels. Safety is enhanced and efficacy maintained if the serum levels are kept between 0.5 and 0.9 ng/ml (67,68). As with aldosterone antagonists, particular care should be taken to monitor electrolytes and renal function.

The combination of hydralazine and nitrates was the first vasodilator therapy to have definite benefit for heart failure (69) but was shown subsequently to be inferior to ACE-inhibition (70). The combination of the two agents gives both preload and afterload reduction. This results in symptomatic improvement and an antiremodeling effect with associated modest mortality reduction. The combination is difficult to sustain chronically because the side effect profile is poor and it must be taken four times per day to attain full effect. Due to the perceived lower benefit of ACE-inhibition in African Americans, a fixed dose combination (BiDi1) was tested as additional therapy over and above standard treatment in the A-Heft trial (71) and found to be beneficial. Whether the effect carries over to others is not known. Occasionally this combination has been added to patients who have hemodynamic evidence of inadequate vasodilation despite maximal conventional dosing of standard therapy and found to be effective. Its most frequent use, however, is as alternative therapy for those who cannot tolerate renin-angiotensin inhibition of any kind (8,59).

CASE PRESENTATION

The patient continued to do well. A repeat echocardiogram was performed approximately 4 months after the patient had achieved full-dose therapy. The patient felt he had now returned back to his baseline functional capacity, was working full-time, did not have significant fatigue at the end of the day, and was back to riding his bicycle about 15 minutes per day after work. He was again able to walk up four flights of stairs to his business. The echocardiogram, however, revealed only modest improvement in ejection fraction from 10% to 20%. The left ventricle remained markedly enlarged and spherical. His filling characteristics, however, had improved from a restrictive pattern at presentation to a Type I diastolic dysfunction pattern, consistent with substantial reduction in filling pressures. Right ventricular function had also improved considerably. The right ventricle was now almost normal in function, with only mild enlargement noted. Pulmonary pressures remained elevated with a peak estimated pulmonary artery (PA) pressure of 49 mmHg. Consultation with the electrophysiology team was strongly recommended to the patient for placement of a defibrillator and also consideration of a bi-ventricular pacing device, even though he was symptomatically markedly improved. The patient, however, declined placement of the defibrillator, primarily because he was still paying off the very large deductible from his initial hospitalization. He said he wanted to wait until several more months had passed to see if his ventricle showed further signs of improvement. He was started on 25 mg of spironolactone. At a return visit 4 months later, he continued to feel well, continued to work full-time, but was told that his consulting contract would not be renewed after the job was completed in another 4 months. He again was advised to have a defibrillator device placed but again declined. Two months later he died suddenly in his apartment.

CONCLUSION

This is the story of a real patient and illustrates most of the typical evaluation and decision making that occurs over the natural history of heart failure due to a non-ischemic cardiomyopathy. It also shows the limitations of our current therapy. Many patients have a more robust response to medical therapy; others do not. The remaining cases presented in this book show variations on this basic theme of heart failure and the different approaches needed to optimize therapy.

REFERENCES

1. Mant J, Doust J, Roalfe A, et al. Systematic review and individual patient data meta-analysis of diagnosis of heart failure, with modelling of implications of different diagnostic strategies in primary care. *Health Technol Assess.* 2009;13(32):1–207; iii.
2. McKee PA, Castelli WP, McNamara PM, et al. The natural history of congestive heart failure: the Framingham study. *N Engl J Med.* 1971;285(26):1441–1446.
3. Drazner MH, Hellkamp AS, Leier CV, et al. Value of clinician assessment of hemodynamics in advanced heart failure: the ESCAPE trial. *Circ Heart Fail.* 2008;1(3):170–177.
4. Madias JE. The resting electrocardiogram in the management of patients with congestive heart failure: established applications and new insights. *Pacing Clin Electrophysiol.* 2007;30(1):123–128.
5. Kamath SA, Meo Neto JP, Canham RM, et al. Low voltage on the electrocardiogram is a marker of disease severity and a risk factor for adverse outcomes in patients with heart failure due to systolic dysfunction. *Am Heart J.* 2006;152(2):355–361.
6. Madias JE, Agarwal H, Win M, et al. Effect of weight loss in congestive heart failure from idiopathic dilated cardiomyopathy on electrocardiographic QRS voltage. *Am J Cardiol.* 2002;89(1):86–88.
7. Dickstein K, Cohen-Solal A, Filippatos G, et al. ESC Guidelines for the diagnosis and treatment of acute and chronic heart failure 2008: the Task Force for the Diagnosis and Treatment of Acute and Chronic Heart Failure 2008 of the European Society of Cardiology. Developed in collaboration with the Heart Failure Association of the ESC (HFA) and endorsed by the European Society of Intensive Care Medicine (ESICM). *Eur Heart J.* 2008;29(19):2388–2442.
8. Jessup M, Abraham WT, Casey DE, et al. writing on behalf of the 2005 Guideline Update for the Diagnosis and Management of Chronic Heart Failure in the Adult Writing Committee. 2009 focused update: ACCF/AHA guidelines for the diagnosis and management of heart failure in adults: a report of the American College of Cardiology/American Heart Association Task Force on Practice Guidelines. *J Am Coll Cardiol.* 2009;53(15):1343–1382.
9. Januzzi JL, Jr. The role of natriuretic peptide testing in guiding chronic heart failure management: review of available data and recommendations for use. *Arch Cardiovasc Dis.* 2012;105(1):40–50.
10. Maisel AS, Krishnaswamy P, Nowak RM, et al. Rapid measurement of B-type natriuretic peptide in the emergency diagnosis of heart failure. *N Engl J Med.* 2002;347(3):161–167.
11. Januzzi JL, Jr, Camargo CA, Anwaruddin S, et al. The N-terminal Pro-BNP investigation of dyspnea in the emergency department (PRIDE) study. *Am J Cardiol.* 2005;95(8):948–954.
12. Bettencourt P, Azevedo A, Pimenta J, et al. N-terminal-pro-brain natriuretic peptide predicts outcome after hospital discharge in heart failure patients. *Circulation.* 2004;110(15):2168–2174.
13. Logeart D, Thabut G, Jourdain P, et al. Predischarge B-type natriuretic peptide assay for identifying patients at high risk of readmission after decompensated heart failure. *J Am Coll Cardiol.* 2004;43(4):635–641.
14. Felker GM, Hasselblad V, Hernandez AF, et al. Biomarker-guided therapy in chronic heart failure: a meta-analysis of randomized controlled trials. *Am Heart J.* 2009;158(3):422–430.
15. Berger R, Moertl D, Peter S, et al. N-terminal pro-B-type natriuretic peptide-guided, intensive patient management in addition to multidisciplinary care in chronic heart failure a 3-arm, prospective, randomized pilot study. *J Am Coll Cardiol.* 2010;55(7): 645–653.
16. Moinuddin MJ, Figueredo V, Amanullah AM. Infiltrative diseases of the heart. *Rev Cardiovasc Med.* 2010;11(4):218–227.
17. Raju H, Alberg C, Sagoo GS, et al. Inherited cardiomyopathies. *BMJ.* 2011;343:d6966.
18. Gersh BJ, Maron BJ, Bonow RO, et al. 2011 ACCF/AHA guideline for the diagnosis and treatment of hypertrophic cardiomyopathy: executive summary: a report of the American College of Cardiology Foundation/American Heart Association Task Force on Practice Guidelines. *Circulation.* 2011;124(24): 2761–2796.
19. Marcus FI, McKenna WJ, Sherrill D, et al. Diagnosis of arrhythmogenic right ventricular cardiomyopathy/dysplasia: proposed modification of the Task Force Criteria. *Eur Heart J.* 2010;31(7):806–814.
20. Vasan RS, Larson MG, Benjamin EJ, et al. Congestive heart failure in subjects with normal versus reduced left ventricular ejection fraction: prevalence and mortality in a population-based cohort. *J Am Coll Cardiol.* 1999;33(7):1948–1955.
21. Lang RM, Badano LP, Tsang W, et al. EAE/ASE recommendations for image acquisition and display using three-dimensional echocardiography. *J Am Soc Echocardiogr.* 2012;25(1):3–46.
22. Lang RM, Bierig M, Devereux RB, et al. Recommendations for chamber quantification. *Eur J Echocardiogr.* 2006;7(2):79–108.
23. Mor-Avi V, Lang RM, Badano LP, et al. Current and evolving echocardiographic techniques for the quantitative evaluation of cardiac mechanics: ASE/EAE consensus statement on methodology and indications endorsed by the Japanese Society of Echocardiography. *J Am Soc Echocardiogr.* 2011;24(3):277–313.
24. Brieke A, DeNofrio D. Right ventricular dysfunction in chronic dilated cardiomyopathy and heart failure. *Coron Artery Dis.* 2005;16(1):5–11.
25. Gupta S, Khan F, Shapiro M, et al. The associations between tricuspid annular plane systolic excursion (TAPSE), ventricular dyssynchrony, and ventricular interaction in heart failure patients. *Eur J Echocardiogr.* 2008;9(6):766–771.
26. Grayburn PA, Appleton CP, DeMaria AN, et al. Echocardiographic predictors of morbidity and mortality in patients with advanced heart failure: the Beta-blocker Evaluation of Survival Trial (BEST). *J Am Coll Cardiol.* 2005;45(7):1064–1071.
27. Ghio S, Gavazzi A, Campana C, et al. Independent and additive prognostic value of right ventricular systolic function and pulmonary artery pressure in patients with chronic heart failure. *J Am Coll Cardiol.* 2001;37(1):183–188.
28. Sun JP, James KB, Yang XS, et al. Comparison of mortality rates and progression of left ventricular dysfunction in patients with idiopathic dilated cardiomyopathy and dilated versus nondilated right ventricular cavities. *Am J Cardiol.* 1997;80(12):1583–1587.
29. Suh IW, Song JM, Lee EY, et al. Left atrial volume measured by real-time 3-dimensional echocardiography predicts clinical outcomes in patients with severe left ventricular dysfunction and in sinus rhythm. *J Am Soc Echocardiogr.* 2008;21(5):439–445.
30. Matsumoto K, Tanaka H, Okajima K, et al. Relation between left ventricular morphology and reduction in functional mitral regurgitation by cardiac resynchronization therapy in patients with idiopathic dilated cardiomyopathy. *Am J Cardiol.* 2011;108(9):1327–1334.
31. Cleland JG, Daubert JC, Erdmann E, et al. The effect of cardiac resynchronization on morbidity and mortality in heart failure. *N Engl J Med.* 2005;352(15):1539–1549.
32. John Sutton MG, Plappert T, Abraham WT, et al. Effect of cardiac resynchronization therapy on left ventricular size and function in chronic heart failure. *Circulation.* 2003;107(15):1985–1990.
33. Rosario LB, Stevenson LW, Solomon SD, et al. The mechanism of decrease in dynamic mitral regurgitation during heart failure treatment: importance of reduction in the regurgitant orifice size. *J Am Coll Cardiol.* 1998;32(7):1819–1824.

34. Lowes BD, Gill EA, Abraham WT, et al. Effects of carvedilol on left ventricular mass, chamber geometry, and mitral regurgitation in chronic heart failure. *Am J Cardiol*. 1999;83(8):1201–1205.
35. Capomolla S, Febo O, Gnemmi M, et al. Beta-blockade therapy in chronic heart failure: diastolic function and mitral regurgitation improvement by carvedilol. *Am Heart J*. 2000;139(4):596–608.
36. Pino PG, Galati A, Terranova A. Functional mitral regurgitation in heart failure. *J Cardiovasc Med (Hagerstown)*. 2006;7(7):514–523.
37. Kirkpatrick JN, Vannan MA, Narula J, et al. Echocardiography in heart failure: applications, utility, and new horizons. *J Am Coll Cardiol*. 2007;50(5):381–396.
38. Sorrell VL, Reeves WC. Noninvasive right and left heart catheterization: taking the echo lab beyond an image-only laboratory. *Echocardiography*. 2001;18(1):31–41.
39. Stein JH, Neumann A, Marcus RH. Comparison of estimates of right atrial pressure by physical examination and echocardiography in patients with congestive heart failure and reasons for discrepancies. *Am J Cardiol*. 1997;80(12):1615–1618.
40. Nagueh SF, Appleton CP, Gillebert TC, et al. Recommendations for the evaluation of left ventricular diastolic function by echocardiography. *J Am Soc Echocardiogr*. 2009;22(2):107–133.
41. Yusuf S, Zucker D, Peduzzi P, et al. Effect of coronary artery bypass graft surgery on survival: overview of 10-year results from randomised trials by the Coronary Artery Bypass Graft Surgery Trialists Collaboration. *Lancet*. 1994;344(8922):563 –570.
42. Allman KC, Shaw LJ, Hachamovitch R, et al. Myocardial viability testing and impact of revascularization on prognosis in patients with coronary artery disease and left ventricular dysfunction: a meta-analysis. *J Am Coll Cardiol*. 2002;39(7):1151–1158.
43. Bax JJ, van der Wall EE, Harbinson M. Radionuclide techniques for the assessment of myocardial viability and hibernation. *Heart*. 2004;90(Suppl 5):v26–v33.
44. Rizzello V, Poldermans D, Biagini E, et al. Prognosis of patients with ischaemic cardiomyopathy after coronary revascularisation: relation to viability and improvement in left ventricular ejection fraction. *Heart*. 2009;95(15):1273–1277.
45. Schuster A, Morton G, Chiribiri A, et al. Imaging in the management of ischemic cardiomyopathy: special focus on magnetic resonance. *J Am Coll Cardiol*. 2012;59(4):359–370.
46. Velazquez EJ, Williams JB, Yow E, et al. Long-term survival of patients with ischemic cardiomyopathy treated by coronary artery bypass grafting versus medical therapy. *Ann Thorac Surg*. 2012;93(2):523–530.
47. Tsuyuki RT, Shrive FM, Galbraith PD, et al. Revascularization in patients with heart failure. *CMAJ*. 2006;175(4):361–365.
48. Phillips HR, O'Connor CM, Rogers J. Revascularization for heart failure. *Am Heart J*. 2007;153(4 Suppl):65–73.
49. Velez M, Westerfeldt B, Rahko PS. Why it pays for hospitals to initiate a heart failure disease management program. *Dis Manage Health Outcomes*. 2008;16:155–173.
50. Felker GM, Lee KL, Bull DA, et al. Diuretic strategies in patients with acute decompensated heart failure. *N Engl J Med*. 2011;364(9):797–805.
51. Flather MD, Yusuf S, Kober L, et al. Long-term ACE-inhibitor therapy in patients with heart failure or left-ventricular dysfunction: a systematic overview of data from individual patients. ACE-Inhibitor Myocardial Infarction Collaborative Group. *Lancet*. 2000;355(9215):1575–1581.
52. Clinical outcome with enalapril in symptomatic chronic heart failure; a dose comparison. The NETWORK Investigators. *Eur Heart J*. 1998;19(3):481–489.
53. Rochon PA, Sykora K, Bronskill SE, et al. Use of angiotensin-converting enzyme inhibitor therapy and dose-related outcomes in older adults with new heart failure in the community. *J Gen Intern Med*. 2004;19(6):676–683.
54. Ryden L, Armstrong PW, Cleland JG, et al. Efficacy and safety of high-dose lisinopril in chronic heart failure patients at high cardiovascular risk, including those with diabetes mellitus. Results from the ATLAS trial. *Eur Heart J*. 2000;21(23):1967–1978.
55. Testani JM, Kimmel SE, Dries DL, et al. Prognostic importance of early worsening renal function after initiation of angiotensin-converting enzyme inhibitor therapy in patients with cardiac dysfunction. *Circ Heart Fail*. 2011;4(6):685–691.
56. Bangalore S, Kumar S, Messerli FH. Angiotensin-converting enzyme inhibitor associated cough: deceptive information from the Physicians' Desk Reference. *Am J Med*. 2010;123(11):1016–1030.
57. Granger CB, McMurray JJ, Yusuf S, et al. Effects of candesartan in patients with chronic heart failure and reduced left-ventricular systolic function intolerant to angiotensin-converting-enzyme inhibitors: the CHARM-Alternative trial. *Lancet*. 2003;362(9386): 772–776.
58. Konstam MA, Neaton JD, Dickstein K, et al. Effects of high-dose versus low-dose losartan on clinical outcomes in patients with heart failure (HEAAL study): a randomised, double-blind trial. *Lancet*. 2009;374(9704):1840–1848.
59. Lindenfeld J, Albert NM, Boehmer JP, et al. Executive Summary: HFSA 2010 Comprehensive Heart Failure Practice Guideline. *J Card Fail*. 2010;16(6):475–539.
60. Zannad F, McMurray JJ, Krum H, et al. Eplerenone in patients with systolic heart failure and mild symptoms. *N Engl J Med*. 2011;364(1):11–21.
61. Pitt B, Remme W, Zannad F, et al. Eplerenone, a selective aldosterone blocker, in patients with left ventricular dysfunction after myocardial infarction. *N Engl J Med*. 2003;348(14):1309–1321.
62. Pitt B, Zannad F, Remme WJ, et al. The effect of spironolactone on morbidity and mortality in patients with severe heart failure. Randomized Aldactone Evaluation Study Investigators. *N Engl J Med*. 1999;341(10):709–717.
63. Juurlink DN, Mamdani MM, Lee DS, et al. Rates of hyperkalemia after publication of the Randomized Aldactone Evaluation Study. *N Engl J Med*. 2004;351(6):543 –551.
64. Foody JM, Farrell MH, Krumholz HM. beta-Blocker therapy in heart failure: scientific review. *JAMA*. 2002;287(7):883–889.
65. Gattis WA, O'Connor CM, Gallup DS, et al. Predischarge initiation of carvedilol in patients hospitalized for decompensated heart failure: results of the Initiation Management Predischarge: Process for Assessment of Carvedilol Therapy in Heart Failure (IMPACT-HF) trial. *J Am Coll Cardiol*. 2004;43(9):1534 –1541.
66. Fonarow GC, Abraham WT, Albert NM, et al. Carvedilol use at discharge in patients hospitalized for heart failure is associated with improved survival: an analysis from Organized Program to Initiate Lifesaving Treatment in Hospitalized Patients with Heart Failure (OPTIMIZE-HF). *Am Heart J*. 2007;153(1):82–11.
67. Rathore SS, Curtis JP, Wang Y, et al. Association of serum digoxin concentration and outcomes in patients with heart failure. *JAMA*. 2003;289(7):871–878.
68. Ahmed A, Rich MW, Love TE, et al. Digoxin and reduction in mortality and hospitalization in heart failure: a comprehensive post hoc analysis of the DIG trial. *Eur Heart J*. 2006;27(2): 178–186.
69. Cohn JN, Archibald DG, Ziesche S, et al. Effect of vasodilator therapy on mortality in chronic congestive heart failure. Results of a Veterans Administration Cooperative Study. *N Engl J Med*. 1986;314(24):1547–1552.

70. Cohn JN, Johnson G, Ziesche S, et al. A comparison of enalapril with hydralazine-isosorbide dinitrate in the treatment of chronic congestive heart failure. *N Engl J Med*. 1991;325(5):303–310.

71. Taylor AL, Ziesche S, Yancy C, et al. Combination of isosorbide dinitrate and hydralazine in blacks with heart failure. *N Engl J Med*. 2004;351(20):2049 –2057.

72. Fonseca C, Sarmento PM, Minez A, et al. Comparative value of BNP and NT-proBNP in diagnosis of heart failure. *Rev Port Cardiol*. 2004;23(7–8):979–991.

73. Morrison LK, Harrison A, Krishnaswamy P, et al. Utility of a rapid B-natriuretic peptide assay in differentiating congestive heart failure from lung disease in patients presenting with dyspnea. *J Am Coll Cardiol*. 2002;39(2):202–209.

74. Mueller T, Gegenhuber A, Dieplinger B, et al. Capability of B-type natriuretic peptide (BNP) and amino-terminal proBNP as indicators of cardiac structural disease in asymptomatic patients with systemic arterial hypertension. *Clin Chem*. 2005;51(12):2245–2251.

2

Patient With Heart Failure Following a Large Myocardial Infarction

JANE E. WILCOX AND WILLIAM G. COTTS

CASE PRESENTATION

A 52–year-old African American woman with a past medical history significant for hypertension and hyperlipidemia presented to her local hospital with 1 hour of chest pain. Her vital signs were 98.9°F, heart rate 90 beats/minute, blood pressure 140/90 mmHg, and she was tachypneic with a respiratory rate of 24 breaths/minute. On physical exam she appeared anxious and uncomfortable. Her lungs were clear. Heart exam revealed a regular rate and rhythm with no murmurs, S3, or S4. Her electrocardiogram (**Figure 2-1**) was significant for prominent ST segment elevations in the anterior leads. She was given aspirin, oxygen, and heparin and was taken immediately to the coronary catheterization suite for the diagnosis of ST-segment elevation myocardial infarction.

She underwent primary percutaneous intervention with a drug eluting stent for a thrombosis in a long lesion in the proximal segment of the left anterior descending (LAD) artery (**Figure 2-2**, cath films). During the procedure, she became short of breath and hypotensive with systolic blood pressure of 70 mmHg. An intra-aortic balloon pump (IABP) was placed for cardiogenic shock that enhanced coronary perfusion during diastole and reduced afterload during systole.

Primary percutaneous coronary intervention (PCI) is the preferred reperfusion strategy for ST-elevation myocardial infarction (STEMI) when it can be performed in a timely manner by experienced personnel. Patients with acute myocardial infarction accompanied by pulmonary edema or cardiogenic shock (systolic blood pressure less than 90 mmHg, pulmonary capillary wedge pressure (PCWP) greater than 15 mmHg) have a high in-hospital mortality rate of up to 60% (1) and there is a significant reduction in mortality with IABP therapy (2). The Should We Emergently Revascularize Occluded Coronaries for Cardiogenic Shock (SHOCK) trial provides the rationale for emergent revascularization in patients with acute myocardial infarction (AMI) complicated by cardiogenic shock. In this trial, a low number needed to treat (NNT) of eight patients had to receive coronary revascularization (via PCI or coronary artery bypass grafting [CABG]) to prevent one death at 6 months.

CASE PRESENTATION

A Swan-Ganz pulmonary artery catheter (PAC) was placed for hemodynamic monitoring and she was taken to the Coronary Care Unit (CCU). Upon arrival to the CCU she was found to have the following hemodynamic parameters: central venous pressure (CVP) 20 mmHg, pulmonary artery systolic/diastolic pressure (PAS/PAD) 50 mmHg/21 mmHg, pulmonary artery mean (PAM) pressure 31 mmHg, PCWP 21 mmHg, cardiac output (CO) 5 L/min, cardiac index (CI) 2.5 L/min/m^2. Essentially, her hemodynamics showed elevated filling pressures from an ischemic left ventricle, and her CO was improved by the IABP. Her systemic venous oxygen saturation was measured at 55% suggesting inadequate supply of oxygen in relation to tissue demands (3).

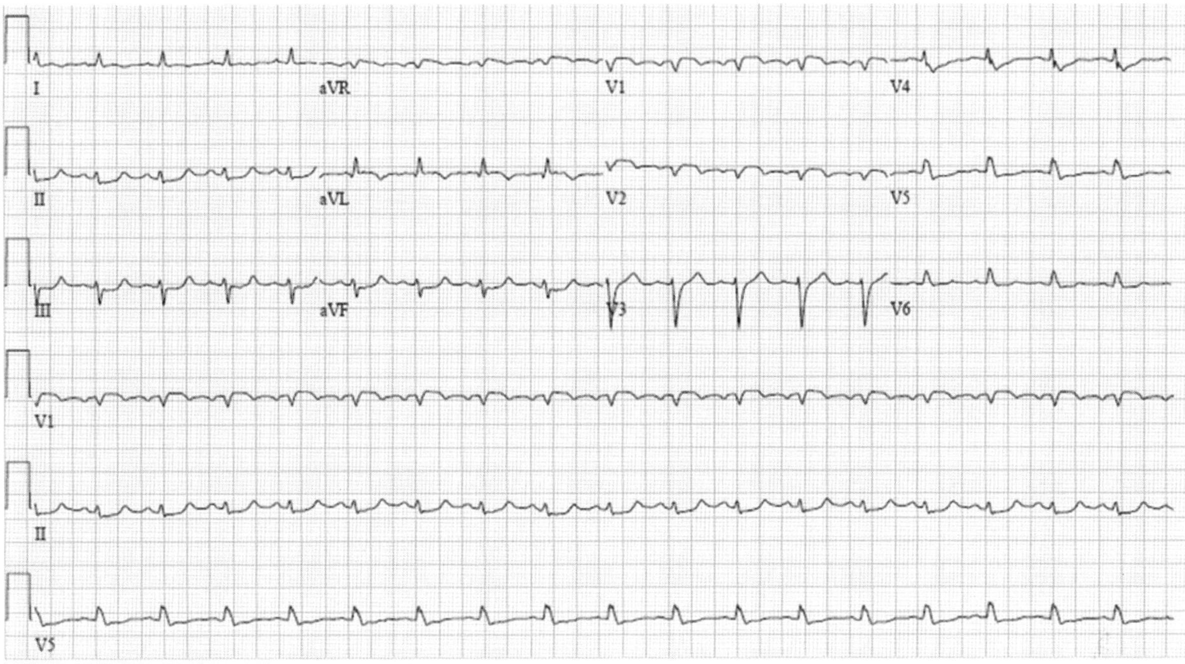

Figure 2-1
Initial ECG with anterior precordial ST elevation and reciprocal changes in the inferior leads. Low voltage is also demonstrated. The findings, while subtle, are consistent with an anterior wall myocardial infarction.

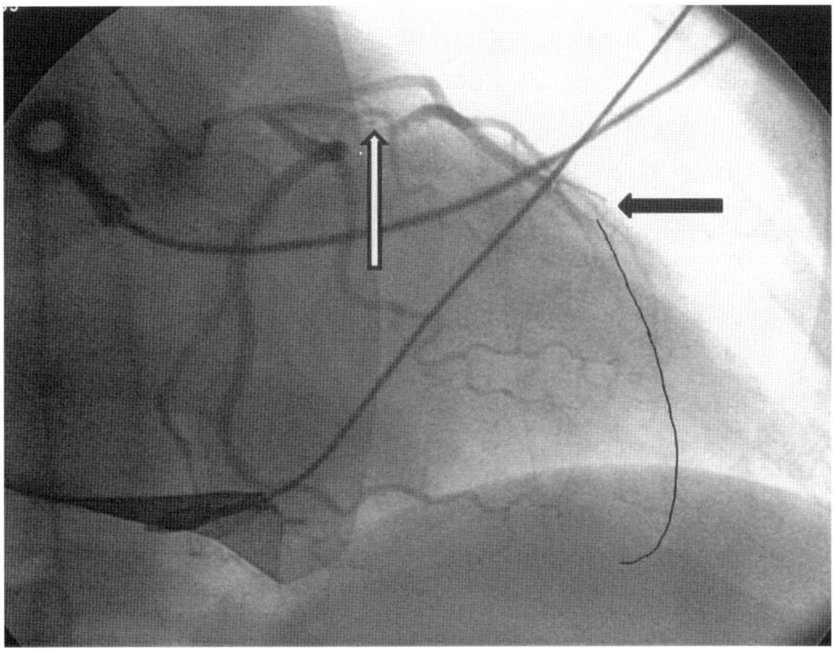

Figure 2-2
Left heart catheterization with mid left anterior descending artery culprit lesion (solid arrow) and proximal left anterior descending 95% stenosis (open arrow). The thin red line shows the downstream course of the artery beyond the occlusion.

A low systemic venous oxygen saturation in patients with AMI portends a worse overall prognosis (4). The indication for invasive hemodynamic monitoring in this case was considered to be AMI associated with cardiogenic shock necessitating IABP placement. While the Evaluation study of congestive heart failure and pulmonary artery catheterization effectiveness (ESCAPE) trial (5) demonstrated that the addition of a PAC does not decrease mortality in patients admitted for heart failure exacerbations, the PAC is indicated in the setting of acute hemodynamic compromise.

CASE PRESENTATION

Continuous hemodynamic support was achieved overnight with the IABP therapy. Improved forward flow allowed for effective diuresis and her subsequent PCWP was 15 mmHg and CI improved to 2.8 L/min/m^2. The patient's mean arterial blood pressure remained stable at greater than 65 mmHg, which allowed for the IABP to be weaned from 1:1 (inflation/deflation of the balloon with each cardiac cycle) to 2:1 and then finally 3:1 and removed. To mitigate the risk of embolic events with an intra-aortic device in place, the patient was anticoagulated with heparin during this time period.

POST-MYOCARDIAL INFARCTION CARE

CASE PRESENTATION

Our patient continued to do well clinically after removal of the IABP, which allowed the CCU team to focus on post–myocardial infraction (MI) care, with particular attention to potential complications in this vulnerable time period. She remained on telemetry to monitor for electrical abnormalities.

Bradyarrhythmias, including heart block (more common with right coronary artery lesions) and tachyarrhythmias including ventricular tachycardia (VT), occur in up to 15% of MIs (6). Accelerated idioventricular rhythm (AIVR) is found in up to 40% of patients who are continuously monitored post-MI and represents reperfusion in most patients (7). Mechanical complications post-MI can be devastating. They include: mitral regurgitation, either due to complete or partial papillary muscle rupture; free wall rupture of the left ventricle, which occurs in 1% to 4.5% of AMI patients (8); and septal rupture, or acute ventricular septal defect (VSD), which has been reported to be about half as common as free wall rupture and typically occurs 3 to 5 days after an acute MI. VSDs may, however, develop within the first 24 hours or as late as 2 weeks (9).

CASE PRESENTATION

No valvular abnormalities were noted on a two-dimensional echocardiogram with Doppler that was performed on our patient. Overall, left ventricular (LV) function was moderately reduced at 35% to 40%, stemming from a "hypokinetic" anterior wall. A large LV thrombus was associated with this area and intravenous heparin was begun as a bridge to chronic warfarin therapy (**Figure 2-3**).

In 1998, the GISSI-3 study demonstrated that the highest rate of occurrence of LV thrombus formation was found among patients with anterior AMI and an EF less than 40% (10). Current available data are mixed regarding prophylactic anticoagulation to prevent LV thrombus in patients with anterior wall MI (11). Prospective randomized trials are needed to

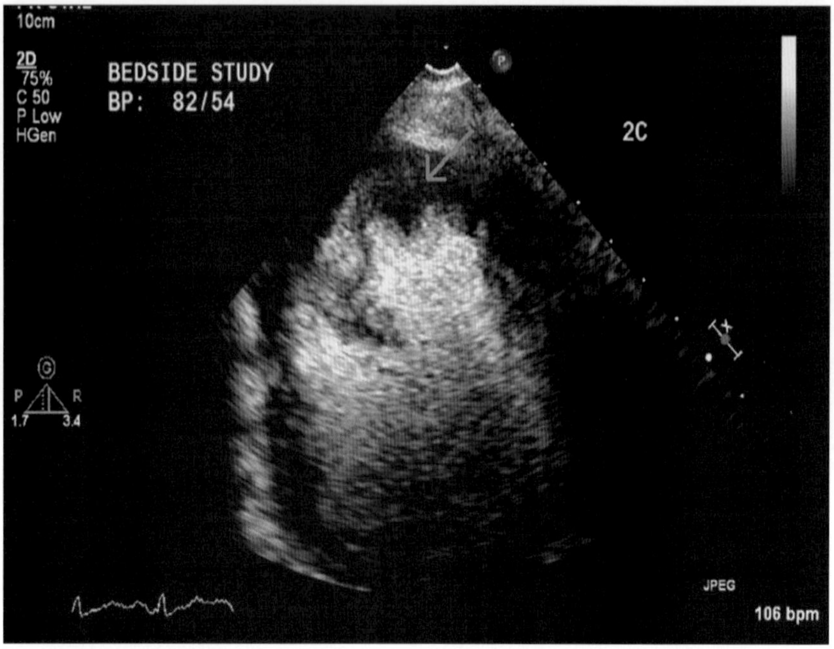

Figure 2-3
Echocardiogram showing left ventricular apical thrombus.

determine the optimal strategy for preventing this serious adverse outcome.

Post-MI care is often divided into secondary prevention and risk stratification. Secondary prevention, which focuses on diagnosing and treating existing disease in its early stages before it leads to significant morbidity, can be accomplished with (a) pharmacotherapy and (b) screening for comorbid conditions that contribute to coronary artery disease (CAD) and heart failure mortality. When an MI is complicated by LV dysfunction, tertiary prevention (reducing negative consequences from established disease) must be utilized as well. Pharmacotherapy and device therapies are the cornerstones of treatment. To stay within the scope of this book, this chapter will focus on post MI patients with reduced LV systolic function as compared to those with preserved LV function.

According to current ACC/AHA guidelines (12), this patient was started on anti-neurohormonal therapies known to reduce mortality post-MI; beta blockers and angiotensin-converting enzyme (ACE) inhibitors should be started without delay once the patient is clinically stable. Captopril and metoprolol tartate are reasonable choices due to their short half-lives. However, once a tenuous patient is stable (or this is not an issue), the nonselective beta-blocker and α1-blocker carvedilol is preferred. The Comparison of carvedilol and metoprolol on clinical outcomes in patients with chronic heart failure in the Carvedilol or Metoprolol European Trial (COMET) showed a 20% reduction in mortality in heart failure patients treated with carvedilol versus metoprolol tartrate. Our patient was started at 6.25 mg BID of carvedilol in the hospital, increased to 12.5 mg BID the day prior to discharge. The target dose of carvedilol is 25 mg BID that can be titrated as an outpatient. An alternative beta-blocker that was shown to reduce mortality by 34% in the MERIT-HF trial is metoprolol succinate (XL or extended release). The salient point of either drug is appropriate outpatient dosage. Clinicians should aim for target doses used in clinical trials, either 25 mg BID of carvedilol or 200 mg of metoprolol XL.

Dual antiplatelet therapy with aspirin/thienopyridine ADP-receptor antagonist (eg, clopidogrel or prasugrel) was initiated immediately based on data from Clopidogrel as Adjunctive Reperfusion Therapy (CLARITY)–Thrombolysis in Myocardial Infarction (TIMI) CLARITY-TIMI and TRITON-TIMI 38 trials (13,14). An alternative nonthienopyridine antagonist of the platelet P2Y12 ADP receptor is ticagrelor, which can be used as an alternative to clopidogrel or prasugrel, and was shown to reduce all cause mortality when compared with clopidogrel in the Platelet inhibition and patient outcomes, Ticagrelor versus Clopidogrel in Patients with Acute Coronary Syndromes (PLATO) trial (15). There was a trend toward harm in the North American subgroup associated with major bleeding that was thought to be secondary to higher aspirin dosages. Therefore, aspirin 81 mg should be used in conjunction with ticagrelor, and based on the Double-dose versus standard-dose clopidogrel and high-dose versus low-dose aspirin in individuals undergoing percutaneous coronary intervention for acute coronary syndromes (CURRENT OASIS 7) trial, 81 mg of aspirin is just as effective as 325 mg, but with a trend toward reduced bleeding (16).

Our patient was also discharged on atorvastatin 80 mg. Based on the Pravastatin or Atorvastatin Evaluation and Infection Therapy (PROVE-IT) and the Myocardial Ischemia Reduction with Acute Cholesterol Lowering (MIRACL) trials, the ACC/AHA guidelines carry a class I recommendation for statins to be administered in the acute setting of a MI (17,18).

The landmark Eplerenone, a selective aldosterone blocker, in patients with left ventricular dysfunction after myocardial infarction (EPHESUS) trial evaluated the use of aldosterone blockade with eplerenone added to optimal medical therapy for acute myocardial infarction in patients with LV dysfunction. EPHESUS demonstrated a reduction in morbidity and mortality in the eplerenone group (19). This was corroborated in a recent meta-analysis that showed a 20% reduction in all-cause mortality with the use of aldosterone blockade in patients with heart failure post-MI (20). As this benefit is not observed when eplerenone is initiated after 7 days (21), it is critical to begin eplerenone early in these patients. Our patient's complete list of discharge medications are listed in **Table 2-1**.

Postdischarge Care: The Vulnerable Period

In this patient with a recent anterior wall MI and reduced LV function with a mural thrombus, it is imperative to ensure that she is receiving all appropriate therapies prior to discharge to reduce her chances for admission for heart failure. She was discharged home with a follow-up in cardiology clinic in 2 weeks; important considerations to maximize medical and device therapy should be performed at this visit.

CASE PRESENTATION

First Follow-up Visit

At her 2 week follow-up visit, our patient was seen in cardiology clinic. Assessment of (a) volume status, (b) symptoms, and (c) appropriate use of guideline-based therapies should

Table 2-1
Discharge Dedication Regime

MEDICATION	DISCHARGE DOSE	FOLLOW-UP CLINIC DOSE AT 2 WEEKS	TARGET DOSE
Atorvastatin	80 mg q day	80 mg q day	80 mg q day (fixed dose per PROVE-IT trial)
Carvedilol	12.5 mg BID	12.5 mg BID (limited by blood pressure)	25 mg BID
Captopril/Lisinopril	6.25 mg TID captpril changed to l0 mg lisinopril q day	20 mg q day lisinopril	40 mg q day lisinopril
Aspirin	325 mg q day	81 mg q day	81–325 mg q day
Clopidogrel	75 mg q day	75 mg q day	75 mg q day
Eplerenone	25 mg q day	25 mg q day (limited by potassium levels)	50 mg q day
Warfarin (for LV thrombus)	5 mg, goal INR 2–3	goal INR 2–3	goal INR 2–3

Note: LV = left ventriclar

be part of this visit in all postdischarge patients. Overall, she was feeling much better, but still with low levels of energy. She appeared euvolemic, with minimal elevation in her jugular venous pulse (JVP) and no rales on lung exam. Her medications were increased as blood pressure and renal function/electrolytes allowed (specifically potassium levels). Follow-up clinic medication doses are listed in **Table 2-1**. She was also referred to "cardiac rehab" at this visit. Exercise-based cardiac rehabilitation is associated with an approximate 30% reduction in overall mortality and a 50% reduction in reinfarction post-MI. Despite this, cardiac rehabilitation remains an underused tool for secondary prevention post-MI (22).

In patients with chronic heart failure, the risk of death is greatest in the early period after discharge after a hospitalization for heart failure and is directly related to the duration and frequency of heart failure hospitalizations. These findings suggest a role for increased surveillance in the early postdischarge period of greatest vulnerability after a heart failure admission (23). Although patients with acute heart failure have improvement in symptoms during hospitalization, the postdischarge rehospitalization rate and mortality within 60 to 90 days remain as high as 30% and 15%, respectively (24).

At the first follow-up appointment from the hospital (as in the case with our patient) or at the first visit to establish care as an outpatient, a systematic and comprehensive evaluation should occur. There are many evidenced-based therapies that are underutilized in the community caring for heart failure patients. The Improving Evidence-Based Care for Heart Failure in Outpatient Cardiology Practices: Primary Results of the Registry to Improve Heart Failure Therapies in the Outpatient Setting (IMPROVE-HF) cohort demonstrated that a practice-based performance improvement intervention implemented in *outpatient cardiology* or *multispecialty practices* increases the use of guideline-recommended care for eligible patients (25). *Referral to a comprehensive clinic* or implementing a practice-based intervention may improve the use of beta-blockers, aldosterone antagonists, cardiac resynchronization therapy (CRT), implantable cardioverter-defibrillator (ICD), and heart failure education (25).

CASE PRESENTATION

Three Month Follow-up Visit

In our patient, a critical component of the post-AMI discharge plan involved follow-up in clinic for repeat Left Ventricular Ejection Fraction (LVEF) assessment. Due to varied increases in LVEF in response to neurohormonal medical therapy, the guidelines recommend that ICD placement occur at least 40 days post-MI with an LVEF less than or equal to 35%, and New York Heart Association (NYHA) functional Class II or III symptoms. In patients with a non-ischemic etiology for heart failure, the standard of care is to allow a sufficient time period (generally 60–90 days) for uptitration to maximal doses of medications. During this time, providers can assess for comorbidities that affect survival (ie, cancer or end-stage lung disease), as the benefit of ICD therapy is not apparent until after 1 year (26), and may only be harmful if implanted in such individuals. As she was committed to warfarin therapy (in addition to aspirin and clopidogrel) due to the large LV mural thrombus, repeat echocardiography for assessment of overall LV function and thrombus resolution was done at 3 months post discharge.

CASE PRESENTATION

She did have an ICD placed for primary prevention of SCD approximately 3 months after her AMI, as her LVEF was now estimated to be 25% to 30% at that time. Medications should also be uptitrated to evidence based doses as previously mentioned. Our patient also had a cardiac MRI (CMR) at this visit, which showed a large area of scar (evidenced by greater than 50% thickness gadolinium contrast-enhanced myocardium) in the entire LV anterior wall (**Figure 2-4**). The lack of significant viable myocardium may be important for both patients and clinicians in prognosis and potential for recovery, which is addressed in future sections.

Over the next several months, this patient was admitted multiple times to outside hospitals for symptoms of acute heart failure, mostly with pulmonary congestion, weight gain, and lower extremity edema.

Acute heart failure can present with different signs and symptoms and precipitating events, often multifactorial in nature, and are varied and should be identified and treated. Observational data has demonstrated that ischemic events (including MI, 27), atrial fibrillation (27), and worsening valvular disease (28) are mechanisms associated with a substantial number of readmissions leading to exacerbation of and progression of heart failure and death (29). Noncardiac comorbidities, including acute kidney injury, acute respiratory infections, and medication and dietary noncompliance are potential triggers for readmission as well. Gheorghiade and Braunwald have proposed a six-axis model for initial assessment of factors that should be considered in patients presenting with acute heart failure syndromes. These are: clinical severity, systolic blood pressure (SBP), heart rate and rhythm, precipitants, comorbidities, and de novo or chronic heart failure (**Figure 2-5**).

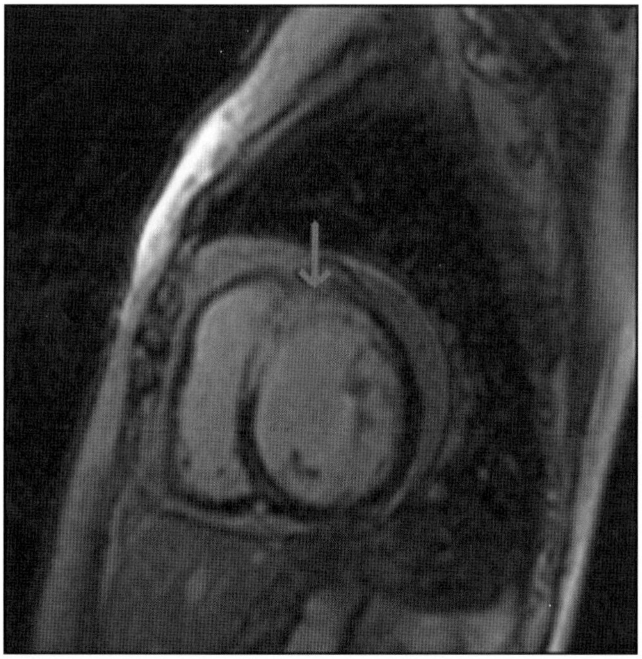

Figure 2-4
Short axis view of the cardiac MRI showing minimal viability in anterior wall (arrow). This was true from base to apex.
Source: From reference 82.

RISK STRATIFICATION

Hospitalization for heart failure independently portends a poor prognosis (30,31) and the in-hospital mortality rate is variable among heart failure patients ranging from 0.4% to 28.0%. To better risk stratify these patients several studies have developed models of risk prediction (29,32–36). The Get with the Guidelines (GWTG) heart failure risk score uses commonly available clinical variables to predict in-hospital mortality and has been shown to be a validated tool for risk stratification. Additionally, the tool is applicable to patients with preserved left ventricular systolic function. The mortality risk score calculator is available online and includes age, systolic blood pressure, blood urea nitrogen, heart rate, sodium, chronic obstructive lung disease (COPD), and nonblack race; all factors are predictive of in-hospital mortality. The predicted and observed probabilities of in-hospital mortality varies across deciles (range of 0.4% to 9.7%) in the GWTG study (**Figure 2-6**; 36)

Vital sign and laboratory data obtained on hospital admission are easily obtained and can prognosticate risk. In the Acute Decompensated Heart

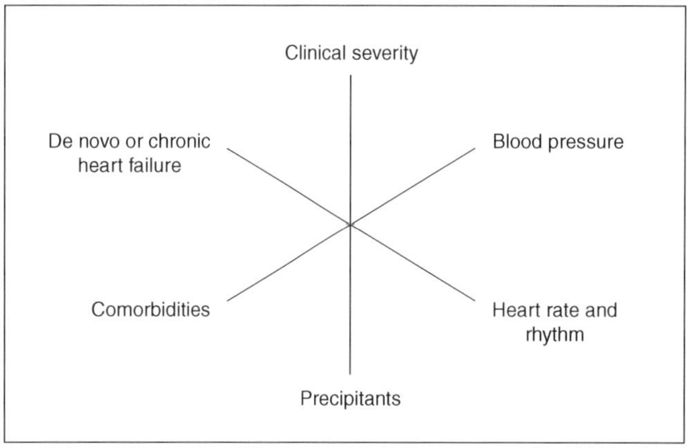

Figure 2-5
Six-axis approach to evaluation of acute heart failure patients.
Source: adapted from Gheorghiade and Braunwald. JAMA. 2011;305(16):1702-1703.

Systolic BP	Points
50-59	28
60-69	26
70-79	24
80-89	23
90-99	21
100-109	19
110-119	17
120-129	15
130-139	13
140-149	11
150-159	9
160-169	8
170-179	6
180-189	4
190-199	2
≥200	0

BUN	Points
≤9	0
10-19	2
20-29	4
30-39	6
40-49	8
50-49	9
60-69	11
70-79	13
80-89	15
90-99	17
100-109	19
110-119	21
120-129	23
130-139	25
140-149	27
≥150	28

Sodium	Points
≤130	4
1131	3
132	3
133	3
134	2
135	2
136	2
137	1
138	1
≥139	0

Age	Points
≤19	0
20-29	3
30-39	6
40-49	8
50-59	11
60-69	14
70-79	17
80-89	19
90-99	22
100-109	25
≥110	28

Heart Rate	Points
≤79	0
180-84-	1
85-89	3
90-94	4
95-99	5
100-104	6
≥105	8

Black Race	Points
Yes	0
No	3

COPD	Points
Yes	2
No	0

Total Score	Probability of Death
0-33	<1%
34-50	1-5%
51-57	>5-10%
58-61	>10-15%
62-65	>15-20%
66-70	>20-30%
71-74	>30-40%
75-78	>40-50%
≥79	>50%

Figure 2-6
The Get With the Guidelines Heart Failure (GWTG-HF) risk score system for in-hospital mortality.
Source: From reference 36.

Failure National Registry (ADHERE), mortality rates were as low as 1.8% in the low-risk patient group to 28% in the highest risk group. The single best predictor for mortality was high admission levels of blood urea nitrogen (greater than or equal to 43 mg/dL [15.35 mmol/L]), followed by low admission SBP (less than 115 mmHg), and then by elevated levels of serum creatinine (greater than or equal to 2.75 mg/dL [243.1 μmol/L]; 35).

COMORBIDITIES

Renal Failure

Comorbidities confer a significantly increased mortality risk even in patients with an overall high mortality risk due to heart failure; this is especially true in older individuals (37,38). Effective risk stratification can influence clinical decision making. Therefore, the medical team should initiate in-hospital screening for comorbidities that may affect prognosis. Particular attention to serum creatinine and glomerular filtration rate (GFR) during and after hospitalization is important for long-term outcomes (39,40). Chronic kidney disease (CKD) is associated with an increased risk for all major cardiovascular (CV) events after MI, particularly among patients with an estimated GFR less than 45 mL/min. In a recent randomized clinical trial, the ACE inhibitor captopril resulted in a substantial reduction of CV events in patients with CKD, and to a lesser extent in patients with normal kidney function (41).

Diabetes

Additionally, the presence of diabetes mellitus (DM) increases overall mortality risk in patients with AMI and LV dysfunction even after controlling for other known risk factors (42,43). Patients treated with insulin have a particularly high risk (43). A normal HbA1C of 5.3% excluded DM in our patient (44). Although she is relatively young at 52 years old, it is important to consider age when risk stratifying the patient with AMI. Heart failure after AMI is associated with poor outcomes especially in elderly patients, even when receiving appropriate background medical therapy (45).

Blood Pressure

Blood pressure is another nonmodifiable prognostic factor similar to age. Gheorghiade et al demonstrated that blood pressure is an independent predictor of morbidity and mortality in patients with heart failure; relative hypotension (SBP less than 120 mmHg) upon hospital admission portends a poor prognosis despite medical therapy (24). In addition to age, loss of weight, or leanness are also associated with poor prognosis in chronic heart failure (46). This is known typically as "cardiac cachexia."

Anemia and Iron Deficiency

Anemia is an additional predictor of poor outcomes in the heart failure population. The Organized Program to Initiate Lifesaving Treatment in Patients with Heart Failure (OPTIME-HF) investigators studied data from over 48,000 patients at 259 hospitals and demonstrated that one quarter of individuals were moderately to severely anemic (hemoglobin 5 to 10.7 g/dl). Anemic patients were more likely to be older, Caucasian, women, have renal dysfunction, preserved systolic function, and less likely to be receiving ACE inhibitors and beta blocker (BB) at discharge. Lower hemoglobin was associated with more readmissions at 90 days (33.1% vs. 24.2%) and mortality (4.8% vs. 3.0%, lowest vs. highest quartile) in hospitalized patients with heart failure (all $P < .0001$; 47).

Functional iron deficiency may be the result of chronic inflammation in chronic illness such as malignancy, chronic infectious diseases, chronic kidney disease, and chronic heart failure (48). The Ferric carboxymaltose in patients with heart failure and iron deficiency (FAIR-HF) trial demonstrated that treatment with IV ferric carboxymaltose in patients with chronic heart failure and iron deficiency, *with or without anemia*, improves symptoms, functional capacity, and quality of life. Additionally, there were no significant side effects (49). Erythropoiesis-stimulating agents have been investigated extensively in the past few years and might be of benefit in patients with heart failure and anemia. However, concerns have arisen regarding the safety of erythropoiesis-stimulating agents in patients with chronic kidney disease. The Reduction of Events With Darbepoetin Alfa in Heart Failure Trial (RED-HF) study will show whether use of darbepoetin alfa in anemic patients with chronic heart failure will reduce all cause mortality or hospitalization for heart failure (50).

Lung Disease and Sleep Disordered Breathing

COPD is associated with a poorer survival in heart failure patients. In the study of the Norwegian heart failure registry involving individuals with reduced EF (less than 40%), COPD independently predicted death along with other factors including increased age, creatinine, NYHA Class III/IV, and diabetes (51).

Sleep disordered breathing (SDB) is very common among heart failure patients. The prevalence ranges from 24% to 76% (52,53). There are two types of sleep disorders, obstructive sleep apnea (OSA) where the oropharyngeal musculature collapses the upper airway, and central sleep apnea (CSA), which occurs when the brain stem fails to stimulate breathing (54). SDB is not just associated with heart failure, but OSA may contribute to the development and progression of heart failure by inducing repetitive cycles of apnea-induced hypoxia. This leads to surges in sympathetic tone and increased blood pressure, as well as increased production of reactive oxygen species and inflammatory mediators. Increased sympathetic activity can elevate systemic vascular resistance, leading to increased left ventricular afterload, and subsequent myocardial oxygen demand (54,55). Untreated OSA in heart failure patients is associated with increased mortality independent of other risk factors (54). In contrast to OSA, CSA is often a result of heart failure (56). The Canadian Continuous Positive Airway Pressure (CPAP) for Patients with CSA and Heart Failure Trial (CANPAP; 57) showed that CPAP had no effect on heart transplant (HT)-free survival; however, in a secondary analysis when SBD was adequately treated, LVEF and transplant-free survival were increased (56). Future studies are needed to determine whether treating SDB reduces morbidity and mortality. Due to the high prevalence of SBD in the heart failure population, all patients should be screened and the diagnosis requires nocturnal polysomnography (58).

SOCIAL DETERMINANTS IN HEART FAILURE

Mental Health

In addition to physical health, an individual's mental health can affect prognosis. Depression and cognitive function are closely related to heart failure prognosis, with lower LVEF and memory dysfunction predicting mortality. Poorer global cognitive score (as determined by the minimental status score), working memory (most predictive), psychomotor speed, and executive function have also been shown to be significant predictors (59). Interestingly, although worsened cognitive function may predict heart failure outcomes, cognitive deficits have not been shown to mediate the relationship between heart failure severity and health-related quality of life (HRQL; 60). Quality of life (QOL) has been recently shown to be mediated mostly by the following predictors: (a) low baseline QOL (low admission Kansas City Cardiomyopathy score); (b) high B-type natriuretic peptide (BNP); (c) hyponatremia; (d) tachycardia; (e) hypotension; (f) absence of beta-blocker therapy; and (g) history of diabetes mellitus and arrhythmia (61).

Racial Disparities

Studies have demonstrated a disproportionate burden of heart failure in African American patients, with greater prevalence of heart failure and higher rates of heart failure hospitalization compared with whites (62–65). The etiology of these disparities is likely multifactorial, related in part to worse outpatient management, access to care, socioeconomic status, and health literacy. In a recent study by Chaudry et al, black race was strongly associated with worse health literacy and all measures of poor access to care in unadjusted analyses. After adjusting for demographics, noncardiac comorbidity, social support, insurance status, and socioeconomic status (income and education), the odds of black race associated with reduced health literacy was twofold higher than white individuals. Cost as a deterrent to seeking health care and absence of a medical home (OR 1.76 and 1.55 respectively) were also notable differences (65).

POTENTIAL FOR CARDIAC FUNCTION RECOVERY

Both inpatient and outpatient management of heart failure patients should be comprehensive and include a direct assessment of the myocardium and targets for potential recovery. Specifically, an assessment of viability should be made in these patients. Myocardial viability has been shown to be an important prognostic marker in patients with CAD and LV dysfunction (66–68), with multiple studies demonstrating that the presence of myocardial viability predicts LV functional recovery in patients with CAD and low LVEF (69–71). "Hibernating myocardium" has been clinically useful in selecting patients whose chronic contractile myocardial dysfunction improves following coronary revascularization (70–77). Cleland and colleagues (78) showed that improved LV function was linearly associated with the volume of hibernating myocardium, and in a meta-analysis, Allman and colleagues (79) found a strong association between myocardial viability on noninvasive testing and improved survival after revascularization in patients with CAD and LV dysfunction. A recent substudy of the surgical treatment of ischemic heart failure (STICH) trial found that the extent of viable myocardium by dobutamine echocardiography, single-photon emission computed tomography (SPECT), or both in patients with heart failure with reduced LVEF due to CAD, who were candidates for surgical revascularization, was a univariate predictor of mortality and heart failure events, but failed to hold true after multivariable adjustment (80). A potential reason for this finding is that all viable but dysfunctional myocardium may not recover with revascularization. If the myocardium is irreversibly remodeled, it may be nonrecoverable with current available therapies. More research is needed in this area, especially with regard to predictors of improvement in LV function. A recent post hoc analysis of the IMPROVE-HF cohort demonstrated that almost one-third of outpatients had a dramatic improvement in LVEF (from 24.5% to 46.2%, 92% relative improvement) over 2 years. Multivariate analysis revealed female sex, no prior MI, non-ischemic heart failure etiology, and no digoxin use were associated with greater than 10% improvement in LVEF (81). Myocardial viability and its potential for recovery are likely future targets for therapy. There are many modalities available to assess for myocardial viability; the various sensitivities and specificities are displayed in **Figure 2-7** (82). *As previously mentioned, our patient had a CMR that showed a large area of scar (**Figure 2-4**). These CMR findings did not suggest that revascularization would be of major benefit to her.* Bello and colleagues showed that gadolinium-enhanced CMR predicts the response in LV function and remodeling (83). The amount of dysfunctional but viable myocardium by CMR is an independent predictor of the percent increase in EF expected after revascularization. Patients with significant scarring are unlikely to improve (83).

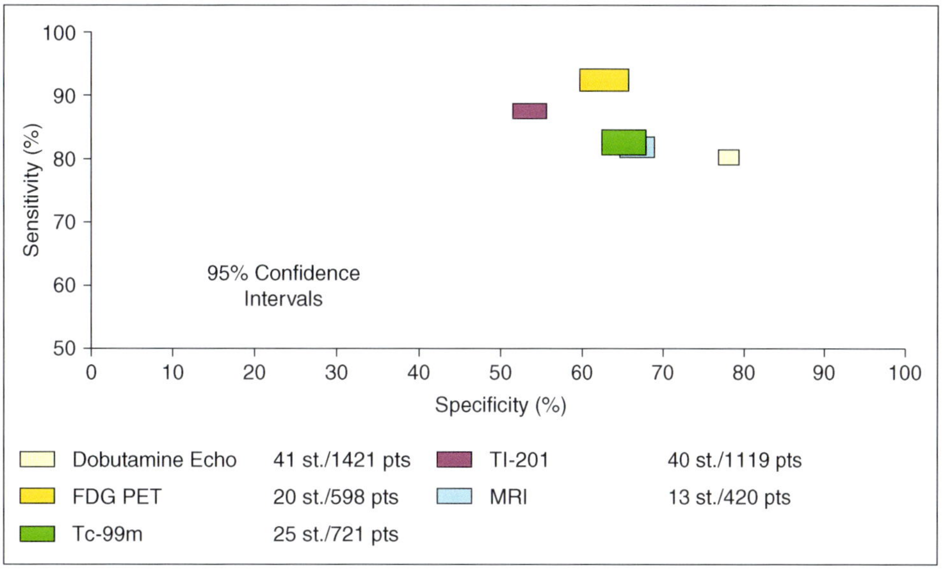

Figure 2-7

Relative sensitivities and specificities of the various modalities currently used for myocardial ischemia and myocardial viability assessment. For sensitivity, positron emission tomography (PET) is most sensitive ($P < .05$) versus other modalities. For specificity, echocardiography (Echo) is superior versus other modalities ($P < .05$).

Note: pts = patients; st = number of studies; Tc-99m = technitium nuclear studies; Tl-201 = thallium 201 studies.

DEVICE THERAPIES FOR HEART FAILURE

CASE PRESENTATION

This patient was referred for outpatient echocardiography for reassessment of LV function to determine if she would be a candidate for CRT and ICD therapy, and to evaluate if her LV thrombus had resolved after warfarin therapy.

Ventricular dyssynchrony has been associated with increased mortality in heart failure patients (84–86). CRT consists of atrial synchronized pacing of the left ventricle by an electrode, usually placed via the coronary sinus in order to achieve more synchronous contraction between the left ventricle and right ventricle (87). This dyssynchrony of contractile function is frequently present in heart failure patients with intraventricular conduction abnormalities (eg, left bundle branch blocks) manifested by a prolonged QRS. This leads to hemodynamic compromise of the left ventricle due to suboptimal ventricular filling (88).

There is excellent evidence (level of A in the guidelines, based on randomized controlled trials) that patients with LVEF of less than or equal to 35%, in sinus rhythm, and NYHA functional Class III or ambulatory Class IV symptoms despite being maximized on optimal medical therapy and who have evidence of cardiac dyssynchrony (defined as a QRS duration greater than or equal to 120 ms, although those patients with QRS prolongation of greater than 150 ms appear to derive the most benefit), should receive CRT, with or without an ICD, unless contraindicated (89–95). Clinical trials have shown that these patients derive significant benefit from this therapy, resulting in a reduction of risk of heart failure hospitalizations and death, in addition to improvement in functional status (89,95,96). One of these landmark studies, the Cardiac Resynchronization-Heart Failure (CARE-HF), demonstrated that even without concomitant ICD, the use of CRT reduced the risk of heart failure hospitalization and mortality by 37% (hazard ratio (HR) = 0.63, $P < .001$, 16% absolute reduction). Similarly, in the Comparison of Medical Therapy, Pacing, and Defibrillation in Heart Failure (COMPANION) trial, CRT alone reduced the risk of death from or hospitalization for heart failure by 34% ($P < .002$) and by 40% in the CRT-D group ($P < .001$ for the comparison with the medical therapy group).

Patients with non-ischemic cardiomyopathy (NICM) are more likely to respond to CRT when compared with ICM, and have improved outcomes (97). This finding underscores the importance of myocardial substrate, viability, and the potential for recovery in response to current medical and device therapies.

This patient had a narrow QRS without a left bundle branch block (LBBB) (**Figure 2-1**) and therefore did not meet criteria for CRT. It has been postulated that although female patients encounter similar, if not greater benefit from CRT implantation (98), they may be less likely to accept devices. In the IMPROVE-HF trial only 35% of indicated female patients initially had a CRT device at baseline. After 24 months, this improved to 65% suggesting that improved provider awareness can increase utilization rates and therefore reduce patient morbidity and mortality (25).

Currently, the guidelines indicate the use of CRT to NYHA Class II, III, and ambulatory Class IV patients, as new data have extended this to less symptomatic populations. NYHA Class I or II patients may receive substantial clinical benefits from CRT-D as well. Zareba and colleagues have recently demonstrated that heart failure patients with an EF less than or equal to 30% and a LBBB experience a reduction in heart failure progression and a reduction in the risk of ventricular tachyarrhythmias. This was not observed in patients with a right bundle branch block (RBBB) or other intraventricular conduction delays (99). The use of an ICD in combination with CRT should be based on the indications for ICD therapy (100).

Defibrillator Therapy

There is strong clinical trial evidence that ICD therapy is indicated for primary prevention of sudden cardiac death to reduce total mortality in patients with non-ischemic cardiomyopathy or heart failure due to ischemic heart disease (26, 94, 95,101–104). The benefit of ICD implantation was first noted in the Multicenter Automatic Defibrillator Implantation Trial II (MADIT-II). In patients with a prior MI and LV dysfunction (EF less than 30%), prophylactic ICD implantation improved survival during an average follow-up of 20 months. Mortality rates were 19.8% in the conventional-therapy group compared to 14.2% in the ICD group. Multiple studies have supported this finding and ICD benefit is similar in NYHA Class I to III heart failure patients with NICM as demonstrated by the Defibrillators in Non-Ischemic Cardiomyopathy Treatment Evaluation (DEFINITE) trial (103).

If patients with prior MI or chronic ischemic heart disease are "on the cusp" of an indication for ICD (ie, an estimated EF of 37%), a reasonable option is to risk stratify patients with an electrophysiology study. If sustained ventricular tachyarrhythmias can be induced, the risk of sudden death in these patients ranges from 5% to 6% per year, therefore can be improved with ICD implantation (105).

The balance of potential risks and benefits of ICD implantation is complex and must be discussed in great detail with each individual patient. Providers must inform and educate patients that ICD therapy may decrease his or her risk of sudden death, but this may not represent increased QOL or decreased total mortality (106). Patients should understand the expectations and limitations of ICD therapy (including lead fracture and inappropriate shocks) which, while rare, can significantly affect QOL. Additionally, providers should address cessation of ICD therapy or "turning off the shock-box" with patients who develop significant comorbidities that affect short-term survival.

CASE PRESENTATION

Refractory Heart Failure: Clinical Presentation at 6 Months

Six months after her initial anterior wall MI, she presented to our institution for refractory heart failure symptoms and evaluation for advanced therapies for heart failure. She was now NYHA Class IV(107), where any physical activity brings on discomfort and symptoms occur at rest, and ACC Stage D (108), with advanced disease requiring hospital-based support, HT, or palliative care. She had been re-hospitalized recently despite being compliant with her medical regimen and very strict sodium (less than 1000 mg/daily) and fluid restriction (less than 1L daily). She underwent right heart catheterization (RHC) as part of her advanced therapy workup.

Pulmonary Hypertension in Heart Failure

Determination of pulmonary hypertension and filling pressures is especially important in this population and often affects therapeutic options. Pulmonary hypertension (PH) is defined as any condition that leads to a PAM pressure of greater than or equal to 25 mmHg at rest (109,110). The current World Health Organization classification system is as follows (111): (a) pulmonary arterial hypertension (PAH); (b) PH due to left-sided heart disease; (c) PH due to lung diseases causing hypoxemia such as COPD or OSA; (d) chronic thromboembolic disease; and (e) miscellaneous (including sarcoidosis). PH is a very common comorbidity among heart failure patients, with prevalence estimates between 60% and 80%, and is associated with high morbidity and mortality (112,113). PH seen in heart failure is generally caused by chronically elevated left atrial pressure (LAP), which can be secondary to reduced systolic function, diastolic dysfunction, or significant valvular disease such as mitral regurgitation. However, the categories of PH do not exist in silos, and often times an individual heart failure patient may have multiple causes of PH, for example secondary to pulmonary venous congestion and OSA.

The gold standard for diagnosing PH remains a direct measurement of PA pressures and cardiac output by RHC; however, echocardiography is a useful noninvasive modality to screen for PH. The estimated velocity of the tricuspid regurgitant jet can estimate PA systolic pressure (114). If the PA systolic pressure is 35 to 45 mmHg, PH is "mild" and "moderate" at 46 to 60 mmHg, and "severe" if greater than 60 mmHg (114). A recent meta-analysis found that the summary sensitivity and specificity of echocardiography for diagnosing PH was 83% (95% CI 73–90) and 72% (95% CI 53–85; n = 12), respectively (115). So, echo can be a useful initial assessment, but RHC is still necessary for both diagnostic and therapeutic reasons in these patients.

Clinical Manifestations and Pathophysiology Class II PH

Patients often have concomitant PH due to left-sided heart disease and present with typical heart failure symptoms such as dyspnea on exertion, exertional angina, and when severe, volume overload, hepatic congestion, and signs of right-sided heart failure. Chronic sustained LAP elevation translates backward to the pulmonary capillaries and leads to a cascade of adverse anatomical and functional events. There are two major components of PH secondary to left heart failure: (a) hydrostatic and (b) vasoreactive. The pulmonary vasculature bed normally is highly distensible and is a low pressure, low resistance system. Large increases in blood flow may cause only a minimum increase in PAM pressure due to the large capacitance. Chronically elevated LV end-diastolic pressure (reflected in LAP) increases hydrostatic pressure on the pulmonary vasculature. At some critical point, the compensatory mechanism is overcome and PAM pressure increases first with exercise and then at rest. West et al coined this term "alveolar capillary stress failure" to describe the fragmentation of the alveolar–capillary membrane during mechanical injury (116). This is generally a reversible phenomenon. If this is sustained, capillaries undergo more structural changes including thickening of the basal lamina, and proliferation of reticular and elastic fibrils. Impaired pulmonary vascular smooth muscle relaxation is mostly due to endothelial dysfunction in heart failure patients. The endothelial local control of vasomotility is primarily based on a balanced release of nitric oxide (NO) and endothelin-1 (ET-1). This balance has been the target for therapies in heart failure patients with PH (116).

CASE PRESENTATION

Upon arrival to the hospital her blood pressure was 82/60 mmHg with a heart rate of 92 beats/min. A narrow pulse pressure with a relatively high heart rate is indicative of a low output state despite the fact that the patient appeared comfortable and was in no apparent distress. She had minimal pulmonary crackles, an S3 heart sound, and trace lower extremity edema. Her JVP was to the angle of her jaw at 45 degrees. Gentle diuresis was attempted overnight with 20 IV lasix and she underwent RHC the following day, which revealed a CVP of 12 mmHg, PAS/PAD 84/34 mmHg, PAM of 53 mmHg, and PCWP of 28 mmHg. Her low output state was confirmed by an estimated CI of 1.66 (L/min/m^{-}) and a mixed venous saturation of 46%. Her measured transpulmonary gradient (TPG = PAM-PCWP) was 25 mmHg and calculated pulmonary vascular resistance (PVR) was [(TPG/CO) x 80] 664 dynes*sec/cm^5. Normal values for TPG and PVR are less than 10 mmHg and less than 130 dynes*sec/cm5 respectively.

Pulmonary Hypertension in Heart Transplant

The extent of left-sided PH is an important determinant of morbidity and mortality in patients with heart failure (113,118) and development of right ventricle failure is an important concern for patients being evaluated for HT. Data from the International Society of Heart Transplantation registry indicate that right ventricular dysfunction accounts for 50% of all cardiac complications and 19% of early deaths in this patient population (119,120).

This has led to the assessment of pulmonary arterial reaction to vasodilators prior to heart transplantation, to select those patients who are more likely to survive the subsequent right heart strain after heart transplantation and also to indicate which agents might be useful in their postoperative management. Early data from Stanford University using nitroprusside to reverse PH has helped to risk stratify patients and created a framework for transplantation decisions, which is still used in part today. They found that patients with a PVR greater than 2.5 Wood units measured at baseline study had a higher 3-month mortality rate (17.9%) versus those with resistance less than or equal to 2.5 units (6.9%). Additionally, those whose PVR could be reduced to less than or equal to 2.5 units with nitroprusside (without a drop in blood pressure) had a 3-month mortality rate of only 3.8% (121).

Our patient underwent "reversibility" testing, where pulmonary pressures are measured after initiation of a vasodilator, such as nitroprusside, adenosine, or inhaled NO. Only 10% to 20% of patients have a positive response to this test, achieving a reduction in PAM by at least 10 mmHg with the PAM pressure decreasing to 40 mmHg or less, accompanied by a normal or high cardiac output. If all three of these conditions are met, patients are more likely to respond to calcium channel blocker therapy for Class I PH (122).

In the past, patients with an elevated PVR greater than 2.5 Woods units have often been excluded from transplantation. Oral phosphodiesterases and mechanical support devices have recently challenged this paradigm. Small studies have suggested that chronic sildenafil use in heart failure patients with PH, who may otherwise have been excluded from transplant, has been shown to be safe and effective in reducing an elevated TPG and PVR and allows for a successful tranpslantation (123).

CASE PRESENTATION

A RHC demonstrated no reversibility with inhaled NO in our patient, and a persistently elevated PAM of around 50 mmHg. She was worked up for additional causes for PH, including thromboembolic disease, autoimmune disease, and intrinsic lung disease, all of which were negative. She was started on the oral phosphodiesterase inhibitor, sildenafil, at 10 mg three times daily and uptitrated to 60 mg daily dosing. She was also started on the inotropic agent milrinone in the hospital due to her low-output state. It was determined she would be high risk for right ventricular failure post-HT and therefore the heart failure surgeons were consulted to discuss mechanical support with a left ventricular assist device (LVAD).

Left Ventricular Assist Device Therapy

LVADs have demonstrated improved survival in patients, both as a bridge to transplant (BTT) and as destination therapy (DT) when patients may not be transplant candidates. The device type began as a pulsatile pump (mimicking the natural action of the heart), but now continuous flow pumps have replaced pulsatile pumps as the preferred technology.

The Randomized Evaluation of Mechanical Assistance for the Treatment of Congestive Heart Failure (REMATCH) trial done in 2001 randomized patients to the pulsatile HeartMate (by Thoratec) or optimal medical control in nontransplant candidates. One-year survival rates were 52% in the device group and 25% in the medical-therapy group ($P = .002$). At 2 years, the HeartMate patient's survival rate was 23% compared with 8% in the medical group ($P = .09$).

In 2009, the HEARTMATE II trial demonstrated that the axial flow pump technology is clearly superior to pulsatile flow LVADs in DT patients. Two-year survival was more than double in the continuous flow group (58% vs. 24%), and the smaller continuous flow pump had a lower likelihood of disabling stroke (from pump thrombosis) or pump reoperation/replacement (124). A postmarketing study confirmed the original study findings in a real-world setting and was approved by the FDA for bridge to transplant in January 2010 (125). The Evaluation of the HeartWare Left Ventricular Assist Device for the Treatment of Advanced Heart Failure (ADVANCE) trial had a noninferiority primary endpoint of the even smaller Heartware device (**Figure 2-8**) when compared with HeartMate II (**Figure 2-8**) and is currently being studied in DT patients.

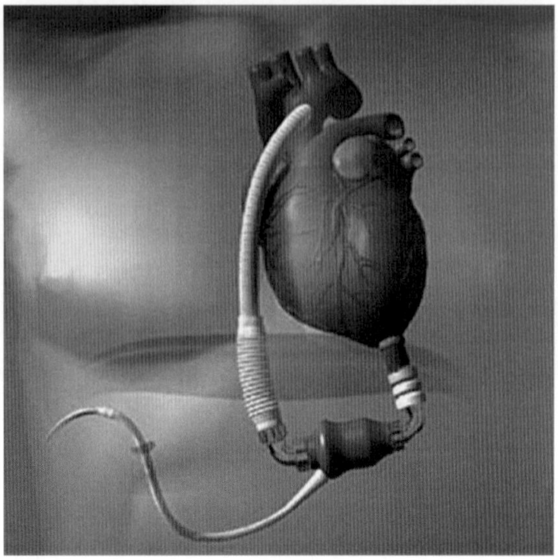

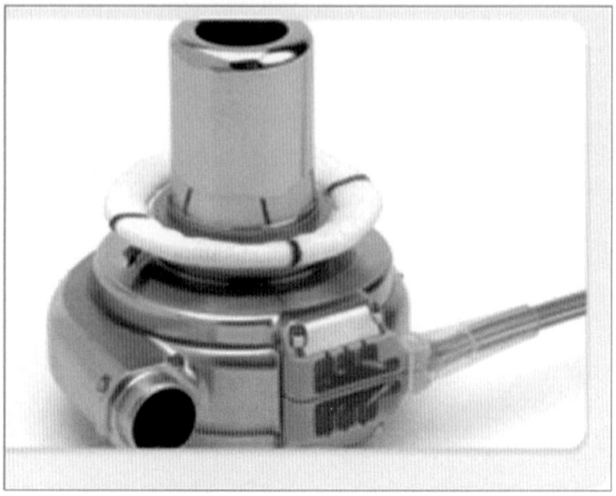

Figure 2-8
The HeartMate II and Heartware devices.

CASE PRESENTATION

Chronic ventricular unloading with LVAD therapy has been shown to normalize pulmonary pressures and thus allow a patient to be a possible HT candidate (126). This strategy has been termed "bridge to decision" therapy. A multidisciplinary meeting was held with our patient and options were reviewed. If her PVR decreased after LVAD therapy, she would be listed for transplant, and if not she would have the LVAD as DT. The team considered home inotrope therapy as an option; however, this is only a reasonable strategy as a BTT if the waiting time is expected to be short (less than 100 days; 127).

The Outcomes of a Prospective Trial of Intravenous Milrinone for Exacerbations of Chronic Heart Failure (OPTIME-CHF) demonstrated that the routine use of IV milrinone as an adjunct to standard therapy to treat hospitalized patients with exacerbations of chronic heart failure is not recommended; however, patients with acutely decompensated heart failure or evidence of tissue hypoperfusion (as in the case of our patient) were not included in this trial (128).

A substantial number of patients with longer waiting times may end up needing LVAD therapy if inotropes are not enough support. The Interagency Registry For Mechanical Circulatory Support (INTERMACS; 1), is a database on all patients with a mechanical circulatory support device since 2006, and is the result of a collaborative effort between the National Heart, Lung, and Blood Institute (NHLBI), the Food and Drug Administration (FDA), the Center for Medicaid and Medicare Services (CMS), and the advanced heart failure/mechanical circulatory support professional community. Patients are entered into the system with regard to their clinical status at the time of implantation and given an INTERMACS score (see **Table 2-2**; 129). The classification system ranges from 1, the "crash and burn patient," to 7, the NYHA Class III patient "living comfortably with meaningful activity limited to mild physical exertion." This is clearly a broad range of patients, and most patients who currently receive LVAD therapy are INTERMACS Class I. However, a recent study suggests that LVAD therapy in less acutely decompensated patients (ie, more "stably dependent" or "sliding on intrope patients") actually had longer survival and shorter lengths of stay compared with lower INTERMACS score patients (130). The Evaluation of VAD Intervention Before Inotropic Therapy (REVIVE-IT) trial is currently studying this question in higher INTERMACS patients.

One important decision facing the team was determining the need for right ventricular support with a biventricular VAD (BiVAD). Risk score calculators are available, but the salient features in this evaluation include the presence of right ventricular dysfunction on echo, a PAS pressure of less than 50 mmHg, and a low right ventricular stroke work index (RVSWI) of less than 450 mmHg·ml/m^2. This is predictive of right ventricle failure and may predict who will need biventricular support (131,132). Our patient did not meet any of these criteria.

Table 2-2
Interagency Registry for Mechanically Assisted Circulatory Support (INTERMACS) Levels

PROFILE	PROFILE NAME	DESCRIPTION
1	Critical Cardiogenic Shock	Life threatening hypotension despite escalating inotropic support and critical organ hypoperfusion.
2	Progressive Decline	Declining function despite IV inotropic support. Worsening renal function, nutritional depletion.
3	Stable Inotrope Dependant	Stable blood pressure, organ function, nutrition, symptoms. Continuous IV inotropic support or temporary circulatory support—cannot be weaned off.
4	Resting Symptoms	Can be stabilized at normal volume status but has daily symptoms of congestion at rest or with minimal activities of daily living.
5	Exertion Intolerant	No symptoms at rest or with activities of daily living. All other activities can cause symptoms of congestion. Frequently has refractory volume overload.
6	Exertion Limited	Comfortable at rest with no fluid overload. Can do activities of daily living and other low level activities but fatigue after a few minutes.
7	Advanced NYHA III	Placeholder for the future. No recent fluid overload events, becomes symptomatic after mild physical exertion.

Source: Adapted from reference 128.

CASE PRESENTATION

She underwent implantation with a HeartMate II device (**Figure 2-8**) and after 6 months of LVAD therapy, a repeat RHC was performed (**Figure 2-9**), which revealed a CVP of 7 mmHg, PAS/PAD 31/11 mmHg with PAM of 20 mmHg, and PCWP of 7 mmHg. Mixed venous saturation was 78% and the patient was feeling well and able to do more activities of daily living. She was now functional NYHA Class II to III. As her PVR had improved, she was listed for cardiac transplantation and was successfully transplanted in August of 2010.

Approximately 2,300 HTs are performed in the United States each year. With over five million Americans suffering with heart failure, and the aging population, the supply demand ratio cannot be met with HT alone. The future of heart failure should be aimed at preventative measures to reduce the incidence of heart failure, novel therapies targeted at viable yet dysfunctional myocardium and predictors of improvement, and increased utilization of mechanical support devices as destination therapy and also as mechanisms of reverse remodeling and recovery (133).

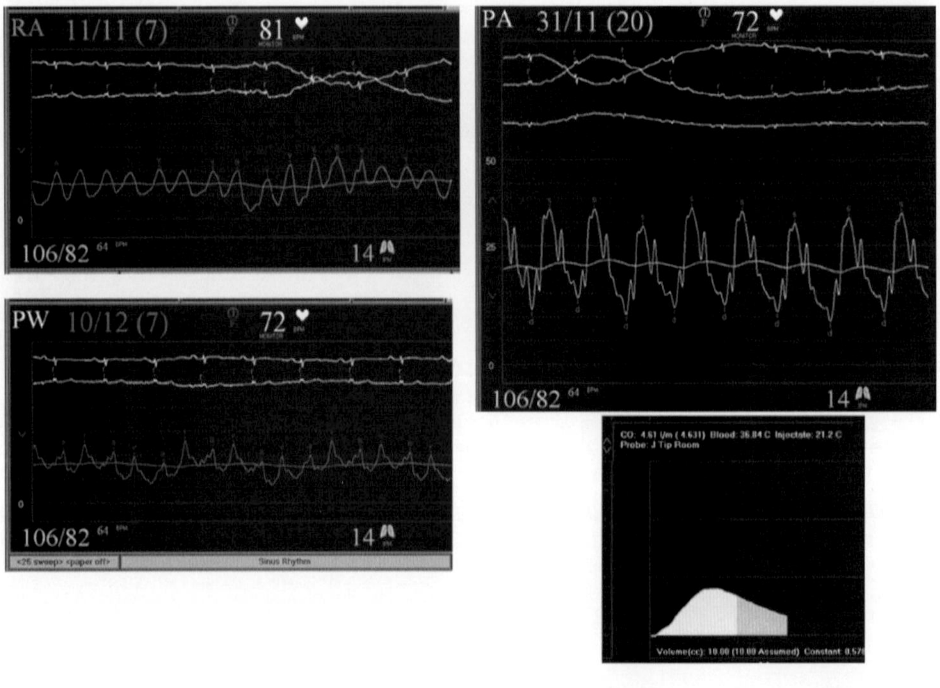

Figure 2-9
Post left ventricular assist device hemodynamics, which are now markedly improved after 6 months of therapy.

Note: Upper left panel: right atrial (RA) pressures, mean 7 mmHg.
Upper right panel: pulmonary artery (PA) pressures, 30/11 with a mean of 20 mmHg.
Lower left panel: pulmonary wedge pressure (PW), mean 7.
Lower right panel: cardiac output determination. Cardiac output was 4.6 L/min.

REFERENCES

1. Killip T, 3rd, Kimball JT. Treatment of myocardial infarction in a coronary care unit. A two year experience with 250 patients. *Am J Cardiol.* 1967;20:457–464.
2. Bahekar A, Singh M, Singh S, et al. Cardiovascular outcomes using intra-aortic balloon pump in high-risk acute myocardial jnfarction with or without cardiogenic shock: a meta-analysis. *J Cardiovasc Pharmacol Ther.* 2012;17(1):44–56.
3. Mims BC. Physiologic rationale of Sv-O_2 monitoring. *Crit Care Nurs Clin North Am.* 1989;1:619–628.
4. Kyff JV, Vaughn S, Yang SC, Raheja R, Puri VK. Continuous monitoring of mixed venous oxygen saturation in patients with acute myocardial infarction. *Chest.* 1989;95:607–611.
5. Binanay C, Califf RM, Hasselblad V, et al. Evaluation study of congestive heart failure and pulmonary artery catheterization effectiveness: the ESCAPE trial. *JAMA.* 2005;294:1625–1633.
6. Volpi A, Cavalli A, Santoro L, Negri E. Incidence and prognosis of early primary ventricular fibrillation in acute myocardial infarction—results of the Gruppo Italiano per lo Studio della Sopravvivenza nell'Infarto Miocardico (GISSI-2) database. *Am J Cardiol.* 1998;82:265–271.

7. Antman EM, Anbe DT, Armstrong PW, et al. ACC/AHA guidelines for the management of patients with ST-elevation myocardial infarction; A report of the American College of Cardiology/American Heart Association Task Force on Practice Guidelines (Committee to Revise the 1999 Guidelines for the Management of patients with acute myocardial infarction). *J Am Coll Cardiol.* 2004;44:E1–E211.

8. Solodky A, Behar S, Herz I, et al. Comparison of incidence of cardiac rupture among patients with acute myocardial infarction treated by thrombolysis versus percutaneous transluminal coronary angioplasty. *Am J Cardiol.* 2001;87:1105–1108; A9.

9. Figueras J, Alcalde O, Barrabes JA, et al. Changes in hospital mortality rates in 425 patients with acute ST-elevation myocardial infarction and cardiac rupture over a 30-year period. *Circulation.* 2008;118:2783–2789.

10. Chiarella F, Santoro E, Domenicucci S, Maggioni A, Vecchio C. Predischarge two-dimensional echocardiographic evaluation of left ventricular thrombosis after acute myocardial infarction in the GISSI-3 study. *Am J Cardiol.* 1998;81:822–827.

11. Udell JA, Wang JT, Gladstone DJ, Tu JV. Anticoagulation after anterior myocardial infarction and the risk of stroke. *PLoS One*;5:e12150.

12. Antman EM, Anbe DT, Armstrong PW, et al. ACC/AHA guidelines for the management of patients with ST-elevation myocardial infarction—executive summary: a report of the American College of Cardiology/American Heart Association Task Force on Practice Guidelines (Writing Committee to Revise the 1999 Guidelines for the Management of Patients With Acute Myocardial Infarction). *Circulation.* 2004;110:588–636.

13. Chua D, Lo C, Babor EM. Addition of clopidogrel to aspirin and fibrinolytic therapy for myocardial infarction. *N Engl J Med.* 2005;352:2647–2648; author reply -8.

14. Wiviott SD, Braunwald E, McCabe CH, et al. Prasugrel versus clopidogrel in patients with acute coronary syndromes. *N Engl J Med.* 2007;357:2001–2015.

15. Wallentin L, Becker RC, Budaj A, et al. Ticagrelor versus clopidogrel in patients with acute coronary syndromes. *N Engl J Med.* 2009;361:1045–1057.

16. Mehta SR, Bassand JP, Chrolavicius S, et al. Dose comparisons of clopidogrel and aspirin in acute coronary syndromes. *N Engl J Med.* 2010;363:930–942.

17. Cannon CP, Braunwald E, McCabe CH, et al. Intensive versus moderate lipid lowering with statins after acute coronary syndromes. *N Engl J Med.* 2004;350:1495–1504.

18. Schwartz GG, Olsson AG, Ezekowitz MD, et al. Effects of atorvastatin on early recurrent ischemic events in acute coronary syndromes: the MIRACL study: a randomized controlled trial. *JAMA.* 2001;285:1711–1718.

19. Pitt B, Remme W, Zannad F, et al. Eplerenone, a selective aldosterone blocker, in patients with left ventricular dysfunction after myocardial infarction. *N Engl J Med.* 2003;348:1309–1321.

20. Ezekowitz JA, McAlister FA. Aldosterone blockade and left ventricular dysfunction: a systematic review of randomized clinical trials. *Eur Heart J.* 2009;30:469–477.

21. Adamopoulos C, Ahmed A, Fay R, et al. Timing of eplerenone initiation and outcomes in patients with heart failure after acute myocardial infarction complicated by left ventricular systolic dysfunction: insights from the EPHESUS trial. *Eur J Heart Fail.* 2009;11:1099–1105.

22. Lawler PR, Filion KB, Eisenberg MJ. Efficacy of exercise-based cardiac rehabilitation post-myocardial infarction: a systematic review and meta-analysis of randomized controlled trials. *Am Heart J.* 2011;162:571–584; e2.

23. Solomon SD, Dobson J, Pocock S, et al. Influence of nonfatal hospitalization for heart failure on subsequent mortality in patients with chronic heart failure. *Circulation.* 2007;116:1482–1487.

24. Gheorghiade M, Abraham WT, Albert NM, et al. Systolic blood pressure at admission, clinical characteristics, and outcomes in patients hospitalized with acute heart failure. *JAMA.* 2006;296:2217–2226.

25. Fonarow GC, Albert NM, Curtis AB, et al. Improving evidence-based care for heart failure in outpatient cardiology practices: primary results of the Registry to Improve the Use of Evidence-Based Heart Failure Therapies in the Outpatient Setting (IMPROVE HF). *Circulation* 2010;122:585–596.

26. Mark DB, Nelson CL, Anstrom KJ, et al. Cost-effectiveness of defibrillator therapy or amiodarone in chronic stable heart failure: results from the Sudden Cardiac Death in Heart Failure Trial (SCD-HeFT). *Circulation.* 2006;114:135–142.

27. Khand AU, Gemmell I, Rankin AC, Cleland JG. Clinical events leading to the progression of heart failure: insights from a national database of hospital discharges. *Eur Heart J.* 2001;22:153–164.

28. Harinstein ME, Flaherty JD, Fonarow GC, et al. Clinical assessment of acute heart failure syndromes: emergency department through the early post-discharge period. *Heart.* 2011;97:1607–618.

29. Abraham WT, Fonarow GC, Albert NM, et al. Predictors of in-hospital mortality in patients hospitalized for heart failure: insights from the Organized Program to Initiate Lifesaving Treatment in Hospitalized Patients with Heart Failure (OPTIMIZE-HF). *J Am Coll Cardiol.* 2008;52:347–356.

30. Fonarow GC, Peacock WF, Horwich TB, et al. Usefulness of B-type natriuretic peptide and cardiac troponin levels to predict in-hospital mortality from ADHERE. *Am J Cardiol.* 2008;101:231–237.

31. Gheorghiade M, Abraham WT, Albert NM, et al. Relationship between admission serum sodium concentration and clinical outcomes in patients hospitalized for heart failure: an analysis from the OPTIMIZE-HF registry. *Eur Heart J.* 2007;28:980–988.

32. Felker GM, Leimberger JD, Califf RM, et al. Risk stratification after hospitalization for decompensated heart failure. *J Card Fail.* 2004;10:460–466.

33. Pocock SJ, Wang D, Pfeffer MA, et al. Predictors of mortality and morbidity in patients with chronic heart failure. *Eur Heart J.* 2006;27:65–75.

34. Brophy JM, Dagenais GR, McSherry F, Williford W, Yusuf S. A multivariate model for predicting mortality in patients with heart failure and systolic dysfunction. *Am J Med.* 2004;116:300–304.

35. Fonarow GC, Adams KF, Jr, Abraham WT, Yancy CW, Boscardin WJ. Risk stratification for in-hospital mortality in acutely decompensated heart failure: classification and regression tree analysis. *JAMA.* 2005;293:572–580.

36. Peterson PN, Rumsfeld JS, Liang L, et al. A validated risk score for in-hospital mortality in patients with heart failure from the American Heart Association get with the guidelines program. *Circ Cardiovasc Qual Outcomes.* 2010;3:25–32.

37. Ahluwalia SC, Gross CP, Chaudhry SI, et al. Impact of comorbidity on mortality among older persons with advanced heart failure. *J Gen Intern Med.* 2012;27(5):513–519.

38. Ahluwalia SC, Gross CP, Chaudhry SI, Leo-Summers L, Van Ness PH, Fried TR. Change in comorbidity prevalence with advancing age among persons with heart failure. *J Gen Intern Med.* 2011; 26:1145–1151.

39. Manjunath G, Tighiouart H, Ibrahim H, et al. Level of kidney function as a risk factor for atherosclerotic cardiovascular outcomes in the community. *J Am Coll Cardiol.* 2003;41:47–55.

40. Wright RS, Reeder GS, Herzog CA, et al. Acute myocardial infarction and renal dysfunction: a high-risk combination. *Ann Intern Med.* 2002;137:563–570.

41. Tokmakova MP, Skali H, Kenchaiah S, et al. Chronic kidney disease, cardiovascular risk, and response to angiotensin-converting enzyme

inhibition after myocardial infarction: the Survival And Ventricular Enlargement (SAVE) study. *Circulation*. 2004;110:3667–3673.

42. Vaccaro O, Eberly LE, Neaton JD, Yang L, Riccardi G, Stamler J. Impact of diabetes and previous myocardial infarction on long-term survival: 25-year mortality follow-up of primary screenees of the Multiple Risk Factor Intervention Trial. *Arch Intern Med*. 2004;164:1438–1443.
43. Murcia AM, Hennekens CH, Lamas GA, et al. Impact of diabetes on mortality in patients with myocardial infarction and left ventricular dysfunction. *Arch Intern Med*. 2004;164:2273–2279.
44. Kilpatrick ES, Bloomgarden ZT, Zimmet PZ. International Expert Committee report on the role of the A1C assay in the diagnosis of diabetes: response to the International Expert Committee. *Diabetes Care*. 2009;32:e159; author reply e60.
45. White HD, Aylward PE, Huang Z, et al. Mortality and morbidity remain high despite captopril and/or Valsartan therapy in elderly patients with left ventricular systolic dysfunction, heart failure, or both after acute myocardial infarction: results from the Valsartan in Acute Myocardial Infarction Trial (VALIANT). *Circulation*. 2005;112:3391–3399.
46. Pocock SJ, McMurray JJ, Dobson J, et al. Weight loss and mortality risk in patients with chronic heart failure in the candesartan in heart failure: assessment of reduction in mortality and morbidity (CHARM) programme. *Eur Heart J*. 2008;29:2641–250.
47. Young JB, Abraham WT, Albert NM, et al. Relation of low hemoglobin and anemia to morbidity and mortality in patients hospitalized with heart failure (insight from the OPTIMIZE-HF registry). *Am J Cardiol*. 2008;101:223–230.
48. von Haehling S, Anker MS, Jankowska EA, Ponikowski P, Anker SD. Anemia in chronic heart failure: Can we treat? What to treat? *Heart Fail Rev*. Epub date 10/7/2011.
49. Anker SD, Comin Colet J, Filippatos G, et al. Ferric carboxymaltose in patients with heart failure and iron deficiency. *N Engl J Med*. 2009;361:2436–2448.
50. McMurray JJ, Anand IS, Diaz R, et al. Design of the Reduction of Events with Darbepoetin alfa in Heart Failure (RED-HF): a Phase III, anaemia correction, morbidity-mortality trial. *Eur J Heart Fail*. 2009;11:795–801.
51. De Blois J, Simard S, Atar D, Agewall S. COPD predicts mortality in HF: the Norwegian Heart Failure Registry. *J Card Fail*. 2010;16: 225–229.
52. Somers VK, White DP, Amin R, et al. Sleep apnea and cardiovascular disease: an American Heart Association/American College of Cardiology Foundation Scientific Statement from the American Heart Association Council for High Blood Pressure Research Professional Education Committee, Council on Clinical Cardiology, Stroke Council, and Council on Cardiovascular Nursing. *J Am Coll Cardiol*. 2008;52:686–717.
53. Hiestand DM, Britz P, Goldman M, Phillips B. Prevalence of symptoms and risk of sleep apnea in the US population: Results from the national sleep foundation sleep in America 2005 poll. *Chest*. 2006;130:780–786.
54. Chowdhury M, Adams S, Whellan DJ. Sleep-disordered breathing and heart failure: focus on obstructive sleep apnea and treatment with continuous positive airway pressure. *J Card Fail*. 2010;16:164–174.
55. Bradley TD, Floras JS. Obstructive sleep apnoea and its cardiovascular consequences. *Lancet*. 2009;373:82–93.
56. Arzt M, Floras JS, Logan AG, et al. Suppression of central sleep apnea by continuous positive airway pressure and transplant-free survival in heart failure: a post hoc analysis of the Canadian Continuous Positive Airway Pressure for Patients with Central Sleep Apnea and Heart Failure Trial (CANPAP). *Circulation*. 2007;115:3173–180.
57. Kaneko Y, Floras JS, Usui K, et al. Cardiovascular effects of continuous positive airway pressure in patients with heart failure and obstructive sleep apnea. *N Engl J Med*. 2003;348:1233–1241.
58. Farre R, Montserrat JM, Navajas D. Noninvasive monitoring of respiratory mechanics during sleep. *Eur Respir J*. 2004;24: 1052–1060.
59. Pressler SJ, Kim J, Riley P, Ronis DL, Gradus-Pizlo I. Memory dysfunction, psychomotor slowing, and decreased executive function predict mortality in patients with heart failure and low ejection fraction. *J Card Fail*. 2010;16:750–760.
60. Pressler SJ, Subramanian U, Kareken D, et al. Cognitive deficits and health-related quality of life in chronic heart failure. *J Cardiovasc Nurs*. 2010;25:189–198.
61. Allen LA, Gheorghiade M, Reid KJ, et al. Identifying patients hospitalized with heart failure at risk for unfavorable future quality of life. *Circ Cardiovasc Qual Outcomes*. 2011;4:389–398.
62. Dries DL, Exner DV, Gersh BJ, Cooper HA, Carson PE, Domanski MJ. Racial differences in the outcome of left ventricular dysfunction. *N Engl J Med*. 1999;340:609–616.
63. Yancy CW. Heart failure in African Americans: a cardiovascular engima. *J Card Fail*. 2000;6:183–186.
64. Yancy CW. Heart failure in African Americans. *Am J Cardiol*. 2005;96:3i–12i.
65. Chaudhry SI, Herrin J, Phillips C, et al. Racial disparities in health literacy and access to care among patients with heart failure. *J Card Fail*. 2011; 17:122–127.
66. Cigarroa CG, deFilippi CR, Brickner ME, Alvarez LG, Wait MA, Grayburn PA. Dobutamine stress echocardiography identifies hibernating myocardium and predicts recovery of left ventricular function after coronary revascularization. *Circulation*. 1993;88:430–436.
67. Bristow MR, Gilbert EM, Abraham WT, et al. Carvedilol produces dose-related improvements in left ventricular function and survival in subjects with chronic heart failure. MOCHA Investigators. *Circulation*. 1996;94:2807–2816.
68. Schinkel AF, Poldermans D, Vanoverschelde JL, et al. Incidence of recovery of contractile function following revascularization in patients with ischemic left ventricular dysfunction. *Am J Cardiol*. 2004;93:14–17.
69. Ross J, Jr. Myocardial perfusion-contraction matching. Implications for coronary heart disease and hibernation. *Circulation*. 1991;83:1076–1083.
70. Di Carli MF, Asgarzadie F, Schelbert HR, et al. Quantitative relation between myocardial viability and improvement in heart failure symptoms after revascularization in patients with ischemic cardiomyopathy. *Circulation*. 1995;92:3436–3444.
71. Packer M, Antonopoulos GV, Berlin JA, Chittams J, Konstam MA, Udelson JE. Comparative effects of carvedilol and metoprolol on left ventricular ejection fraction in heart failure: results of a meta-analysis. *Am Heart J*. 2001;141:899–907.
72. Rahimtoola SH. The hibernating myocardium. *Am Heart J*. 1989;117:211–221.
73. Rahimtoola SH. The hibernating myocardium in ischaemia and congestive heart failure. *Eur Heart J*. 1993;14(Suppl A):22–26.
74. Rahimtoola SH. From coronary artery disease to heart failure: role of the hibernating myocardium. *Am J Cardiol*. 1995;75:16E–22E.
75. Rahimtoola SH. Hibernating myocardium: a brief article. *Basic Res Cardiol*. 1995;90:38–40.

76. Rahimtoola SH. Clinical aspects of hibernating myocardium. *J Mol Cell Cardiol.* 1996;28:2397–2401.

77. Rahimtoola SH, La Canna G, Ferrari R. Hibernating myocardium: another piece of the puzzle falls into place. *J Am Coll Cardiol.* 2006;47:978–980.

78. Cleland JG, Pennell DJ, Ray SG, et al. Myocardial viability as a determinant of the ejection fraction response to carvedilol in patients with heart failure (CHRISTMAS trial): randomised controlled trial. *Lancet.* 2003;362:14–21.

79. Allman KC, Shaw LJ, Hachamovitch R, Udelson JE. Myocardial viability testing and impact of revascularization on prognosis in patients with coronary artery disease and left ventricular dysfunction: a meta-analysis. *J Am Coll Cardiol.* 2002;39:1151–1158.

80. Bonow RO, Maurer G, Lee KL, et al. Myocardial viability and survival in ischemic left ventricular dysfunction. *N Engl J Med.* 2011; 364:1617–625.

81. Wilcox JE, Fonarow GC, Yancy CW, et al. Factors associated with improvement in ejection fraction in clinical practice among patients with heart failure: findings from IMPROVE HF. *Am Heart J.*163:49–56; e2.

82. Schinkel AF, Bax JJ, Poldermans D, Elhendy A, Ferrari R, Rahimtoola SH. Hibernating myocardium: diagnosis and outcomes. *Curr Probl Cardiol.* 2007;32:375–340.

83. Bello D, Shah DJ, Farah GM, et al. Gadolinium cardiovascular magnetic resonance predicts reversible myocardial dysfunction and remodeling in patients with heart failure undergoing beta-blocker therapy. *Circulation.* 2003;108:1945–1953.

84. Shamim W, Francis DP, Yousufuddin M, et al. Intraventricular conduction delay: a prognostic marker in chronic heart failure. *Int J Cardiol.* 1999;70:171–178.

85. Xiao HB, Roy C, Fujimoto S, Gibson DG. Natural history of abnormal conduction and its relation to prognosis in patients with dilated cardiomyopathy. *Int J Cardiol.* 1996;53:163–170.

86. Unverferth DV, Magorien RD, Moeschberger ML, Baker PB, Fetters JK, Leier CV. Factors influencing the one-year mortality of dilated cardiomyopathy. *Am J Cardiol.* 1984;54:147–152.

87. Blanc JJ, Etienne Y, Gilard M, et al. Evaluation of different ventricular pacing sites in patients with severe heart failure: results of an acute hemodynamic study. *Circulation.* 1997;96:3273–3277.

88. Xiao HB, Lee CH, Gibson DG. Effect of left bundle branch block on diastolic function in dilated cardiomyopathy. *Br Heart J.* 1991;66:443–447.

89. Cleland JG, Daubert JC, Erdmann E, et al. The effect of cardiac resynchronization on morbidity and mortality in heart failure. *N Engl J Med.* 2005;352:1539–1549.

90. Higgins SL, Hummel JD, Niazi IK, et al. Cardiac resynchronization therapy for the treatment of heart failure in patients with intraventricular conduction delay and malignant ventricular tachyarrhythmias. *J Am Coll Cardiol.* 2003;42:1454–1459.

91. Abraham WT. Cardiac resynchronization therapy for heart failure: biventricular pacing and beyond. *Curr Opin Cardiol.* 2002;17: 346–352.

92. Abraham WT. Cardiac resynchronization therapy is important for all patients with congestive heart failure and ventricular dyssynchrony. *Circulation.* 2006;114:2692–2698; discussion 8.

93. Abraham WT, Young JB, Leon AR, et al. Effects of cardiac resynchronization on disease progression in patients with left ventricular systolic dysfunction, an indication for an implantable cardioverter-defibrillator, and mildly symptomatic chronic heart failure. *Circulation.* 2004;110:2864–2868.

94. Young JB, Abraham WT, Smith AL, et al. Combined cardiac resynchronization and implantable cardioversion defibrillation in advanced chronic heart failure: the MIRACLE ICD Trial. *JAMA.* 2003;289:2685–2694.

95. Bristow MR, Saxon LA, Boehmer J, et al. Cardiac-resynchronization therapy with or without an implantable defibrillator in advanced chronic heart failure. *N Engl J Med.* 2004;350:2140–150.

96. Moss AJ, Hall WJ, Cannom DS, et al. Cardiac-resynchronization therapy for the prevention of heart-failure events. *N Engl J Med.* 2009;361:1329–1338.

97. Solomon SD, Foster E, Bourgoun M, et al. Effect of cardiac resynchronization therapy on reverse remodeling and relation to outcome: multicenter automatic defibrillator implantation trial: cardiac resynchronization therapy. *Circulation.* 2010;122:985–992.

98. Arshad A, Moss AJ, Foster E, et al. Cardiac resynchronization therapy is more effective in women than in men: the MADIT-CRT (Multicenter Automatic Defibrillator Implantation Trial with Cardiac Resynchronization Therapy) trial. *J Am Coll Cardiol.* 2011;57:813–820.

99. Zareba W, Klein H, Cygankiewicz I, et al. Effectiveness of Cardiac Resynchronization Therapy by QRS Morphology in the Multicenter Automatic Defibrillator Implantation Trial-Cardiac Resynchronization Therapy (MADIT-CRT). *Circulation.* 2011; 123:1061–1072.

100. Jessup M, Abraham WT, Casey DE, et al. 2009 focused update: ACCF/AHA Guidelines for the Diagnosis and Management of Heart Failure in Adults: a report of the American College of Cardiology Foundation/American Heart Association Task Force on Practice Guidelines: developed in collaboration with the International Society for Heart and Lung Transplantation. *Circulation.* 2009;119:1977–2016.

101. Moss AJ, Zareba W, Hall WJ, et al. Prophylactic implantation of a defibrillator in patients with myocardial infarction and reduced ejection fraction. *N Engl J Med.* 2002;346:877–883.

102. Hohnloser SH, Kuck KH, Dorian P, et al. Prophylactic use of an implantable cardioverter-defibrillator after acute myocardial infarction. *N Engl J Med.* 2004;351:2481–2488.

103. Kadish A, Dyer A, Daubert JP, et al. Prophylactic defibrillator implantation in patients with nonischemic dilated cardiomyopathy. *N Engl J Med.* 2004;350:2151–2158.

104. Packer DL, Prutkin JM, Hellkamp AS, et al. Impact of implantable cardioverter-defibrillator, amiodarone, and placebo on the mode of death in stable patients with heart failure: analysis from the sudden cardiac death in heart failure trial. *Circulation.* 2009;120:2170–2176.

105. Klein HU, Reek S. The MUSTT study: evaluating testing and treatment. *J Interv Card Electrophysiol.* 2000;4(Suppl 1):45–50.

106. Stewart GC, Weintraub JR, Pratibhu PP, et al. Patient expectations from implantable defibrillators to prevent death in heart failure. *J Card Fail.* 2010;16:106–113.

107. Hunt SA, Abraham WT, Chin MH, et al. ACC/AHA 2005 Guideline Update for the Diagnosis and Management of Chronic Heart Failure in the Adult: a report of the American College of Cardiology/American Heart Association Task Force on Practice Guidelines (Writing Committee to Update the 2001 Guidelines for the Evaluation and Management of Heart Failure): developed in collaboration with the American College of Chest Physicians and the International Society for Heart and Lung Transplantation: endorsed by the Heart Rhythm Society. *Circulation.* 2005;112:e154–e235.

108. Kossman CE. Nomenclature and criteria for the diagnosis of cardiovascular diseases. *Circulation.* 1964;30:321–325.

109. Simonneau G, Galie N, Rubin LJ, et al. Clinical classification of pulmonary hypertension. *J Am Coll Cardiol*. 2004;43:5S–12S.

110. McLaughlin VV, Archer SL, Badesch DB, et al. ACCF/AHA 2009 expert consensus document on pulmonary hypertension a report of the American College of Cardiology Foundation Task Force on Expert Consensus Documents and the American Heart Association developed in collaboration with the American College of Chest Physicians; American Thoracic Society, Inc.; and the Pulmonary Hypertension Association. *J Am Coll Cardiol*. 2009;53:1573–1619.

111. McLaughlin VV. Classification and epidemiology of pulmonary hypertension. *Cardiol Clin*. 2004;22:327–341; v.

112. Ghio S, Gavazzi A, Campana C, et al. Independent and additive prognostic value of right ventricular systolic function and pulmonary artery pressure in patients with chronic heart failure. *J Am Coll Cardiol*. 2001;37:183–188.

113. Abramson SV, Burke JF, Kelly JJ, Jr, et al. Pulmonary hypertension predicts mortality and morbidity in patients with dilated cardiomyopathy. *Ann Intern Med*. 1992;116:888–895.

114. Dokainish H, Nguyen JS, Bobek J, Goswami R, Lakkis NM. Assessment of the American Society of Echocardiography-European Association of Echocardiography guidelines for diastolic function in patients with depressed ejection fraction: an echocardiographic and invasive haemodynamic study. *Eur J Echocardiogr*. 12:857–864.

115. Janda S, Shahidi N, Gin K, Swiston J. Diagnostic accuracy of echocardiography for pulmonary hypertension: a systematic review and meta-analysis. *Heart*. 97:612–622.

116. West JB, Mathieu-Costello O. Vulnerability of pulmonary capillaries in heart disease. *Circulation*. 1995;92:622–631.

117. Katz SD, Balidemaj K, Homma S, Wu H, Wang J, Maybaum S. Acute type 5 phosphodiesterase inhibition with sildenafil enhances flow-mediated vasodilation in patients with chronic heart failure. *J Am Coll Cardiol*. 2000;36:845–851.

118. Guglin M, Khan H. Pulmonary hypertension in heart failure. *J Card Fail*. 2010;16:461–474.

119. Goland S, Czer LS, Kass RM, et al. Pre-existing pulmonary hypertension in patients with end-stage heart failure: impact on clinical outcome and hemodynamic follow-up after orthotopic heart transplantation. *J Heart Lung Transplant*. 2007;26:312–318.

120. Butler J, Stankewicz MA, Wu J, et al. Pre-transplant reversible pulmonary hypertension predicts higher risk for mortality after cardiac transplantation. *J Heart Lung Transplant*. 2005;24:170–177.

121. Costard-Jackle A, Fowler MB. Influence of preoperative pulmonary artery pressure on mortality after heart transplantation: testing of potential reversibility of pulmonary hypertension with nitroprusside is useful in defining a high risk group. *J Am Coll Cardiol*. 1992;19:48–54.

122. Sitbon O, Humbert M, Jais X, et al. Long-term response to calcium channel blockers in idiopathic pulmonary arterial hypertension. *Circulation*. 2005;111:3105–3111.

123. Jabbour A, Keogh A, Hayward C, Macdonald P. Chronic sildenafil lowers transpulmonary gradient and improves cardiac output allowing successful heart transplantation. *Eur J Heart Fail*. 2007;9:674–677.

124. Slaughter MS, Rogers JG, Milano CA, et al. Advanced heart failure treated with continuous-flow left ventricular assist device. *N Engl J Med*. 2009;361:2241–2251.

125. Starling RC, Naka Y, Boyle AJ, et al. Results of the post-U.S. Food and Drug Administration-approval study with a continuous flow left ventricular assist device as a bridge to heart transplantation: a prospective study using the INTERMACS (Interagency Registry for Mechanically Assisted Circulatory Support). *J Am Coll Cardiol*. 2011;57:1890–1898.

126. Nair PK, Kormos RL, Teuteberg JJ, et al. Pulsatile left ventricular assist device support as a bridge to decision in patients with end-stage heart failure complicated by pulmonary hypertension. *J Heart Lung Transplant*. 2010;29:201–208.

127. Assad-Kottner C, Chen D, Jahanyar J, et al. The use of continuous milrinone therapy as bridge to transplant is safe in patients with short waiting times. *J Card Fail*. 2008;14:839–843.

128. Cuffe MS, Califf RM, Adams KF, Jr, et al. Short-term intravenous milrinone for acute exacerbation of chronic heart failure: a randomized controlled trial. *JAMA*. 2002;287:1541–1547.

129. Interagency Registry for Mechanically Assisted Circulatory Support. Available at www.intermacs.org. Accessed December 11, 2012.

130. Boyle AJ, Ascheim DD, Russo MJ, et al. Clinical outcomes for continuous-flow left ventricular assist device patients stratified by pre-operative INTERMACS classification. *J Heart Lung Transplant*. 30:402–407.

131. Fitzpatrick JR, 3rd, Frederick JR, Hsu VM, et al. Risk score derived from pre-operative data analysis predicts the need for biventricular mechanical circulatory support. *J Heart Lung Transplant*. 2008;27:1286–1292.

132. Matthews JC, Koelling TM, Pagani FD, Aaronson KD. The right ventricular failure risk score a pre-operative tool for assessing the risk of right ventricular failure in left ventricular assist device candidates. *J Am Coll Cardiol*. 2008;51:2163–2172.

133. Birks EJ, George RS, Hedger M, et al. Reversal of severe heart failure with a continuous-flow left ventricular assist device and pharmacological therapy: a prospective study. *Circulation*. 2011;123:381–390.

3

Tako-Tsubo (Stress) Cardiomyopathy

SCOTT W. SHARKEY

CASE PRESENTATION

A 56-year-old woman presented to the emergency department by ambulance because of acute chest heaviness and shortness of breath. The patient had a history of upper gastrointestinal hemorrhage and had experienced melena earlier in the day. Her coronary risk factor profile included active cigarette smoking and hypertension.

Emergency Department Course

On initial examination, the patient was alert, acutely ill, and dyspneic. The blood pressure was 72/60 mmHg and heart rate 138 beats per minute (sinus tachycardia). The jugular venous pressure was normal, the lung fields were clear. Cardiac examination revealed regular tachycardia without murmur. There was no peripheral edema. Stool was guaic positive.

An ECG revealed sinus tachycardia and ST-segment elevation in leads V3–V6 consistent with acute anterior myocardial infarction (**Figure 3-1**). Chest x-ray showed normal heart size and clear lung fields. The initial troponin I was 0.02 ng/ml, hemoglobin 10.8 g/dl, and creatinine 0.63 mg/dl.

The emergency department diagnosis was acute anterior myocardial infarction due to left anterior descending coronary artery (LAD) occlusion and treatment was started with clopidogrel, aspirin, and IV heparin. A beta-blocker was withheld because of hypotension. The patient was transferred to a tertiary care hospital for emergency coronary angiography and percutaneous coronary intervention. During transport, the patient developed cardiogenic shock.

Cardiac Catheterization

In the cardiac catheterization lab, the patient required intubation, mechanical ventilation, and placement of an intra-aortic balloon pump. IV phenylephrine was used to further support systolic blood pressure. Coronary angiography demonstrated widely patent coronary arteries. A left ventriculogram demonstrated severe left ventricular systolic dysfunction with ejection fraction 20% and pronounced "apical ballooning" (**Video 3-1;** to view the video, please visit http://www.demosmedpub.com/video/?vid=829). The left ventricular end-diastolic pressure was 25 mmHg. A diagnosis of acute tako-tsubo (stress) cardiomyopathy (TTC) was established. A bedside two-dimensional echocardiogram confirmed severe left ventricular systolic dysfunction with "apical ballooning," left ventricular outflow tract obstruction, and severe mitral regurgitation (**Video 3-2A and B**; to view the videos, please visit http://www.demosmedpub.com/video/?vid=830 and http://www.demosmedpub.com/video/?vid=831). The left ventricular outflow tract gradient could not be measured because of signal overlap with the mitral regurgitation jet. Right ventricular contraction was normal.

Hospital Course

The patient was transferred to the ICU. A repeat hemoglobin was 5 g/dl, consistent with acute gastrointestinal hemorrhage (the presumed stressor for the TTC). Emergency endoscopy demonstrated an actively bleeding gastric antral ulcer with visible vessel, which was treated with epinephrine injection and clipping. The patient was transfused and anticoagulation was discontinued.

Subsequent laboratory testing demonstrated peak troponin of 1.62 ng/ml and peak brain natriuretic peptide of 1,040 pg/ml. On hospital day three, an echocardiogram demonstrated

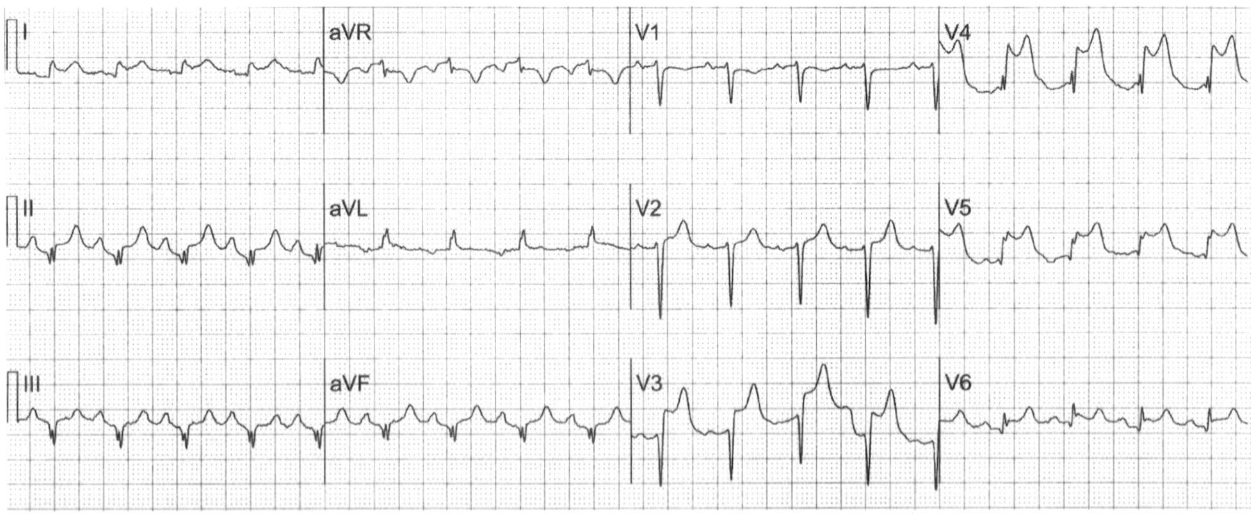

Figure 3-1
Admission ECG shows sinus tachycardia and ST-segment elevation in leads V3-V6, I, and II.

persistent left ventricular dysfunction (ejection fraction 30%) with left ventricular thrombus. Anticoagulation with heparin and warfarin was initiated while monitoring the patient for recurrent gastrointestinal hemorrhage. Over the next several days, the patient improved. Phenylephrine infusion was discontinued, the intra-aortic balloon pump was removed, and the patient was extubated.

Cardiac magnetic resonance imaging (CMR) demonstrated left ventricular apical ballooning without mycocardial infarction (no delayed hyperenhancement after gadolinium injection). Three discrete left ventricular thrombi were identified. There was no clinical evidence of cerebral embolism. Anticoagulation was continued.

A follow-up echocardiogram demonstrated improvement in left ventricular ejection fraction from 30% to 35%, with resolution of left ventricular outflow tract obstruction, and improvement in the degree of mitral regurgitation from severe to moderate. Long acting metoprolol 12.5 mg and lisinopril 2.5 mg were initiated. Follow-up ECG demonstrated appearance of deep symmetric T-wave inversion and QT interval lengthening (**Figure 3-2**). The patient was discharged.

Outpatient Course

At initial visit, 4 weeks postdischarge, the patient was significantly improved. A repeat echocardiogram showed resolution of "apical ballooning," improvement in left ventricular ejection fraction to 55%, and disappearance of left ventricular thrombus. Despite normal left ventricular ejection fraction, an electrocardiogram (ECG) showed persistence of T-wave inversion. Warfarin, beta-blocker, and angiotensin converting enzyme inhibitor were discontinued.

TTC is a newly recognized cardiomyopathy with an acute onset, characterized by a distinctive left ventricular contraction profile, a predilection for middle aged and older women, an antecedent stressor, and reversibility. While uncommon (perhaps 5%–10% of women with suspected acute coronary syndrome), the prevalence of this cardiomyopathy is increasing now that it is more widely recognized. In the early stages, TTC is indistinguishable from an acute coronary syndrome and can be complicated by significant congestive heart failure.

APPROACH TO THE PATIENT

Patients with TTC typically present to the emergency department with sudden onset of chest discomfort or shortness of breath. The ECG usually shows ischemic changes (50% of TTC patients have ST-segment elevation identical to that of acute anterior myocardial infarction from LAD occlusion). In other cases, widespread T-wave inversion or anterior Q waves are present. The initial troponin is elevated in 90% of TTC patients, although the peak troponin is usually substantially lower than that with acute coronary syndrome. In the typical TTC patient, the peak troponin T is 0.6 ng/ml. The disparity between a minor troponin elevation and marked acute left ventricular systolic dysfunction is due to myocardial stunning without significant myocardial infarction.

The seasoned clinician may suspect TTC because of its predilection for women and its association with an antecedent stressful event. The stressor may be either physical (40%–45% of patients), such as acute infection or surgical procedure, or emotional (40%–45% of patients), such as a heated argument or grief from the death of a family member. Respectful questioning of the patient and family with regard to social stress is necessary to uncover some emotional triggers. We now recognize this cardiomyopathy

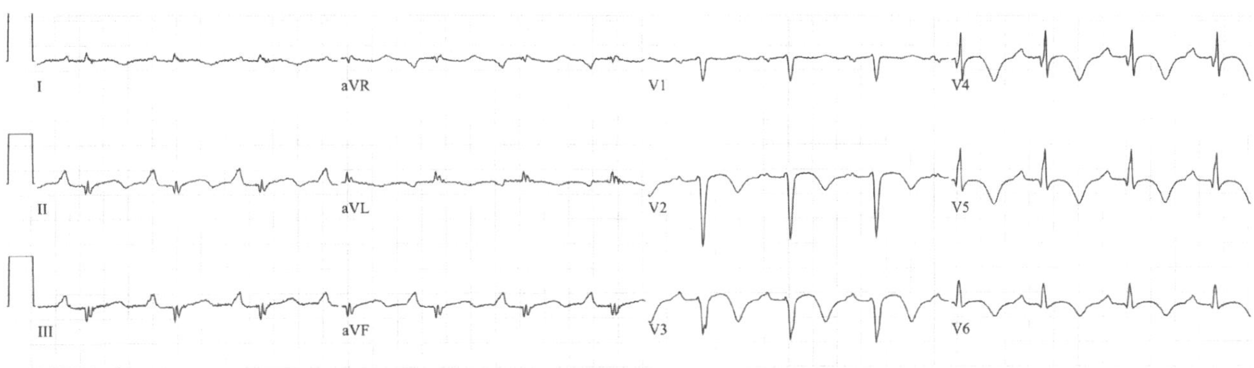

Figure 3-2
Follow-up ECG shows T-wave inversion in leads V2–V6 with significant QT interval lengthening (QTc = 531 msec). R wave voltage is reduced in leads V2–V5.

occurs spontaneously (no overt stressor) in about 10% of patients, therefore the name "stress cardiomyopathy" is misleading.

IMAGING

An urgent coronary angiogram and left ventriculogram is necessary to differentiate TTC from acute coronary syndrome. It is quite acceptable to treat the patient with suspected TTC as you would a patient with acute coronary syndrome until the diagnosis is verified. A two-dimensional echocardiogram is necessary even in the patient who has had a left ventriculogram to assess for left ventricular outflow tract obstruction, mitral valve regurgitation, left and right ventricular thrombus, and right ventricular dysfunction. Three unique patterns of abnormal left ventricular contraction (ballooning) occur in patients with TTC (**Videos 3-3–3-5;** to view the videos, please visit the following respective links; http://www.demosmedpub.com/video/?vid=832; http:/www.demosmedpub.com/video/?vid=833; http://www.demosmedpub.com/video/?vid=834). The left ventricular "apical ballooning" pattern was the first described, is currently the most common, occurring in about 75% of patients, and is considered a hallmark of this cardiomyopathy. More recently, the "mid-ventricular ballooning" pattern has been recognized as occurring in a substantial minority of patients (approximately 25%). Recognition of the mid-ventricular ballooning pattern is increasing. A third pattern, "inverted ballooning," is rarely encountered. Each contraction pattern is, in general, distinct from that caused by obstructive coronary artery disease and can be recognized by careful examination of imaging modalities including two-dimensional echocardiography, left ventriculography, and CMR. A note of caution, the apical ballooning pattern of TTC can resemble the wall motion abnormality caused by an acute coronary syndrome in the distribution of a "wrap around" left anterior descending coronary artery, and the inverted ballooning pattern can resemble the wall motion abnormality caused by acute myocarditis. In uncertain cases, CMR with gadolinium contrast is valuable because delayed hyperenhancement (a marker for scar) is very rarely present in TTC, yet frequently present in a vascular distribution (acute coronary syndrome) or patchy distribution (acute myocarditis).

In about 25% of cases, right ventricular contraction is also abnormal, typically involving the apical one-third to one-half of the chamber, and best appreciated on echocardiography (apical four chamber view) or CMR (**Video 3-6**; to view the video, please visit http://www.demosmedpub.com/video/?vid=835). Right ventricular involvement can occur with either left ventricular apical ballooning or mid-ventricular ballooning and is associated with a lower left ventricular ejection fraction. Right ventricular thrombus may be present. The hemodynamic importance of abnormal right ventricular contraction in TTC is not known.

HOSPITAL MANAGEMENT

During the first 24 hours, I recommend the patient be confined to either an ICU or telemetry unit depending on hemodynamic status and comorbid conditions. Traditionally, these patients have been treated with a beta-blocker and an angiotensin converting enzyme inhibitor in the same way as a patient with left ventricular dysfunction from acute myocardial infarction. Whether these drugs improve the prognosis of this acute cardiomyopathy is unknown, since left ventricular function typically improves spontaneously. Beta-blockers and angiotensin converting enzyme inhibitors (in standard doses) do not prevent either occurrence or recurrence of TTC (about 20% of patients are receiving these drugs at presentation). In my practice, I have continued these drugs until the left ventricular function has returned to normal (generally 2–6 weeks). Aspirin and clopidogrel are not necessary since this is not an acute coronary event. In the presence of right or left ventricular thrombus (discussed below), IV heparin followed by warfarin anticoagulation is appropriate. Hospital mortality is low (2%–3%) and may be either cardiac (cardiogenic shock or ventricular fibrillation) or from a comorbid condition (cancer or severe lung disease). Death to due cardiac rupture has been reported.

CONGESTIVE HEART FAILURE

Congestive heart failure complicates TTC in an important number of patients and ranges in severity from radiographic pulmonary congestion to cardiogenic shock. B-type natriuretic peptide (BNP) levels are often substantially elevated and well above those observed with acute coronary syndrome. The average BNP for a patient with TTC may be three to four times that of a patient with acute coronary syndrome. Keep in mind, the BNP peak may not occur until 48 hours. Heart failure is in part caused by left ventricular systolic dysfunction (the median left ventricular ejection fraction is 30%), which is significantly below that observed with acute anterior myocardial infarction due to LAD occlusion. Myocardial edema within the abnormally contracting myocardium is common (best evaluated on CMR), and might contribute to heart failure by reducing left ventricular compliance and thereby increasing left ventricular filling pressure.

As illustrated by this patient, congestive heart failure can be aggravated by left ventricular outflow tract obstruction due to systolic anterior mitral leaflet motion. This is an uncommon but well-documented complication of TTC, occurring in 5% to 10% of cases and typically observed in the subset of patients with the apical ballooning contraction pattern. In general, left ventricular outflow tract obstruction completely resolves once left ventricular contraction recovers. Persistence of left ventricular outflow tract obstruction and systolic anterior mitral leaflet motion should raise consideration for coexisting hypertrophic cardiomyopathy.

Also illustrated by this patient, significant mitral valve regurgitation is yet another influence on congestive heart failure. Systolic anterior mitral leaflet motion and left ventricular outflow tract obstruction, resulting in elevated left ventricular systolic wall stress with improper mitral leaflet coaptation, leads to important mitral regurgitation. The typical murmur of mitral regurgitation may be obscured by the murmur of left ventricular outflow tract obstruction. Significant mitral valve regurgitation can also occur without systolic anterior mitral leaflet motion and may be caused by coexisting conditions such as mitral annular calcification.

Mild congestive heart failure (typically pulmonary congestion) can be treated with furosemide. Patients with hypotension or cardiogenic shock will require more aggressive measures including IV inotropic drugs and/or insertion of an intra-aortic balloon pump. In my experience, these patients respond well to IV catecholamine drugs including dopamine, phenylephrine (used in this patient), and norepinephrine. The use of these drugs may seem counterintuitive, since the popular explanation for TTC involves catecholamine mediated cardiotoxicity. Nonetheless, in physiologic doses, catecholamine drugs are effective treatment for hypotension in this cardiomyopathy. Whether a non-catecholamine drug, such as vasopressin, is superior has not been established. For more profound hypotension, an intra-aortic balloon pump is effective. Some investigators have raised concern that an intra-aortic balloon pump might worsen left ventricular outflow tract obstruction by reducing left ventricular cavity size, although this has not been an issue in my experience.

VENTRICULAR THROMBUS

Akinetic segments within the left or right ventricle provide a substrate for ventricular thrombus formation (**Figure 3-3**). As illustrated by this patient, thrombi can be multiple and in locations different from that observed in acute myocardial infarction caused by coronary artery occlusion. These thrombi can be the source of both systemic and pulmonary embolism. Therefore, absent major hemorrhage, it is reasonable to initially treat patients with tako-tsubo cardiomyopathy with IV heparin. In my practice, I have reserved warfarin for those patients with documented ventricular thrombus and have continued this treatment until ventricular contraction has returned to normal.

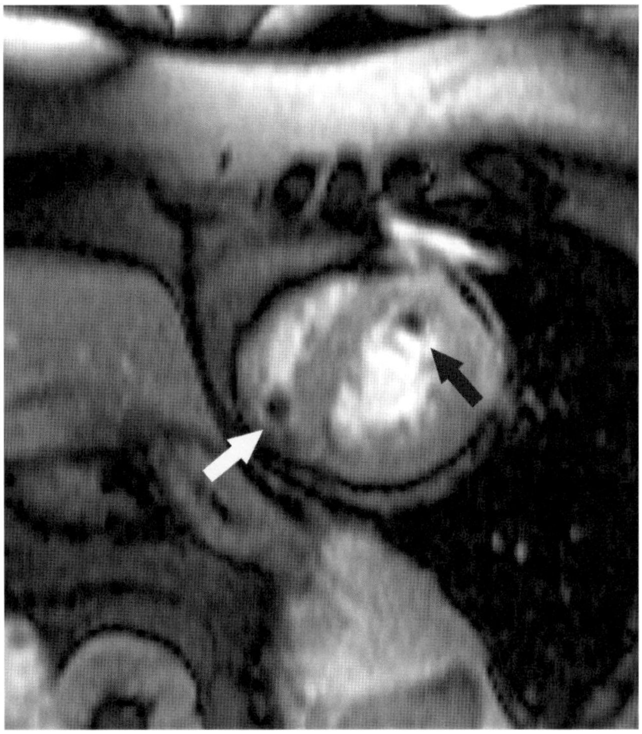

Figure 3-3
Cross sectional cardiac MRI shows right ventricular (white arrow) and left ventricular (black arrow) thrombi.

ARRHYTHMIA AND ECG EVOLUTION

Despite significant acute left ventricular dysfunction, clinically important ventricular arrhythmias are quite uncommon in TTC. Ventricular fibrillation is rare, unpredictable, and sometimes fatal. The most common serious ventricular arrhythmia in TTC is Torsade de pointes ventricular tachycardia, occurring in the setting of significant QT interval prolongation (**Figure 3-4**). An ECG hallmark of TTC is progressive T-wave inversion and QT interval prolongation evolving over the course of several days. Torsade de pointes occurs in a very small number of patients even though the QT interval may exceed 500 msec. Patients with bradycardia, heart block, or variable heart rate (as with atrial fibrillation) seem to be more vulnerable. Because the QT interval lengthening is a delayed process, I advocate monitoring these patients until the time of hospital discharge and avoiding drugs that might further prolong the QT interval. I am especially cautious in those patients with bradycardia (heart rate below 60 beats/minute).

Atrial fibrillation either on admission or during hospitalization is occasionally present, as might be expected in this older aged population. Standard treatment of atrial fibrillation is appropriate including cardioversion or rate control and anticoagulation.

POSTHOSPITAL MANAGEMENT

At 1 month postdischarge, I repeat an echocardiogram to verify recovery of left ventricular contraction (occasionally recovery will be longer). Complete recovery of left ventricular systolic function is a hallmark of TTC and persistent left ventricular dysfunction should raise concern for a different or coexisting cardiomyopathy. In my opinion, it is safe and reasonable to discontinue beta-blocker, angiotensin converting enzyme inhibitor, and anticoagulation once left ventricular ejection fraction has returned to normal.

The recurrence rate of TTC is about 5% during a 5-year interval. Recurrences may be multiple (I am aware of a patient with three well-documented recurrences) and are not prevented by standard doses of beta-blockers, angiotensin converting enzyme inhibitors, calcium channel blockers, or nitrates. About 85% of patients with TTC are alive at 3 years after initial diagnosis, with mortality usually from underlying noncardiac condition such as cancer or chronic obstructive pulmonary disease. Longer term outcome has not yet been established and will be influenced by age and comorbid conditions.

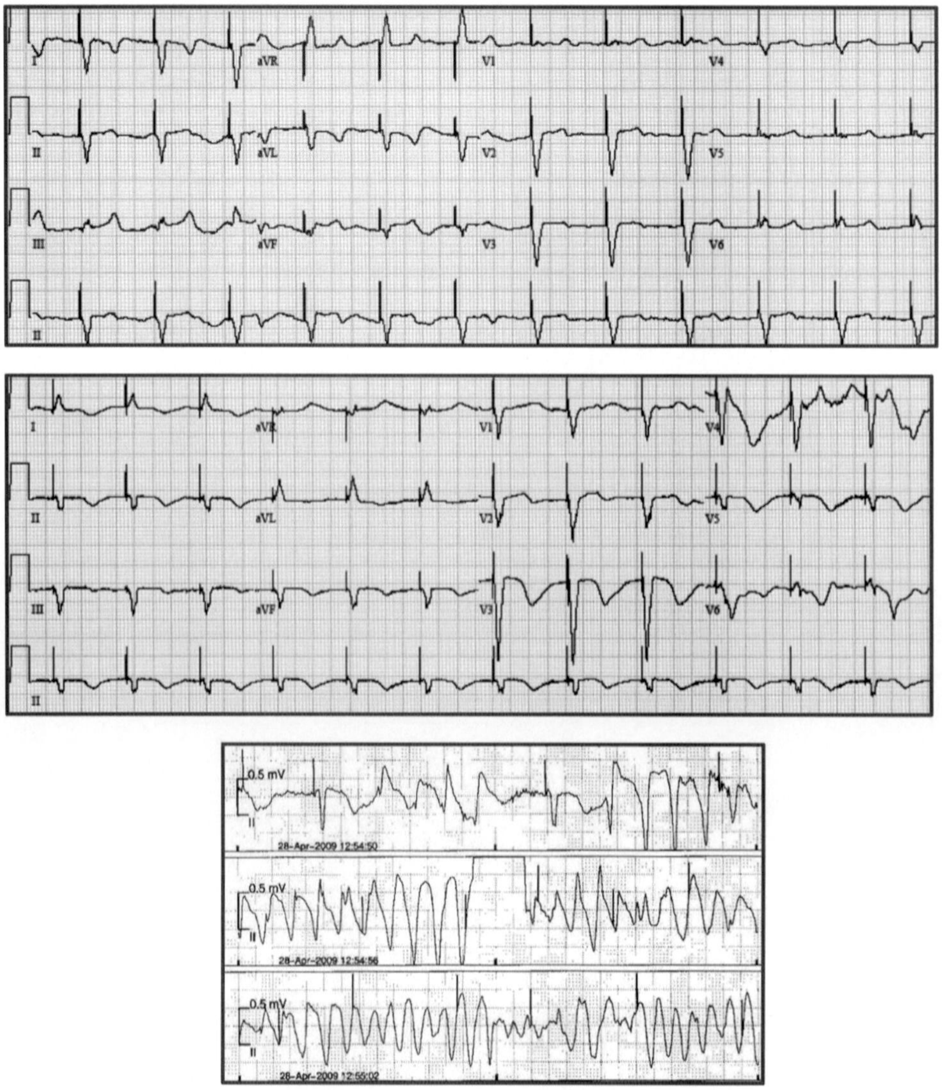

Figure 3-4
Serial ECGs and rhythm strip in a patient with tako-tsubo cardiomyopathy and complicated by torsade de pointes. (Top) Initial ECG shows ventricular paced rhythm and underlying atrial fibrillation (QTc = 485 msec). (Middle) Follow-up ECG shows ventricular paced rhythm with T-wave inversion in leads V3–V6 and significant QT interval lengthening (QTc = 624 msec). (Bottom) Occurrence of torsade de pointes ventricular tachycardia requiring cardioversion.

BIBLIOGRAPHY

Bybee KA, Prasad A. Stress-related cardiomyopathy syndromes. *Circulation.* 2008;118(4):397–409.

Dote K, Sato H, Tateishi H, et al. Myocardial stunning due to simultaneous multivessel coronary spasms: a review of 5 cases [Japanese]. *J Cardiol.* 1991;21(2):203–214.

Eitel I, von Knobelsdorff-Brenkenhoff F, Bernhardt P, et al. Clinical characteristics and cardiovascular magnetic resonance findings in stress (takotsubo) cardiomyopathy. *JAMA.* 2011;306(3):277–286.

El Mahmoud R, Mansencal N, Pilliere R, et al. Prevalence and characteristics of left ventricular outflow tract obstruction in tako-tsubo syndrome. *Am Heart J.* 2008;156(3):543–548.

Elesber AA, Prasad A, Bybee KA, et al. Transient cardiac apical ballooning syndrome: prevalence and clinical implications of right ventricular involvement. *J Am Coll Cardiol.* 2006;47(5):1082–1083.

Hurst RT, Askew JW, Reuss CS, et al. Transient midventricular ballooning syndrome: a new variant. *J Am Coll Cardiol.* 2006;48(3):579–583.

Kurisu S, Sato H, Kawagoe T, et al. Tako-tsubo-like left ventricular dysfunction with ST-segment elevation: a novel cardiac syndrome mimicking acute myocardial infarction. *Am Heart J.* 2002;143(3):448–455.

Madhavan M, Borlaug BA, Lerman A, et al. Stress hormone and circulating biomarker profile of apical ballooning syndrome (takotsubo cardiomyopathy): insights into the clinical significance of B-type natriuretic peptide and troponin levels. *Heart.* 2009;95(17):1436–1441.

Park JH, Kang SJ, Song JK, et al. Left ventricular apical ballooning due to severe physical stress in patients admitted to the medical ICU. *Chest*, 2005; 128(1), 296–302.

Pavin D, Le Breton H, Daubert C. Human stress cardiomyopathy mimicking acute myocardial syndrome.[see comment]. *Heart*, 1997; 78(5), 509–511.

Sharkey SW, Lesser JR, Zenovich AG, et al. Acute and reversible cardiomyopathy provoked by stress in women from the united states. *Circulation*. 2005;111(4):472–479.

Sharkey SW, Shear W, Hodges M, et al. Reversible myocardial contraction abnormalities in patients with an acute noncardiac illness. *Chest*. 1998;114(1):98–105.

Sharkey SW, Windenburg DC, Lesser JR, et al. Natural history and expansive clinical profile of stress (tako-tsubo) cardiomyopathy. *J Am Coll Cardiol*. 2010;55(4):333–341.

Tsuchihashi K, Ueshima K, Uchida T, et al. Transient left ventricular apical ballooning without coronary artery stenosis: a novel heart syndrome mimicking acute myocardial infarction. angina pectoris-myocardial infarction investigations in Japan [see comment]. *J Am Coll Cardiol*. 2001;38(1):11–18.

Wittstein IS, Thiemann DR, Lima JA, et al. Neurohumoral features of myocardial stunning due to sudden emotional stress. *N Engl J Med*. 2005;352(6):539–548.

4

Atrial Fibrillation and Cardiomyopathy With Heart Failure

ANJALI VAIDYA AND MARIELL JESSUP

INTRODUCTION

Atrial fibrillation is an increasingly prevalent condition affecting millions of adults. In the ATRIA (AnTicoagulation and Risk Factors In Atrial fibrillation) study, 1% of adults had atrial fibrillation, and this increased with age. Seventy percent of adults with atrial fibrillation were over the age of 65, and almost half were at least 75 years old (1). Similar findings were reported from the Framingham Heart Study, with a lifetime risk of atrial fibrillation of 25% in men and women over the age of 40 (2). The morbidity associated with atrial fibrillation is significant, leading to stroke, other systemic thromboembolism, bleeding as a complication of anticoagulation therapy, and functional limitations due to symptoms of dyspnea, fatigue, and palpitations. In addition to the significant morbidity associated with atrial fibrillation, this arrhythmia has also been described as a possible independent risk factor for mortality in certain populations, including older adults and those with concomitant cardiovascular disease such as ischemic heart disease and heart failure (3–5). The intersection between atrial fibrillation and heart failure represents an increasingly common problem and is the subject of this chapter.

The Framingham Heart Study demonstrated the epidemiologic relationship between heart failure and atrial fibrillation and coexistence of these two important phenomena in 2003. In patients who developed atrial fibrillation without underlying structural heart disease or heart failure, 3.3% of these patients per year went on to develop heart failure (6). There are a number of potential mechanisms by which atrial fibrillation leads to heart failure. Chronic and persistent tachycardia with this abnormal rhythm can lead to a rate-related cardiomyopathy. The neurohormonal activation associated with atrial fibrillation promotes elevated circulating levels of norepinephrine and angiotensin II, also known to contribute to sodium retention, volume overload, and heart failure. Finally, the loss of atrial-ventricular synchrony can limit adequate ventricular filling, affecting stroke volume and cardiac output. The inverse relationship is also true between heart failure and atrial fibrillation. In the Framingham Heart Study, one out of five patients who had developed heart failure without prior atrial fibrillation went on to develop atrial fibrillation over a mean follow-up of 4 years (6).

Although controversial, there is some data to suggest that atrial fibrillation may be an independent risk factor for mortality in heart failure patients. In the Candesartan in Heart failure-Assessment of Reduction in Mortality and morbidity (CHARM) trials, 7,599 patients with heart failure were enrolled. Of these patients, nearly 20% had atrial fibrillation at the onset of the study. After nearly 40 months of follow-up, atrial fibrillation was shown to be associated with increased all-cause mortality (24% vs. 14%) in patients with heart failure who had both reduced and preserved systolic function (7). Similar findings were demonstrated in the Studies of Left Ventricular Dysfunction (SOLVD) trial, in which atrial fibrillation was present in approximately 6% of the 6,517 enrolled patients who were followed over 3 years. Atrial fibrillation was found to be a predictor of mortality in this large population of patients with left ventricular dysfunction, ranging from asymptomatic to New York Heart Association (NYHA) functional Class III (34% vs. 23%; 8). Despite this compelling evidence, there are other reported studies that have demonstrated no significant association between atrial fibrillation and mortality in select heart failure populations. The largest of these are the Vasodilator Heart Failure Trials (V-HeFTs), which in total included 1,427 patients, of whom 14% had atrial fibrillation. At 2 years of follow-up, there was no significant difference in either mortality or hospitalization in those patients with atrial fibrillation (9).

What follows are a series of cases that illustrate atrial fibrillation coexisting with heart failure, highlighting important areas of the clinical evaluation, diagnostic approaches, and management strategies.

CASE 1: ATRIAL FIBRILLATION AS A RESULT OF PATIENT NONCOMPLIANCE

FM is a 72-year-old male with a history of nonischemic cardiomyopathy, a left ventricular ejection fraction (LVEF) of 45%, and severe obstructive sleep apnea. He has been managed with intermittent continuous positive airway pressure (CPAP) at night, beta blocker and ace-inhibitor therapy, and occasional diuretic use. He admitted poor adherence with both his CPAP therapy and his oral medications; after a month off treatment, he reported worsening exertional dyspnea, orthopnea, paroxysmal nocturnal dyspnea, and lower extremity edema. A 6-minute walk test revealed a drop from 421 m, performed 4 months ago, to his present performance of 302 m. A repeat echocardiogram revealed an LVEF of 30%. His volume overload was thought to be related to progressive left ventricular dysfunction and sleep disordered breathing, associated with nocturnal hypoxia, activating peripheral chemoreceptors and the sympathetic nervous system. He subsequently developed palpitations and was noted to have new onset atrial fibrillation with a ventricular response rate of 103 beats per minute (**Figure 4-1**).

It is important, with the onset of new atrial fibrillation, to search for an etiology, or precipitating cause (10). There are many etiologic possibilities, and these should be considered dependent on the relevant factors of the individual patient (**Table 4-1**). In this particular case, an elevation in left atrial pressure due to progressive volume overload and systolic dysfunction was identified as the most likely cause. FM was managed with

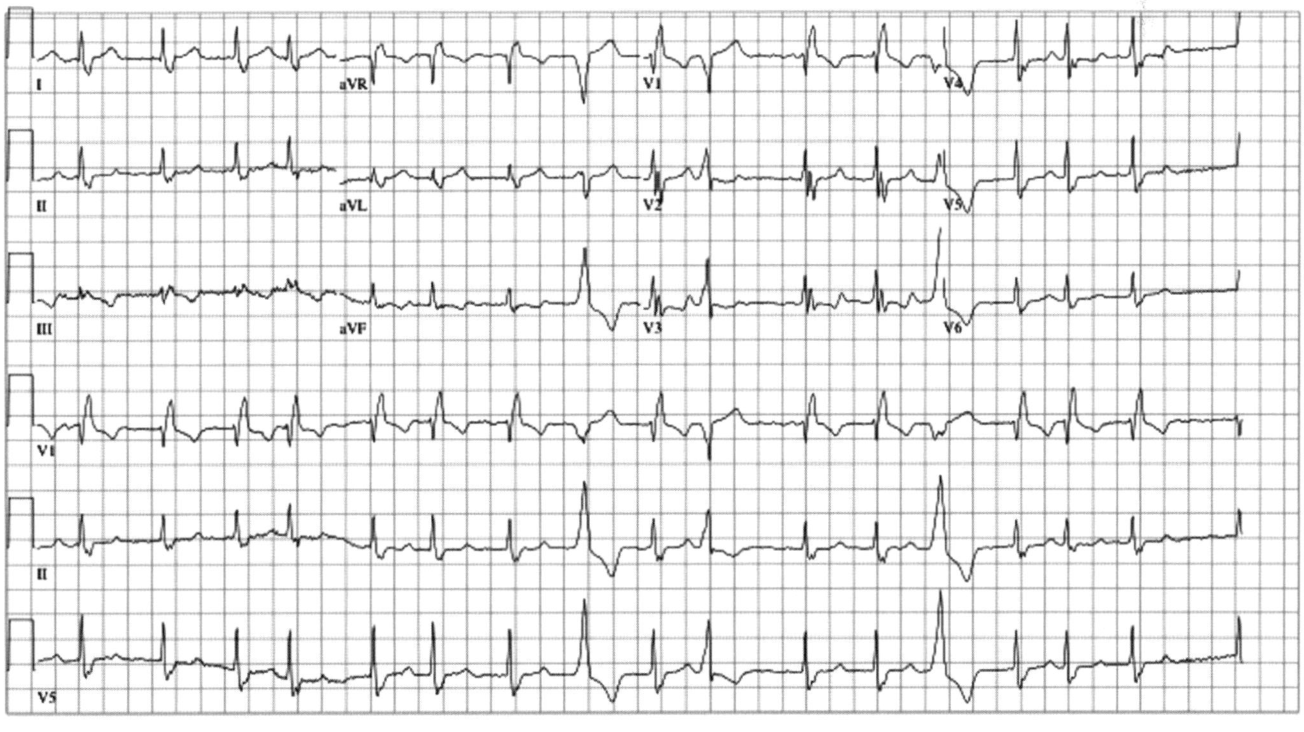

Figure 4-1
Electrocardiogram demonstrating atrial fibrillation with rapid ventricular response and premature ventricular contraction.

Table 4-1
Etiologies and Factors Predisposing Patients to Atrial Fibrillation

Electrophysiological abnormalities
- Enhanced automaticity (focal AF)
- Conduction abnormality (reentry)

Atrial pressure elevation
- Mitral or tricuspid valve disease
- Myocardial disease (primary or secondary, leading to systolic or diastolic dysfunction)
- Semilunar valvular abnormalities (causing ventricular hypertrophy)
- Systemic or pulmonary hypertension (pulmonary embolism) Intracardiac tumors or thrombi

Atrial ischemia
- Coronary artery disease

Inflammatory or infiltrative atrial disease
- Pericarditis
- Amyloidosis
- Myocarditis
- Age-induced atrial fibrotic changes

Drugs
- Alcohol
- Caffeine

Endocrine disorders
- Hyperthyroidism
- Pheochromocytoma

Changes in autonomic tone
- Increased parasympathetic activity
- Increased sympathetic activity

Primary or metastatic disease in or adjacent to the atrial wall

Postoperative
- Cardiac, pulmonary, or esophageal

Congenital heart disease

Neurogenic
- Subarachnoid hemorrhage
- Nonhemorrhagic, major stroke

Idiopathic (lone AF)

Familial AF

Note: AF = fibrillation.

Source: Borrowed with permission from Fuster V, Rydén LE, Cannom DS, et al. 2011 ACCF/AHA/HRS focused updates incorporated into the ACC/AHA/ESC 2006 guidelines for the management of patients with atrial fibrillation: a report of the American College of Cardiology Foundation/American Heart Association Task Force on Practice Guidelines. *Circulation*. 2011;123:e269–e367.

re-initiation of appropriate heart failure medical therapy including beta blocker, angiotensin converting enzyme inhibitor, and diuretic, and CPAP for his sleep disordered breathing. With this therapy, his heart rate was more optimally controlled, although his rhythm remained as atrial fibrillation.

The decision to manage patients with systolic heart failure and atrial fibrillation with rate versus rhythm control is a complicated one without clear evidence to support one strategy over another. Up until recently, subsets of larger studies looking at this issue in populations with atrial fibrillation but not selected for the comorbidity of heart failure were relied upon to extrapolate data relevant to patients with heart failure. These included large and influential trials such as Danish Investigations of Arrhythmia and Mortality ON Dofetilide (DIAMOND; 11), Rate Control versus Electrical (RACE) cardioversion (12), and most recently, Atrial Fibrillation Follow-up Investigation of Rhythm Management (AFFIRM; 13). The AFFIRM trial is especially notable as a recent landmark trial that addressed the issue of rate versus rhythm control. A total of 4,060 patients over the age of 65 were randomized to rhythm control (in which antiarrhythmic drugs were chosen by the treating physician, supplemented by electrical cardioversion as necessary) or rate control (with a goal resting heart rate less than 80 beats per minute and, after a 6-minute walk, less than 110 beats per minute). The primary end point was all-cause mortality. After 3.5 years of follow-up, there was no significant difference in mortality between the two groups of rate versus rhythm control. The results of this large, multicenter, randomized trial have greatly influenced clinical practice guidelines for the management of atrial fibrillation. However, it is imperative to note that the majority of patients enrolled in this study did not have heart failure. In fact, only 4.8% of the patients were noted to have cardiomyopathy, and the mean LVEF was 55%. Moreover, analyses of prespecified subgroups showed that rate control resulted in better outcomes for those patients *without* heart failure and those with an LVEF greater than or equal to 50% (13).

More recently, the Atrial Fibrillation and Congestive Heart Failure (AF-CHF) study addressed the same issue specifically within a population of heart failure patients (14) This trial enrolled 1,376 patients with atrial fibrillation and symptoms of systolic heart failure with an LVEF less than 35%. They were randomized to either rate control with beta blocker therapy, or rhythm control with antiarrhythmic medications, including dofetilide, sotalol, or amiodarone. After a mean follow-up of 37 months, there was no significant difference between the two groups in the primary outcome of cardiovascular mortality.

Based on the current available data regarding this important issue, the strategy of rhythm versus rate control must be made based on individual case details. Rhythm control involves the use of antiarrhythmic drugs, which can have significant side effects, especially in the elderly. For this reason, rate control may be a preferred strategy in those who are easily able to achieve and maintain rate control without antiarrhythmic drugs and in those who are not limited by symptoms of atrial fibrillation even while well rate-controlled. Beta blockers and judicious use of digoxin can be effective and safe in achieving rate control. Nondihydropyridine calcium channel blockers (such as diltiazem and verapamil), however, have negative inotropic effects and may suppress myocardial contractility; this may be detrimental in systolic heart failure, and these drugs should be avoided in patients with a low LVEF (15). Many patients, however, will remain significantly symptomatic despite rate control, or suffer from hemodynamic compromise related to loss of atrial systolic function. Similarly, many patients will not be able to achieve adequate rate control despite aggressive use of medical therapy such as beta blockers and digoxin. In these patients, rhythm control is often the preferred method of choice in the management of atrial fibrillation.

In our index case, patient FM continued to have symptoms of fatigue and palpitations despite improvement in his overall volume status and a functional increase in his 6-minute walk distance up to 354 meters. Even with management of his heart failure and titration of beta blocker therapy to a resting heart rate of 74 beats per minute and an exertional heart rate of 108 beats per minute, an electrical cardioversion was performed in conjunction with initiation of amiodarone therapy. Notably, 8 weeks later, while in normal sinus rhythm, a repeat echocardiogram revealed an improvement in his LVEF to 55%.

CASE 2: ATRIAL FIBRILLATION CAUSING TACHYCARDIA-MEDIATED CARDIOMYOPATHY

MK is a 60-year-old male with a history of hypertension, hyperlipidemia, an oligodendroglioma status post resection and radiation therapy, and paroxysmal atrial fibrillation first diagnosed during a colonoscopy 2 years prior to presentation. He developed progressive dyspnea on exertion approximately 3 months previously that lead to an acute worsening of his symptoms after 1 week and an ultimate visit to a local emergency department. He was found to have atrial fibrillation with a rapid ventricular response of 150 to 160 beats per minute, and was told that he was in "heart failure." He was treated with IV furosemide and heparin. An echocardiogram revealed a LVEF of 30% with a mildly dilated left ventricle of 5.9 cm at end diastole and no significant valvular abnormalities. One year prior to this presentation, he had an echocardiogram that revealed an LVEF of 60%.

The initial evaluation of this newly diagnosed cardiomyopathy included a left heart catheterization with coronary angiography. This revealed a 30% stenosis of his left anterior descending artery, and otherwise mild luminal irregularities throughout the remainder of his coronary arteries. In addition, thyroid function was normal. He was managed with warfarin, metoprolol succinate (for rate control and his underlying cardiomyopathy), and lisinopril. He was readmitted 12 weeks later with palpitations and dyspnea, and found to have atrial fibrillation with a resting heart rate of 130 beats per minute and a systolic blood pressure of 70 mm Hg. On exam, he had a jugular venous pressure of 16 cm water, a laterally displaced apical impulse, a S3 gallop, rales, and bilateral lower extremity edema. A repeat echocardiogram revealed LVEF of 10% to 15% (**Figure 4-2**). He was treated with further diuresis and digoxin was added to his regimen for added effects of rate control and inotropic support. Upon optimization of his hemodynamics and volume status with appropriate heart failure therapy, a dual chamber implantable cardioverter defibrillator was implanted prior to discharge.

During his subsequent appointment in the office, he reported feeling well but with mild dyspnea and persistent palpitations. The question was raised again as to the etiology of his cardiomyopathy, as ischemia had been ruled out with angiography. At rest, it was noted that MK had a heart rate of 105 beats per minute, despite metoprolol and digoxin therapy. His physical examination revealed a jugular venous pressure of 5 cm water, an irregularly irregular heartbeat, no murmurs, and a nondisplaced apical impulse. He had no rales, his abdomen was soft and nondistended, and he had no lower extremity

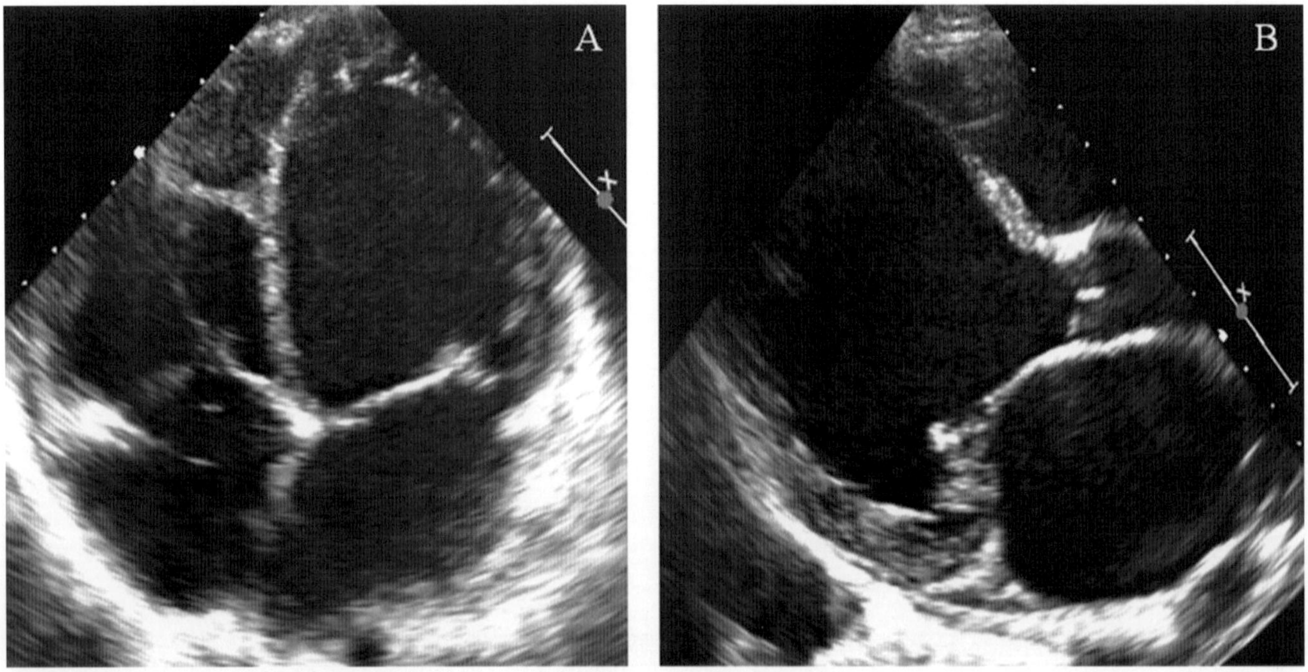

Figure 4-2
Echocardiogram of tachycardia-mediated cardiomyopathy. (A) Apical four-chamber view. (B) Parasternal long axis view.

edema, with intact distal pulses and warm extremities. His electrocardiogram revealed atrial fibrillation with nonspecific T wave abnormalities. Upon interrogation of his defibrillator, he was noted to have persistent atrial fibrillation since implantation of the device with ventricular rates frequently as high as 180 beats per minute. At this time, having ruled out ischemia, endocrinopathy, and other toxic exposures for a cardiomyopathy, it was thought that MK likely had a tachycardia-induced cardiomyopathy.

This diagnosis is a common and important one to recognize, as management of the tachycardia with adequate rate or rhythm control may have a profound impact on improving left ventricular function. To establish this diagnosis, it is important to first identify other possible etiologies for a patient's cardiomyopathy, including but not limited to ischemic heart disease, endocrinopathy, toxin exposures, infectious etiologies, or myocarditis. In one study of over two hundred patients with heart failure associated with atrial fibrillation, the presumed diagnosis for the cardiomyopathy was a tachycardia-mediated cardiomyopathy in nearly 30% of cases (16). Patients who already have implanted devices such as pacemakers or implantable cardioverter defibrillators have the advantage of easily determining the burden of arrhythmia and tachycardia by device interrogation. In patients who do not already have such implantable electronic devices, use of a Holter monitor or event recorder can be a valuable diagnostic strategy to determine what percentage of time a patient has atrial fibrillation and what is the range of heart rate with both rest and exertion.

In the systolic heart failure population, strategies for the management of rhythm versus rate control suggest that the approach of rhythm control may be more effective, likely due to the greater chance of achieving heart rate control. One study followed patients with chronic atrial fibrillation and presumed tachycardia-mediated cardiomyopathy for a mean follow-up of nearly 5 months. After cardioversion, the mean LVEF improved from 32% to 53%. At 1 year, the LVEF remained normal in those who maintained sinus rhythm; however, the LVEF fell to abnormal levels once again in those who had recurrent atrial fibrillation (17).

Rhythm control for atrial fibrillation in the heart failure population is a strategy that requires meticulous observation of the patient. If this approach is undertaken, it is with the use of antiarrhythmic drugs. The American Heart Association/American College of Cardiology/Heart Rhythm Society guidelines from 2011 recommend using either amiodarone or dofetilide as first-line agents in the strategy of rhythm control with patients experiencing atrial fibrillation and heart failure (10). Both drugs are Class III antiarrhythmic drugs that block potassium channels and prolong repolarization, action potential duration, and the refractory period. Similarly, the European Society of Cardiology recommends amiodarone, though did not suggest dofetilide as initial management (18). It is well recognized that amiodarone is associated with a variety of toxicities, including thyroid, liver, lung, skin, and neurologic effects. These adverse effects must be monitored closely in any patient on chronic amiodarone therapy. However, amiodarone has the advantage of having little negative inotropic effect, and despite having the pharmacologic properties described above, less incidence of QT prolongation or proarrhythmia compared to others in its same class. One study examined four trials of low-dose (less than 400 mg daily) amiodarone for a minimum of 1 year in patients with underlying heart failure or myocardial infarction and noted that there were no cases of torsade de pointes in nearly 750 patients (19). Another advantage of amiodarone is its intrinsic beta blocking activity, so that if atrial fibrillation does recur, it is often accompanied by a well-controlled ventricular response rate due to increased refractoriness of the atrioventricular (AV) node. The Congestive Heart Failure Survival Trial of Antiarrhythmic Therapy (CHF-STAT) demonstrated another potential benefit from amiodarone in the use of heart failure patients with LVEF less than or equal to 40% and greater than 10 ventricular premature beats per hour. A subset analysis of 103 of the patients in this trial who had atrial fibrillation were randomly assigned to amiodarone or to placebo. In the amiodarone group, 31% converted back to sinus rhythm (compared to 8% of the placebo group). There was also a 20% reduction in the mean ventricular response rate compared to placebo. Those on amiodarone and who converted to sinus rhythm had a lower mortality than those who remained in atrial fibrillation (20).

The Danish Investigations of Arrhythmia and Mortality ON Dofetilide—Congestive Heart Failure (DIAMOND-CHF) and Danish Investigations of Arrhythmia and Mortality ON Dofetilide—Myocardial Infarction (DIAMOND-MI) trials examined the use of dofetilide in patients with left ventricular dysfunction and atrial fibrillation or atrial flutter (21). Those receiving dofetilide had a 59% chance of converting to sinus rhythm as compared to 34% of the patients receiving placebo. In addition, those patients receiving dofetilide and who converted to sinus rhythm had a 79% chance of maintaining this rhythm at 1 year as compared to 42% of those who had converted with placebo. The DIAMOND-CHF trial, which included over 1,500 patients with symptomatic heart failure, demonstrated safety with the use of this drug in the heart failure population. Moreover, mortality was lower in those patients in whom sinus rhythm was restored and maintained—with a risk ratio of 0.44. Notably, the risk of mortality increased as the corrected QT interval increased (risk ratio of 0.4 when QTc is less than 429 milliseconds and risk ratio of 1.3 when QTc interval is greater than 479 milliseconds). Importantly, torsade de pointes is the most notable side effect of dofetilide seen in 3.3% of patients. The majority of episodes occurred within the first 3 days of use, thus requiring inpatient telemetry monitoring for the initiation of this drug (22).

It is important to note that dronedarone, a compound similar to amiodarone in chemical structure and action (but without the iodine moieties that are thought to be related to amiodarone-induced toxicity) is contraindicated in heart failure with a NYHA Class III or IV functional status, and is also not recommended for NYHA Class II with a recent exacerbation. This was found in the Antiarrhythmic Trial with Dronedarone in Moderate to Severe CHF Evaluating Morbidity Decrease (ANDROMEDA) trial, which included patients with symptomatic heart failure and severe left ventricular systolic dysfunction (LVEF < 35%). ANDROMEDA was discontinued early due to increased incidence of death in the dronedarone group (8.1% vs. 3.8%) during a short, median follow-up of only 2 months (23). Another Class III antiarrhythmic drug that should be used with caution in the heart failure population is sotalol. The risk of QT prolongation and torsades de pointes is significant with this drug. It also requires inpatient initiation and telemetry monitoring. The additional beta blocking property of this drug, when added to other beta blockers used for the management of left ventricular dysfunction, can add to the syndrome of heart failure in patients who may already be decompensated related to atrial arrhythmia and volume overload with underlying structural heart disease (24).

Class IC antiarrhythmic drugs are sodium channel blockers that inhibit Phase 0 depolarization. Flecainide and propafenone fall into this category of drugs, and because they dissociate from the sodium channel (and hence become ineffective) during diastole, they have a greater effect at faster heart rates, when less time is spent in diastole. For this reason, the Class IC agents have been used widely in supraventricular tachyarrhythmias. However, these drugs are also associated with a risk for increased adverse events in heart failure. They have a negative inotropic effect that can worsen heart failure, especially in those with NYHA Class III or IV functional class (25). Propafenone is associated with a significant increase in pulmonary capillary wedge pressure, systemic vascular resistance, pulmonary vascular resistance, and decline in cardiac output, and should be completely avoided in patients with overt heart failure. It is thought to be safe if used with caution and with close monitoring in those with mildly decreased left ventricular systolic function and no signs of overt heart failure (26,27). Note that ischemic heart disease must be ruled out, either with coronary angiography or stress testing, prior to the use of Class IC agents, due to the increased risk of sudden cardiac death in this population (28).

Although antiarrhythmic drug therapy is generally the first-line approach for rhythm control in atrial fibrillation, it often does not achieve long-term success, and invasive, long-term measures need to be considered. The pulmonary veins are the site of origin of atrial rhythm, and electrical isolation of these abnormal foci can be achieved with radiofrequency catheter ablation (29,30). One study specifically compared pulmonary vein isolation for atrial fibrillation in patients with left ventricular dysfunction (LVEF < 45%) as compared to those with normal systolic function (29). In the 1 year following radiofrequency catheter ablation, in those who were not maintained on antiarrhythmic drug therapy, there was an equal maintenance of sinus rhythm between the patients with normal LVEF and those with LVEF less than 45%. In those who were maintained on antiarrhythmic drug therapy, 78% of those with left ventricular dysfunction and 84% of those without ventricular dysfunction were successfully maintained in sinus rhythm. Among the group with systolic dysfunction, the mean NYHA functional class dropped from 2.3 to 1.4 with significant improvements in quality of life and exercise time. In addition to sinus rhythm maintenance and functional class improvements, the group with the reduced left ventricular function improved LVEF from a mean percentage of 35% to 56%, and most of this improvement was within the first 3 months after ablation.

For patients who are not successful with medical therapy for rate control and rhythm control, an alternative to radiofrequency catheter ablation to isolate the pulmonary veins is ablation of the atrioventricular node with subsequent implantation of a permanent pacemaker. In patients with heart failure, right ventricular pacing can lead to further ventricular dysfunction via ventricular dyssynchrony, especially when pacing is present greater than 40% of the time. For this reason, after AV nodal ablation and an expectation for a much higher degree of ventricular pacing, cardiac resynchronization therapy (CRT) with biventricular pacing should be considered (31). Similarly, for patients with heart failure who may be considered for CRT, those with atrial fibrillation may also benefit from radiofrequency ablation of the AV node to prevent the high rates of native conduction overriding that of the ventricular pacemaker and reduce the benefit of the resynchronization (32).

CASE 3: ATRIAL FIBRILLATION COMPLICATING INFILTRATIVE CARDIOMYOPATHY WITH PRESERVED LEFT VENTRICULAR EJECTION FRACTION—AMYLOIDOSIS

LD is a 67-year-old male who presented with a stroke that was thought to be either ischemic or embolic in nature. Despite neurologic recovery, he subsequently reported exertional fatigue and was noted to have a new diagnosis of atrial fibrillation. An echocardiogram revealed normal LVEF, diastolic dysfunction, moderate left ventricular hypertrophy with asymmetric septal hypertrophy, biatrial enlargement, and mild pulmonary hypertension by concomitant Doppler estimation. A diagnosis of presumed hypertrophic nonobstructive cardiomyopathy was made, and he was managed with beta blocker and diuretic therapy. Despite rate control with beta blocker therapy, he remained profoundly symptomatic with severe exertional fatigue walking across the room and continued lower extremity edema. His atrial fibrillation was then managed with attempted medical cardioversion with flecainide and subsequently with sotalol, without sustained maintenance of sinus rhythm. A repeat echocardiogram revealed preserved left ventricular systolic function but the patient had now developed severe, increased biventricular wall thickness, severe right ventricular dysfunction, severe diastolic dysfunction with a restrictive transmitral inflow pattern, and worsening pulmonary hypertension with a Doppler estimated pulmonary artery systolic pressure of 105 mm Hg (**Figure 4-3**). His physical exam revealed a blood pressure of 118/68 mm Hg, heart rate of 67 beats per minute, jugular venous pressure of 20 cm of water with abdominojugular reflux, S4 gallop, murmur of mitral regurgitation, decreased breath sounds at the right base consistent with a pleural effusion, and warm lower extremities with moderate symmetric bilateral lower extremity edema.

Given the constellation of severe biventricular wall thickening, restrictive cardiomyopathy, and pleural effusion, he was evaluated for amyloidosis. Serum and urine protein electrophoreses revealed light chains and a subsequent bone marrow biopsy revealed 35% plasma cells. A fat pad biopsy was strongly positive with Congo red stain, consistent with the diagnosis of primary AL light chain amyloidosis. Treatment was initiated with bortezamib and dexamethasone, followed by addition of lenalidomide. Meanwhile, increasing diuretic therapy was needed for continued extremity edema.

LD suffered from persistent atrial fibrillation despite uptitration of antiarrhythmic medications. He underwent pulmonary vein isolation with radiofrequency ablation; after 3 months, he had recurrent atrial fibrillation again and was referred for a repeat radiofrequency catheter ablation. Despite

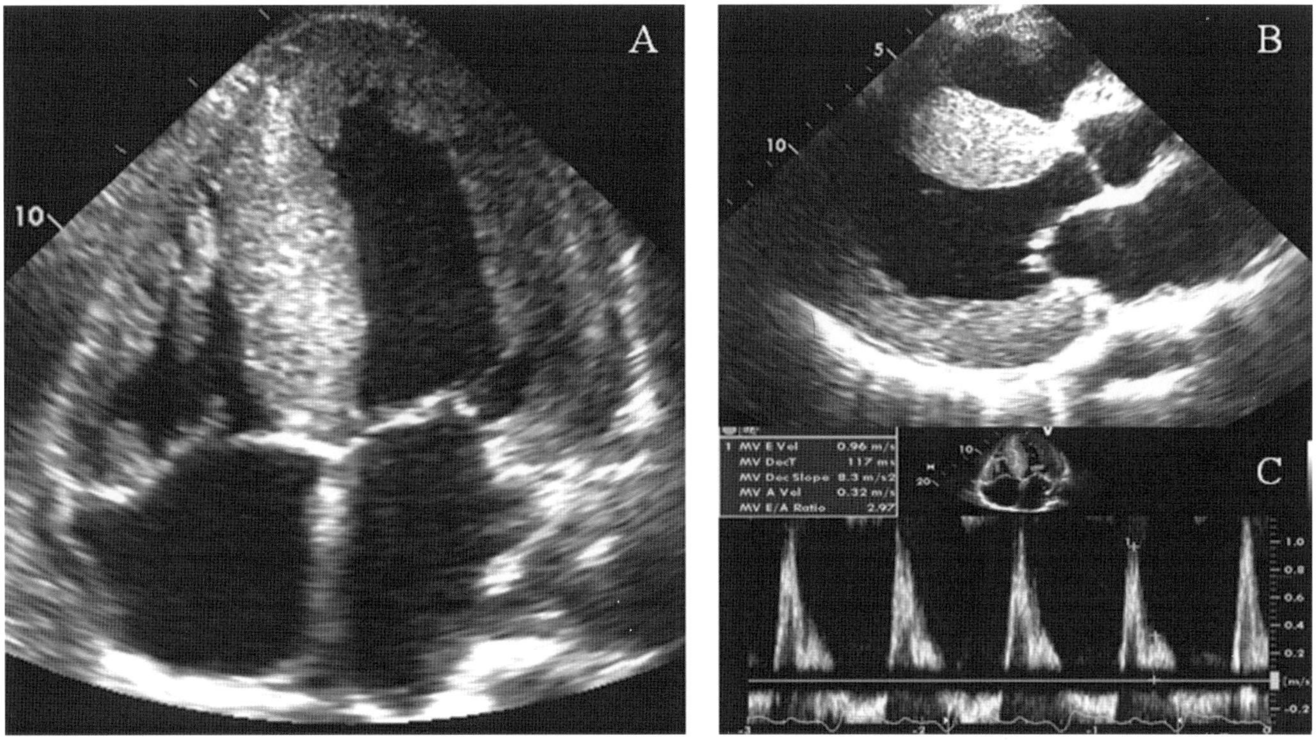

Figure 4-3
Echocardiogram of cardiac amyloidosis. (A) Apical four-chamber view. (B) Parasternal long axis view. (C) Restrictive inflow Doppler.

this second ablation and continuous antiarrhythmic medical therapy with flecainide, he continued to have persistent atrial fibrillation. At this point, due to the failed attempt at rhythm control, antiarrhythmic therapy was discontinued and the focus of his management for atrial fibrillation was switched toward rate control with uptitration of his beta blocker (metoprolol succinate) as tolerated.

This case highlights additionally important areas to consider in the management of atrial fibrillation in heart failure. Unlike the previously described cases, this case represents atrial fibrillation occurring in the presence of an infiltrative cardiomyopathy with a preserved ejection fraction. Atrial fibrillation is a common entity seen in left ventricular diastolic dysfunction. One study included nearly 900 patients over the age of 65 years old and followed them for 4 years. Patients with abnormal diastolic function were found to have an increased risk of developing atrial fibrillation compared to those without diastolic dysfunction (33). Management of patients with heart failure with preserved ejection fraction and atrial fibrillation is, in general, similar to those with abnormal systolic function with regard to rate control and rhythm control strategies. One notable difference, however, is the use of nondihydropyridine calcium channel blockers. In systolic dysfunction, this class of agents should be avoided due to its negative inotropic effects. In patients with preserved systolic function and heart failure with atrial fibrillation, this class can be more safely used. In fact, nondihydropyridine calcium channel blockers, such as verapamil and diltiazem, can be beneficial in those with hypertrophic cardiomyopathy by decreasing contractility and subsequent improvement in obstructive gradients within the left ventricular cavity and outflow tract (34).

In addition, the profoundly important issue of anticoagulation must be addressed in all patients with atrial fibrillation, especially those patients considered at higher risk such as those with heart failure. Most patients who have heart failure with atrial fibrillation meet the criteria to be treated with anticoagulation to lower the risk of a cardiac source of systemic embolus. This holds true for those with left ventricular systolic dysfunction and those with preserved LVEF. The case presented here represents a subset of heart failure patients thought to be at even higher risk for intracardiac thrombus formation, as amyloid infiltration of the myocardium results in mechanically dysfunctional atria with stasis, even when in sinus rhythm. This can be demonstrated by diminished atrial strain, decreased a-wave Doppler velocities on mitral valve inflow, and decreased tissue Doppler velocities of the mitral valve annulus in patients with amyloidosis in sinus rhythm (35). The most commonly used risk model to determine the need for anticoagulation is the CHADS2 score, a simple model incorporating five clinical risk factors that has been validated in a number of different patient populations (36). More recently, a modified version has been named the CHA2DS2-VASc score (37).

The choice of antithrombotic agent to use is worth discussing, given the current range of available options, including antiplatelet and antithrombotic drugs. Antiplatelet drugs such as aspirin and clopidogrel have been studied in patients with atrial fibrillation for prevention of thromboembolic stroke. Warfarin has been shown to be more effective in prevention when compared to aspirin alone, aspirin in combination with clopidogrel, or when using low-dose warfarin in combination with aspirin (38). As a result, aspirin alone is thought to be reasonable therapy for primary prevention of stroke only in patients thought to be low risk for thromboembolism. Notably, this is generally not the case for patients with a history of heart failure. More recently, the use of oral direct thrombin inhibitors has been studied as an alternative to warfarin therapy, appealing in strategy primarily due to the lack of continuous monitoring needed with these regimens. Rivaroxaban was shown, in the Rivaroxaban Once daily oral direct factor Xa inhibition Compared with vitamin K antagonism for prevention of stroke and Embolism Trial in Atrial Fibrillation (ROCKET AF), to be noninferior to warfarin with regard to prevention of stroke and systemic embolism and showed a significantly lower rate of intracranial and fatal bleeding (39). Similarly, the Randomized Evaluation of Long-term anticoagulation therapY (RE-LY) trial studied the safety and efficacy of dabigatran compared to warfarin in a study involving over 18,000 patients with nonvalvular atrial fibrillation. After 2 years median follow-up, dabigatran was found to be noninferior at a low dose, and superior at a high dose, to warfarin in prevention of stroke or systemic embolism. Dabigatran also had lower bleeding complications than warfarin, with the exception of extracranial bleeding on high dose dabigatran in the elderly subgroup. It is now used frequently as a substitute for warfarin therapy, as there is no need for monitoring and has less drug and dietary interactions. Despite these advantages, however, when being used, the prescriber must take into consideration the higher cost, the twice daily dosing, and the lack of a reversing agent (40).

SUMMARY

With the growing epidemic of heart failure, (41,42) management strategies aimed at targeting all aspects of the underlying etiology and associated comorbidities are critically important to reduce the significant hospitalization rate and mortality associated with this syndrome. One of the most common comorbidities is atrial fibrillation, both as a mechanism for the development of heart failure, and as a complication secondary to it. A thorough evaluation is necessary of each patient who presents with new heart failure as well as new atrial fibrillation, as both syndromes are closely related to one another. Regarding management, there is not compelling evidence to universally recommend rhythm versus rate control; however, individual patients may require one strategy over the other. Within the realm of rhythm control, there are many challenges in the choice of antiarrhythmic drugs in patients with heart failure; issues such as structural heart disease, overt and decompensated heart failure signs and symptoms, and underlying ischemic heart disease pose significant limitations in the safety of many of these drugs. Invasive methods of rhythm control using radiofrequency catheter ablation, such as pulmonary vein isolation or atrioventricular node ablation with insertion of a permanent pacemaker, may serve as useful strategies in patients who are unable to achieve adequate rate or rhythm control with drug therapy alone. Finally, the issue of antithrombotic therapy is another important aspect of management for the prevention of systemic thromboembolism. Individual patient factors such as risk for thromboembolism, adherence to a daily or twice daily regimen, drug–drug interactions, and risk for bleeding, must be considered as physicians choose between aspirin, warfarin, or newer oral direct thrombin inhibitors. Atrial fibrillation and heart failure are, indeed, dual epidemics and their respective management must ultimately consider the looming specter of the other disease.

REFERENCES

1. Go AS, Hylek EM, Phillips KA, et al. Prevalence of diagnosed atrial fibrillation in adults: national implications for rhythm management and stroke prevention: the Anticoagulation and Risk Factors in Atrial Fibrillation (ATRIA) Study. *JAMA*. May 9, 2001;285(18):2370–2375.
2. Lloyd-Jones DM, Wang TJ, Leip EP, et al. Lifetime risk for development of atrial fibrillation: the Framingham Heart Study. *Circulation*. August 31, 2004;110(9):1042–1046.
3. Crenshaw BS, Ward SR, Granger CB, et al. Atrial fibrillation in the setting of acute myocardial infarction: the GUSTO-I experience. Global Utilization of Stretokinase and TPA for Occluded Coronary Arteries. *J Am Coll Cardiol*. August, 1997;30(2):406–413.
4. Eldar M, Canetti M, Rotstein Z, et al. Significance of paroxysmal atrial fibrillation complicating acute myocardial infarction in the thrombolytic era. SPRINT and Thrombolytic Survey Groups. *Circulation*. Match 17, 1998;97(10):965–970.
5. Conen D, Chae CU, Glynn RJ, et al. Risk of death and cardiovascular events in initially healthy women with new-onset atrial fibrillation. *JAMA*. May 25, 2011;305(20):2080–2087.
6. Wang TJ, Larson MG, Levy D, et al. Temporal relations of atrial fibrillation and congestive heart failure and their joint influence on mortality: the Framingham Heart Study. *Circulation*. June 17, 2003;107(23):2920–2925.
7. Olsson LG, Swedberg K, Ducharme A, et al. Atrial fibrillation and risk of clinical events in chronic heart failure with and without left ventricular systolic dysfunction: results from the Candesartan in Heart failure-Assessment of Reduction in Mortality and morbidity (CHARM) program. *J Am CollCardiol*. May 16, 2006;47(10):1997–2004.
8. Dries DL, Exner DV, Gersh BJ, et al. Atrial fibrillation is associated with an increased risk for mortality and heart failure progression in patients with asymptomatic and symptomatic left ventricular systolic dysfunction: a retrospective analysis of the SOLVD trials. Studies of Left Ventricular Dysfunction. *J Am CollCardiol*. September, 1998;32(3):695–703.
9. Carson PE, Johnson GR, Dunkman WB, et al. The influence of atrial fibrillation onprognosis in mild to moderate heart failure. The V-HeFT Studies. The V-HeFT VA Cooperative Studies Group. *Circulation*. June, 1993;87(6 Suppl):VI102–VI110.
10. Wann LS, Curtis AB, January CT, et al. 2011 ACCF/AHA/HRS focused update on the management of patients with atrial fibrillation (updating the 2006 guideline): a report of the American College of Cardiology Foundation/American Heart Association Task Force on Practice Guidelines. *Circulation*. January 4, 2011;123(1):104–123.
11. Pedersen OD, Søndergaard P, Nielsen T, et al. Atrial fibrillation, ischaemic heart disease, and the risk of death in patients with heart failure. *Eur Heart J*. December, 2006;27(23):2866–2870.
12. Hagens VE, Crijns HF, Van Veldhuisen DJ, et al. Rate control versus rhythm control for patients with persistent atrial fibrillation with mild to moderate heart failure: results from the Rate Control versus Electrical cardioversion (RACE) study. *Am Heart J*. June, 2005;149(6):1106–1111.
13. Wyse DG, Waldo AL, DiMarco JP, et al. Atrial Fibrillation Follow-up Investigation of Rhythm Management (AFFIRM) Investigators. A comparison of rate and rhythm control in patients with atrial fibrillation. *N Engl J Med*. December 5, 2002;347(23):1825–1833.
14. Roy D, Talajic M, Nattel S, et al. Rhythm control versus rate control for atrial fibrillation and heart failure. *N Engl J Med*. June 19, 2008;358(25):2667–2677.
15. Gillis AM, Verma A, Talajic M, et al. CCS Atrial Fibrillation Guidelines Committee. Canadian Cardiovascular Society atrial fibrillation guidelines 2010: rate and rhythm management. *Can J Cardiol*. January–February, 2011;27(1):47–59.
16. Fujino T, Yamashita T, Suzuki S, et al. Characteristics of congestive heart failure accompanied by atrial fibrillation with special reference to tachycardia-induced cardiomyopathy. *Circ J*. June, 2007;71(6):936–940.
17. Kleny JR, Sacrez A, Facello A, et al. Increased in radionuclide left ventricular ejection fraction after cardioversion of chronic atrial fibrillation in idiopathic dilated cardiomyopathy. *Eur Heart J*. September, 1992;13(9):1290–1295.
18. European Heart Rhythm Association; European Association for Cardio-Thoracic Surgery. Camm AJ, Kirchhof P, Lip GY, et al. Guidelines for the management of atrial fibrillation: the Task Force for the Management of Atrial Fibrillation of the European Society of Cardiology (ESC). *Eur Heart J*. October, 2010;31(19):2639–2429.
19. Vorperian VR, Havighurst TC, Miller S, et al. Adverse effects of low dose amiodarone: a meta-analysis. *J Am CollCardiol*. September, 1997;30(3):791–798.
20. Deedwania PC, Singh BN, Ellenbogen K, et al. Spontaneous conversion and maintenance of sinus rhythm by amiodarone in patients with heart failure and atrial fibrillation: observations from the veterans affairs congestive heart failure survival trial of antiarrhythmic therapy (CHF-STAT). The Department of Veterans Affairs CHF-STAT Investigators. *Circulation*. December 8, 1998;98(23):2574–2579.
21. Pedersen OD, Bagger H, Keller N, et al. Efficacy of dofetilide in the treatment of atrial fibrillation-flutter in patients with reduced left ventricular function: a Danish investigations of arrhythmia and mortality on dofetilide (diamond) substudy. *Circulation*. July 17, 2001;104(3):292–296.
22. Torp-Pedersen C, Møller M, Bloch-Thomsen PE, et al. Dofetilide in patients with congestive heart failure and left ventricular dysfunction. Danish Investigations of Arrhythmia and Mortality on Dofetilide Study Group. *N Engl J Med*. September 16, 1999;341(12):857–865.
23. Køber L, Torp-Pedersen C, McMurray JJ, et al. Increased mortality after dronedarone therapy for severe heart failure. *New Engl J Med*. June 19, 2008;358(25):2678–2687.
24. Lehmann MH, Hardy S, Archibald D, et al. Sex difference in risk of torsade de pointes with d,l-sotalol. *Circulation*. November 15, 1996;94(10):2535–2541.
25. Kjekshus J, Bathen J, Orning OM, et al. A double-blind, crossover comparison of flecainide acetate and disopyramide phosphate in the treatment of ventricular premature complexes. *Am J Cardiol*. February 27, 1984;53(5):72B–78B.
26. Brodsky MA, Allen BJ, Abate D, et al. Propafenone therapy for ventricular tachycardia in the setting of congestive heart failure. *Am Heart J*. October, 1985;110(4):794–799.
27. Baker BJ, Dinh H, Kroskey D, et al. Effect of propafenone on left ventricular ejection fraction. *Am J Cardiol*. November 14, 1984;54(9):20D–22D.
28. Echt DS, Liebson PR, Mitchell LB, et al. Mortality and morbidity in patients receiving encainide, flecainide, or placebo. The Cardiac Arrhythmia Suppression Trial. *N Engl J Med*. 1991; 324(12):781.
29. Hsu LF, Jaïs P, Sanders P, et al. Catheter ablation for atrial fibrillation in congestive heart failure. *N Engl J Med*. December 2, 2004;351(23):2373–2383.
30. Chen MS, Marrouche NF, Khaykin Y, et al. Pulmonary vein isolation for the treatment of atrial fibrillation in patients with impaired systolic function. *J Am CollCardiol*. March 17, 2004;43(6):1004–1009.

31. Sweeney MO, Hellkamp AS, Ellenbogen KA, et al. Adverse effect of ventricular pacing on heart failure and atrial fibrillation among patients with normal baseline QRS duration in a clinical trial of pacemaker therapy for sinus node dysfunction. *Circulation*. June 17, 2003;107(23):2932–2937.

32. Gasparini M, Regoli F, Galimberti P, et al. Cardiac resynchronization therapy in heart failure patients with atrial fibrillation. *Europace*. November, 2009;11(Suppl 5):v82–v86.

33. Tsang TS, Gersh BJ, Appleton CP, et al. Left ventricular diastolic dysfunction as a predictor of the first diagnosed nonvalvular atrial fibrillation in 840 elderly men and women. *J Am CollCardiol*. November 6, 2002;40(9):1636–1644.

34. Bonow RO, Dilsizian V, Rosing DR, et al. Verapamil-induced improvement in left ventricular diastolic filling and increased exercise tolerance in patients with hypertrophic cardiomyopathy: short- and long-term effects. *Circulation*. October, 1985;72(4): 853–864.

35. Modesto KM, Dispenzieri A, Cauduro SA, et al. Left atrial myopathy in cardiac amyloidosis: implications of novel echocardiographic techniques. *Eur Heart J*. January, 2005;26(2):173–179.

36. Gage BF, Waterman AD, Shannon W, et al. Validation of clinical classification schemes for predicting stroke: results from the National Registry of Atrial Fibrillation. *JAMA*. January 13, 2001;285(22):2864–2870.

37. Pieri A, Lopes TO, Gabbai AA. Stratification with CHA2DS2-VASc score is better than CHADS2 score in reducing ischemic stroke risk in patients with atrial fibrillation. *Int J Stroke*. October, 2011;6(5):466.

38. vanWalraven C, Hart RG, Singer DE, et al. Oral anticoagulants vs aspirin in nonvalvular atrial fibrillation: an individual patient meta-analysis. *JAMA*. November 20, 2002;288(19):2441–2448.

39. Patel MR, Mahaffey KW, Garg J, et al. Rivaroxaban versus warfarin in nonvalvular atrial fibrillation. *N Engl J Med*. September 8, 2011;365(10):883–891.

40. Connolly SJ, Ezekowitz MD, Yusuf S, Eikelboom J, Oldgren J, Parekh A, Pogue J, Reilly PA, et al..RE-LY. Dabigatran versus warfarin in patients with atrial fibrillation. *N Engl J Med*. 2009;361(12):1139

41. Lloyd-Jones D, Adams RJ, Brown TM, et al. et al. Heart disease and stroke statistics—2010 update: a report from the American Heart Association. *Circulation*, February 23, 2010;121(7):e46–e215.

42. McMurray JJ, Petrie MC, Murdoch DR, et al. Clinical epidemiology of heart failure: public and private health burden. *Eur Heart J*. December, 1998;19(Suppl P):P9–P16.

5

Heart Failure With Preserved Ejection Fraction (HFPEF): A Common Sense Approach

VINAY THOHAN, EBERE CHUCKWU, BRANDON DRAFTS, AND MANRIQUE ALVAREZ

INTRODUCTION

To develop appropriate diagnostic and treatment strategies for cardiovascular syndromes, it is imperative to have an understanding of the pathophysiologic underpinnings that lead from specific diseases to individual patient morbidity and mortality. For example, the disease progression of atherosclerosis to acute coronary syndrome is well established and treatment strategies to address each aspect along the spectrum are now evidence-based mainstays. However, while syndromes may be labeled as one clinical entity, they are truly a constellation of multiple comorbidities conspiring to render patients symptomatic, often leading to disease progression. This basic paradigm is still an oversimplification of heart failure with a preserved ejection fraction (HFPEF) where the relative influence of comorbidities, genetic background, and temporal injury along with an incomplete understanding of a unifying disease state are all relevant gaps in knowledge. Irrespective of these gaps in knowledge, clinicians are faced with the real world challenge of diagnosing and treating patients with HFPEF. In short, physicians must be able to articulate a coherent understanding of HFPEF, define a process for evaluating patients, and initiate a treatment algorithm that is specific for individual patients and emphasizes modalities that curb disease progression.

HFPEF EPIDEMIOLOGY

Heart failure is among the only cardiovascular diseases that are rising in incidence, prevalence, and attributable deaths (**Figure 5-1**). It accounts for roughly $40 billion in annual U.S. health expenditures, with greater than three quarters of this amount distributed to inpatient costs, and it is the single largest inpatient expenditure for health among those over the age of 65 (1–3). Incident heart failure doubles between the decades from 65 to 85 and since HFPEF is demographically a disease of the elderly, a greater proportion of heart failure later in life is attributed to HFPEF (**Figure 5-2**). With an estimated 10,000 people in the United States turning 65 years old every day until 2030, we are expected to face epidemic numbers of HFPEF in the decades to come (4). Population-based analysis and well-characterized functional assessments have demonstrated that HFPEF is just as limiting to functional capacity and longevity as HFREF (**Figures 5-3, 5-4; 5-12**). Contrary to this description is that clinical trials for HFPEF often enroll populations with lower mortality and morbidity (13,14). These observations are not

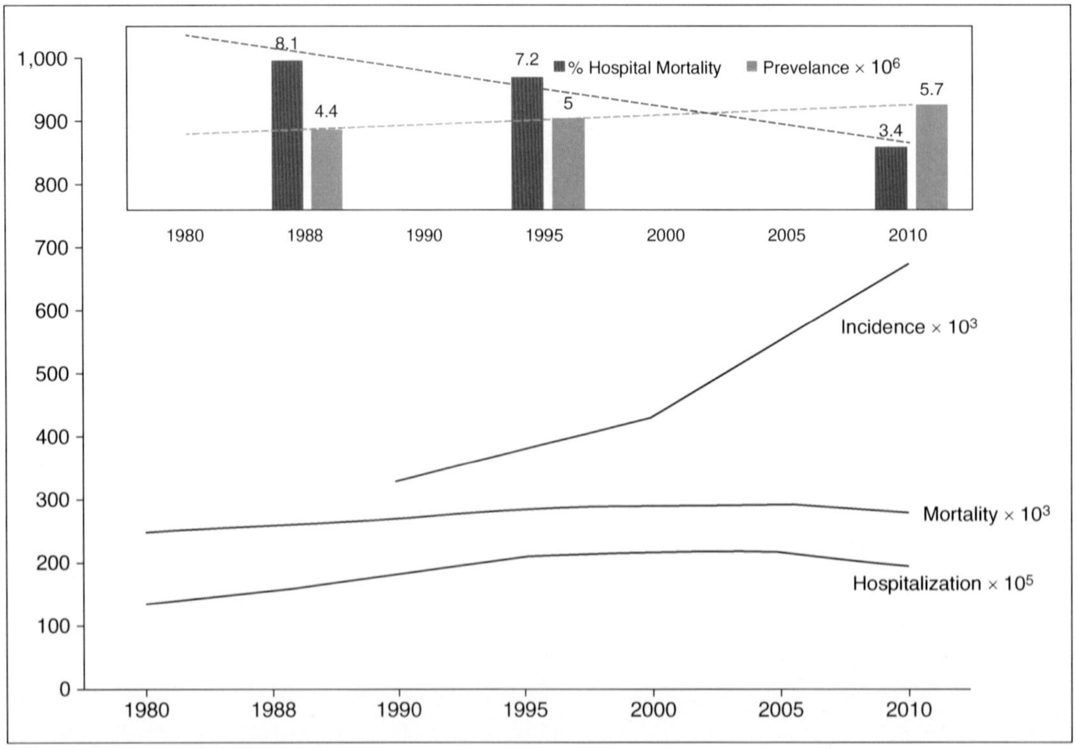

Figure 5-1

Thirty-year U.S. trends in heart failure.

Note: Total numbers of hospitalizations and overall mortality appears to have reached a plateau in the most recent data. Compounded by a reduction of inpatient hospital mortality (8.1% to 3.4%), this has resulted in an overall increase in both incidence and prevalence. Estimates for 2012 indicate that 6.6 million people in the U.S. will suffer from heart failure.

Source: Adapted from references 4, 63, 64, and 162.

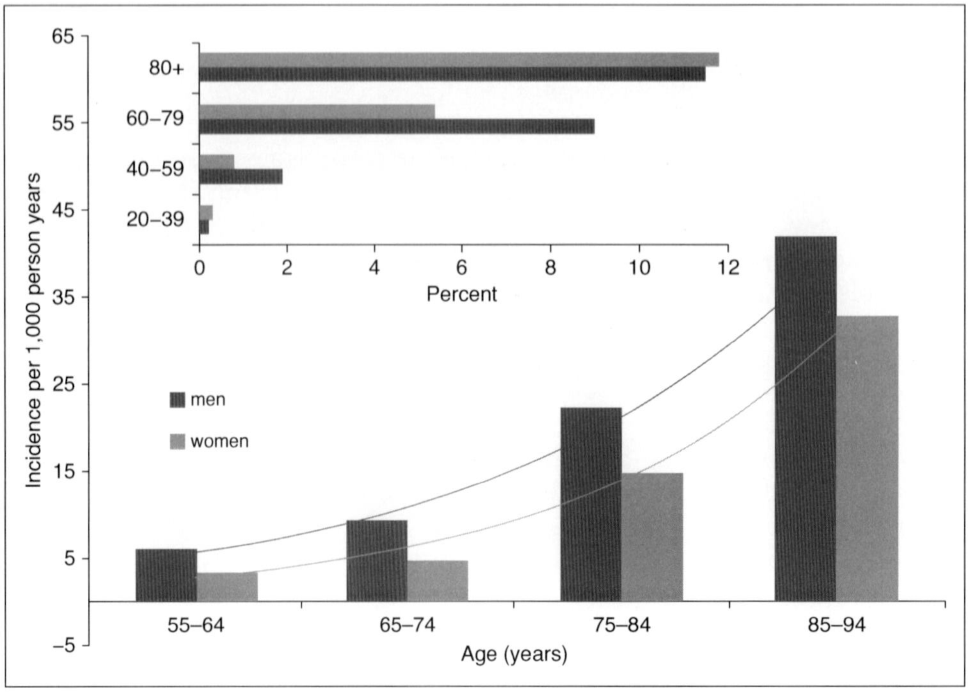

Figure 5-2

Age and gender distribution for heart failure in the United States.

Note: The incidence per 1,000 patient years among men and women in the United States increases most acutely between the sixth and eighth decade of life. The inset shows that the percentage of men and women suffering with heart failure is greater than 10% by the age of 80.

Source: Adapted from references 4, 63, 64, and 162.

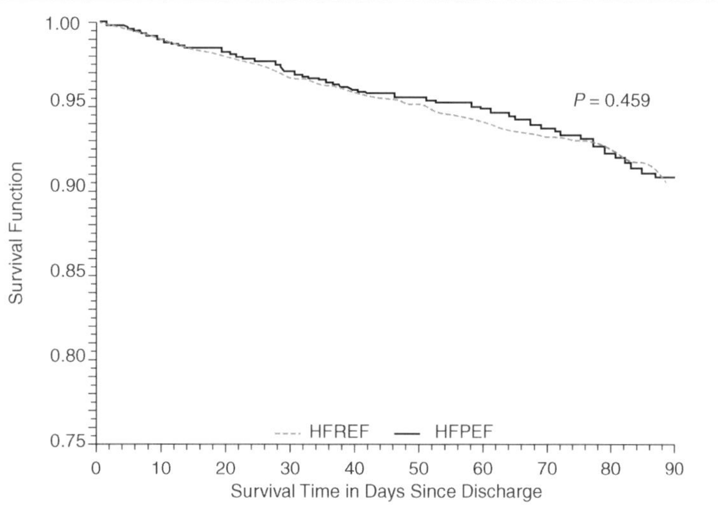

	Day 0	Day 30	Day 60	Day 90
HFPEF	2294	2188	1994	469
HFREF	2604	2471	2195	441

Figure 5-3
Kaplan Meir analysis of survival after hospitalization for heart failure among patients with HFREF and HFPEF (modified from OPTIMIZE-HF; 9).
Note: Community-based data demonstrates equivalently poor survivorship after hospitalized with HF irrespective of ejection fraction.

CPX test variables	Control (mean EF = 54) (n = 28)	HFREF (mean EF = 31) (n = 28)	HFPEF (mean EF = 60) (n = 59)
Workload, W	83 (4.4)	47 (3.3)	58 (3.4)
Time, s	637 (35)	352 (26)	449 (28)
Heart rate, beats/min	143 (4.5)	127 (3.3)	129 (3.5)
Blood pressure, mm Hg			
Systolic	168 (6)	163 (5)	182 (5)
Diastolic	88 (3)	83 (2)	88 (2)
Pulse pressure, mm Hg	82 (5)	81 (4)	97 (5)
Respiratory rate, breaths/min	29 (2)	34 (1)	34 (1)
Relative VO_2, mL/kg per min	19.9 (0.7)	13.1 (0.5)	14.2 (0.5)
Absolute VO_2, mL/min	1421 (58)	970 (44)	1165 (45)
Oxygen pulse, mL/beat	10.0 (0.5)	7.8 (0.3)	8.9 (0.4)
VCO_2, mL/min	1606 (70)	1046 (52)	1262 (54)
VE/VCO_2 ration	36 (1.00)	41 (1.03)	39 (0.93)
Breathing reserve	0.58 (0.03)	0.58 (0.02)	062 (0.02)
Respiratory exchange ration	1.16 (0.02)	1.10 (0.02)	1.09 (0.02)
Peak lactate, mmol/L	6.19 (0.60)	3.87 (0.34)	4.44 (0.35)
ATvenVO_2, mL/min-kg	11.5 (0.4)	8.7 (0.3)	9.1 (0.3)
6-minute walk, ft	1802 (87)	1356 (58)	1430 (60)

Figure 5-4
Comprehensive cardiopulmonary exercise testing among well characterized groups of patients with HFPEF, HFREF, and age matched controls demonstrating equivalent measures of functional limitations, regardless of ejection fraction, and significantly impaired exercise capacity as compared with controls (119).

solely reconciled by the competing risks associated with age alone and heart failure in the elderly identifies a clinical scenario with a compendium of traditionally noncardiovascular concerns that impact health. Older patients are often physically frail and emotionally isolated, with varying degrees of cognitive deficits and psychosocial challenges. These factors must be included in any diagnostic strategy and incorporated into novel therapeutic options to truly improve health. The aforementioned comorbidities are often not discussed, much less targeted in traditional clinical trial strategies (15–17). It is not surprising that to date no large-scale clinical trial has meaningfully changed the practice of HFPEF and that all are neutral with regard to mortality endpoints (14).

This chapter attempts to provide a clinically based understanding of the pathophysiology associated with HFPEF, with an emphasis on conventionally available diagnostic and common sense therapeutic strategies. We will highlight the central role of imaging technologies, specifically Doppler echocardiography as it pertains to guiding diagnosis and treatment opportunities. Case-based clinical judgment, applied to available evidence-based strategies, will be discussed to underscore treatment and address the prospect for future investigations.

PATHOPHYSIOLOGY

HFPEF generally presents with a constellation of cardiopulmonary symptoms in the presence of near normal measures of ejection fraction (note: finer measures of systolic function are abnormal but may not be diagnostically obvious or clinically reported). Therefore, several diseases, both cardiac and noncardiac, must be excluded when dealing with what is classically considered HFPEF. **Table 5-1** provides a differential diagnosis of illnesses that may present

Table 5-1
Cardiovascular, Clinical, and Echocardiographic Features Associated With Various Diseases That Comprise a Differential Diagnosis for HFPEF

	CARDIOVASCULAR AND CLINICAL FINDINGS	ECHOCARDIOGRAM
Pericardial		
Effusion	Dyspnea, orthopnea, hypotension, pulses paradox, elevated neck veins, clear lungs	> 2 cm echo free space, RV/RA compression, respiratory variation RV/LV filling
Constrictive	Fatigue, weight loss, ascites, o/w similar to effusion	Pericardial thick/small effusion, discordance RV/LV filling, preserved annualar TD-velocity
Valvular		
Aortic stenosis	Angina, syncope, SEM, soft or solitary S2, delayed and diminished carotid upstroke	Calcification, limited excursion, doppler gradient mean > 40, peak > 4 m/s, AVA < 1 cm
Aortic regurgitation	Diastolic murmur, dynamic precordium, increased pulse pressure	Dilated ventricle, vena contracta > 0.6 cm
Mitral stenosis	Diastolic murmur, opening snap, increased P2	LA enlargement, limited excursion, Doppler gradient mean > 10, AVA < 1.0 cm
Mitral regurgitation	Holo-systolic murmur (absent if acute), increased P2, pulmonary edema	Flail segment, ruptured chordea or perforation Vena contracta > 0.7 cm, systolic reversal pulmonary veins, EROA > 0.4 cm
Infiltrative (Multi-System)		
Amyloidosis	Biventricular failure, ECG voltage discordance, atrial errythmia, hyotension, neurologic, renal and vascular abnormalities	Ventricular hypertrophy, bi-atrial enlargement, bright valves Restrictive ventricular filling
Hemochromatosis	Atrial and ventricular arrythmia	Nonspecific
Fabry's disease	Neurologic and renal abnormalities	See description of amyloid
Metabolic		
Anemia	Tachycardia, systolic murmur, dynamic precordium, S4	Nonspecific
Hyperthyroid	Tachycardia, systolic murmur, dynamic precordium, S4, arrhythmia	Right side chamber enlargement

(Continued)

Table 5-1 *(Continued)*
Cardiovascular, Clinical, and Echocardiographic Features Associated With Various Diseases That Comprise a Differential Diagnosis for HFPEF

	CARDIOVASCULAR AND CLINICAL FINDINGS	ECHOCARDIOGRAM
Physiologic		
Pregnancy	Tachycardia, systolic murmur, dynamic precordium, S4	Left atrial and ventricular enlargement
Developmental		
Hypertrophic cardiomyopathy	Angina, syncope, SEM, bifid carotid upstroke	Variable locations of hypertrophy, restrictive LV filling and abnormal TDI velocities
LV noncompaction	Incidental	Variable pattern of compacted vs noncompacted myocardium

Note: AVA = ; LV = left ventricular; RA = right atrial; RV = right ventricular; TDI = Tissue Doppler Index.

with many of the clinical features of HFPEF in the presence of a normal ejection fraction (pericardial, valvular, infiltrative, metabolic, physiologic, or developmental). While specific diastolic abnormalities are present in each of these conditions, therapeutic interventions are generally targeted at the specific putative process and/or systemic illness and not diastolic abnormalities per se. Therefore, these illnesses are not included in this chapter but only mentioned to remind clinicians of their importance in the differential diagnosis of HFPEF.

NOMENCLATURE

Central to the understanding of any disease state is a consistent moniker of the phenotype. The last 25 years has seen an evolution of the terminology used to describe this condition and most recently investigators have settled on two names: HFPEF and diastolic heart failure (DHF). DHF describes the dominant physiologic concerns pertaining to patients who are afflicted with this variety of heart failure; it is also true that subtle systolic abnormalities coexist, and similar diastolic abnormalities are evident in reduced systolic heart function (18–21). While cardiovascular specialists and cardiac physiologists may have an adequate understanding of the nuanced differences among various forms of heart failure, and can rapidly distinguish a physiologic disturbance of myocardial properties rendering diastolic dysfunction and the syndrome of heart failure (19,22–29), most clinicians, facing the constellation of signs and symptoms of heart failure, and objective abnormalities (eg, invasive catheterization or Doppler echocardiogram) indicating or even labeled as "diastolic dysfunction," may not be able to reconcile that the patient in front of them is *not* suffering from DHF. Similarly, patients with aforementioned clinical conditions (see **Table 5-1**) also have diastolic dysfunction, thereby adding to the confusion surrounding the term DHF. HFPEF makes no assertions about diastolic function (although specific measures of diastolic function are indeed abnormal) and encompasses a phenotype that includes those with subtle systolic abnormalities (30–35). HFPEF includes a variety of traditionally noncardiovascular concerns (age, gender, anemia, renal insufficiency, etc.) that impart clinical risk and does not rely solely on a description of myocardial physiology as the proposed target of intervention. Therefore, we will refer to this clinical condition as HFPEF.

NORMAL DIASTOLE PHYSIOLOGY

Normal diastole comprises approximately two-thirds of the entire cardiac cycle at resting heart rates, beginning shortly after peak systole and ending just prior to the initiation of electrical depolarization of the ventricular myocardium, signaling the next systolic contraction (**Figure 5-5**). Diastole, unlike what the name implies, is far from the simple passive filling of the heart, and like systole is dependent on a well-orchestrated series of intracellular processes and dependent voltage gated ion channels, high-energy phosphate metabolism, and the ordered transit of several elements—chief of which include calcium, sodium, and potassium. In fact, several orders of magnitude in calcium concentration must be removed from the cytoplasmic space and sequestered back into the sarcoplasmic reticulum at the completion of systole to allow efficient diastole. This process is mediated chiefly by the sarcoplasmic reticulum ATPase and the efficiency of this enzyme can be altered to fit physiologic conditions through site specific phosphorolation. Relaxation results in a rapid fall in intracardiac pressure from peak systole to a point where the pressure falls below that of the left atrium. Once the mitral valve opens, a rapid transit of blood into the ventricles ensues, a process that initially is mediated by suction and later dependant on ventricular compliance. Suction and more extensively compliance are related to the intrinsic viscoelastic properties of the myocardium. While these properties typically cannot be modulated beat to beat as can relaxation, they can be altered by structural changes that render the myocardium more or less complaint. Abnormalities of relaxation, suction, and compliance are the hallmarks of early cardiovascular injury from a wide range of specific disease states. The final stage of normal diastole is atrial contraction and the volume delivered accounts for approximately 10% of total ventricular diastolic filling. Diastolic abnormalities effecting normal ventricular relaxation impair early rapid filling of the heart, relegating filling to occur later in diastole, with greater dependence on atrial contraction. Thus, some of the early Doppler echocardiographic changes associated with diastolic dysfunction are prolongation of the isovolumetric relaxation time, reduction in early filling velocity (E-wave), and increases in atrial filling velocity (A-wave). Up to 30% of total ventricular filling volume may be accounted for by atrial contraction. Diastole and its individual components can be modulated over a wide range of cardiovascular demands with the goals of timely, efficient cardiac filling and maintenance of low intracardiac pressures. Maladaptive changes in diastole mediated by a variety of diseases are often the first manifestations of cardiovascular injury and are ubiquitously present among patients with overt heart failure.

ABNORMALITIES OF DIASTOLE WITH HFPEF

It has been established through invasive and more commonly noninvasive techniques, that the myocardium of patients with HFPEF has demonstrable abnormalities that impair relaxation, suction, and compliance; each integral aspects of normal diastolic function (24,26,27,36–40). These abnormalities, compounded by vascular stiffness and redistribution of intravascular blood volume, renders the heart unable to fill under normal physiologic low pressures either at rest or, more relevant to HFPEF, with activity

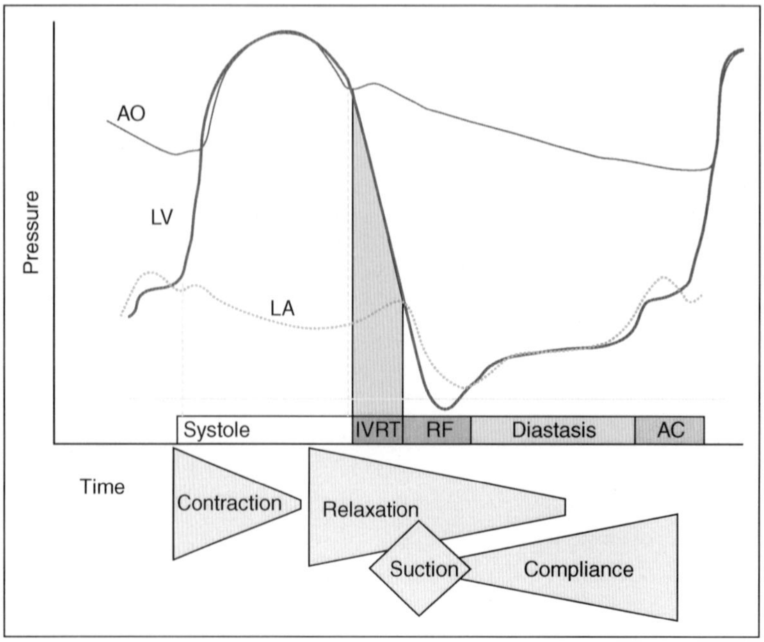

Figure 5-5
The physiologic considerations during diastole are represented by the pressure and time relationship. Patients with HFPEF have abnormal measures of various diastolic components including relaxation, suction and compliance. Abnormalities of diastolic parameters result in the inability to modulate LV filling efficiently during cardiovascular stress (hypertension, tachycardia, volume overload, etc.) and cardiopulmonary symptoms ensue from a rise in LA- pressure.

Note: AO = aortic; AC = atrial contraction; IVRT = isovolumetric relaxation time; LA = left atrial; LV = left ventricle; RF = rapid filling.

(24,41,42). When these changes in higher filling pressures are temporally sustained and transmitted to the pulmonary circuit, heart failure symptoms ensue (**Figure 5-6**). Sporadic elevations in diastolic pressure may be clinically tolerated but undoubtedly stimulate many of the myocardial stress responses that further exacerbate interstitial and myocyte remodeling (43). The remodeling process is complex and still evolving, but when cellular signaling initiated by elevated filling pressures is sustained by chronic cardiovascular diseases (hypertension [HTN], diabetes mellitus [DM], coronary artery disease [CAD] etc.; 15,44–48) it becomes deleterious and specific myocardial changes occur that alter the viscoelastic properties of the heart (25,36,49). Some examples of changes that have been studied include: altered content and constituency of interstitial collagen (50–53), impaired cellular energetics through altered calcium transit (54–56), changed isoforms of sarcomeric proteins with reduced elastic recoil (57), and deleterious inflammatory stress responses (58–60). These changes are present with various forms of cardiac injury and they are not sufficient to illicit the clinical syndrome of HFPEF, but simply provide the substrate of diastolic dysfunction.

Therefore, the most important axiom in communicating information to consulting physicians about the pathophysiology of HFPEF is:

> Diastolic dysfunction does NOT equate to (diastolic) heart failure.

This axiom is worthy of emphasis since it appears to be a recurrent point of confusion among consulted and consulting physicians. Most contemporary echocardiographic studies perform comprehensive Doppler assessments and subsequent reports often comment on diastolic function; the phrase "diastolic dysfunction is present by Doppler" is often stated. This designation only provides a noninvasive description of the filling characteristics of the heart; it in no way confirms or excludes HFPEF. Indeed, many cross-sectional analyses of older patient populations have demonstrable abnormalities of diastolic function without overt clinical heart failure (20,61). Stated simply, patients can have abnormalities of diastolic filling without having heart failure symptoms. However, *all patients* with symptomatic heart failure will have abnormalities of diastolic filling.

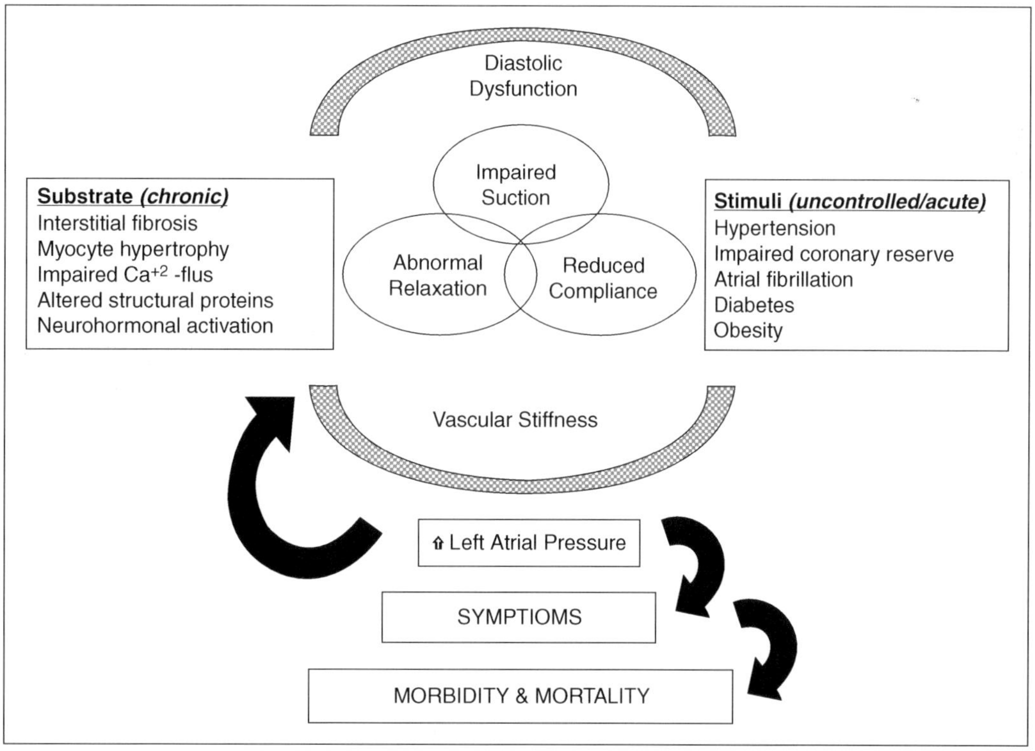

Figure 5-6
A conceptual model of HFPEF. Temporally sustained myocardial injuries illicit interstitial and myocyte remodeling, resulting in diastolic dysfunction. These changes, compounded by age dependant vascular stiffness, provide the appropriate milieu for HFPEF. Either acute or uncontrolled stimuli lead to elevation of LAP. When elevation in LAP are sufficient to cause pulmonary congestion, symptomatic heart failure ensues (at rest or with exercise) leading to hospitalization and death.

Source: Adapted from reference 14.

Superimposed on the substrate of diastolic dysfunction are the ever more prevalent stimuli of hypertension, impaired coronary reserve, atrial fibrillation, diabetes, altered fluid homeostasis and vascular tone, and obesity. Each of these stimuli conspires, often cumulatively, to drive individuals with proportionally greater alterations in diastolic performance, subtle reductions in systolic performance, toward the clinical syndrome of heart failure. It is often sufficient to temporally reduce individual stimuli to improve symptoms but it is likely inadequate to reverse the substrate using a single targeted approach. Therefore, multimodal interventions to patient care must include a keen understanding of the factors associated with HFPEF; targeting those conditions that are most responsible for acute deterioration and then tailoring chronic therapies in order to truly address disease progression.

The American College of Cardiology (ACC)/American Heart Association (AHA)/Heart Failure Society of America (HFSA)/European Society of Cardiology (ESC) each have guideline statements for chronic heart failure (inclusive of HFPEF) and in 2009 the European Study Group on Diastolic Heart Failure addressed a comprehensive diagnostic strategy for HFPEF (**Figure 5-7**; 62–65). Unlike chronic systolic heart failure, HFPEF does not have definitive strategies to reduce mortality. Despite a wide spectrum of primarily pharmaceutical-based strategies to address HFPEF, no treatment has demonstrated a survival advantage (13,14,40). However, medical interventions have pointed toward improvements in other endpoints including rehospitalization, exercise tolerance, and quality of life measures (66–68). Therapies for HFPEF thus far have been relegated to the treatment of comorbidities in an effort to influence disease progression. The lack of clinical efficacy for a mortality endpoint with the use of standard heart failure therapy has fueled a debate contending that HFPEF is either a separate clinical disease or does not fall within the spectrum of heart failure diseases (28,29). While these debates help to shape the form and content of future academic endeavors, clinicians are faced daily with the vexing task of caring for an ever-growing population of those who are afflicted with HFPEF. In an effort to maintain clinical

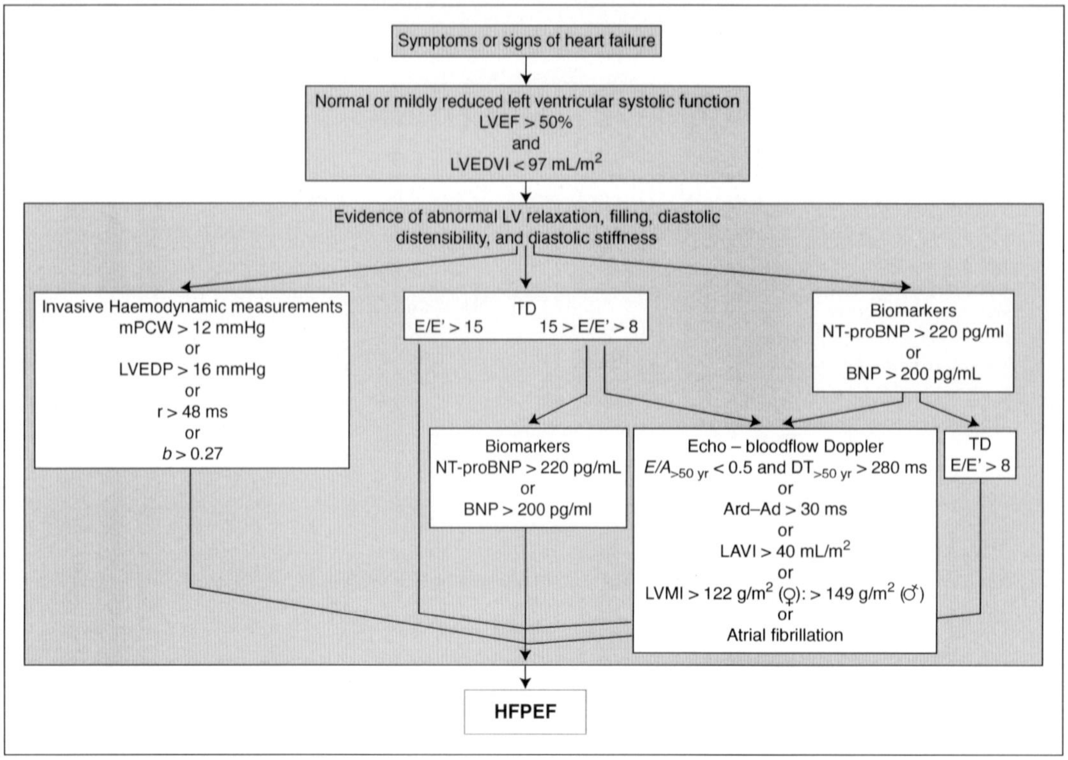

Figure 5-7
EDHF group paradigm for the diagnosis of HFPEF.

Note: This criteria requires both the presence of the heart failure syndrome and objective measures of cardiac diastolic performance and/or cardiac remodeling. A = late (atrial) mitral inflow velocity; Ard-Ad = time difference in atrial wave of pulmonary venous flow and mitral A; b = modulus for compliance; BNP = b-type naturetic peptide; NT-proBNP = n-terminal pro b-type naturetic peptide; E = early mitral inflow velocity; E' = early mitral annular tissue Doppler velocity; LVEDP = left ventricular end diastolic pressure; LVEDVI = left ventricular end diastolic volume index; LVEF = left ventricular ejection fraction; mPCWP = mean pulmonary capillary wedge pressure; τ = time constant for relaxation.

relevance we will present a case; though fictional, it is not unlike the many patients that clinicians often provide care. While no single case can encompass all the nuances of HFPEF, we will employ a temporal follow-up of one example that will serve to demonstrate some of the unique challenges of HFPEF.

CASE PRESENTATION

A 75-year-old African American woman with long-standing hypertension, obesity, and remote history of non-Hodgkin's lymphoma previously treated with both anthracycline-based chemotherapy and abdominal radiotherapy in the 1980s, was diagnosed with heart failure. She had complaints of decreased energy, exertional dyspnea, and occasional paroxysms of nocturnal dyspnea over the last several months. A physical exam was remarkable for elevated neck veins (12 cm), nonpalpable cardiac point of maximal impulse, negative S3 without murmurs, and Grade 2 peripheral edema. She was noted to have Grade 1 hypertension despite compliance with amlodipine 10 mg daily and was initiated on hydrochlorthiazide 25 mg daily.

DEFINITION AND DIAGNOSIS OF HFPEF

The diagnosis of HFPEF requires both the presence of the heart failure syndrome, near normal measures of cardiac systolic function, and demonstrable diastolic abnormalities. Our patient certainly has some of the signs and symptoms associated with the heart failure syndrome (**Figure 5-8**); however, no assessment of cardiac structure, function, or hemodynamics were obtained to either confirm heart failure or distinguish between HFPEF and heart failure with a reduced ejection fraction (HFREF). Exertional dyspnea, decreased energy, and edema are commonly associated with a variety of noncardiac illnesses, for example anemia, hypothyroidism, chronic obstructive pulmonary disease, pulmonary hypertension, and sleep apnea, to name a few. In this case, a comprehensive Doppler echocardiogram would have been instructive in diagnosing or narrowing the cause of cardiopulmonary symptoms. A comprehensive two-dimensional

Framingham	Boston	European Society
<u>**MAJOR CRITERIA**</u>	<u>**CATEGORY I: History**</u>	1. Symptoms of heart failure (at rest or during exercise)
Paroxysmal nocturnal dyspnea/ orthopnea	Rest dyspnea (4 pts)	
Neck vein distension	Orthopnea (4 pts)	
Rales	Paroxysmal nocturnal dyspnea (3 pts)	2. Objective evidence of cardiac dysfunction (at rest)
Cardiomegaly	Dyspnea on walking on level (2 pts)	
Acute pulmonary edema	Dyspnea on climbing (1 pt)	
S3 gallop	<u>**CATEGORY II: Physical examination**</u>	3. Response to treatment directed towards heart failure (in cases where diagnosis is in doubt)
Increased venous pressure>16cm water	Heart rate abnormality (1-2pts)	
Circ.time > 25 sec	Jugular venous pressure elevation (1-2 pts)	
Hepatojugular reflux	Lung crackles (1-2pts)	***Criteria 1 and 2 should be fulfilled in all cases***
<u>**MINOR CRITERIA**</u>	Wheezing (3 pts)	
Ankle edema	Third heart sound (3 pts)	
Night cough	<u>**CATEGORY III: Chest radiography**</u>	
Dyspnea on exertion	Alveolar pulmonary edema (4 pts)	
Hepatomegaly	Interstitial pulmonary edema (3 pts)	
Pleural effusion	Bilateral pleural effusions (3 pts)	
Vital capacity decreased 1/3 from maximum	Cardiothoracic ratio >0.50 (3 pts)	
	Upper-zone flow redistribution (2 pts)	
Tachycardia rate of >120/min)	***Definite HEART FAILURE 8-12 pts***	
<u>**MAJOR OR MINOR CRITERION**</u>	***Possible 5-7 pts***	
and wt loss>4.5 kg in 5 days with therapy	***Unlikely 4 pts or less***	
HEART FAILURE = present with 2 major or 1 major and 2 minor criteria		

Figure 5-8
Three contemporary criteria for the diagnosis of heart failure syndrome.

Note: The European Society of Cardiology criteria require the clinical syndromes as well as the presence of objective cardiac dysfunction.

Source: Adapted from 65, 163, and 164.

echocardiogram (2DE) with Doppler carries a Class I indication for the evaluation of heart failure. The European standard for diagnosing HFPEF would require objective assessment of cardiac structure and function (both systolic and diastolic). Other clinically directed evaluations that would be helpful in narrowing the differential diagnosis and assisting in targeting therapy would include: complete blood count, basic metabolic panel, thyroid function studies, electrocardiogram (ECG), pulmonary artery catheterization (PAC) and lateral chest x-ray, and a B-type naturetic peptide (BNP). We caution readers on the indiscriminate application of biomarkers such as BNP in the absence of a clinical syndrome. While elevated BNP does carry risk in a variety of disease states (69), it loses sensitivity and specificity for the diagnosis of heart failure unless used in the presence of clinically relevant cardiopulmonary symptoms. Furthermore, there is a wide range of "normal" BNP published in the literature and changes in BNP have been observed with age, gender, race, body habitus, and renal function to name a few (70). Based on the evaluation presented in this case thus far, a diagnosis of HFPEF cannot be confirmed.

CASE CONTINUATION

Two weeks later, she presented to an outside hospital (OSH) with worse fatigue, weakness, hypotension (blood pressure = 90/55 mmHg), elevated creatinine (2.6 g/dL) compared with baseline (1.5 g/dL), and a low potassium 2.5 mg/dL. The hospitalist service held her antihypertensive agents and she received 1 L IV normal saline along with potassium supplementation. Her renal function improved and she was discharged home within 48 hours of admission with amlodipine 10 mg daily.

PHYSIOLOGICAL CONSIDERATION OF HFPEF

Hypotension is an uncommon presenting or predisposing clinical concern for HFPEF. In fact, the Acute Decompensated Heart Failure National Registry (ADHERE) Database registry found only 1% of patients admitted with heart failure and a preserved systolic function were hypotensive (SBP less than or equal to 90; 71). The clinical response to diuretic-based antihypertensive regimen (thiazide diuretic) in this case can be used to highlight an underlying physiologic principal among patients with HFPEF. Invasive hemodynamic data indicate a steep-end diastolic pressure volume relationship where small changes or even redistribution of effective volume (ie, preload) can have profound effects on intracardiac hemodynamics (21,24,36,39,72). The reduction in preload associated with diuretic therapy among patients with clinically evident volume congestion should result in reduction of end-diastolic pressure, decrease of pulmonary venous congestion, and improvements in peripheral edema (**Figure 5-9**; 72,73). However, dehydration and subsequent impairments in endorgan perfusion would stimulate physiologic responses designed to augment cardiac output. Acute responses would include tachycardia (chronotropy) and an increase in contractility (inotropy); with chronotropy generally accounting for most of the increase in cardiac output. It is well established that HFPEF patients have impaired chronotropic response to exercise (7,60,74–76). Thus, in volume contracted states, chronotropic incompetence may worsen endorgan perfusion (as seen in the present case). The ideal hemodynamic state would be one where endorgan perfusion was maintained without a substantial rise in intracardiac pressures at rest or more importantly with activity. This concept poses a challenge for patients with HFPEF who have steep end-diastolic pressure volume relationships at physiologic relevant volumes states and operational stiffness (inverse of compliance; 27,49). Therefore, impaired diastolic performance limits the heart's capacity to modulate filling to maintain low intracardiac pressures at the disparate volume states, effectively narrowing the sweet spot for euvolumia. If the volume state is too high then one may face a rise in intracardiac pressure and if too low then impairment of systemic perfusion may ensue. Finding the right balance may require frequent clinical evaluation, titration of medical therapy, and periodic objective assessments of cardiac performance.

CASE CONTINUATION

Seven days later she awoke with acute shortness of breath, requiring emergency medical services, and intubation enroute to the emergency department. She was admitted to the coronary care unit with hypertensive emergency (BP = 210/110 mmHg) and pulmonary edema. Laboratory data revealed Bun/Cr = 48/2.7, BNP of 1309, hemoglobin = 10.2, and normal liver and thyroid function studies. The 12-lead ECG demonstrated new onset atrial fibrillation, ventricular rate of 132 beats per minute, and nonspecific T wave changes (**Figures 5-10A** and **5-10B**). She was acutely treated with IV diuretics, diltiazem, and nitrates. She underwent transesophageal echocardiogram (TEE) directed cardioversion and was extubated within 24 hours. Her cardiac biomarkers demonstrated peak elevation of troponin I = 2.1 before cardioversion.

(A)

	Hemodynamic data
Heart rate (BPM)	98
RA (m)	14 mmHg
RV (s/ed)	64/16 mmHg
PA (m)	66/33 (43) mmHg
PCWP (m)	23 mmHg
Ao (s/d/m)	166/98/110 mmHg
LV	176/30 mmHg
Fick CO (l/min)	5.38
Fick CO (l/min/m2)	2.31

(B)

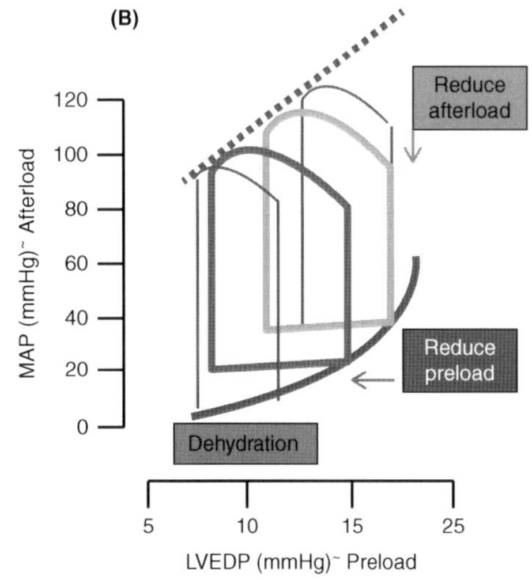

Figure 5-9
(A) Hemodynamic data for HFPEF demonstrates elevated aortic, central venous, and left ventricular end diastolic pressures (case). Cardiac output and index at a heart rate of 98 are within normal limits. (B) Conceptually, targeting reductions in afterload (MAP) and preload (LVEDP) while maintaining same contractility (dashed line) would result in increased stroke work (area circumscribed by the shapes). Diuretics are the mainstay of reducing preload, while afterload reduction generally requires individualized therapy based on patient specific clinical factors. Note further reduction preload (dehydration) can cause reduction in stroke work and systemic perfusion (note shape lowest on the afterload/preload relationship).

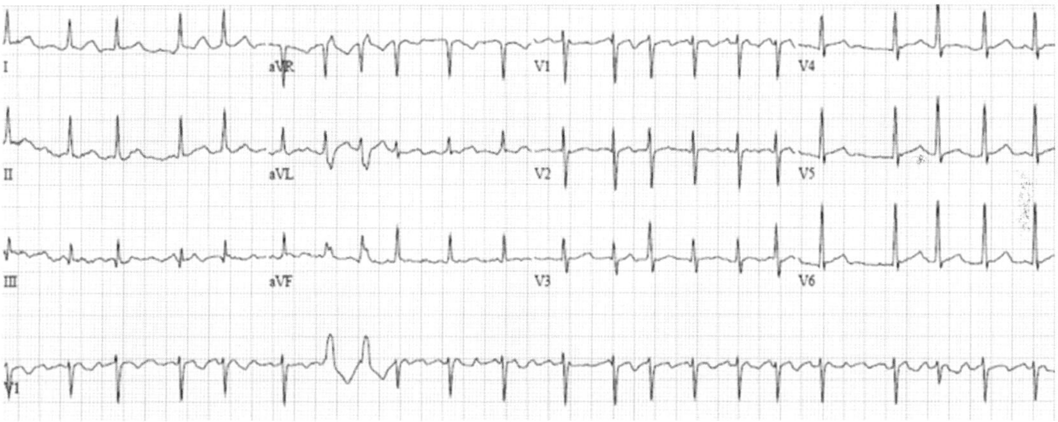

(A)

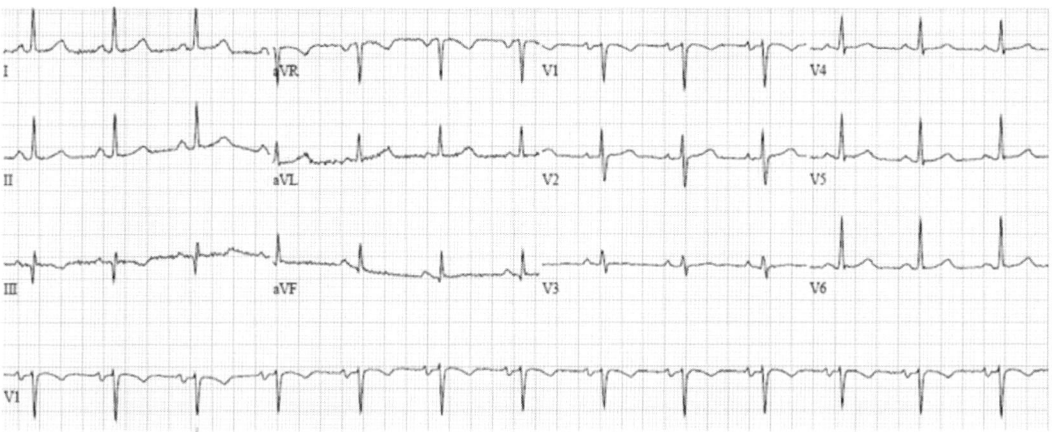

(B)

Figure 5-10
(A) ECG on initial presentation. (B) ECG after cardioversion.

ACUTE PRESENTATION, EVALUATION, AND MANAGEMENT OF HFPEF

The acute clinical presentations of both HFPEF and HFREF are identical and as such are indistinguishable by bedside physical examination, laboratories, or chest radiographs even among experienced clinicians (14,26,27). While clinical presentation may be identical irrespective of heart failure type, HFPEF patients are usually older, more often women with hypertension and atrial fibrillation as compared with HFREF patients (**Table 5-2**). Symptoms can vary from progressive effort intolerance (shortness of breath on exertion) to flash pulmonary edema as our case demonstrates (9,71,73,77). The later usually occurs in the presence of other comorbidities such as uncontrolled hypertension, ischemia, and tachycardia that can be associated with atrial fibrillation, infection, and anemia (15,77), Hypertension with left ventricular hypertrophy (LVH) is the most common associative finding with HFPEF and contributes to observed deleterious effects of increased left ventricular wall stress, impaired relaxation, decreased compliance, and chronically elevated filling pressures (45,46). Among patients in sinus rhythm, where atrial contraction may contribute up to 30% of left ventricular filling, the aforementioned physiologic abnormalities may be tolerated (78,79). The loss of atrial contribution to ventricular filling (ie, atrial fibrillation) compounded by rapid heart rates, result in shorter diastolic filling time; thereby resulting in elevated cardiac filling pressure and heart failure symptoms. (**Figure 5-9**). Often, greater diastolic abnormalities require greater dependency of sinus rhythm to maintain low symptom states. For example, among patients who suffer with amyloidosis of the heart, which represents the most extreme aspects of diastolic abnormalities (relaxation and especially compliance), the presence of atrial fibrillation is not well tolerated clinically and often represents the end-stage phenotype with death occurring in weeks to months (80,81). Additionally, any physiologic condition (eg, pain, anemia, hypoxia, ischemia, etc.) associated with tachycardia can lead to reductions in diastolic filling time and may influence the management of acute and chronic HFPEF. The maintenance of normal sinus rhythm has not been associated with long-term mortality benefits as compared with a rate control strategy (82). However, TEE assisted cardioversion in the case presented resulted in both a rapid control of tachycardia and restored the physiologic benefits of sinus rhythm.

Generally, the management of acute heart failure syndromes begins with clinical diagnostic strategies to assess volume and perfusion status. We advocate the Forrester classification, a framework that works well for either HFPEF or HFREF (**Figure 5-11**). Most hospitalized patients with heart failure syndromes are classified as volume expanded with normal perfusion (9,71). While no standard has been established for the optimal management of acute heart failure (either HFREF or HFPEF), the mainstays of therapy for Forrester Class III should include volume

Table 5-2
Data Modified From ADHERE Registry (71)

	HFPEF	HFREF
Age (yrs)	73.9	69.8
Women (%)	62	40
African American (%)	17	22
Hypertension (%)	77	69
Edema (%)	69	63
Rales (%)	69	67
Dyspnea at rest (%)	34	34
SBP > 140 mmHg (%)	61	44
AFIB (%)	21	17
VT (%)	3	11
LOS (days)	4.9	5.0
Mortality (%)	2.8	3.9
Asymptomatic (%)		55

Note: The prototypic HFREF patient is an older Caucasian race woman with hypertension. Registry data indicates equivalent clinical markers of edema, rales, and dyspnea at rest. While atrial fibrillation as opposed to ventricular tachyarrhythmias are more common with HFPEF, despite equivalent LOS, mortality appears to be lower in patients admitted with HFPEF.

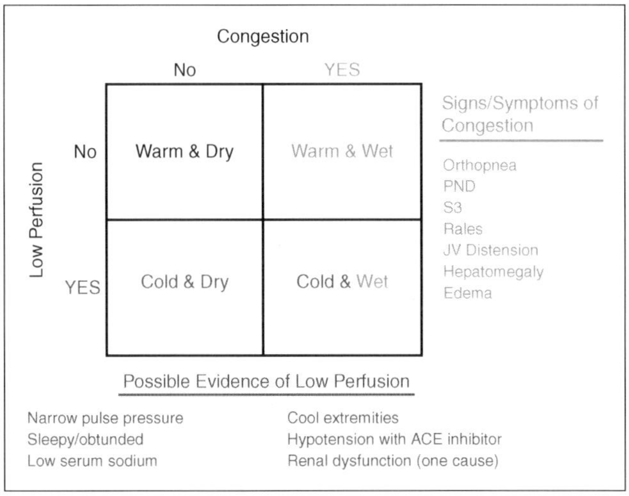

Figure 5-11
Initial presentation of HF can be evaluated using the modified Forrestor classification (165). The clinical evaluation of congestion and perfusion allows practitioners to segregate patients into three broad categories. Those presenting with a warm and wet phenotype are the most common initial presentation for heart failure (HFPEF = 91%, HFREF = 72%).

reduction (generally IV diuretics) and vasodilation. The choice of vasodilators is varied but since many patients with HFPEF have renal dysfunction, we generally advocate the use of agents with limited acute effects on renal function. The use of IV nitrate infusion in the case presented has several distinct advantages including: arterial and venous dilation thereby reducing both afterload and preload respectively, improved coronary flow reserve thereby reducing ischemia, and the ease of titration with a wide dose range and predictable side effect profile (83). Alternative methods to modulate nitric oxide pathways include IV nitroprusside and nesiritide, which have specific restrictions, narrowing dosing curve and toxicities that limit their ease of use (**Figure 5-9**). Simultaneously, clinicians should evaluate and attempt to reverse precipitating factors that may have contributed to acute deterioration. We advocate a focus on arrhythmia, ischemia, hypoxia, and anxiety/pain. Supplemental oxygen therapy followed by escalation to noninvasive positive pressure ventilation and intubation with ventilatory support should be based on the severity of the clinical condition. Opiod-based analgesia has of late been questioned in the management of a variety of cardiovascular conditions; however, when judiciously applied for heart failure syndromes, it can be very effective. While the acquisition of 2DE with Doppler is not required for the management of acute heart failure syndromes, it can be crucial when either the volume status of the patient is uncertain or the patients present with a clinical picture consistent with cardiogenic shock (84–87).

CASE CONTINUATION

A 2DE revealed moderate left ventricular hypertrophy, mildly enlarged atria, normal systolic function, Grade 3 diastolic dysfunction, and moderate pulmonary hypertension without significant valvular or pericardial abnormalities. A myocardial perfusion imaging study revealed reversible anterior wall defect and a right and left heart catheterization was performed. No significant angiographic coronary artery disease was noted and hemodynamic data is presented in **Figure 5-9**.

CURRENT DIAGNOSTIC CRITERIA FOR HFPEF

The European Society of Cardiology Study Group on Diastolic Heart Failure has proposed that the diagnosis of HFPEF requires the demonstration of three essential components:

1. Presence of signs or symptoms of congestive heart failure (**Figure 5-8**).
2. Presence of normal or mildly abnormal left ventricular systolic function (defined as an LVEF greater than 50% and left ventricular end diastolic volume index of less than 97 mL/m^2).
3. Presence of left ventricular diastolic dysfunction (abnormal left ventricular relaxation, filling, or stiffness). This can be detected noninvasively (transthoracic echocardiogram) or invasively (cardiac catheterization).

However, Zile et al demonstrated in a small, clinically well-characterized cohort of individuals who underwent comprehensive cardiovascular testing, that nearly all had at least one abnormality of diastolic function, thus leading authors to surmise that objective measures of diastolic function are confirmatory and not required in the definition of HFPEF. While this conclusion may hold true in well-characterized populations, most patient presentations are much more heterogeneous, and the central question is not whether specific measures of diastolic function are abnormal, but rather, whether these abnormalities have contributed to the presenting cardiopulmonary symptoms (See Axiom 1). In this regard, the evaluation of central hemodynamics, specifically elevations of diastolic cardiac filling pressures with left and right heart catheterization, may be required. The invasive nature of catheterization does not lend itself to immediate use and widespread application. Therefore, 2DE with comprehensive Doppler assessment has supplanted invasive approaches for the assessment of cardiac structure as well as systolic and diastolic function (84–87). Additionally, echo Doppler effectively excludes other cardiac disease that may present with heart failure and a normal ejection fraction (eg, pericardial, myocardial or valvular heart diseases). Measures of ejection fraction (typically less than 40%) help assign risk, and are used to initiate specific guideline based medical and device strategies. Echocardiography, particularly three-dimensional assessments, accurately assess cardiac chamber volume and mass that may evolve as important risk factors across the spectrum of patients with HFPEF. For example, atrial volume enlargement, presumably the results of chronic elevations of ventricular pressures among patients with HFPEF, has been identified as an independent prognostic risk factor (20,88).

DOPPLER ECHOCARDIOGRAPHY AND HFPEF

Arguably the most valuable information gleaned from echocardiography is ascertained by a comprehensive Doppler assessment of diastole. Importantly, Doppler assessments allow the noninvasive evaluation of specific diastolic parameters and accurately estimate measures of central hemodynamics (85,87,89–91). Temporally, diastole is inversely related to heart rate and can range from 0.6–0.2 seconds in duration. High frequency Doppler techniques have sample rates on the order of 10 ms and do not require multibeat sampling with reconstruction algorithms or stitching of sampled data to analyze diastolic parameters, as are necessary with other noninvasive imaging modalities. Generally speaking, a combination of Doppler methods are used to characterize diastole, assess hemodynamics, and prognosticate outcome over a wide range of cardiovascular conditions (37,44,84,92,93). The most frequently applied Doppler methods are pulsed wave Doppler of the inflow of the mitral valve and pulmonary veins, tissue Doppler imaging of the mitral annulus, and color M-mode flow propagation velocity of the mitral inflow (the latter will not be discussed in this chapter). The technical aspects of a comprehensive Doppler assessment of diastole, including specifics on image acquisition, can be found in the American Society of Echocardiography consensus statement on assessment of Diastolic Function (94). Common diastolic variables and the specific Doppler patterns obtained with these techniques help clinicians understand diastole (**Figure 5-12**). One should always remember that data obtained from these techniques are temporally related (to be precise it is *beat specific*) and dependant on the hemodynamic state at the time the echo Doppler was performed. Thus, a true understanding of diastole relies on integrating echo Doppler data with patient clinical status. Finally, many of the Doppler diastolic abnormalities found among HFPEF patients can also be noted with patients who suffer with acute or chronic valvular heart diseases, pericardial disease, and physiologic conditions such as pregnancy or anemia (see **Table 5-1**).

The cellular events leading to normal diastole generally start shortly after peak systole and precede aortic valve closure. Following aortic valve closure, left ventricular pressure declines rapidly and once it falls below that of the left atrium, results in mitral valve opening. The time between closure of the aortic valve and the opening of the mitral valve is known as the isovolumic relaxation time (IVRT) and can accurately be measured using pulsed wave Doppler analysis. With the mitral valve open and continued left ventricular pressure decline, a rapid transit of blood from the left atrium to the left ventricle in early diastole ensues, mediated by the suction and the relative gradient between the two chambers, known as rapid or early filling. The velocity of blood conventionally assessed by pulsed wave Doppler at the mitral valve leaflet tips is proportional to flow and is called the E-wave (early). Once the majority of blood volume has been transmitted the left ventricular pressure increases and the gradient between the left atrium and left ventricle decreases, resulting in a deceleration of blood velocity. The deceleration time, a measure obtained from the down slope of the E-wave, reflects this interaction and has been most closely related to left ventricular chamber compliance. (84) The last phase of diastole is mediated by atrial contraction; the Doppler assessment of which is obtained by PW interrogation at the mitral valve leaflet and is known as the A-wave. The velocities and time relationships described with PW Doppler techniques are load dependant, meaning that physiologic changes in preload can alter values leading to uncertainty between normal and abnormal patterns. Fortunately, each of the preceding events and timing intervals can also be interrogated with tissue Doppler techniques that assess myocardial motion by filtering for low velocity Doppler signals, such as those created by the movement of the myocardium. Since these events require high frequency sampling, generally a small sample volume at the mitral annulus is used for interrogation. The annular tissue Doppler peak early wave velocity (e-prime or e′), unlike the E-wave, is a relatively load independent measure and is related to measures of relaxation. Perhaps the most

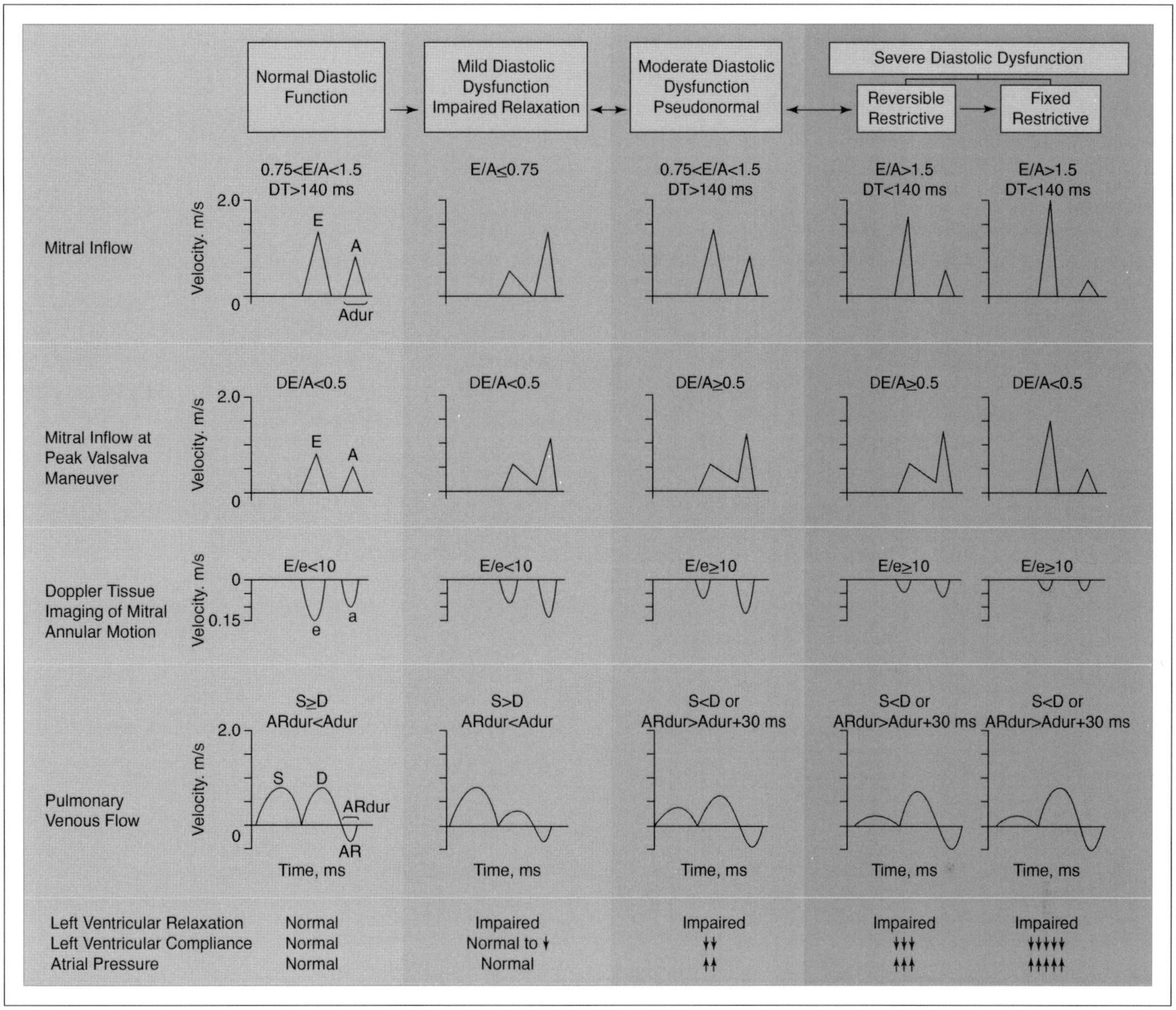

Figure 5-12
Comprehensive assessment of diastolic function by Doppler echocardiography (61). The ratio of the trans-mitral E wave velocity and mitral annular tissue Doppler velocity (E/e') is predictive of mean left atrial pressure.

seminal and clinically relevant observation over the last 20 years of research in the field of diastology has been the proven direct relationship between preload (mean left atrial pressure [LAP]) and the ratio of the pulsed wave and tissue Doppler assessment of early filling (E/e'). Specific linear regression equations have been developed to accurately estimate mean LAP and research has reproduced this relationship over a wide range of cardiac disorders. This simple tool (ie, E/e') allows clinicians to attribute cardiopulmonary symptoms to objective measures of intracardiac pressure, and can thus be used to manage care. The use of E/e' ratio has been advocated as a criteria used to diagnose HFPEF (65,95). Several important caveats do exist when using this ratio. First, TDI at the mitral annulus can be measured in a variety of views, most commonly at the medial and lateral annulus from the apical four chamber view, with the lateral velocity being higher (85,91,93). Investigators have suggested that the mean value be used for HFPEF and a ratio of E/e' less than eight indicates normal left ventricular filling pressures, while values above 15 indicates elevated left ventricular filling pressures. Intermediate values require integrating the information obtained with other parameters of diastolic function and remodeling in the assessment of LAP. Second, the E/e' ratio loses accuracy for mean LAP in patients with atrial fibrillation and often cannot be used with significant mitral stenosis or mechanical prosthetic mitral valves. (96) Finally, it is worth noting that TDI assessment of annular velocities can aid in the distinction between pericardial constriction and myocardial restrictive diseases; both can present with clinical heart failure and a normal ejection fraction. Among patients with constrictive pericarditis, the pericardium forms a restraint to lateral myocardial expansion; thus, during diastole, the left ventricular filling is mostly by a longitudinal motion of the heart, resulting in a normal medial e′, which is often higher than the lateral e′ (97,98).

Additional information can be gleaned from interrogation of the pulmonary vein flow pattern. In sinus rhythm, three distinct wave forms are visualized (systolic-S, diastolic-D, A wave reversal-AR). Under conditions of normal LAP the peak velocity of the S wave is larger than the D wave. As LAP increases S wave velocity diminishes, D wave velocity increases and AR becomes more prominent. Elevated LAP can be confidently diagnosed by comprehensive Doppler techniques when the S/D ratio is less than 1 and AR duration is 30 ms longer than the mitral A wave duration (89).

CASE CONTINUATION

The patient was continued on intermittent IV diuretics for the next 2 days, started on an angiotensin receptor blocker, and was discharged on Day 4. She presented to her primary care provider within 2 weeks of hospital discharge in a wheelchair with persistent complaints of fatigue, lethargy, poor appetite, and mild edema. Her laboratories including BUN/Cr, potassium, and hemoglobin were near baseline and a BNP was 305 ng/dL. Hospital records reviewed indicated that she received no education on heart failure management (ie, dietary discretion, vital sign monitoring, or signs/symptoms alerts), there was no evaluation of her mobility, and she did not understand her medications.

HOSPITAL TO HOME CHALLENGES IN HFPEF

Rehospitalization rates among patients with heart failure clinical syndrome are alarmingly high, irrespective of LVEF, and have garnered the scrutiny of national regulatory agencies and third-party payers (3). In 2013, hospitals with higher than standard 30-day readmission rates will face reductions in Medicare reimbursements for heart failure care. Readmission rates in several large population based studies approach 50% at 6 months. Patients with HFPEF are more often readmitted with noncardiovascular causes and compared with HFREF patients more often die from noncardiovascular causes (**Figure 5-13** and **5-14**; 3,11,99,100). The case presented exemplifies several factors involved with the care of individuals with HFPEF.

First, evidence-based treatments of acute heart failure (especially HFPEF) are not standardized and while the most recent ACC/AHA guideline statements have added a separate section with recommendations for "the hospitalized patient," nearly all Class I recommendations carry an expert consensus level of evidence (ie, large-scale randomized clinical trial supporting recommendations are lacking). Second, the fragmentation of modern medical care among hospitalized patient is most obvious when caring for acute exacerbations of chronic illnesses such as heart failure. Episodic care models have resulted in medical systems that can deliver adept, efficient patient throughput in the hospital setting while not necessarily improving overall health. As a result, transitions have been a centerpiece of many care models with the creation of multidisciplinary teams charged with optimizing patient experience

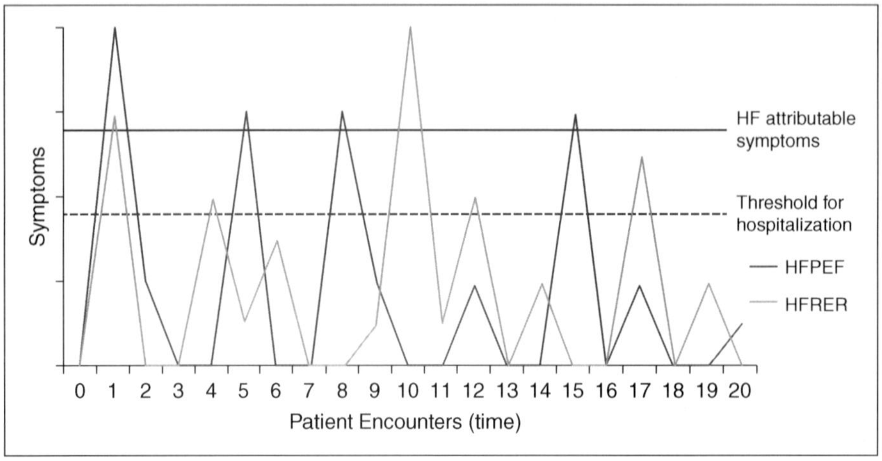

Figure 5-13
A proposed clinical trajectory of patients with either HFPEF or HFREF. Note both groups have equivalent numbers of hospitalizations (HFPEF = 5 vs. HFREF = 4); however, the HF attributable symptoms are proportionally different (HFPEF = 2/5 vs. HFREF = 4/4), thus indicating a lower HF attributable cause for hospitalization in HFPEF patients.

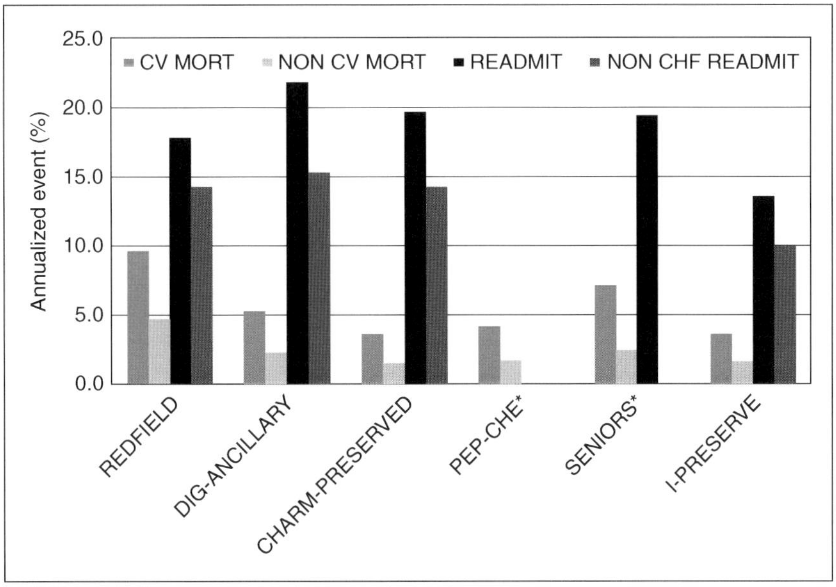

Figure 5-14

Annualized events among five major clinical trials enrolling patients with HFPEF (see text for references). Redfield data represents a large longitudinal clinical registry.

Note: While mortality and readmission rates varied in each clinical experience, approximately half of the deaths and three-quarters of the readmits were not related to cardiovascular or heart failure causes respectively. (*indicates incomplete data available).

and care while improving health. In the case presented, the initial hospitalization and subsequent medication changes may have provided the stimuli for the second hospitalization for pulmonary edema; recall, while the care was appropriate for dehydration, it did result in the discontinuation of diuretics and reduction of antihypertensive medications. Additionally, there were no assessments of functional capacity and, we would surmise, no heart failure education. Similarly, while one may argue the empiric treatments for decompensated heart failure during the second hospitalization, there was also no mention of functional assessment at the time of discharge, no formal education process, and no evaluation of the home environment, elements of care that can be the focus of multidisciplinary care teams. Among the 18 Class I recommendations in the ACC/AHA guidelines for a hospitalized patient only three carried a B level of evidence, among which only one applies to all forms of heart failure (irrespective of LVEF): *a post-discharge system of care to facilitate transition*. In fact, among the more consistent markers of readmission were comorbidities and the lack of clinical follow-up within 30 days (99,101). Hospital systems with an integrated care program and early access to transitions to home programs best practice models of care and are advocated by the ACC/AHA, and evidence-based data support this intervention (63).

Third, patients with HFPEF truly signify a high-risk population of predominantly elderly patients with a constellation of traditional cardiovascular and nontraditional factors that influence health and prognosis (102). Patients with HFPEF are often physically frail and emotionally isolated, with varying degrees of cognitive deficits and psychosocial challenges (16,103). The fact is underscored by both clinical trials and large-scale longitudinal studies that have demonstrated that patients with HFPEF indeed have a poor prognosis, comparable to those with HFREF; however, the cause specific morbidity and mortality is generally noncardiovascular (**Figure 5-14**; 13,14,17).

CASE CONTINUATION

She was readmitted to the geriatric service for failure to thrive and consideration of palliative care. Her polypharmacy was pruned when she was found to be using three separate sleep aids, two nonsteroidal anti-inflammatories, and a codeine-based analgesic (which was making her nauseous). She was evaluated by a multidisciplinary team comprised of a nutritionist, physical therapist, and social worker. She participated with physical therapy, which focused on gait stability and mobility, and despite dietary restrictions, her appetite improved. The social work evaluation revealed that she was widowed 2 years ago, socially isolated, and lived in a single-level home without a working telephone. She was also found to be functionally illiterate and could not read the labels on her medications without assistance. While in the hospital she underwent evaluation of nocturnal oxygen desaturation and bradycardia, which revealed severe obstructive sleep apnea and CPAP therapy was initiated. Her medical therapy was optimized to include candesartan, furosimide, and aldactone (once daily dosing regimens) with resulting excellent control of blood pressure. She was discharged with home health to live with her daughter and enrolled in an outpatient heart failure program that continued to focus on both exercise and heart failure education. She was seen 7 days after hospitalization in a Heart Failure to Home, hospital based clinic where medications, laboratory, physical exam, and access to primary care/cardiology was confirmed. When she returned to her primary care physician 2 weeks later she was coherent, conversant, and understood her medications and dietary restrictions. She was participating with rehabilitation and importantly did not have symptoms of fatigue, breathlessness, or signs of edema. The geriatric social worker helped to socially reintegrate this patient by enrolling her into a local senior center.

BEYOND HOSPITAL TO HOME TRANSITIONS IN CARE

The multidisciplinary team model of care deployed in this case has been effectively used for a number of chronic illnesses including cancer, HIV, and solid organ transplantation. Patients with HFPEF are equally complex. They have, on average, five noncardiac comorbidities that render those with HFPEF a limited multiorgan reserve. They are usually taking a litany of prescription and over-the-counter medications, each with side effects and drug/drug interactions, making pharmacologic management challenging. Some, as in the case presented, have cognitive impairment and emotional isolation. These factors are compounded by the rapid transit from inpatient to outpatient services leading to fragmented care. Additionally, many patients experience hastily arranged and poorly planned discharges to a narrow range of outpatient options where home health care is underutilized and community support is thin. It is obvious when evaluating this demographic, why no single intervention (medical or device) has reduced mortality among those with HFPEF and only a few have demonstrated improvements in well defined surrogate endpoints. The creation of multidisciplinary teams to care for the breadth of complexity faced with patients who suffer with HFPEF is an approach that has not yet been tested in clinical trials.

Beyond the social and community resources that must be leveraged to assist in transition of care and reintegration of patients back to the home environment, clinicians must be able to target the comorbidities associated with HFPEF. Foremost is the treatment of hypertension, and while there are a wealth of treatment options available, specific drug classes have been investigated and some may prove to have distinct clinical advantages. The target goal for blood pressure should follow traditional Joint National Committee on Prevention (JNC)–7 guidelines (104). Some argue that the macro- and microstructural changes observed in the hearts of patients with HFPEF are an end-stage phenotype of years of poorly controlled hypertension (43,45,46,68,105,106). However, in addition to hypertension, patients with HFREF often suffer with multiple comorbidities including diabetes, chronic renal insufficiency, atrial fibrillation, obesity, impaired coronary reserve, and chronic obstructive pulmonary diseases to name a few. Therefore, the specific choice of antihypertensive therapy should be guided by a balance between the specific antihypertensive agent and its chronic effects on the aforementioned comorbidities. **Table 5-3** provides a common sense approach to the various classes of agents in the context of treating hypertension and HFPEF. Compliance with therapies can be optimized using once daily medication dosing, intermittent monitoring of side effect profiles, and frequent clinical assessments.

TARGETED THERAPIES FOR HFPEF

Renin Angiotensin Aldosterone System

Activation of the Renin Angiotensin Aldosterone System (RAAS) system promotes development of the substrate for HFPEF through its direct myocardial effects including: myocyte hypertrophy and interstitial fibrosis (32,51,59,107–109). Additionally, the RAAS is disregulated among patients with hypertension, diabetes, renal insufficiency, coronary disease, and atrial fibrillation (66,108–111). Hence, the rationale for a potential role for agents that attenuate these pathways have been studied in patients with HFPEF. A number of randomized clinical trials have targeted RAAS, the results of which are included in the following section.

The Perindopril in Elderly People with Chronic Heart Failure (PEP-CHF) study (112) randomized 850 patients with chronic heart failure to perindopril 4 mg per day or placebo. The primary endpoint was a composite of all-cause mortality and unplanned heart failure related hospitalization with a minimum follow-up of 1 year. Results revealed no significant differences

Table 5-3
Proposed Class of Chronic Medical Therapy for HFPEF Based on the Presence of Commonly Associated Medical Comorbidities

	ACE-I/ARB	DIURETIC	BETA-BLOCKERS	CALCIUM CHANNEL BLOCKERS	ALDOSTERONE ANTAGONIST	NITRATES
DMII	+	–	–	/	/	/
AFIB	+	/	+	+	/	/
CKD	+	/	/	/	–	/
CAD	+	/	+	+	/	+
Obesity	+	+	–	+	/	/
COPD	/	/	–	/	/	/

Note: The symbols indicate beneficial, neutral, and negative effects on disease states with chronic therapy (labeled +, /, - respectively). On balance, ACE-I or ARB have sustained beneficial effects on most cardiovascular conditions and should be considered as an initial treatment options.

in the primary endpoints at 1-year follow-up, which may be partly due to the low-event rate in the study as well as a high rate of discontinuation of blinded therapy (28% of the perindopril group and 26% of the placebo group at 1 year). Nevertheless, post hoc analysis revealed a decrease in hospitalization for heart failure (P = .033), improvement in functional class (P < .030), and 6-minute corridor walk distance (P = .011) had improved in those assigned to perindopril.

The Candersatan in Heart Failure: Assessment of Reduction in Mortality and Morbidity-Preserved (CHARM-Preserved) study randomized 3,023 patients to candesartan 32 mg or placebo. The primary endpoint was cardiovascular death or admission to hospital for chronic heart failure (CHF). Results reveal that there was no significant difference in the primary endpoint at a median follow-up period of 36 months. As with the PEP-CHF trial, candesartan nonsignificantly reduced hospitalization for heart failure.

The two studies evaluating the role of Irbesartan in HFPEF were the Irbesartan in Heart Failure with Preserved Ejection Fraction (I-PRESERVE) study (113) and Hong Kong diastolic heart failure (114). I-PRESERVE was a multinational effort that randomized 4,028 patients to irbesartan or placebo with a mean follow-up of 49 months for clinical cardiovascular endpoints including death and hospitalization, while the Hong Kong diastolic heart failure study evaluated a highly select group of 150 patients comparing irbesartan or ramipril with a background of diuretic therapy for quality of life endpoints. Neither trial achieved a statistically significant benefit with irbesartan.

While mechanistic studies and small clinical trials using spironolactone to attenuate the effects of aldosterone appear to signal benefit, no large randomized clinical trial has established a role for this type of therapy in HFPEF (115–117). A large randomized National Institutes of Health (NIH)–funded clinical trial entitled the Treatment of Preserved Cardiac Function with an Aldosterone Antagonist (TOPCAT) hopes to address this very important question (118).

Sympathetic Nervous System

Sustained neurohormonal activiation is a pathologic hallmark of heart failure. Kitzman and colleagues demonstrated that HFPEF patients, as compared with age-matched controls, have dramatic up-regulation of a variety of neurohormones with levels that are similar to disease matched SHF cohorts (119). Similarly, elevations of neurohormones among patients with HFPEF are associated with disease severity, exercise intolerance, and other measures of cardiovascular outcome (5,7,60). Chronic upregulation of the sympathetic nervous system mediated through interactions of norepinephrine and various adrenergic receptors, is well characterized in a number of cardiovascular disease states including: hypertension, left ventricular hypertrophy, ischemic heart disease, atrial fibrillation, and systolic heart failure. In fact, beta-blockers are the cornerstone for the treatment of each of these comorbidities of HFPEF and are a Class I indication for patients with ACC/AHA Stage B, C, and D heart failure (63,64). A true large-scale clinical investigation of beta adrenergic receptor blocker therapy has not been conducted in HFPEF; however, several smaller studies are worthy of mention.

The Study of the Effects of Nebivolol Intervention on Outcomes and Rehospitalization in Seniors with Heart Failure (SENIORS) study randomized 2,128 heart failure patients aged over 70, regardless of LVEF, to 10 mg of nebivolol, a beta-1 selective blocker, or placebo. The primary outcome was a composite of all cause mortality or time to cardiovascular hospital. Less than 250 patients had an LVEF greater than 50% and no statistical benefit in the primary endpoint was observed in this subgroup while the overall population did demonstrate a favorable effect from nebivolol (120).

The Swedish Doppler Echocardiographic (SWEDIC) study evaluated the effects of carvedilol versus placebo in 97 patients with diastolic heart failure. The primary endpoint was a change in four selected echo variables at 6 months. Results revealed no significant improvements in the composite score for diastolic dysfunction (121). Paradoxically, only patients in the placebo group appeared to have a signal toward subjective clinical benefit. As noted in a prior section of this chapter, HFPEF patients may have chronotropic incompetence and the addition of beta-blocker agents may contribute to symptoms during exertion (122,123).

Miscellaneous Therapy

The hallmark of symptomatic heart failure is congestion and among the more common therapies for both acute and chronic congestive heart failure are diuretics and nitrates. Examination of the ADHERE database comprising greater than 50,000 patients hospitalized with HFPEF revealed 64% of patients were using diuretic therapy prior to hospitalization, 91% of initial therapies included IV diuretics, and 79.5% of patients were discharged with oral diuretic therapy. While only 18% of patients with decompensate HFPEF were initiated on IV vasodilators, in 61% of cases these were categorized as nitroglycerine, and the remainder were largely treated with nesiritide (71). Both diuretics and vasodilators have pharmacologic properties that result in reduction of central vascular congestion predominantly through a combination of afterload and preload reductions. Additionally, improved venous capacitance may assist in shifting left ventricular performance toward a more compliant portion of the pressure–volume relationship. While no randomized trial has studied the role of these agents in HFPEF, they are recommended by the ACC/AHA/HFSA guidelines for use in HFPEF (63,64). As noted by the case discussion, careful monitoring of diuretic therapy is warranted so as not to precipitate volume contraction and hypoperfusion (**Figure 5-9B**).

HFPEF is a disease state described as having a near normal ejection fraction; however, subtle measures of systolic performance, and particularly, exercise induced systolic difference compared with normal age-matched controls have been demonstrated (22,35,122,124–126). Additionally, evaluation of select populations in prospective trials may provide further insight. A subgroup analysis of the Digitalis Investigational Group (DIG) trial with preserved EF (LVEF greater than 45%) demonstrated no differences in the primary study endpoints of mortality from cardiovascular causes and hospitalization for heart failure. However, there was a trend toward decreased hospitalization for heart failure counterbalanced by increases in hospitalization for unstable angina (127). Therefore, among patients in sinus rhythm with relatively preserved ejection fraction the use of digoxin is not advocated.

Perhaps the most undertreated comorbidity associated with HFPEF is sleep disordered breathing (SDB) and is worthy of mention since the most common variant, obstructive sleep apnea, is associated with intense neurohormonal activation, resistant hypertension, atrial fibrillation, worsening clinical heart failure, impaired quality of life, and increased mortality (128–132). Among several prospective cohorts of well-characterized ambulatory outpatients with heart failure, the prevalence of SDB ranged from 69% to 80% and 40% to 62% had obstructive sleep apnea (OSA; 133,134). Additionally, among 395 consecutive acutely decompensated HFPEF patients who had not previously been tested for SDB, the incidence of SDB was 75% with 57% having OSA. Potential intersections between the pathologic changes associated with OSA and HFPEF include periodic nocturnal hypoxia, decreased preload, increased afterload, reduced diastolic transmural pressure gradient, and chronic neurohormonal activition. Therefore, the management of OSA may attenuate the difficulty associated with controlling comorbidities and subsequent symptoms of HFPEF (128,129). However, it is important to note that while the use of continuous positive airway pressure (CPAP) has been demonstrated in small studies to improve cardiovascular function and other surrogate endpoints, there have been no trials conducted specifically in HFPEF populations (135–137).

Among the most consistent and common symptoms related by patients with HFPEF is exercise intolerance leading to reductions in quality of life and physical frailty (16,138,139). Physiologic factors that limit exercise capacity range from chronotropic incompetence, inability to recruit cardiac output, impaired peripheral skeletal muscle function, the degree of diastolic dysfunction, and abnormal exercise induced central filling pressures (6,75,76,122,124–126,139). A corollary to these observations is that exercise training has demonstrable benefits in each of these same factors and can be considered as a therapeutic intervention that has impacts on a wide range of cardiopulmonary disorders, notwithstanding the known comorbidities of HFPEF (138,139). Edelmann et al has demonstrated that randomly assigning 64 patients (2:1 randomization) with HFPEF to supervised graded exercise training resulted in objective improvements of Doppler assessments of diastolic function, cardiopulmonary exercise capacity, cardiac remodeling, and quality of life measures (140). These data are yet to be reproduced in a larger population of HFPEF patients. However, the largest study to date evaluating the impact of exercise training among patients with heart failure (LVEF less than 40%) found that diastolic dysfunction correlated stronger with exercise capacity than LVEF and among those subjects randomized to exercise training, consistent improvements in cardiopulmonary testing, quality of life, and reduction in heart failure hospitalization were noted; the mortality endpoint in this study was not statistically different between the two groups (141–143). Additionally, the Heart Failure And a Controlled Trial Investigating Outcomes of Exercise Training (HF ACTION) trial also demonstrated the safety of exercise training in an ambulatory heart failure population with a mean LVEF equal to 25% and, therefore, the clinical trial design could be expanded to include a HFPEF population, where extracardiac skeletal muscle factors leading to frailty may play a significant role in overall event rates.

EMERGING THERAPIES FOR HFPEF

The quest for targeted treatment options for HFPEF has been spurned by the lack of mortality benefit observed in clinical trials with traditional heart failure therapies. (14) Simultaneously, novel research has pushed our understanding of heart failure and the seminal role that diastole plays irrespective of heart function. In fact, while demographic data and measures of cardiac remodeling point toward two distinct patterns when describing heart failure as either reduced or preserved ejection fraction, it is also true that these apparent disparate illnesses are indistinguishable on acute clinical presentation and both have equally limiting chronic cardiopulmonary limitations (7,9,18,29,119,144,145), leading to the concept that *all symptoms of heart failure* (irrespective of cardiac function) are due to the inability to maintain low cardiac filling pressures either at rest or more importantly among those that suffer with HFPEF, with exertion (6,39,87,124,126,146,147).

Sildenafil is a Type-5 phosphodiesterase inhibitor (PDE-5i), and while its clinical development has been for erectile dysfunction, the mechanism of action, observed clinical effects, and safety profile in patients with a wide range of cardiovascular diseases has lead to its evaluation for HFPEF. Specifically, downstream effects of PDE-5i resulting from guanosine monophosphate inhibition and nitric oxide production have been associated with reversal LVH secondary to pressure overload in mice models (83,148). Additionally, PDE-5i has demonstrated improvements in diastolic parameters and measures of remodeling in a small randomized trial among patients with systolic heart failure (149). Currently, a multicenter randomized trial evaluating the effectiveness of sildenafil for the improvement of health outcomes and exercise ability in subjects with HFPEF (The RELAX Study) is underway (150).

Chronotropic incompetence and failure of the classic Frank Starling mechanism to augment cardiac output has been described as a major factor in the pathophysiology in patients with HFPEF (7,122,124,145,151). Additionally, regional and temporal dyssynchrony assessed by tissue Doppler and 2D–speckled tracking echocardiography has been observed among patients with hypertensive and diastolic dysfunction as well as those with HFPEF (30,152–154). These facts have lead to the concept that intracardiac pacemaker strategies including biventricular pacemakers may have therapeutic potential for the treatment of HFPEF. Data from 266 patients with systolic heart failure who received biventricular pacemakers found that baseline diastolic dyssynchrony was not only more common than systolic dyssynchrony but also predicted response as characterized by an improved LVEF greater than 15% (155). The Restoration of Chronotropic Competence in Heart Failure Patients with Normal Ejection Fraction (RESET) study is a multicenter study evaluating the effect of atrial pacing on functional capacity and quality of life measures among patients with HFPEF (156). The question of whether rate responsive biventricular pacing would be a strategy for HFPEF is awaiting further study.

Collagen type, content, and constituency among patients with HFPEF have been evaluated serologically and at the myocardial unstructural level (40,115,157). The differential activation of metalloproteinases (MMP) mediated by tissue inhibitors of MMP (TIMP), along with the neurohormonal activation of myofibroblasts, have yielded insight into the changes in extracellular matrix among patients with HFPEF (32,36,52,53,109,157). The net effects of these changes include transition from more compliant and less fibrillar forms of collagen is to stiffer varieties; resulting in less compliant cardiac chambers (36,50,53). Among the nonenzymatic changes that can occur with chronic hemodynamic injury to long-term structural proteins such as collagen is cross-linking by advanced glycation endproducts (AGE). Collagen AGE accumulation at the level of the heart and vasculature has been associated with the phenotype of HFPEF (158–160). Little et al advanced the theoretical concept of AGE and HFPEF by utilizing Alagebrium (ALT-711), a small molecule with the capacity to break AGE. This small pilot study of 23 patients demonstrated a 16-week course of ALT-711 in a well-characterized HFPEF patient population, and demonstrated reductions in left ventricular mass by MRI, improvements in ECHO Doppler surrogates of diastolic function (filling and relaxation), and better quality of life measures (161). Larger randomized studies are needed to confirm this intriguing finding.

CONCLUSION

HFPEF is the end product of a number of temporally episodic and sustained comorbidities that tax the aging cardiovascular system until the syndrome of heart failure ensues. HFPEF signifies an exceptional high-risk population of predominantly elderly people who, in addition to multiple poorly controlled comorbidities, frequently face the challenges of social isolation, cognitive deficits, and frailty. With more than 10,000 people turning 65 years old daily until the year 2030, the face of heart failure will change to reflect the HFPEF demographic and health care systems must respond accordingly. Currently heart failure is the leading inpatient cost for Centers for Medicare and Medicaid Services (CMS) and has been targeted one measure of health care delivery with penalties for hospitals with higher than average readmission rate beginning in 2013. Currently, no therapies have demonstrated convincing mortality benefits for patients with HFPEF and guidelines have emphasized symptom control and management of hypertension with a diuretic based medical regimen. While discrete strides have been made to understand the changes associated with cardiac structure and function, a unifying physiology is lacking. It is clear that the final common pathway to cardiopulmonary symptoms arise from objective abnormalities of diastolic function resulting in elevations of central circulatory pressures. The extent to which therapies help target and attenuate the progression of comorbidities to the development of overt heart failure will likely determine incidence and disease outcomes of patients with HFPEF. We advocate a targeted comprehensive echocardiogram with Doppler approach to patients with a HFPEF syndrome as well as a focus toward both cardiovascular and noncardiovascular therapies. The future for HFPEF treatment will depend on bending the ever growing curve of multiple comorbidities in an aging population, developing a unifying preclinical model for investigation, and approaching new modes of care delivery as well as novel targets for therapeutic interventions.

REFERENCES

1. Dunlay SM, Shah ND, Shi Q, Morlan B, VanHouten H, Long KH, Roger VL. Lifetime costs of medical care after heart failure diagnosis. *Circ Cardiovasc Qual Outcomes*. 2011;4:68–75.
2. Roger VL. The heart failure epidemic. *Int J Environ Res Public Health*. 2010;7:1807–1830.
3. Jencks SF, Williams MV, Coleman EA. Rehospitalizations among patients in the Medicare fee-for-service program. *N Engl J Med*. 2009;360:1418–1428.
4. Aging population statistics. Federal Interagency Forum on Aging Related Statistics. 2011. Ref Type: Internet Communication
5. Farr MJ, Lang CC, Lamanca JJ, Zile MR, Francis G, Tavazzi L, et al. Cardiopulmonary exercise variables in diastolic versus systolic heart failure. *Am J Cardiol*. 2008;102:203–206.
6. Guazzi M, Myers J, Peberdy MA, Bensimhon D, Chase P, Arena R. Cardiopulmonary exercise testing variables reflect the degree of diastolic dysfunction in patients with heart failure-normal ejection fraction. *J Cardiopulm Rehabil Prev*. 2010;30:165–172.
7. Kitzman DW, Higginbotham MB, Cobb FR, Sheikh KH, Sullivan MJ. Exercise intolerance in patients with heart failure and preserved left ventricular systolic function: failure of the Frank-Starling mechanism. *J Am Coll Cardiol*. 1991;17:1065–1072.
8. Bhatia RS, Tu JV, Lee DS, Austin PC, Fang J, Haouzi A, Gong Y, Liu PP. Outcome of heart failure with preserved ejection fraction in a population-based study. *N Engl J Med*. 2006;355:260–269.
9. Fonarow GC, Stough WG, Abraham WT, Albert NM, Gheorghiade M, Greenberg BH, et al. Characteristics, treatments, and outcomes of patients with preserved systolic function hospitalized for heart

failure: a report from the OPTIMIZE-HF Registry. *J Am Coll Cardiol.* 2007;50:768–777.

10. Sherazi S, Zareba W. Diastolic heart failure: predictors of mortality. *Cardiol J.* 2011;18:222–232.
11. Dunlay SM, Redfield MM, Weston SA, Therneau TM, Hall LK, Shah ND, Roger VL. Hospitalizations after heart failure diagnosis a community perspective. *J Am Coll Cardiol.* 2009;54:1695–1702.
12. Edelmann F, Stahrenberg R, Polzin F, Kockskamper A, Dungen HD, Duvinage A et al. Impaired physical quality of life in patients with diastolic dysfunction associates more strongly with neurohumoral activation than with echocardiographic parameters: quality of life in diastolic dysfunction. *Am Heart J.* 2011;161:797–804.
13. Kitzman DW. Understanding results of trials in heart failure with preserved ejection fraction: remembering forgotten lessons and enduring principles. *J Am Coll Cardiol.* 2011;57:1687–1689.
14. Thohan V, Patel S. The challenges associated with current clinical trials for diastolic heart failure. *Curr Opin Cardiol.* 2009;24: 230–238.
15. Marechaux S, Six-Carpentier MM, Bouabdallaoui N, Montaigne D, Bauchart JJ, Mouquet F, et al. Prognostic importance of comorbidities in heart failure with preserved left ventricular ejection fraction. *Heart Vessels.* 2011:26:313–320.
16. Murad K, Kitzman DW. Frailty and multiple comorbidities in the elderly patient with heart failure: implications for management. *Heart Fail Rev.* 2011. Sep;17(4–5):581–8. doi: 10.1007/s10741-011-9258-y.
17. Kitzman DW. Outcomes in patients with heart failure with preserved ejection fraction: it is more than the heart. *J Am Coll Cardiol.* 2012;59:1006–1007.
18. Chatterjee K, Massie B. Systolic and diastolic heart failure: differences and similarities. *J Card Fail.* 2007;13:569–576.
19. De Keulenaer GW, Brutsaert DL. Systolic and diastolic heart failure: different phenotypes of the same disease? *Eur J Heart Fail.* 2007;9:136–143.
20. Abhayaratna WP, Marwick TH, Smith WT, Becker NG. Characteristics of left ventricular diastolic dysfunction in the community: an echocardiographic survey. *Heart.* 2006;92:1259–1264.
21. Baicu CF, Zile MR, Aurigemma GP, Gaasch WH. Left ventricular systolic performance, function, and contractility in patients with diastolic heart failure. *Circulation.* 2005;111:2306–2312.
22. Sanderson JE, Fraser AG. Systolic dysfunction in heart failure with a normal ejection fraction: echo-Doppler measurements. *Prog Cardiovasc Dis.* 2006;49:196–206.
23. Brutsaert DL. Cardiac dysfunction in heart failure: the cardiologist's love affair with time. *Prog Cardiovasc Dis.* 2006;49:157–181.
24. Garcia MJ. Left ventricular filling. *Heart Fail Clin.* 2008;4:47–56.
25. Zile MR, Baicu CF, Gaasch WH. Diastolic heart failure—abnormalities in active relaxation and passive stiffness of the left ventricle. *N Engl J Med.* 2004;350:1953–1959.
26. Zile MR, Brutsaert DL. New concepts in diastolic dysfunction and diastolic heart failure: Part II: causal mechanisms and treatment. *Circulation.* 2002;105:1503–1508.
27. Zile MR, Brutsaert DL. New concepts in diastolic dysfunction and diastolic heart failure: Part I: diagnosis, prognosis, and measurements of diastolic function. *Circulation.* 2002;105:1387–1393.
28. Borlaug BA, Redfield MM. Diastolic and systolic heart failure are distinct phenotypes within the heart failure spectrum. *Circulation.* 2011;123:2006–2013.
29. De Keulenaer GW, Brutsaert DL. Systolic and diastolic heart failure are overlapping phenotypes within the heart failure spectrum. *Circulation.* 2011;123:1996–2004.
30. Wang J, Khoury DS, Yue Y, Torre-Amione G, Nagueh SF. Preserved left ventricular twist and circumferential deformation, but depressed longitudinal and radial deformation in patients with diastolic heart failure. *Eur Heart J.* 2008;29:1283–1289.
31. Yu CM, Zhang Q, Yip GW, Lee PW, Kum LC, Lam YY, Fung JW. Diastolic and systolic asynchrony in patients with diastolic heart failure: a common but ignored condition. *J Am Coll Cardiol.* 2007;49:97–105.
32. Yamamoto K, Mano T, Yoshida J, Sakata Y, Nishikawa N, Nishio M, et al. ACE inhibitor and angiotensin II type 1 receptor blocker differently regulate ventricular fibrosis in hypertensive diastolic heart failure. *J Hypertens.* 2005;23:393–400.
33. Carluccio E, Biagioli P, Alunni G, Murrone A, Leonelli V, Pantano P, et al. Advantages of deformation indices over systolic velocities in assessment of longitudinal systolic function in patients with heart failure and normal ejection fraction. *Eur J Heart Fail.* 2011;13:292–302.
34. Carerj S, La Carrubba S, Antonini-Canterin F, Di SG, Erlicher A, Liguori E, et al. The incremental prognostic value of echocardiography in asymptomatic stage a heart failure. *J Am Soc Echocardiogr.* 2010;23:1025–1034.
35. Yip GW, Zhang Q, Xie JM, Liang YJ, Liu YM, Yan B, et al. Resting global and regional left ventricular contractility in patients with heart failure and normal ejection fraction: insights from speckle-tracking echocardiography. *Heart.* 2011;97:287–294.
36. van HL, Borbely A, Niessen HW, Bronzwaer JG, van d, V, Stienen GJ, et al. Myocardial structure and function differ in systolic and diastolic heart failure. *Circulation.* 2006;113:1966–1973.
37. Lester SJ, Tajik AJ, Nishimura RA, Oh JK, Khandheria BK, Seward JB. Unlocking the mysteries of diastolic function: deciphering the Rosetta Stone 10 years later. *J Am Coll Cardiol.* 2008;51:679–689.
38. Aizawa Y, Sakata Y, Mano T, Takeda Y, Ohtani T, Tamaki S, et al. Transition from asymptomatic diastolic dysfunction to heart failure with preserved ejection fraction: roles of systolic function and ventricular distensibility. *Circ J.* 2011;75:596–602.
39. Borlaug BA, Kass DA. Invasive hemodynamic assessment in heart failure. *Heart Fail Clin.* 2009;5:217–228.
40. Borlaug BA, Paulus WJ. Heart failure with preserved ejection fraction: pathophysiology, diagnosis, and treatment. *Eur Heart J.* 2011;32:670–679.
41. Borlaug BA, Melenovsky V, Redfield MM, Kessler K, Chang HJ, Abraham TP, Kass DA. Impact of arterial load and loading sequence on left ventricular tissue velocities in humans. *J Am Coll Cardiol.* 2007;50:1570–1577.
42. Borlaug BA, Kass DA. Ventricular-vascular interaction in heart failure. *Cardiol Clin.* 2011;29:447–459.
43. Udelson JE, Konstam MA. Ventricular remodeling fundamental to the progression (and regression) of heart failure. *J Am Coll Cardiol.* 2011;57:1477–1479.
44. Wachtell K, Palmieri V, Gerdts E, Bella JN, Aurigemma GP, Papademetriou V, et al. Prognostic significance of left ventricular diastolic dysfunction in patients with left ventricular hypertrophy and systemic hypertension (the LIFE Study). *Am J Cardiol.* 2010;106:999–1005.
45. Leite-Moreira AF, Correia-Pinto J, Gillebert TC. Diastolic dysfunction and hypertension. *N Engl J Med.* 2001;344:1401.
46. Lapu-Bula R, Ofili E. Diastolic heart failure: the forgotten manifestation of hypertensive heart disease. *Curr Hypertens Rep.* 2004;6:164–170.
47. Dinh W, Lankisch M, Nickl W, Gies M, Scheyer D, Kramer F, et al. Metabolic syndrome with or without diabetes contributes to left ventricular diastolic dysfunction. *Acta Cardiol.* 2011;66:167–174.

48. From AM, Scott CG, Chen HH. The development of heart failure in patients with diabetes mellitus and pre-clinical diastolic dysfunction a population-based study. *J Am Coll Cardiol.* 2010;55:300–305.
49. John JM, Haykowsky M, Brubaker P, Stewart K, Kitzman DW. Decreased left ventricular distensibility in response to postural change in older patients with heart failure and preserved ejection fraction. *Am J Physiol Heart Circ Physiol.* 2010;299:H883–H889.
50. Martos R, Baugh J, Ledwidge M, O'Loughlin C, Conlon C, Patle A, et al. Diastolic heart failure: evidence of increased myocardial collagen turnover linked to diastolic dysfunction. *Circulation.* 2007;115:888–895.
51. Nishikawa N, Yamamoto K, Sakata Y, Mano T, Yoshida J, Miwa T, et al. Differential activation of matrix metalloproteinases in heart failure with and without ventricular dilatation. *Cardiovasc Res.* 2003;57:766–774.
52. Baicu CF, Stroud JD, Livesay VA, Hapke E, Holder J, Spinale FG, Zile MR. Changes in extracellular collagen matrix alter myocardial systolic performance. *Am J Physiol Heart Circ Physiol.* 2003;284:H122–H132.
53. Zile MR, Desantis SM, Baicu CF, Stroud RE, Thompson SB, McClure CD, et al. Plasma biomarkers that reflect determinants of matrix composition identify the presence of left ventricular hypertrophy and diastolic heart failure. *Circ Heart Fail.* 2011;4:246–256.
54. Coutu P, Hirsch JC, Szatkowski ML, Metzger JM. Targeting diastolic dysfunction by genetic engineering of calcium handling proteins. *Trends Cardiovasc Med.* 2003;13:63–67.
55. Wang W, Metzger JM. Parvalbumin isoforms for enhancing cardiac diastolic function. *Cell Biochem Biophys.* 2008;51:1–8.
56. Lacombe VA, Viatchenko-Karpinski S, Terentyev D, Sridhar A, Emani S, Bonagura JD, et al. Mechanisms of impaired calcium handling underlying subclinical diastolic dysfunction in diabetes. *Am J Physiol Regul Integr Comp Physiol.* 2007;293:R1787–R1797.
57. Radke MH, Peng J, Wu Y, McNabb M, Nelson OL, Granzier H, Gotthardt M. Targeted deletion of titin N2B region leads to diastolic dysfunction and cardiac atrophy. *Proc Nat Acad Sci USA.* 2007;104:3444–3449.
58. Yu CM, Cheung BM, Leung R, Wang Q, Lai WH, Lau CP. Increase in plasma adrenomedullin in patients with heart failure characterised by diastolic dysfunction. *Heart.* 2001;86:155–160.
59. Yamamoto K, Masuyama T, Sakata Y, Doi R, Ono K, Mano T, et al. Local neurohumoral regulation in the transition to isolated diastolic heart failure in hypertensive heart disease: absence of AT1 receptor downregulation and "overdrive" of the endothelin system. *Cardiovasc Res.* 2000;46:421–432.
60. Ladeiras-Lopes R, Ferreira-Martins J, Leite-Moreira AF. Acute neurohumoral modulation of diastolic function. *Peptides.* 2008. doi:10.018. Epub 2008 Nov 5. Review.
61. Redfield MM, Jacobsen SJ, Burnett JC Jr, Mahoney DW, Bailey KR, Rodeheffer RJ. Burden of systolic and diastolic ventricular dysfunction in the community: appreciating the scope of the heart failure epidemic. *JAMA.* 2003;289:194–202.
62. Hunt SA, Abraham WT, Chin MH, Feldman AM, Francis GS, Ganiats TG, et al. ACC/AHA 2005 guideline update for the diagnosis and management of chronic heart failure in the adult: a report of the American College of Cardiology/American Heart Association Task Force on Practice Guidelines (Writing Committee to Update the 2001 Guidelines for the Evaluation and Management of Heart Failure): Developed in Collaboration With the American College of Chest Physicians and the International Society for Heart and Lung Transplantation: Endorsed by the Heart Rhythm Society. *Circulation.* 2005;112:e154–e235.
63. Hunt SA, Abraham WT, Chin MH, Feldman AM, Francis GS, Ganiats TG, et al. 2009 focused update incorporated into the ACC/AHA 2005 Guidelines for the Diagnosis and Management of Heart Failure in Adults: a report of the American College of Cardiology Foundation/American Heart Association Task Force on Practice Guidelines: developed in collaboration with the International Society for Heart and Lung Transplantation. *Circulation.* 2009;119:e391-e479.
64. Lindenfeld J, Albert NM, Boehmer JP, Collins SP, Ezekowitz JA, Givertz MM, et al. HFSA 2010 Comprehensive Heart Failure Practice Guideline. *J Card Fail.* 2010;16:e1–194.
65. Guidelines for the diagnosis of heart failure. The Task Force on Heart Failure of the European Society of Cardiology. *Eur Heart J.* 1995;16:741–751.
66. McMurray JJ: Angiotensin inhibition in heart failure. *J Renin Angiotensin Aldosterone Syst.* 2004;5(Suppl 1):S17–S22.
67. Kim SA, Shim CY, Kim JM, Lee HJ, Choi DH, Choi EY, et al. Impact of left ventricular longitudinal diastolic functional reserve on clinical outcome in patients with type 2 diabetes mellitus. *Heart.* 2011;97:1233–1238.
68. Melenovsky V, Borlaug BA, Rosen B, Hay I, Ferruci L, Morell CH, et al. Cardiovascular features of heart failure with preserved ejection fraction versus nonfailing hypertensive left ventricular hypertrophy in the urban Baltimore community: the role of atrial remodeling/dysfunction. *J Am Coll Cardiol.* 2007;49:198–207.
69. Gopal DJ, Iqbal MN, Maisel A. Updating the role of natriuretic peptide levels in cardiovascular disease. *Postgrad Med.* 2011;123:102–113.
70. Chiong JR, Jao GT, Adams KF, Jr. Utility of natriuretic peptide testing in the evaluation and management of acute decompensated heart failure. *Heart Fail Rev.* 2010;15:275–291.
71. Yancy CW, Lopatin M, Stevenson LW, De MT, Fonarow GC. Clinical presentation, management, and in-hospital outcomes of patients admitted with acute decompensated heart failure with preserved systolic function: a report from the Acute Decompensated Heart Failure National Registry (ADHERE) Database. *J Am Coll Cardiol.* 2006;47:76–84.
72. Holland DJ, Sacre JW, Leano RL, Marwick TH, Sharman JE. Contribution of abnormal central blood pressure to left ventricular filling pressure during exercise in patients with heart failure and preserved ejection fraction. *J Hypertens.* 2011;29:1422–1430.
73. Gandhi SK, Powers JC, Nomeir AM, Fowle K, Kitzman DW, Rankin KM, Little WC. The pathogenesis of acute pulmonary edema associated with hypertension. *N Engl J Med.* 2001;344:17–22.
74. Norman HS, Oujiri J, Larue SJ, Chapman CB, Margulies KB, Sweitzer NK. Decreased cardiac functional reserve in heart failure with preserved systolic function. *J Card Fail.* 2011;17:301–308.
75. Haykowsky MJ, Brubaker PH, John JM, Stewart KP, Morgan TM, Kitzman DW. Determinants of exercise intolerance in elderly heart failure patients with preserved ejection fraction. *J Am Coll Cardiol.* 2011;58:265–274.
76. Brubaker PH, Kitzman DW. Chronotropic incompetence: causes, consequences, and management. *Circulation.* 2011;123:1010–1020.
77. Fukuta H, Little WC. Diagnosis of diastolic heart failure. *Curr Cardiol Rep.* 2007; 9:224–228.
78. Nagarakanti R, Ezekowitz M. Diastolic dysfunction and atrial fibrillation. *J Interv Card Electrophysiol.* 2008;22:111–118.
79. Morris DA, Gailani M, Vaz PA, Blaschke F, Dietz R, Haverkamp W, Ozcelik C. Left atrial systolic and diastolic dysfunction in heart failure with normal left ventricular ejection fraction. *J Am Soc Echocardiogr.* 2011;24:651–662.

80. Tsang W, Lang RM. Echocardiographic evaluation of cardiac amyloid. *Curr Cardiol Rep.* 2010;12:272–276.

81. Selvanayagam JB, Hawkins PN, Paul B, Myerson SG, Neubauer S. Evaluation and management of the cardiac amyloidosis. *J Am Coll Cardiol.* 2007;50:2101–2110.

82. Freudenberger RS, Wilson AC, Kostis JB. Comparison of rate versus rhythm control for atrial fibrillation in patients with left ventricular dysfunction (from the AFFIRM Study). *Am J Cardiol.* 2007;100:247–252.

83. Matter CM, Mandinov L, Kaufmann PA, Vassalli G, Jiang Z, Hess OM. Effect of NO donors on LV diastolic function in patients with severe pressure-overload hypertrophy. *Circulation.* 1999;99: 2396–2401.

84. Little WC, Oh JK. Echocardiographic evaluation of diastolic function can be used to guide clinical care. *Circulation.* 2009;120:802–809.

85. Rivas-Gotz C, Manolios M, Thohan V, Nagueh SF. Impact of left ventricular ejection fraction on estimation of left ventricular filling pressures using tissue Doppler and flow propagation velocity. *Am J Cardiol.* 2003;91:780–784.

86. Wang J, Nagueh SF. Current perspectives on cardiac function in patients with diastolic heart failure. *Circulation.* 2009;119: 1146–1157.

87. Wang J, Nagueh SF. Echocardiographic assessment of left ventricular filling pressures. *Heart Fail Clin.* 2008;4:57–70.

88. Pritchett AM, Mahoney DW, Jacobsen SJ, Rodeheffer RJ, Karon BL, Redfield MM. Diastolic dysfunction and left atrial volume: a population-based study. *J Am Coll Cardiol.* 2005;45:87–92.

89. Nagueh SF. Noninvasive evaluation of hemodynamics by Doppler echocardiography. *Curr Opin Cardiol.* 1999;14:217–224.

90. Nagueh SF, Middleton KJ, Kopelen HA, Zoghbi WA, Quinones MA. Doppler tissue imaging: a noninvasive technique for evaluation of left ventricular relaxation and estimation of filling pressures. *J Am Coll Cardiol.* 1997;30:1527–1533.

91. Dokainish H, Nguyen J, Sengupta R, Pillai M, Alam M, Bobek J, Lakkis N. New, simple echocardiographic indexes for the estimation of filling pressure in patients with cardiac disease and preserved left ventricular ejection fraction. *Echocardiography.* 2010;27:946–953.

92. Yu CM, Sanderson JE, Marwick TH, Oh JK. Tissue Doppler imaging a new prognosticator for cardiovascular diseases. *J Am Coll Cardiol.* 2007;49:1903–1914.

93. Nguyen JS, Lakkis NM, Bobek J, Goswami R, Dokainish H. Systolic and diastolic myocardial mechanics in patients with cardiac disease and preserved ejection fraction: impact of left ventricular filling pressure. *J Am Soc Echocardiogr.* 2010;23: 1273–1280.

94. Nagueh SF, Appleton CP, Gillebert TC, Marino PN, Oh JK, Smiseth OA, et al. Recommendations for the evaluation of left ventricular diastolic function by echocardiography. *J Am Soc Echocardiogr.* 2009;22:107–133.

95. Paulus WJ, Tschope C, Sanderson JE, Rusconi C, Flachskampf FA, Rademakers FE, et al. How to diagnose diastolic heart failure: a consensus statement on the diagnosis of heart failure with normal left ventricular ejection fraction by the Heart Failure and Echocardiography Associations of the European Society of Cardiology. *Eur Heart J.* 2007;28:2539–2550.

96. Okura H, Takada Y, Kubo T, Iwata K, Mizoguchi S, Taguchi H, et al. Tissue Doppler-derived index of left ventricular filling pressure, E/E', predicts survival of patients with non-valvular atrial fibrillation. *Heart.* 2006;92:1248–1252.

97. Ha JW, Oh JK, Ling LH, Nishimura RA, Seward JB, Tajik AJ. Annulus paradoxus: transmitral flow velocity to mitral annular velocity ratio is inversely proportional to pulmonary capillary wedge pressure in patients with constrictive pericarditis. *Circulation.* 2001;104:976–978.

98. Rajagopalan N, Garcia MJ, Rodriguez L, Murray RD, Apperson-Hansen C, Stugaard M, et al. Comparison of new Doppler echocardiographic methods to differentiate constrictive pericardial heart disease and restrictive cardiomyopathy. *Am J Cardiol.* 2001;87:86–94.

99. Hatle L. How to diagnose diastolic heart failure a consensus statement. *Eur Heart J.* 2007;28:2421–2423.

100. Lee DS, Gona P, Albano I, Larson MG, Benjamin EJ, Levy D, et al. A systematic assessment of causes of death after heart failure onset in the community: impact of age at death, time period, and left ventricular systolic dysfunction. *Circ Heart Fail.* 2011;4:36–43.

101. Dokainish H, Zoghbi WA, Lakkis NM, Ambriz E, Patel R, Quinones MA, Nagueh SF. Incremental predictive power of B-type natriuretic peptide and tissue Doppler echocardiography in the prognosis of patients with congestive heart failure. *J Am Coll Cardiol.* 2005;45:1223–1226.

102. Braunstein JB, Anderson GF, Gerstenblith G, Weller W, Niefeld M, Herbert R, Wu AW. Noncardiac comorbidity increases preventable hospitalizations and mortality among Medicare beneficiaries with chronic heart failure. *J Am Coll Cardiol.* 2003;42:1226–1233.

103. Kitzman DW, Daniel KR. Diastolic heart failure in the elderly. *Heart Fail Clin.* 2007;3:437–453.

104. Chobanian AV, Bakris GL, Black HR, Cushman WC, Green LA, Izzo JL, Jr, et al. The Seventh Report of the Joint National Committee on Prevention, Detection, Evaluation, and Treatment of High Blood Pressure: the JNC 7 report. *JAMA.* 2003;289: 2560–2572.

105. Hoenig MR, Bianchi C, Rosenzweig A, Sellke FW. The cardiac microvasculature in hypertension, cardiac hypertrophy and diastolic heart failure. *Curr Vasc Pharmacol.* 2008;6:292–300.

106. Wright JW, Mizutani S, Harding JW. Pathways involved in the transition from hypertension to hypertrophy to heart failure. Treatment strategies. *Heart Fail Rev.* 2008;13:367–375.

107. Wu CK, Tsai CT, Hwang JJ, Luo JL, Juang JJ, Hsu KL, et al. Renin-angiotensin system gene polymorphisms and diastolic heart failure. *Eur J Clin Invest.* 2008;38:789–797.

108. Bernal J, Pitta SR, Thatai D. Role of the renin-angiotensin-aldosterone system in diastolic heart failure: potential for pharmacologic intervention. *Am J Cardiovasc Drugs.* 2006;6:373–381.

109. Yoshida J, Yamamoto K, Mano T, Sakata Y, Nishikawa N, Miwa T, Hori M, Masuyama T. Angiotensin II type 1 and endothelin type A receptor antagonists modulate the extracellular matrix regulatory system differently in diastolic heart failure. *J Hypertens.* 2003;21:437–444.

110. Nishio M, Sakata Y, Mano T, Yoshida J, Ohtani T, Takeda Y, et al. Therapeutic effects of angiotensin II type 1 receptor blocker at an advanced stage of hypertensive diastolic heart failure. *J Hypertens.* 2007;25:455–461.

111. Ohtani T, Ohta M, Yamamoto K, Mano T, Sakata Y, Nishio M, et al. Elevated cardiac tissue level of aldosterone and mineralocorticoid receptor in diastolic heart failure: Beneficial effects of mineralocorticoid receptor blocker. *Am J Physiol Regul.Integr Comp Physiol.* 2007;292:R946–R954.

112. Cleland JG, Tendera M, Adamus J, Freemantle N, Polonski L, Taylor J. The perindopril in elderly people with chronic heart failure (PEP-CHF) study. *Eur Heart J.* 2006;27:2338–2345.

113. Massie BM, Carson PE, McMurray JJ, Komajda M, McKelvie R, Zile MR, et al. Irbesartan in Patients with Heart Failure and Preserved

Ejection Fraction. *N Engl J Med*. 2008. Dec 4;359(23):2456–67. doi: 10.1056/NEJMoa0805450. Epub 2008 Nov 11.

114. Yip GW, Wang M, Wang T, Chan S, Fung JW, Yeung L, et al. The Hong Kong diastolic heart failure study: a randomised controlled trial of diuretics, irbesartan and ramipril on quality of life, exercise capacity, left ventricular global and regional function in heart failure with a normal ejection fraction. *Heart*. 2008;94:573–580.

115. Orea-Tejeda A, Colin-Ramirez E, Castillo-Martinez L, Asensio-Lafuente E, Corzo-Leon D, Gonzalez-Toledo R, et al. Aldosterone receptor antagonists induce favorable cardiac remodeling in diastolic heart failure patients. *Rev Invest Clin*. 2007;59:103–107.

116. Mottram PM, Haluska B, Leano R, Cowley D, Stowasser M, Marwick TH. Effect of aldosterone antagonism on myocardial dysfunction in hypertensive patients with diastolic heart failure. *Circulation*. 2004;110:558–565.

117. Pitt B. The role of mineralocorticoid receptor antagonists (MRAs) in very old patients with heart failure. *Heart Fail.Rev*. 2012;17:573–579.

118. Desai AS, Lewis EF, Li R, Solomon SD, Assmann SF, Boineau R, Clausell N, et al. Rationale and design of the treatment of preserved cardiac function heart failure with an aldosterone antagonist trial: a randomized, controlled study of spironolactone in patients with symptomatic heart failure and preserved ejection fraction. *Am Heart J*. 2011;162:966–972.

119. Kitzman DW, Little WC, Brubaker PH, Anderson RT, Hundley WG, Marburger CT, et al. Pathophysiological characterization of isolated diastolic heart failure in comparison to systolic heart failure. *JAMA*. 2002;288:2144–2150.

120. Flather MD, Shibata MC, Coats AJ, Van Veldhuisen DJ, Parkhomenko A, Borbola J, et al. Randomized trial to determine the effect of nebivolol on mortality and cardiovascular hospital admission in elderly patients with heart failure (SENIORS). *Eur Heart J*. 2005;26:215–225.

121. Bergstrom A, Andersson B, Edner M, Nylander E, Persson H, Dahlstrom U. Effect of carvedilol on diastolic function in patients with diastolic heart failure and preserved systolic function. Results of the Swedish Doppler-echocardiographic study (SWEDIC). *Eur J Heart Fail*. 2004;6:453–461.

122. Borlaug BA, Melenovsky V, Russell SD, Kessler K, Pacak K, Becker LC, Kass DA. Impaired chronotropic and vasodilator reserves limit exercise capacity in patients with heart failure and a preserved ejection fraction. *Circulation*. 2006;114:2138–2147.

123. Brubaker PH, Joo KC, Stewart KP, Fray B, Moore B, Kitzman DW. Chronotropic incompetence and its contribution to exercise intolerance in older heart failure patients. *J Cardiopulm Rehabil*. 2006;26:86–89.

124. Borlaug BA, Nishimura RA, Sorajja P, Lam CS, Redfield MM. Exercise hemodynamics enhance diagnosis of early heart failure with preserved ejection fraction. *Circ Heart Fail*. 2010;3:588–595.

125. Holland DJ, Prasad SB, Marwick TH. Contribution of exercise echocardiography to the diagnosis of heart failure with preserved ejection fraction (HFPEF). *Heart*. 2010;96:1024–1028.

126. Sanderson JE. Exercise echocardiography and the diagnosis of heart failure with a normal ejection fraction. *Heart*. 2010;96:997–998.

127. Ahmed A, Rich MW, Fleg JL, Zile MR, Young JB, Kitzman DW, et al. Effects of digoxin on morbidity and mortality in diastolic heart failure: the ancillary digitalis investigation group trial. *Circulation*. 2006;114:397–403.

128. Kasai T, Bradley TD. Obstructive sleep apnea and heart failure: pathophysiologic and therapeutic implications. *J Am Coll Cardiol*. 2011;57:119–127.

129. Somers VK, White DP, Amin R, Abraham WT, Costa F, Culebras A, et al. Sleep apnea and cardiovascular disease: an American Heart Association/american College Of Cardiology Foundation Scientific Statement from the American Heart Association Council for High Blood Pressure Research Professional Education Committee, Council on Clinical Cardiology, Stroke Council, and Council On Cardiovascular Nursing. In collaboration with the National Heart, Lung, and Blood Institute National Center on Sleep Disorders Research (National Institutes of Health). *Circulation*. 2008;118:1080–1111.

130. Sin DD, Fitzgerald F, Parker JD, Newton GE, Logan AG, Floras JS, Bradley TD. Relationship of systolic BP to obstructive sleep apnea in patients with heart failure. *Chest*. 2003;123:1536–1543.

131. Stevenson IH, Teichtahl H, Cunnington D, Ciavarella S, Gordon I, Kalman JM. Prevalence of sleep disordered breathing in paroxysmal and persistent atrial fibrillation patients with normal left ventricular function. *Eur Heart J*. 2008;29:1662–1669.

132. Johansson P, Arestedt K, Alehagen U, Svanborg E, Dahlstrom U, Brostrom A. Sleep disordered breathing, insomnia, and health related quality of life—a comparison between age and gender matched elderly with heart failure or without cardiovascular disease. *Eur J Cardiovasc Nurs*. 2010;9:108–117.

133. Bitter T, Faber L, Hering D, Langer C, Horstkotte D, Oldenburg O. Sleep-disordered breathing in heart failure with normal left ventricular ejection fraction. *Eur J Heart Fail*. 2009;11:602–608.

134. Herrscher TE, Akre H, Overland B, Sandvik L, Westheim AS. High prevalence of sleep apnea in heart failure outpatients: even in patients with preserved systolic function. *J Card Fail*. 2011;17:420–425.

135. Bradley TD, Floras JS. Sleep apnea and heart failure: Part I: obstructive sleep apnea. *Circulation*. 2003;107:1671–1678.

136. Arzt M, Bradley TD. Treatment of sleep apnea in heart failure. *Am J Respir Crit Care Med*. 2006;173:1300–1308.

137. Bradley TD. Right and left ventricular functional impairment and sleep apnea. *Clin Chest Med*. 1992;13:459–479.

138. Kitzman DW. Exercise training in heart failure with preserved ejection fraction: beyond proof-of-concept. *J Am Coll Cardiol*. 2011;58:1792–1794.

139. Kitzman DW, Groban L. Exercise intolerance. *Cardiol Clin*. 2011;29:461–477.

140. Edelmann F, Gelbrich G, Dungen HD, Frohling S, Wachter R, Stahrenberg R, et al. Exercise training improves exercise capacity and diastolic function in patients with heart failure with preserved ejection fraction: results of the Ex-DHF (Exercise training in Diastolic Heart Failure) pilot study. *J Am Coll Cardiol*. 2011;58:1780–1791.

141. Gardin JM, Leifer ES, Fleg JL, Whellan D, Kokkinos P, Leblanc MH, et al. Relationship of Doppler-Echocardiographic left ventricular diastolic function to exercise performance in systolic heart failure: the HF-ACTION study. *Am Heart J*. 2009;158:S45–S52.

142. Flynn KE, Pina IL, Whellan DJ, Lin L, Blumenthal JA, Ellis SJ, Fine LJ, et al. Effects of exercise training on health status in patients with chronic heart failure: HF-ACTION randomized controlled trial. *JAMA*. 2009;301:1451–1459.

143. O'Connor CM, Whellan DJ, Lee KL, Keteyian SJ, Cooper LS, Ellis SJ, et al. Efficacy and safety of exercise training in patients with chronic heart failure: HF-ACTION randomized controlled trial. *JAMA*. 2009;301:1439–1450.

144. Aronow WS. Epidemiology, pathophysiology, prognosis, and treatment of systolic and diastolic heart failure. *Cardiol Rev*. 2006;14:108–124.

145. Maeder MT, Thompson BR, Brunner-La Rocca HP, Kaye DM. Hemodynamic basis of exercise limitation in patients with heart failure and normal ejection fraction. *J Am Coll Cardiol.* 2010;56:855–863.
146. Prasad A, Hastings JL, Shibata S, Popovic ZB, Arbab-Zadeh A, Bhella PS, et al. Characterization of static and dynamic left ventricular diastolic function in patients with heart failure with a preserved ejection fraction. *Circ Heart Fail.* 2010;3:617–626.
147. Sohn DW, Kim HK, Park JS, Chang HJ, Kim YJ, Zo ZH, et al. Hemodynamic effects of tachycardia in patients with relaxation abnormality: abnormal stroke volume response as an overlooked mechanism of dyspnea associated with tachycardia in diastolic heart failure. *J Am Soc Echocardiogr.* 2007;20:171–176.
148. Paulus WJ, van Ballegoij JJ. Treatment of heart failure with normal ejection fraction: an inconvenient truth! *J Am Coll Cardiol.* 2010;55:526–537.
149. Guazzi M, Vicenzi M, Arena R. Phosphodiesterase 5 inhibition with sildenafil reverses exercise oscillatory breathing in chronic heart failure: a long-term cardiopulmonary exercise testing placebo-controlled study. *Eur J Heart Fail.* 2012;14:82–90.
150. Redfield MM, Borlaug BA, Lewis GD, Mohammed SF, Semigran MJ, Lewinter MM, et al. PhosphdiesteRasE-5 Inhibition to Improve CLinical Status and EXercise Capacity in Diastolic Heart Failure (RELAX) Trial: Rationale and Design. *Circ Heart Fail.* 2012;5:653–659.
151. Little WC, Wesley-Farrington DJ, Hoyle J, Brucks S, Robertson S, Kitzman DW, Cheng CP. Effect of candesartan and verapamil on exercise tolerance in diastolic dysfunction. *J Cardiovasc Pharmacol.* 2004;43:288–293.
152. Wang YC, Hwang JJ, Lai LP, Tsai CT, Lin LC, Katra R, Lin JL. Coexistence and exercise exacerbation of intraleft ventricular contractile dyssynchrony in hypertensive patients with diastolic heart failure. *Am Heart J.* 2007;154:278–284.
153. Wang J, Kurrelmeyer KM, Torre-Amione G, Nagueh SF. Systolic and diastolic dyssynchrony in patients with diastolic heart failure and the effect of medical therapy. *J Am Coll Cardiol.* 2007;49:88–96.
154. Park SJ, Oh JK. Correlation between LV regional strain and LV dyssynchrony assessed by 2D STE in patients with different levels of diastolic dysfunction. *Echocardiography.* 2010;27:1194–1204.
155. Shanks M, Bertini M, Delgado V, Ng AC, Nucifora G, van Bommel RJ, et al. Effect of biventricular pacing on diastolic dyssynchrony. *J Am Coll Cardiol.* 2010;56:1567–1575.
156. Kass DA, Kitzman DW, Alvarez GE. The restoration of chronotropic competence in heart failure patients with normal ejection fraction (RESET) study: rationale and design. *J Card Fail.* 2010;16:17–24.
157. Thohan V, Torre-Amione G, Koerner MM. Aldosterone antagonism and congestive heart failure: a new look at an old therapy. *Curr Opin Cardiol.* 2004;19:301–308.
158. Li SY, Du M, Dolence EK, Fang CX, Mayer GE, Ceylan-Isik AF, et al. Aging induces cardiac diastolic dysfunction, oxidative stress, accumulation of advanced glycation endproducts and protein modification. *Aging Cell.* 2005;4:57–64.
159. Bakris GL, Bank AJ, Kass DA, Neutel JM, Preston RA, Oparil S. Advanced glycation end-product cross-link breakers. A novel approach to cardiovascular pathologies related to the aging process. *Am J Hypertens.* 2004;17:23S–30S.
160. Berg TJ, Snorgaard O, Faber J, Torjesen PA, Hildebrandt P, Mehlsen J, Hanssen KF. Serum levels of advanced glycation end products are associated with left ventricular diastolic function in patients with type 1 diabetes. *Diabetes Care.* 1999;22:1186–1190.
161. Little WC, Zile MR, Kitzman DW, Hundley WG, O'Brien TX, Degroof RC. The effect of alagebrium chloride (ALT-711), a novel glucose cross-link breaker, in the treatment of elderly patients with diastolic heart failure. *J Card Fail.* 2005;11:191–195.
162. Roger VL, Go AS, Lloyd-Jones DM, Benjamin EJ, Berry JD, Borden WB, et al. Heart disease and stroke statistics—2012 update: a report from the American Heart Association. *Circulation.* 2012;125:e2–e220.
163. McKee PA, Castelli WP, McNamara PM, Kannel WB. The natural history of congestive heart failure: the Framingham study. *N Engl J Med.* 1971;285:1441–1446.
164. Carlson KJ, Lee DC, Goroll AH, Leahy M, Johnson RA. An analysis of physicians' reasons for prescribing long-term digitalis therapy in outpatients. *J Chronic Dis.* 1985;38:733–739.
165. Thomas SS, Nohria A. Hemodynamic classifications of acute heart failure and their clinical application: an update. *Circ J.* 2012;76:278–286.

II

Optimizing Therapy for Patients With Chronic Heart Failure

6

Acute Decompensated Heart Failure in the Previously Stable Heart Failure Patient: A Practical Guide to Evaluation and Treatment

ELAINE WINKEL

CASE PRESENTATION

Mr. S is a 65-year-old white male with severe, but well-compensated left ventricular systolic dysfunction from a dilated cardiomyopathy due to long-standing hypertensive heart disease. Heart failure was diagnosed 3 years ago when he presented with exertional dyspnea, abdominal bloating, lower extremity edema, and profound fatigue. An echocardiogram showed severe left ventricular systolic dysfunction with a left ventricular ejection fraction (LVEF) of 30%, and moderate mitral and tricuspid regurgitation. Cardiac catheterization showed normal coronary arteries but elevated filling pressures. He started an angiotensin converting enzyme inhibitor (ACE-I), beta-blocker (BB), and diuretic. His symptoms improved, and for the past 3 years he has been clinically stable with New York Heart Association (NYHA) functional Class II symptoms. He is currently on a medication regimen of lisinopril 40 mg daily, carvedilol 25 mg twice daily, furosemide 40 mg daily, and spironolactone 25 mg daily. An echocardiogram 6 months ago showed an LVEF of 40% and no valvular regurgitation.

He comes to your office today complaining of a 4-week history of progressive fatigue and dyspnea on exertion (DOE), but no paroxysmal nocturnal dyspnea (PND), orthopnea, abdominal bloating, or lower extremity edema. He has no palpitations, chest discomfort, or lightheadedness. Two nights ago he developed severe orthopnea and PND. He faithfully takes his medications, maintains a 2,000 mg sodium restriction, and does not drink alcohol or smoke. Six weeks ago he developed gout in his left foot and was given a nonsteroidal anti-inflammatory drug (NSAID) by his family physician. The gout episode was resolved. He has otherwise felt well.

On exam he is an ill-appearing, elderly white male who is mildly dyspneic and tachypneic at rest. His weight has increased 10 pounds compared with the last visit. The blood pressure is 100/64, pulse 90, and regular and respiratory rate 20. His sclerae are anicteric, the central venous pressure (CVP) is 15 cm at 30 degrees with an abnormal hepatojugular reflux (HJR). The lungs are clear, he has an S3 gallop but no murmurs, and he has tender hepatomegaly. He has no dependent edema, and the skin is warm and dry. An electrocardiogram (ECG) shows a normal sinus rhythm at a rate of 90, with no ischemic changes and no arrhythmia. A chest x-ray shows an enlarged cardiac silhouette, but no increased vascular markings and no effusion.

ACUTE DECOMPENSATED HEART FAILURE

Few problems are as challenging (and frustrating) for the physician as the patient with acutely decompensated heart failure (ADHF). There is little data to guide us since there is no agreed upon definition of ADHF, incomplete knowledge of the pathophysiology of

ADHF, diversity of the heart failure population, and a lack of scientific evidence based guidelines for evaluation and management.

However, the Heart Failure Society of America, the American College of Cardiology, and the American Heart Association have recently addressed these issues by including sections on the evaluation and management of ADHF in their respective heart failure guidelines that provide helpful advice (1,2). Three issues are important in successful treatment of ADHF: (a) establishing etiology; (b) optimal treatment; and (c) preventing readmission. We will talk about each of these in depth.

Practically speaking, ADHF can be defined as either new onset heart failure, or slow to rapid worsening of heart failure symptoms in the previously stable heart failure patient, similar to Mr. S. The diagnosis of ADHF is clinical and based on signs and symptoms; but if there is doubt, a B-type natriuretic peptide (BNP) level can be helpful, especially in patients with comorbid illnesses, such as chronic obstructive pulmonary disease. A careful history and physical examination is crucial, with the caveat that the history is infinitely more helpful than the physical exam. Observational studies report that well-treated patients with heart failure often have minimal or absent physical and radiographic findings of pulmonary congestion, despite significant elevation in pulmonary capillary wedge pressure (3,4). Most ADHF patients present with congestive symptoms, with or without concomitant signs of poor perfusion. It is helpful to assign the patient to a hemodynamic subset based on the history and physical exam. Does the physical exam reveal congestion alone (warm and wet), congestion with poor perfusion (cold and wet), or poor perfusion alone (cold and dry; **Figure 6-1**)?

DETERMINING THE ETIOLOGY

Medication and/or dietary noncompliance, which cause volume overload, have long been considered the causes of ADHF. However, they should be diagnoses of exclusion. Other important causes of ADHF should be considered first and include (a) progression of the original cause of heart failure, (b) comorbid conditions that exacerbate heart failure, (c) ingestion of harmful agents, (d) new or recurrent arrhythmias, (e) pregnancy in females of childbearing age, and finally, (f) medication and/or dietary noncompliance (**Table 6-1**).

Do symptoms suggest new or ongoing myocardial ischemia or arrhythmia? Were any new prescriptions or over-the-counter medications added recently that could have exacerbated heart failure? Are alcohol or illicit drugs factors?

Progression of Disease

Progression of the original cause of heart failure must be in the differential diagnosis of ADHF, especially in patients with ischemic heart disease. An acute coronary syndrome (ACS) can commonly present as worsening heart failure symptoms in the absence of chest discomfort. Rule out an ACS with serial troponin levels and ECGs. After optimizing the heart failure regimen and achieving euvolemia, proceed with evaluation for progression of coronary artery disease (CAD) with either noninvasive testing or cardiac catheterization.

Hypertension is a common cause of left ventricular systolic dysfunction. Uncontrolled hypertension can cause ADHF in a previously stable patient. Review of the patient's home blood pressure record is instructive. Does he take agents known to increase blood pressure? Alcohol, caffeine, and certain over the counter herbals and botanicals can worsen blood pressure control.

Progression of valvular or congenital heart disease is a common cause of ADHF. An echocardiogram can establish progression of stenotic or regurgitant lesions, which may be correctable. Infiltrative cardiomyopathies (sarcoid and amyloid), and familial cardiomyopathies, are also progressive diseases that can cause ADHF.

Alcohol is a direct myocardial depressant and a common cause of cardiomyopathy. Has the patient with alcoholic cardiomyopathy started drinking again?

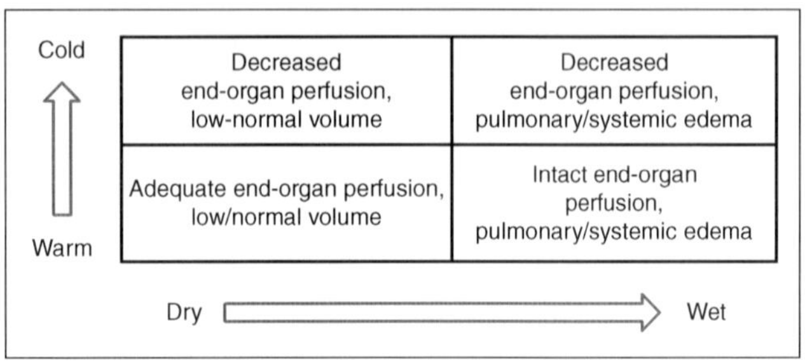

Figure 6-1
Clinical Assessment.

Table 6-1
Precipitating Factors for Acute Decompensated Heart Failure

- Progression of disease
- Myocardial ischemia
- Arrhythmia
- Pacemaker malfunction
- Medical or dietary noncompliance
- Harmful drugs
- Alcohol
- Other comorbid conditions

Comorbid Conditions

Exacerbation of any comorbid condition, such as chronic obstructive pulmonary disease (COPD), diabetes mellitus (DM), or collagen vascular disease can cause ADHF in a previously stable patient. Development of new stresses such as infectious illness, sleep apnea, thyroid disease, or recent surgery or trauma can all cause a stable patient to become unstable.

Arrhythmia, new or recurrent, is a common, but often overlooked cause of ADHF. An ECG, telemetry monitoring, or interrogation of a pacer or implantable cardioverter-defibrillator (ICD) will reveal arrhythmic activity. Is the patient on any antiarrhythmic drugs? Remember that an antiarrhythmic drug can be proarrhythmic. Is the QT interval on EKG prolonged?

Pregnancy must be ruled out in a female patient in her childbearing years, including the early menopausal years.

Medication noncompliance and dietary indiscretion are common causes of ADHF. Ask the patient or family to bring in all medication bottles—prescription and over the counter. Call the patient's pharmacy to see if the medications have been refilled regularly. Talk with the family to ascertain compliance. Perform a careful review of dietary habits, including eating out.

Ingestion of harmful agents, both prescription and over-the-counter medications can exacerbate heart failure. Nonsteroidal anti-inflammatory drugs (5), certain antiarrhythmic drugs, calcium channel blockers, alcohol, and illicit drugs are the "usual suspects." Carefully question the patient and family about recent use of these agents. At times another physician will unknowingly prescribe a medication that can worsen the heart failure state.

CASE PRESENTATION

In Mr. S's case, he has significant CAD risk factors (age, male sex, hypertension); however, cardiac catheterization 3 years ago revealed no CAD. It would be unlikely that CAD would have developed and progressed in so short a time. His blood pressure has been consistently around 100 mmHg systolic at home and in the office in the past 3 years. He denies consumption of alcohol, illicit drugs, and over-the-counter medication. He has no comorbid conditions and has not had an infectious illness, surgery, or trauma recently. Therefore, the cause of his deterioration is fluid retention from the NSAID prescribed recently for gout.

OPTIMAL TREATMENT

Once the diagnosis of ADHF is established, when is hospitalization indicated? Current guidelines suggest hospitalization is recommended when the patient is (a) hypotensive, (b) has worsening renal function, (c) altered mental status, (d) dyspnea or oxygen desaturation at rest, (e) has a hemodynamically significant arrhythmia, and (f) has symptoms suggestive of an acute coronary syndrome. Hospitalization should also be considered for (a) patients with clinically worsened congestion, even in the absence of dyspnea, (b) pulmonary congestion even in the absence of weight gain, (c) associated comorbid conditions, (d) repeated ICD firings, and (e) previously undiagnosed heart failure with signs and symptoms of pulmonary or systemic congestion (**Table 6-2**).

Treatment goals include symptomatic relief of congestion and/or poor cardiac output, attaining euvolemia, correcting precipitating factors, optimizing

Table 6-2
Recommendations for Hospitalizing Patients With ADHF

RECOMMENDATION	CLINICAL STATE
(a) Hospitalization recommended	Severe ADHF: hypotension, worsening renal function, or altered mentation Dyspnea at rest: resting tachypnea or oxygen saturation < 90% Hemodynamically significant arrhythmia, including new onset rapid atrial fibrillation Acute coronary syndromes
(b) Hospitalization strongly considered	Worsened congestion, even without dyspnea Signs & symptoms of pulmonary or systemic congestion, even without weight gain Major electrolyte disturbance Associated comorbid conditions Pneumonia or other infection Pulmonary embolus Uncontrolled diabetic Transient ischemic accident or stroke Repeated ICD firings New heart failure with signs and symptoms of systemic or pulmonary congestion

Note: ADHF = acutely decompensated heart failure; ICD = implantable cardioverter-defibrillator.

oral heart failure therapy, identifying patients who would benefit from coronary revascularization or cardiac resynchronization therapy, identifying thromboembolic risk, heart failure education for the patient and family, and finally, identifying patients who would benefit from a referral to a heart failure disease management program and/or referral to a heart failure cardiologist (1).

Inpatient management should include telemetry monitoring for arrhythmia, daily weights, and strict intake and output measurement. The patient should be on a 2,000 mg sodium restricted diet. A fluid restriction of less than 2 L a day is recommended in patients with moderate hyponatremia (serum sodium less than 130 mEq/L) or to assist with treatment of fluid overload in other patients.

Patients with fluid overload should be given IV rather than oral loop diuretics, since gut congestion likely precludes adequate absorption. Loop diuretics can be administered either as bolus doses or by continuous infusion. ADHF patients are commonly undertreated with diuretics, so doses must be high enough to produce a diuresis that relieves congestion without compromising systemic blood pressure or renal function. Ultrafiltration may be necessary in the diuretic resistant patient. Serum electrolytes and renal function should be measured daily. Normal serum potassium and magnesium levels must be maintained to reduce the likelihood of ventricular arrhythmia.

Hypoxic patients should receive supplemental oxygen. Noninvasive positive pressure ventilation is necessary for severely dyspneic patients. Prophylaxis against venous thromboembolism and pulmonary embolism is necessary.

IV vasodilators, nitroprusside, or nesiritide, are helpful in patients with pulmonary edema or severe hypertension, and in patients with persistent heart failure despite aggressive diuretic therapy. However, these therapies require frequent blood pressure monitoring.

Routine use of IV inotropic agents (milrinone, dobutamine) should be avoided. However, they may be necessary for symptomatic relief in the advanced heart failure patient with concomitant congestion, hypotension, and end-organ dysfunction.

PREVENTING READMISSION

Discharge planning is crucial in preventing readmission for ADHF. Discharge should not be considered until certain criteria are met (**Table 6-3**). Discharge planning should include education about heart failure as a disease, the importance of adherence to a medication regimen and diet, recording of daily weights and vital signs, avoidance of smoking, alcohol, and harmful drugs; expected activity level with a daily exercise regimen, and keeping follow-up appointments.

Hospitalization for ADHF is an important predictor of post-discharge mortality, especially in the first 6 months. Patients enrolled in the OPTIME-CHF trial, a trial of milrinone versus placebo in patients hospitalized for ADHF, had a 10% to 13% 6-month mortality in both groups and a 36% to 42% rate of death or readmission at 6 months (6). These patients represent a high-risk group that needs close, frequent outpatient follow-up. Strong consideration should be given to referral to an Advanced Heart Failure Program.

Table 6-3
Discharge Criteria for Patients With Heart Failure

Recommended for all patients	• Exacerbating factors corrected • Optimal volume status clinically • Transition from intravenous to oral diuretic completed • Patient and family education completed with clear discharge instructions • Ventricular function documented • Smoking cessation counseling initiated • Near optimal pharmacologic therapy achieved, including ACE inhibitor and beta-blocker, or intolerance documented • Follow-up office visit in 7–10 days
Strongly considered for patients with advanced HF or recurrent HF admissions	• Oral medication regimen stable for 24 hours • No IV vasodilator or inotropic agent for 24 hours • Ambulation before discharge to assess functional capacity • Plans for postdischarge management (scale in home, visiting nurse, or telephone follow-up within 3 days after discharge) • Follow up office visit in 7–10 days • Referral to an advanced heart failure management program to see a heart failure cardiologist

Note: ACE = angiotensin converting enzyme.

REFERENCES

1. Lindenfeld J, Albert NM, Boehmer JP, et al. Executive summary: HFSA 2010 comprehensive heart failure practice guideline. *J Card Fail.* 2010;16:475–539.
2. Jessup M, Abraham WT, Casey DE, et al. 2009 focused update: ACCF/AHA Guidelines for the Diagnosis and Management of Heart Failure in Adults: a report of the American College of Cardiology Foundation/American Heart Association Task Force on Practice Guidelines: developed in collaboration with the International Society for Heart and Lung Transplantation. *Circulation.* 2009;119:1977–2016.
3. Mahdyoon H, Klein R, Eyler W, et al. Radiographic pulmonary congestion in end-stage congestive heart failure. *Am J Cardiol.* 1989;63:625–627.
4. Stevenson LW, Perloff JK. The limited reliability of physical signs for estimating hemodynamics in chronic heart failure. *JAMA.* 1989;261:884–888.
5. Gislason GH, Rasmussen JN, Abildstrom SZ, et al. Increased mortality and cardiovascular morbidity associated with use of nonsteroidal anti-inflammatory drugs in chronic heart failure. *Arch Intern Med.* 2009;169:141–149.
6. Cuffe MS, Califf RM, Adams KF, Jr., et al. Short-term intravenous milrinone for acute exacerbation of chronic heart failure: a randomized controlled trial. *JAMA.* 2002;287:1541–1547.

7

Optimizing Heart Failure Management in Idiopathic Non-Ischemic Dilated Cardiomyopathy Complicated by Ventricular Arrhythmia

ROY M. JOHN AND WILLIAM G. STEVENSON

THE CLINICAL PROBLEM

A 48-year-old male presents with progressive shortness of breath over a 3-month period with recent onset of nocturnal dyspnea and orthopnea. He denied chest pain, syncope, or palpitation. There was a history of mild hypertension but no diabetes or renal disease. Family history was unremarkable and there was no history of excess alcohol use. Routine labs, thyroid function tests, and iron studies were normal. Twelve-lead electrocardiogram (ECG) showed left bundle branch block (LBBB). Two-dimensional echocardiography demonstrated global left ventricular dilatation with global left ventricular dysfunction with estimated left ventricular ejection fraction (LVEF) of 30% (**Figure 7-1**, left panel). There was paradoxical septal motion and mild mitral regurgitation. Coronary angiography showed normal left dominant coronary arteries. MRI imaging of the heart showed left ventricular dilation and LVEF consistent with that observed on the echocardiogram, but no evidence of significant infiltrative disease.

Treatment was initiated with diuretics, lisinopril, and carvedilol with relief from acute congestion related symptoms. Dosages of lisinopril and carvedilol were escalated gradually to 20 mg daily and 25 mg bid respectively. However, following hospital discharge, he remained limited with Class III heart failure symptoms. Two months later, he was hospitalized following a syncopal event. The event was witnessed by his wife who described him as abruptly falling to the floor in the kitchen. He was unrousable for a few seconds, following which there was recovery of consciousness with no specific symptoms afterward. He sustained superficial laceration to his forehead during the fall.

A repeat 12-lead ECG showed persistence of LBBB and first-degree atrio-ventricular (AV) block (**Figure 7-2A**). Intracardiac electrophysiological evaluation revealed prolonged atrio-Hisian (AH) interval of 230 msec and His-ventricle (HV) interval of 65 msec. Programmed stimulation of the right ventricle induced a sustained rapid ventricular tachycardia at 220 bpm, which was hemodynamically unstable and required immediate cardioversion to restore sinus rhythm and normal hemodynamic parameters.

An implantable cardioverter-defibrillator (ICD) incorporating cardiac resynchronization therapy (CRT) was implanted. A repeat ECG showed adequate biventricular pacing (**Figure 7-2B**). Lisinopril, carvedilol, and diuretics were continued. Spironolactone 25 mg daily was added. At a follow-up visit 1 month later, he reported considerable improvement in functional capacity. A repeat echocardiogram demonstrated improved left ventricular ejection fraction to 45% and decrease in end systolic left ventricular dimension (**Figure 7-1**, right panel). Two weeks later, the patient returned to clinic to report that he received an ICD shock that awoke him from sleep. Interrogation of the

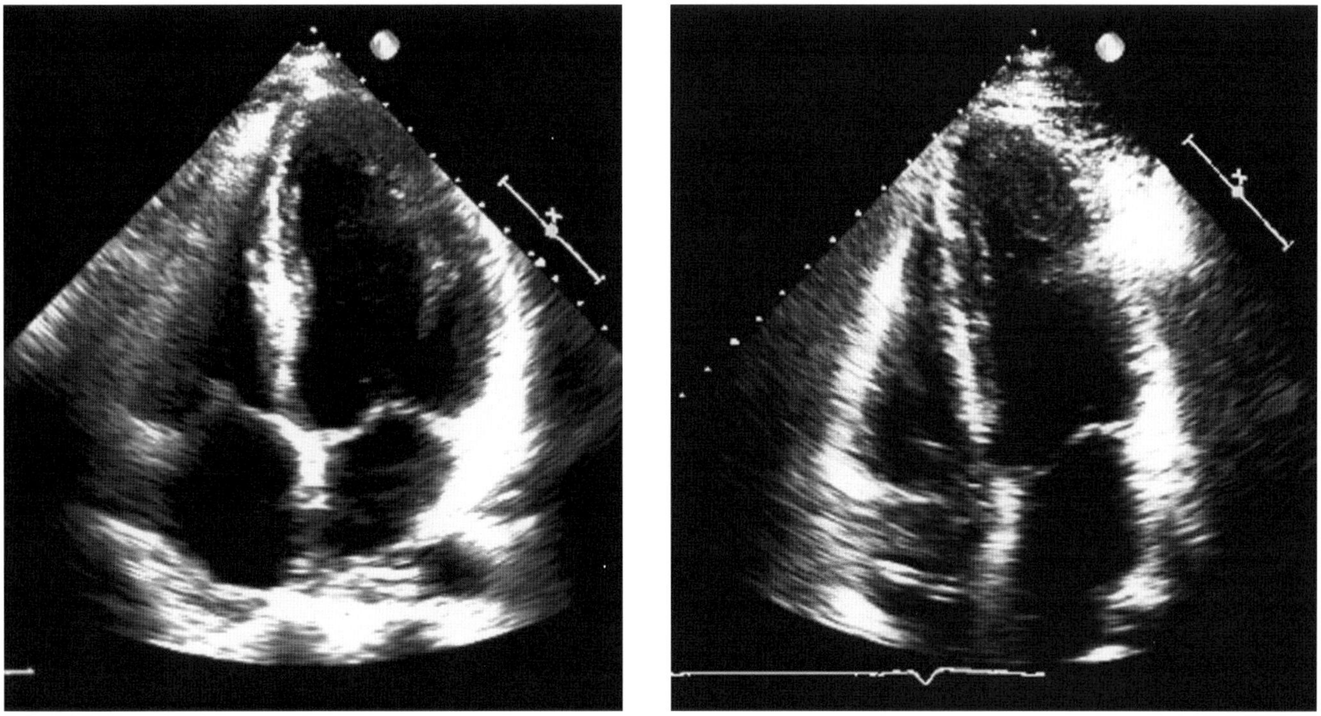

Figure 7-1

Four chamber view of two-dimensional echocardiography in end-systole. The left panel shows images at presentation with heart failure symptoms. There is left ventricular dilatation with left ventricular end systolic diameter of 43 mm. Left ventricular ejection fraction was 35% due to global hypokinesis with dys-sychrony of septal and lateral wall motions. The right panel demonstrates reverse remodeling of the LV with reduction in left ventricular end systolic diameter to 32 mm. Left ventricular ejection fraction had improved to 45%. (See also **Video 7-1A** and **Video 7-1B** by visiting the following links; http://www.demosmedpub.com/video/?vid=836 and http://www.demosmedpub.com/video/?vid=837).

Note: LV = left ventricle.

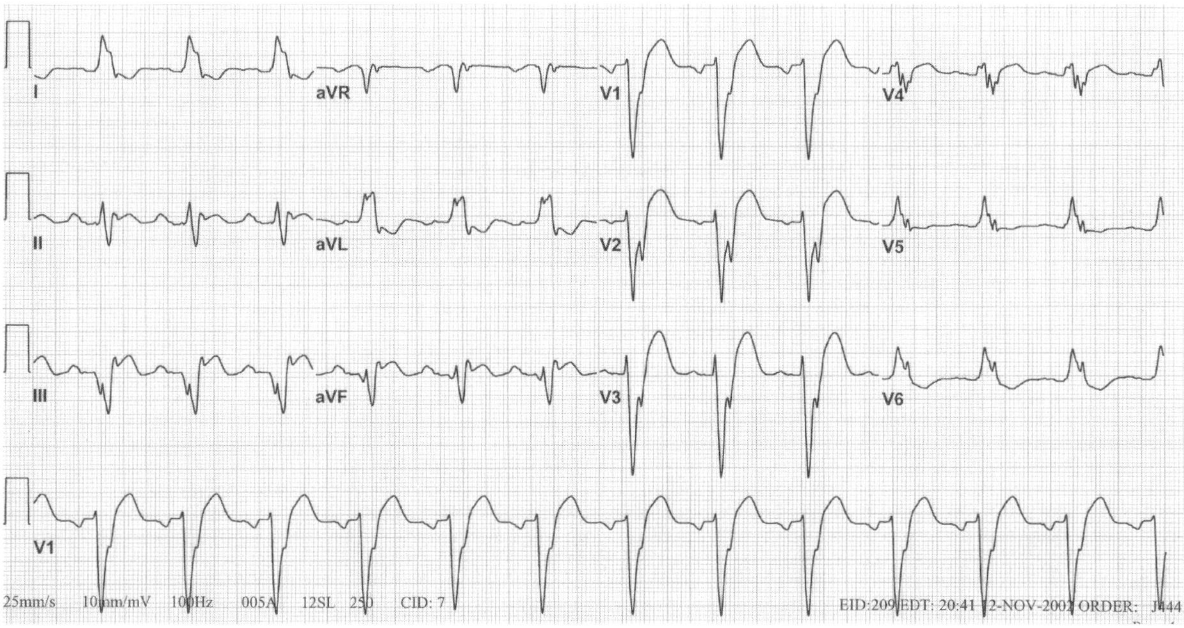

(A)

Figure 7-2

(A) Twelve-lead electrocardiograms at presentation and following biventricular pacing (cardiac resynchronization therapy) are shown. *(Continued)*

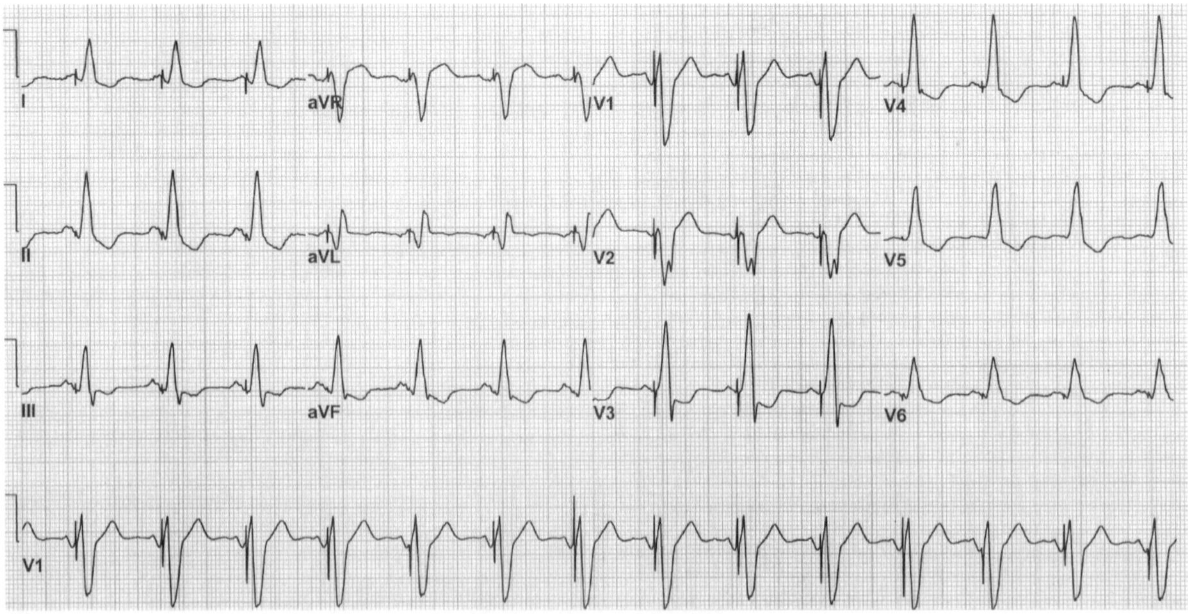

(B)

Figure 7-2 *(Continued)*
(B) The baseline ECG shows left bundle branch block with QRS duration of 200 msec. Figure 7-2B shows atrial synchronized biventricular pacing. The QRS duration has narrowed to 160 msec and there is fusion between left and right ventricular pacing evidenced by prominent R wave in lead V1. Small q wave leads I and aVL suggests early activation of the lateral left ventricular wall.

device confirmed an episode of ventricular tachycardia that was terminated by an ICD shock. Sotalol was commenced in a dose of 120 mg bid and carvedilol was decreased to 12.5 mg bid. He was rehospitalized a month later with two further ICD shocks, both deemed appropriate with prompt conversion of rapid ventricular tachycardia to sinus rhythm (**Figure 7-3**). He is referred for further electrophysiological evaluation.

CASE HIGHLIGHTS

The clinical case described above highlights several aspects of systolic heart failure secondary to an idiopathic non-ischemic dilated cardiomyopathy (NIDCM). After initial evaluation excluded treatable cause such as coronary artery disease, valvular heart disease, sarcoidosis, hemachromatosis, and acute myocarditis, management was directed at acute relief of congestion. Although relief from congestive symptoms was rapidly achieved with diuretics and vasodilators, the patient remained functionally limited. The presence of LBBB and resulting dyssynchrony of ventricular contraction provided an additional avenue for directing therapy to correct mechanical dyssynchrony by implementing CRT. In addition, the patient experienced syncope, a symptom that has major implications for prognosis and treatment in the context of systolic left ventricular dysfunction. Finally, ventricular arrhythmias that trigger ICD shocks are experienced by a significant number of patients with heart failure. Management of these various aspects in patients with NIDCM and heart failure is discussed.

PROBLEM OF QRS WIDENING IN THE HEART FAILURE PATIENT

QRS widening on a surface ECG reflects intraventricular conduction delay. While right bundle branch block (RBBB) is more common as an incidental finding in normal individuals without overt heart disease, LBBB is more common in association with heart disease (1). Prolongation of the QRS (greater than 120 msec) is estimated to occur in approximately 25% to 30% of patients with heart failure. LBBB is almost five times more common than RBBB and is a significant predictor of adverse outcome (2–5). In one study, QRS duration greater than 120 msec had a threefold increase in combined end point of death or cardiac transplantation (6). A stepwise increment in the prevalence of systolic left ventricular dysfunction is observed as QRS complex duration increases progressively over 120 msec (7, 8). In addition, wider QRS has been shown to be associated with a higher prevalence of mitral valve regurgitation (9). Simultaneous activation of the left and right bundles in the normal heart ensures synchronized electromechanical activation of both ventricles with the lateral wall of the left ventricle activated within 20 to 40 msec of septal activation (**Figure 7-4**, left panel).

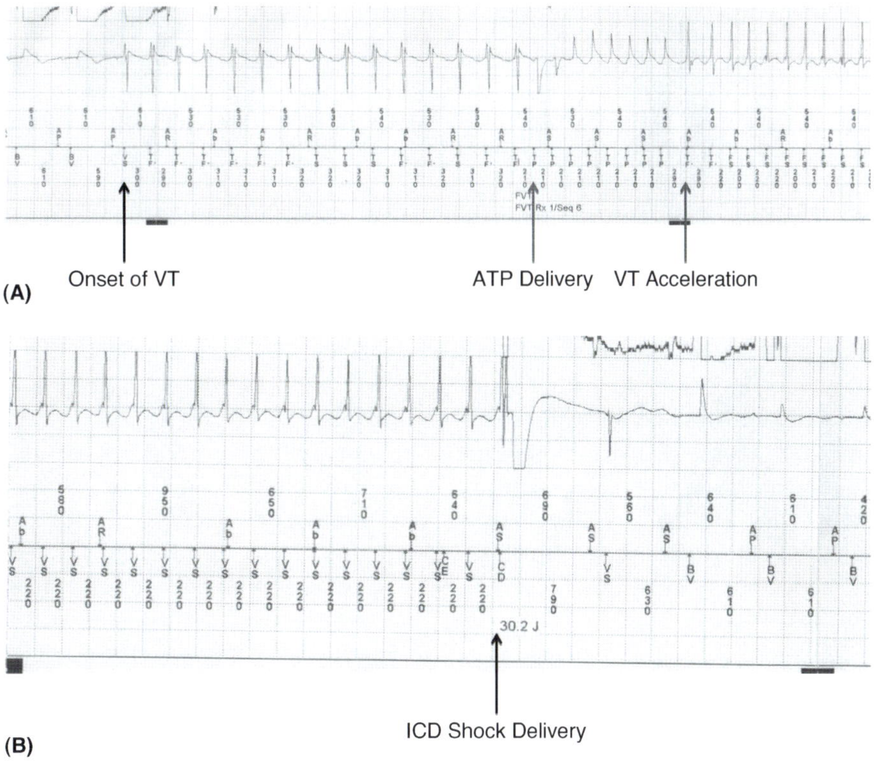

Figure 7-3
Stored electrograms from CRT-D demonstrating sequential therapies for an episode of spontaneous VT. Top to bottom: bipolar electrogram recorded from the right ventricular lead, atrial markers and cycle lengths, and ventricular markers and cycle lengths. The first two complexes in Figure 7-3A are due to atrial pacing (AP) followed by biventricular pacing (BV). The third complex is the onset of a monomorphic VT at a cycle length of 290 to 320 msec (rate 187 to 206 bpm). When detection criteria are met, antitachycardia is delivered at 210 msec in an attempt to terminate the VT by overdrive pacing. However, the train of 8 beats of rapid pacing (TP) fails to terminate VT. The VT is converted to a faster monomorphic VT at cycle length of 220 msec (272 bpm). Figure 7-3B shows detection of the accelerated VT by the ICD and delivery of a 30 J shock with restoration of sinus rhythm (AS followed by VS). CRT is re-established for the second beat of sinus rhythm (BV).

Note: CRT-D = implantable cardioverter defibrillator with cardiac resynchronization therapy; VT = ventricular tachycardia.

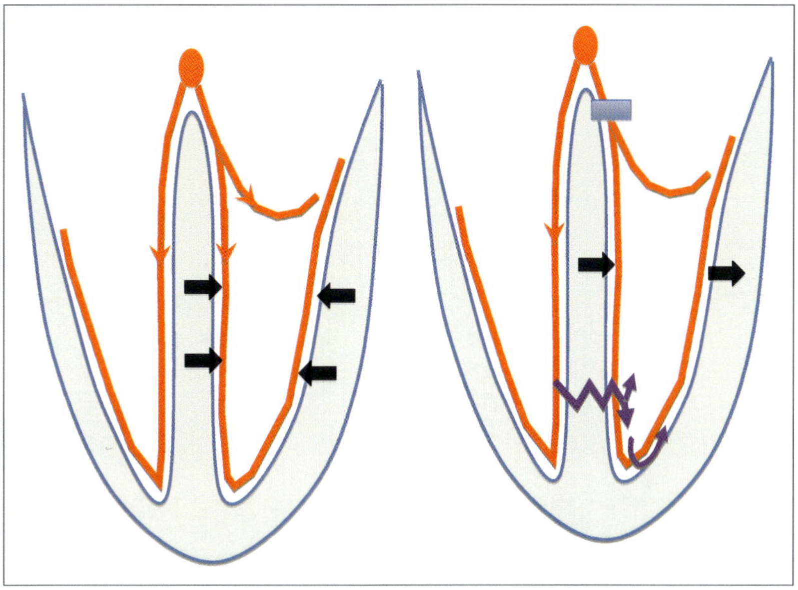

Figure 7-4
Left ventricular electromechanical activation during normal conduction (left panel) and during conduction with LBBB (right panel). Normal intraventricular conduction allows for synchronized activation of the septum and lateral left ventricular wall (black arrows). LBBB delays left ventricular lateral wall activation. The LV is activated transeptally and the impulse travels posteriorly and inferiorly to activate the lateral wall (purple arrows).

Note: LBBB = left bundle branch block; LV = left ventricle.

LBBB completely alters electrical activation of the left ventricle and has been well studied in patients with systolic heart failure using three-dimensional mapping techniques. The activation of the interventricular septum, which is normally left to right, originates on the right side and propagates inferiorly, to the left and slightly anteriorly. From its site of earliest left ventricular breakthrough, activation spreads superiorly and inferiorly reaching the lateral and posterolateral regions by propagating inferiorly around the apex and the inferior wall in a U-shaped activation pattern (**Figure 7-4**, right panel; 10). Activation of the lateral wall can thus be delayed in excess of 100 msec, and usually by 65% to 75% of the total QRS duration (**Figure 7-5**). The resulting left ventricular dysychrony is mechanically inefficient depressing left ventricular ejection fraction and cardiac output. Mitral valve closure is delayed resulting in regurgitation.

ROLE OF CARDIAC RESYNCHRONIZATION

The observation of mechanical dyssynchrony created by abnormal ventricular activation led to the concept of simultaneous biventricular pacing or left ventricular pacing to restore synchronous left ventricular contraction. This "resynchronization" of ventricular activation is achieved by implantating a pacemaker or ICD that, in addition to providing RV pacing, has an additional port for left ventricular pacing. Left ventricular pacing can often be achieved by placing a pacing lead in a left ventricular branch of the coronary sinus for epicardial stimulation (**Figure 7-6**). Rarely, in fewer than 5% of patients, anatomic limitations require that the epicardial lead be placed surgically.

This form of pacing, termed CRT, tends to narrow QRS duration (**Figure 7-2B**), although QRS durations can be variable and narrowing is not always necessary to obtain mechanical benefit from CRT (11). Acute hemodynamic studies of CRT pacing have shown improved left ventricular contractility and cardiac output, an increase in pulse pressure, and a decrease in pulmonary capillary wedge pressure (**Figure 7-7**; 12, 13). These improvements in left ventricular function occur without increasing myocardial oxygen consumption unlike inotropic agents (14). Approximately 70% of patients with adequate CRT pacing will demonstrate persistent echocardiographic improvement in left ventricular ejection fraction and reversal of left ventricular remodeling with reduction in left ventricular chamber dimensions (**Figure 7-1**) over the longer term (15). In addition, mitral regurgitation will be significantly reduced (16).

CRT has been well studied in randomized clinical trials involving over 6,000 patients. Once patients have been treated with optimal medical therapy

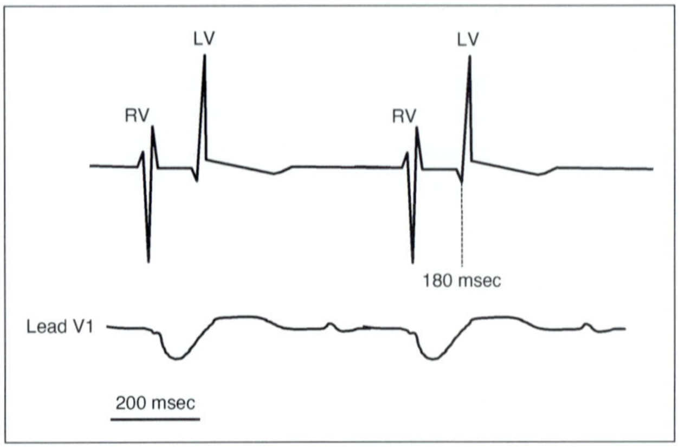

Figure 7-5
Electrogram (top panel) recorded simultaneously from a point of earliest activation in the right ventricular base and latest activation in the left ventricular lateral wall in a patient with NIDCM and LBBB is shown. The conduction time between the two points of recording is markedly prolonged at 180 msec.

Note: LBBB = left bundle branch block; NIDCM = non-ischemic dilated cardiomyopathy.

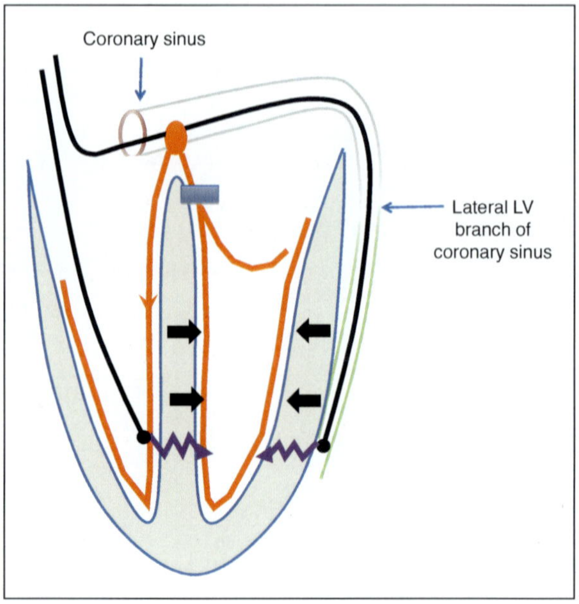

Figure 7-6
A pacing lead in the right ventricle toward the apex and another in a lateral left ventricle branch of the coronary sinus to overlie the epicardium of the LV lateral wall can achieve simultaneous electrical activation (purple arrows) to restore mechanical synchrony and improve left ventricular function.

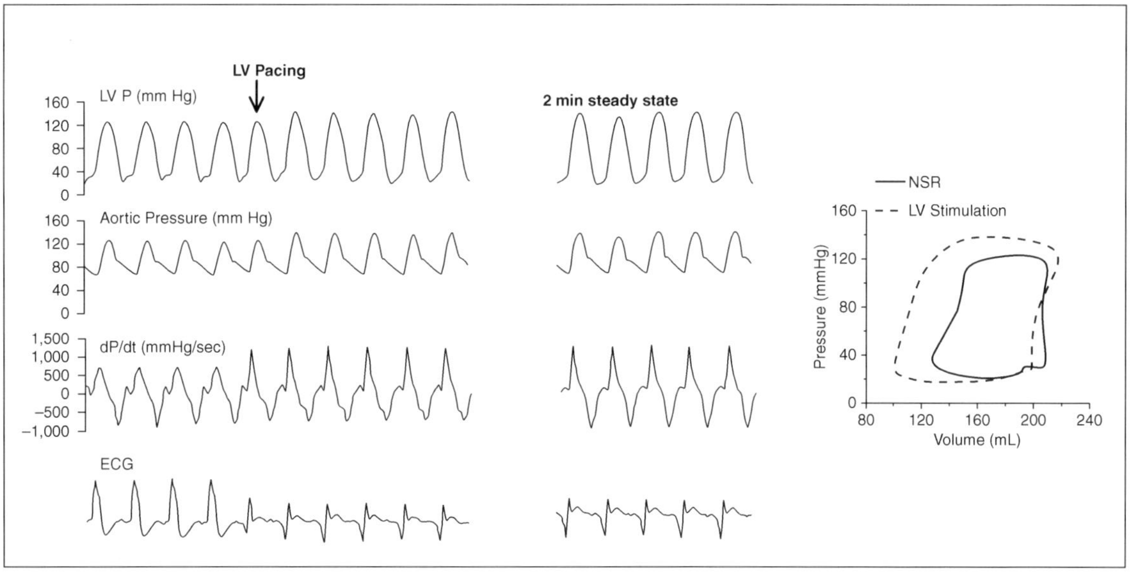

Figure 7-7
Tracings (top to bottom) of left ventricular pressure, aortic pressure, left ventricular maximal dP/dt, and ECG before and after left ventricular stimulation in a patient with NIDCM and LBBB (left panel). Acute increments in left ventricular pressure, aortic pulse pressure, and left ventricular dP/dT are sustained for a 2 minute period of steady state pacing. The left ventricular pressure volume loop (right panel) displays an increase in loop area and width (stroke work and volume, respectively) and a decrease in the end systolic volume with pacing.

Note: LBBB = left bundle branch block; NIDCM = non-ischemic dilated cardiomyopathy.

Source: Reproduced from reference 14.

including beta-blockers and angiotensin converting enzyme blockers or angiotensin receptor blockers, the use of CRT pacing in patients with left ventricular systolic dysfunction with ejection fraction less than 35%, QRS duration greater than 120 msec, and NYHA Class III or IV heart failure symptoms has been shown to improve functional level, quality of life, reduce hospitalization for heart failure, and reduce overall mortality (17–19). Recent trials of CRT in less symptomatic patients (NYHA Class I and II) show a reduction in the composite end point of heart failure hospitalization and death, but mortality reduction is limited to NYHA Class II patients (20–23). Trials have consistently demonstrated reverse remodeling of the ventricles with reduction in ventricular volume and improved ejection fraction in those who respond. It should be recognized that in all but one trial, CRT pacing was combined with an ICD.

In responders, improvement in functional capacity and symptoms occurs early and is usually evident within the first month after successful implantation of a CRT device. However, a third of patients fail to improve (nonresponders). A number of factors may play a role in failures of response to CRT. Loss of CRT pacing may occur when conduction through the AV node arrives before the left ventricular paced impulse occurs, as is particularly a problem during rapid atrial fibrillation (see below). Left ventricular pacing may fail to improve the activation sequence when the left ventricular lead position is inadequate, which is usually a result of unfavorable cardiac anatomy. Abnormal conduction around scars in the left ventricle can also alter activation patterns such that mechanical synchrony proves difficult to achieve. Even with left ventricular pacing, cardiac function may fail to improve due to large areas of infarct related scarred myocardium that cannot be recruited to contract with pacing. In post hoc subgroup analyses of clinical trials, factors associated with the most benefit from CRT are: NIDCM, LBBB, and QRS duration greater than 150 msec. CRT device implantation is more difficult that placement of a non-CRT pacemaker or ICD and complication rates are greater, usually related to the additional manipulations required for the lead and its delivery systems. Lead dislodgement requiring revision is particularly more common (24). Patient selection for this therapy is therefore critical.

Careful follow-up of patients with a CRT device is equally important. The occasional patient may deteriorate after initial response. The possibility of loss of CRT pacing should be an early consideration in such patients, the most common cause being the onset of atrial arrhythmia with rapid native ventricular conduction. Restoration of sinus rhythm and adequate heart rate control often results in recovery of benefit. The use of CRT in patients with persistent or established atrial fibrillation is less well studied than in patients with sinus rhythm. Smaller studies suggest improvement in functional status and quality of life as long as AV nodal conduction can be sufficiently slowed to allow adequate pacing. In a significant number of patients, this will require ablation of the AV node (25, 26).

In a small group of patients (approximately 10%), CRT pacing can lead to deterioration of left ventricular function and functional class (27). This may be related to poor patient selection for such therapy or other, as yet unrecognized factors. If a clear deterioration is documented related to CRT pacing, it is important to consider inactivation of CRT pacing.

SYNCOPE IN NIDCM

Syncope is a common clinical problem and usually cardiovascular in origin. Vasovagal or reflex mechanisms are the predominant causes. When associated with structural heart disease or electrical heart disease, syncope portends a poor prognosis. The frequency of syncope in the heart failure population is not well defined. In the U.S. Carvedilol study, 33% of patients had dizzy spells but only 0.3% had syncope (28). In patients with non-ischemic cardiomyopathy and heart failure, syncope is associated with increased mortality regardless of its origin (29–31). The likely mechanism of increased mortality in the cardiomyopathy patient is ventricular tachycardia, suggesting that the syncopal event is often the result of self-terminating ventricular tachycardia that tends to be recurrent and can subsequently lead to cardiac arrest.

The differential diagnosis of syncope in NIDCM is similar to that in patients without heart disease. They include arrhythmias, orthostatic and drug-induced hypotension, pulmonary embolism, and vasodepressor syncope. However, unless the circumstances excluding an arrhythmia are absolutely clear, such as an episode of orthostasis that occurs during cardiac monitoring, the probability of an arrhythmic etiology is so high that protection against sudden arrhythmic death has to be a serious consideration. There are no diagnostic tests that can reliably determine the risk for sudden death in this population. Impaired ventricular function remains, however, a consistent marker for sudden death risk. Detection of myocardial scar or fibrosis by late gadolinium enhancement on cardiac magnetic resonance imaging has been shown to be associated with higher ventricular arrhythmia event rates (32). Presence of myocardial scars frequently helps in decisions regarding ICD therapy when left ventricular dysfunction is mild. Other noninvasive tests such as signal averaged ECG, heart rate variability, and T-wave alternans lack adequate predictive value to be significantly contributory in management decisions. Intracardiac electrophysiological testing is often performed to define cardiac conduction and the presence of inducible arrhythmias. In NIDCM, however, it is less useful than in patients with prior myocardial infarction, and a negative test does not adequately exclude an arrhythmic etiology and subsequent risk of sudden death (33, 34).

There are no randomized studies to guide the management of syncope in NIDCM. Empiric use of antiarrhythmic drugs such as amiodarone has no proven value. Retrospective data from patients implanted with ICDs show a high rate of appropriate ICD discharges in patients with NIDCM and syncope regardless of outcome of electrophysiological studies (31, 34, 35). Based on these data and high mortality rate for syncope in the context of left ventricular dysfunction and heart failure, the current guidelines recommend the use of an ICD as a Class IIa indication (a reasonable consideration despite the lack of randomized trial data) for unexplained syncope in NIDCM (36).

PREVENTION OF SUDDEN CARDIAC DEATH IN NIDCM

The non-ischemic cardiomyopathies being more hetereogenous in etiology and progression have a more variable prognosis compared to the ischemic cardiomyopathies. The early clinical trials of ICD for sudden death prevention were oriented to patients with coronary artery disease and included few patients with NIDCM. In the presence of advanced heart failure, the risk of ventricular arrhythmia and sudden death appears to parallel those with coronary artery disease with an estimated event rate of 15% to 30% over 3 years (37). The severity of left ventricular dysfunction closely parallels the risk for such arrhythmic events although, as functional class deteriorates, the risk of pump failure gains prominence as the primary cause of death.

For secondary prevention, clinical trials have consistently shown benefit from the use of ICD over antiarrhythmic drugs such as amiodarone (38–40) The role of the ICD for primary prevention of sudden death in NIDCM is less straightforward. Two early small trials limited to NIDCM patients showed no benefit due to a low event rate or inadequate power to reach the end point (41, 42). The DEFINITE trial showed a reduction in arrhythmic mortality but did not reduce total mortality significantly (43). Two subsequent larger studies of patients with Class II to IV heart failure included NIDCM patients as half their study population. The SCD-Heft trial showed a 27% reduction in total mortality for NIDCM patients (44). The COMPANION trial tested the effect of cardiac resynchronization therapy with an ICD or pacemaker in heart failure patients. Once again, ICD patients derived a significant mortality benefit (45).

The current guidelines recommend the use of a prophylactic ICD for patients with chronic heart failure symptoms and left ventricular ejection fraction less than or equal to 35% provided that they are expected to survive more than 1 year with reasonable function (36), CRT should be combined for those with QRS prolongation due to LBBB, particularly when QRS duration is greater than 150 ms, or when frequent right ventricular pacing is anticipated, due to bradyarrhythmias. It should be kept in mind that a significant number of patients with newly diagnosed NIDCM will have improvement in left ventricular function with implementation of medical therapy for heart failure. In the absence of symptoms that suggest dangerous arrhythmia, device implantation should be deferred as medical therapy is initiated for 3 to 6 months, followed by reassessment for consideration of a prophylactic ICD.

MANAGEMENT OF RECURRENT VENTRICULAR ARRHYTHMIAS IN NIDCM

The ICD, while effective for the prevention of sudden death, has no significant role in preventing or suppressing ventricular arrhythmias. The overall incidence of ICD shocks in an ICD recipient is 14% in the first year, the majority being appropriate for ventricular arrhythmias (46). In patients with a history of ventricular tachycardia (VT), shock rates are higher. Although programming changes to implement more aggressive antitachycardia pacing therapies can reduce shock rates, ICD shocks are painful, reduce quality of life, and cause a posttraumatic stress disorder. In addition, ICD shocks are a marker for progressive heart failure and increased mortality (47). Hence, antiarrhythmic drugs and ablation strategies, often in combination, are necessary to suppress recurrences of ventricular arrhythmias. Beta-blockers including sotalol and amiodarone have been shown to reduce ICD shocks (48). However, drug therapy is associated with toxicities that lead to discontinuation in up to a quarter of patients. Further, antiarrhythmic drugs are often inadequate for the prevention of recurrent scar related VT, and arrhythmia breakthrough is common, manifesting as slow incessant VT or multiple recurrences provoking an electrical storm with multiple ICD shocks (49).

For patients, with episodes of monomorphic VT, catheter ablation can markedly reduce arrhythmia recurrences and ICD shocks (50–52). Ablation can be lifesaving when VT is incessant. The greatest experience with VT ablation is in patients with coronary artery disease. Data on ablation in non-ischemic patients are largely limited to single centers, but acute results are comparable although recurrences appear to be more frequent (52,53). Sustained monomorphic VT in the NIDCM patient is usually due to reentry through regions of scar. Although the mechanism is similar to that observed for post–infarct VTs in ischemic cardiomyopathy, the etiology of the scar is probably replacement fibrosis associated with the disease process, rather than infarction. The scar locations are also different, tending to be more perivalvular and often intramural or subepicardial in location (53,54). Percutaneous access to the epicardium for mapping and ablation has increased success rates of VT ablation in this patient population (52).

Findings from electrophysiologic study and catheter ablation of VT in a patient with non-ischemic dilated cardiomyopathy are shown in **Figure 7-8**. Programmed ventricular stimulation induced sustained monomorphic VT (**Figure 7-8**, Panel A). Although the VT rate is only 150 beats/min, blood pressure promptly declined to less than 50 mmHg systolic, and VT was promptly terminated by a burst of pacing (not shown). Despite the fact that the VT was not stable for mapping during VT, ablation could still be performed by identifying the region of the scar that contains the reentry circuit by mapping during sinus rhythm, a process referred to as substrate mapping. **Figure 7-8** Panel B shows a voltage map of the left ventricle created on a three-dimensional electroanatomic mapping system. The colors indicate the peak to peak electrogram amplitude. Purple is normal (greater than 1.5 mV) and blue, green, yellow, and red are progressively lower amplitude, indicative of scar. An area of scar is present in the posterolateral left ventricle adjacent to the mitral annulus. In addition to endocardial mapping via retrograde access, a catheter was also inserted via subxiphoid pericardial puncture into the pericardial space for epicardial mapping. Panels C and D show coronary angiograms taken to identify the relation of the coronary arteries to the epicardial scar location identified by the mapping catheter (yellow arrow). Examination of the electrograms and pacing in this scar region indicated that it contained slowly

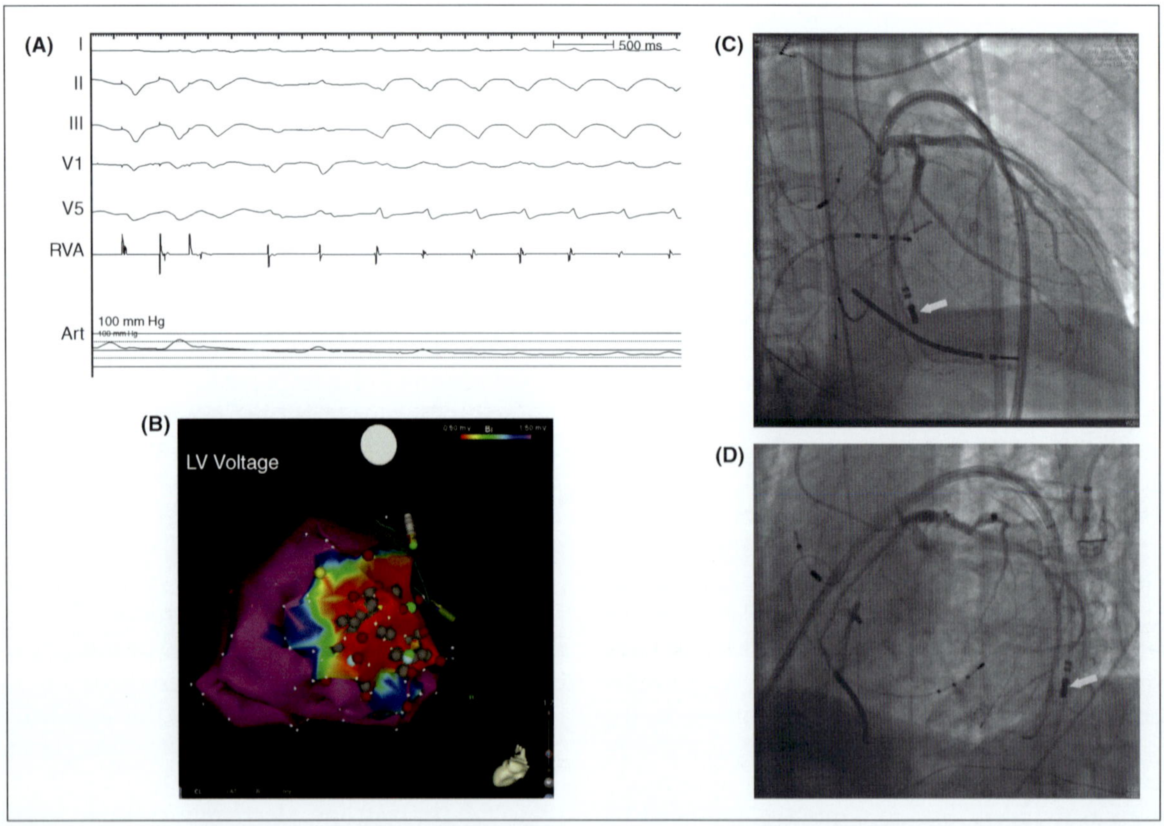

Figure 7-8
Findings from mapping and ablation of sustained monomorphic VT in a patient with NIDCM are shown. Panel A shows initiation of VT by programmed stimulation. Panel B shows the left ventricular endocardial voltage map, with an area of postero-basal scar. The ventricle is viewed from a left posterior oblique position, with mitral annulus at the right and apex toward the left hand side of the figure. Panels C (RAO) and D (LAO) show coronary angiography taken after an ablation catheter has been placed in the pericardial space and positioned at an epicardial, low voltage region in the postero-basal left ventricle (see text for discussion).

Note: LAO = left anterior oblique; NIDCM = non-ischemic dilated cardiomyopathy; RAO = right anterior oblique.

conducting channels that are a likely substrate for VT. Ablation was then performed through that region. The maroon circular tags in Panel B indicate ablation sites. The gray circular tags are areas of dense scar where pacing could not capture myocardial tissue. Ablation abolished the VT shown in Panel A.

SUMMARY

The patient described in the clinical vignette represents a fairly typical pattern of clinical events seen in patients with heart failure and NIDCM. He underwent successful and uncomplicated catheter-based ablation for recurrent ventricular arrhythmias and has remained free of further episodes of VT over a 9-month period of follow-up.

Electrophysiologic abnormalities are important features of the pathophysiology of non-ischemic cardiomyopathies. LBBB delays ventricular activation, causing dyssynchronous activation that further impairs ventricular function. This abnormality can be reversed or improved by CRT. Atrial arrhythmias are common and often require therapy. Atrial arrhythmias can disrupt the application of CRT when AV conduction during rapid atrial fibrillation or flutter prevents appropriate left ventricular pacing. Ventricular arrhythmias are an important cause of sudden death. Syncope is a serious symptom that indicates a high risk of sudden death in this disease. Implantable defibrillators reduce the risk of death, but do not prevent arrhythmias from occurring. Patients who develop sustained ventricular tachycardia usually have areas of scar that have developed within the ventricles. These regions are the substrate for re-entrant VT, which is often refractory to antiarrhythmic drug therapy, and may require catheter ablation. Recognition of the electrophysiologic consequences of cardiomyopathies has important implications for improving heart failure, reducing symptoms, and preventing sudden death.

REFERENCES

1. Rowland DJ. Left and right bundle branch block, left anterior and left posterior hemiblock. *Eur Heart J*. 1984;5(suppl A):A99–A105.
2. Bader H, Garrigue S, Lafitte S, et al. Intra-left ventricular electromechanical asynchrony. A new independent predictor of severe cardiac events in heart failure patients. *J Am Coll Cardiol*. 2004;43:248–256.
3. Juliano S, Fisher SG, Karasik PE, Fletcher RD, Singh SN. QRS duration and mortality in patients with congestive heart failure. *Am Heart J*. 2002;143:1085–1091.
4. Lewinter C, Torp-Pedersen C, Cleland JGF, Keber L. Right and left bundle branch block as predictors of long term mortality following myocardial infarction. *Eur J Heart Fail*. 2011;13: 1349–1354.
5. Baldasseroni S, Opasich C, Gorini M, et al. Left bundle branch block is associated with increated 1-year sudden and total mortality in 5517 outpatients with congestive heart failure: a report from the Italian network on congestive heart failure. *Am Heart J*. 2002;143:398–405.
6. Kalra PR, Sharma R, Shamim W, et al. Clinical characteristics and survival of patients with chronic heart failure and prolonged QRS duration. *J Cardiol*. 2002;86:225–231.
7. Shenkman HJ, Pampati V, Khandelwal AK, et al. Congestive heart failure and QRS duration: establishing prognosis study. *Chest*. 2002;122:528–534
8. Murkofsky RL, Dangas G, Diamond JA, Mehta D, Scheaffer A, Ambrose JA. A prolonged QRS duration on surface electrocardiogram is a specific indicator of left ventricular dysfunction. *J Am Coll Cardiol*. 1998;32:476–482.
9. Sandhu R, Bahler RC. Prevalence of QRS prolongation in a community hospital cohort of patients with heart failure and its relation to left ventricular systolic dysfunction. *Am J Cardiol*. 2004;93:244–246.
10. Auricchio A, Fantoni C, Regoli F, et al. Characterization of left ventricular activation in patients with heart failure and left bundle branch block. *Circulation*. 2004;109:1133–1139.
11. Turner MS, Bleasdale RA, Vienreanu D, et al. Electrical and mechanical components of dyssynchrony in heart failure patients with normal QRS duration and left bundle branch block: impact of left and biventricular pacing. *Circulation*. 2004;109:2544–2549.
12. Kass DA, Chen CH, Curry C, et al. Improved left ventricular mechanics from acute VDD pacing in patients with dilated cardiomyopathy and ventricular conduction delay. *Circulation*. 1999;99:1567–1573.
13. Leclercq C, Cazeau S, Le Breton H, et al. Acute hemodynamic effects of biventricular DDD pacing in patients with end stage heart failure. *J Am Coll Cardiol*. 1998;32:1825–1831.
14. Nelson GS, Berger RD, Fetics BJ, et al. Left ventricular or biventricular pacing improves cardiac function at diminished energy costs in patients with dilated cardiomyopathy and left bundle branch block. *Circulation*. 2000;102:3053–3059.
15. St John Sutton MG, Plappert T, Abraham WT et al. Effect of cardiac resynchronization therapy on left ventricular size and function in chronic heart failure. *Circulation*. 2003;107:1985–1990.
16. Cazeau S, Leclercq C, Lavergne T, Walker S, et al. Effects of multisite biventricular pacing in patients with heart failure and intraventricular conduction delay. *N Engl J Med*. 2001;344:873–880.
17. Cleland JG, Daubert JC, Erdmann E., et al. The effect of of cardiac resynchronization on morbidity and mortality in heart failure. *N Engl J Med*. 2005;353:1539–1549
18. Bristow MR, Saxon LA, Boehmer J, et al. Cardiac resynchronization therapy in with or without an implantable defibrillator in advanced chronic heart failure. *N Engl J Med*. 2004;350: 2140–2150.
19. Abraham WT, Fisher WG, Smith AL, et al. Cardiac resynchronization in chronic heart failure. *N Engl J Med*. 2002;346:1845–1853.
20. Moss AJ, Hall WJ, Cannom DS, et al. Cardiac resynchronization therapy for the prevention of heart failure events. *N Engl J Med*. 2009;361:1329–1338.
21. Tang ASL, Wells GA, Talajic M, et al. Cardiac resynchronization therapy for mild to moderate heart failure. *N Engl J Med*. 2010;363:2385–2395.
22. Daubert C, Gold MR, Abraham WT, et al. Prevention of disease progression by cardiac resynchronization therapy in pateitns with asymptomatic or mildly symptomatic left ventricular dysfunction: insights from the European cohort of the REVERSE (Resynchronization Reverses Remodeling in Systolic Left Ventricular Dysfunction) trial. *J Am Coll Cardiol*. 2009;54:1837–1846.
23. Santangeli P, Di Biase L, Pelargonio G, et al. Cardiac resynchronization therapy in patients with mild heart failure: a systematic review and meta-analysis. *J Interv Card Electrophysiol*. 2011;32:125–135.
24. van Rees JB, de Bie MK, Thijssen J, Borleffs CJ, Schalij MJ, van Erven L. Implantation-related complications of implantable cardioverter-defibrillators and cardiac resynchronization therapy devices: a systematic review of randomized clinical trials. *J Am Coll Cardiol*. August 30, 2011;58(10):995–1000.
25. Upadhyay GA, Choudhry NK, Auricchio A, Ruskin J, Singh JP. Cardiac resynchronization in patients with atrial fibrillation. A meta-analysis of prospective cohort studies. *J Am Coll Cardiol*. 2008;52:1239–1246.
26. Kaszala K, Ellenbogen KA. Role of cardiac resynchronization therapy and atrioventricular junction ablation in patients with permanent atrial fibrillation. *Eur Heart J*. 2011;32:2344–2346.
27. Chung ES, Leon AR, Tavazzi L, et al. Results of the predictors of response to CRT (PROSPECT) trial. *Circulation*. 2008;117:2608–2616.
28. Packer M, Bristow MR, Cohn JN, et al, The effect of carvedilol on morbidity and mortality n patients with chronic heart failure: US Cardvedilol in Heart Failure Study Group. *N Engl J Med*. 1996;334:1349–1355.
29. Singh SK, Link MS, Wang PJ, Homoud M, Estes MNA III. Syncope in the patient with nonischemic dilated cardiomyopathy. *Pacing and Clin Electrophysiol*. 2004;27:97–100
30. Middlekauff HR, Stevenson WG, Stervenson LW, Saon LA. Syncope in advanced heart failure: high risk of sudden death regardless of origin of syncope. *J Am Coll Cardiol*. 1993;21:110–116.
31. Fonarow GC, Feliciano Z, Boyle NG, Knight L, Woo MA, Moriguchi JD, Laks H, Wiener I. Improved survival in patients with non-ischemic advanced heart failure and syncope treated with an implantable cardioverter-defibrillator. *Am J Cardiol*. 2000;85:981–5.
32. Iles L, Pfluger H, Lefkovits L, et al. Myocardial fibrosis predicts appropriate device therapy in patients with implantable cardioverter-defibrillators for primary prevention of sudden cardiac death. *J Am Coll Cardiol*. 2011;57: 821–828.
33. Knight BP, Goyal R, Pelosi F, Flemming M, Horwood L, Morady F, Strickberger SA. Outcome of patients with nonischemic dilated cardiomyopathy and unexplained syncope treated with an implantable defibrillator. *J Am Coll Cardiol*. 1999;33:1964.
34. Russo AM, Verdino R, Schorr C, Nicholas M, Dias D, Hsia H, Callans D, Marchlinski FE. Occurrence of implantable defibrillator events in patients with syncope and nonischemic dilated cardiomyopathy. *Am J Cardiol*. 2001;88:1444–1446.

35. Olshanky B, Poole JE, Johnson G, et al. Syncope predicts outcome of cardiomyopathy patients. Analysis of the SCD-HeFT study. *J Am Coll Cardiol.* 2008;51:1277–1282.
36. Epstein AE, DiMarco JP, Ellenbogen KA, et al. ACC/AHA/HRS 2008 guidelines for device based therapy of cardiac rhythm abnormalities: a report of the American College of Cardiology/American Heart Association Task Force on Practice Guidelines (Writing committee to Revise the ACC/AHA/NASPE 2002 Guideline Update for Implantation of Cardiac Pacemakers and Arntiarrhytmia Devices) developed in collaboration with the American Association for Thoracic Surgery and Society for Thoracic Surgeons. *J Am Coll Cardiol.* 2008;51:e1–e62.
37. Grimm W, Hoffman J, Muller H, Maisch B. Implantable defibrillator event rates in patients with idiopathic dilated cardiomyopathy, nonsustained ventricular tachycardia on Holter and a left ventricular ejection fraction below 30%. *J Am Coll Cardiol.* 2002;39:780–787.
38. The Antiarrhythmics Versus Implantable Defibrillator (AVID) Investigators. A comparison of antiarrhythmic-drug therapy with implantable defibrillators in patients resuscitated from near fatal ventricular arrhythmias. *N Engl J Med.* 1997;337:1576–1583.
39. Connolly SJ, Gent M, Roberts RS, et al. Canadial Implantable Defibrillator Study (CIDS). A randomized trial of the implantable cardioverter defibrillator against amiodarone. *Circulation.* 2000;101:1297–1302.
40. Kuck KH, Cappato R, Siebels J, Ruppel R. for the CASH Investigators. Randomized comparison of antiarrhythmic drug therapy with implantable defibrillator in patients resuscitated from cardiac arrest: the Cardiac Arrest Study Hamburg (CASH). *Circulation.* 2000;102:748–754.
41. Bansch D, Antz M, Boczor S, et al. Primary prevention of sudden cardiac death in idiopathic dilated cardiomyopathy. The Cardiomyopathy Trial (CAT). *Circulation.* 2002;105:1453–1458.
42. Strickberger SA, Hummel JD, Bartlett TG, et al. Amiodarone versus implantable cardioverter defibrillator randomized trial in patients with non-ischemic dilated cardiomyopathy and asymptomatic non-sustained ventricular tachycardia-AMIOVERT. *J Am Coll Cardiol.* 2003;41: 1707–1712.
43. Kadish A, Dyer A, Daubert JP, et al. Prophylactic defibrillator implantation in patients with non-ischemic dilated cardiomyopathy. *New Engl J Med* 2004;350:2151–2158.
44. Bardy GH, Lee KL, Mark DB, et al. Amiodarone or an implantable cardioverter defibrillator for congestive heart failure. *N Engl J Med.* 2005;353:225–237.
45. Bristow MR, Saxon LA, Boehmer J, et al. Cardiac resynchronization therapy with or without an implantable defibrillator in advanced chronic heart failure. N Eng J Med 2004;350: 2140–2150.
46. Saxon LA, Hayes DL, Gilliam FR, et al. Long term outcome after ICD and CRT implantation and influence of remote device follow up: The Altitude Survival Study. *Circulation.* 2010;122: 2359–2367.
47. Poole JE, Johnson GW, Hellkamp AS. Prognostic importance of defibrillator shocks in patients with heart failure. N Engl J Med 2008;359:1009–1017.
48. Connolly SJ, Dorian P, Roberts RS, et al. Comparison of beta-blockers, amiodarone plus beta blockers or sotalol for prevention of shocks from implantable cardioverter defibrillators: the OPTIC study: a randomized trial. JAMA 2006;295:165–171.
49. Credner SC, Klingenheben T, Mauss O, Sticherling C, Hohnloser SH. Electrical storm in patients with transvenous implantable cardioverter-defibrillators: incidence, management and prognostic implications. J Am Coll Cardiol 1998;32:1909–1915.
50. Stevenson WG, Wilber DJ, Natale A, et al. Irrigated radiofrequency catheter ablation guided by electroanatomic mapping for recurrent ventricular tachycardia after myocardial infarction: the multicenter thermacool ventricular tachycardia ablation trial. Circulation 2008;118:2773–2782.
51. Mallidi J, Nadkarani GN, Berger RD, et al. Meta-analysis of catheter ablation as an adjunct to medical therapy for treatment of ventricular tachycardia in patients with structural heart disease. Heart Rhythm 2011;8:503–510.
52. Aliot EM, Stevenson WG, Almendral-Garrote JM, Bogun F, Calkins CH, Delacretaz E, Della Bella P, Hindricks G, Jaïs P, Josephson ME, Kautzner J, Kay GN, Kuck KH, Lerman BB, Marchlinski F, Reddy V, Schalij MJ, Schilling R, Soejima K, Wilber D; EHRA/HRS Expert Consensus on Catheter Ablation of Ventricular Arrhythmias. Heart Rhythm. 2009;6:886–933.
53. Soejima K, Stevenson WG, Sapp JL, Selwyn AP, Couper G, Epstein LM. Endocardial and epicardial radiofrequency ablation of ventricular tachycardia associated with dilated cardiomyopathy: the importance of low-voltage scars. J Am Coll Cardiol. 2004;43:1834.
54. Hsia HH, Callans DJ, Marchlinski FE. Characterization of endocardial electrophysiological substrate in patients with nonischemic cardiomyopathy and monomorphic ventricular tachycardia. Circulation. 2003;108:704.

8

Cardiac Resynchronization Therapy in Heart Failure

ADAM P. PLEISTER AND WILLIAM T. ABRAHAM

INTRODUCTION

Cardiac resynchronization therapy (CRT), or biventricular (BiV) pacing, has emerged over the last several years as a powerful tool in the treatment of heart failure patients. Careful selection of those patients who may benefit from CRT is paramount and must be based on defined criteria to ensure maximum benefit. In this chapter, two "typical" heart failure patients will be presented: one with severe symptoms and systolic dysfunction, and another with a mild-to-moderate presentation of heart failure. A discussion of the current evidence for CRT in heart failure will follow, including clinical trial results and major society guidelines. Based on clinical and diagnostic data, the rationale for or against implantation of a CRT device in the two heart failure patients will be discussed. Further management considerations as well as prognostic features will also be addressed.

CASE PRESENTATION: PATIENT A

Patient A presents as a first-time visit to a general cardiology clinic to establish care. He is a 54-year-old African American male who recently moved from another state and wishes to have all of his cardiac care managed at this clinic. On history, he endorses chronic dyspnea with moderate exertion over the past several months, which he believes may have worsened over the past few weeks. He denies dyspnea at rest. He also reports chronic fatigue and light-headedness with moderate exertion. He admits that he can complete his activities of daily living, although it takes most of his day to do so and it leaves him fatigued. In addition, he reports orthopnea and some mild, bilateral lower extremity edema. He denies chest pain, angina, palpitations, syncope, paroxysmal nocturnal dyspnea (PND), abdominal distension, recent weight changes, or changes in appetite. He further denies depression, anxiety, vision changes, headaches, or any specific gastroenterology or genitourinary symptoms. He reports that he has been compliant with his medication regimen over the past 3 years and that he monitors his weight and blood pressure "a few times a week." He states that his weight has been stable at around 160 pounds and his blood pressure measures in the 110 to 120s systolic and 70 to 80s diastolic. A complete, 12-point review of symptoms is otherwise unremarkable. Further history and examination of his past medical records reveal a previous tobacco smoking history (20 pack-years over a 20-year period; however, he quit 12 years ago). He denies any alcohol or illicit drug use during his lifetime. He has no family history of early (before the age of 65) coronary artery disease, heart failure, sudden cardiac death, arrhythmia, or known cardiomyopathy.

Patient A's medical history is significant for non-ischemic cardiomyopathy diagnosed 3 years ago, with no specific etiology elucidated at that time. His initial left ventricular ejection fraction (LVEF) at the time of diagnosis was less than 10%. He was followed by a cardiologist for some time, but has not seen one in over a year due to his recent move from another state. Further review of records shows a transthoracic echocardiogram (TTE) report from 18 months ago that lists the following: dilated left ventricle, LVEF 20% to 25%, mild mitral regurgitation (MR), and normal right ventricular size and function. A report of a left heart catheterization from 5 years ago notes the following: normal coronary arteries, LVEF 20%, global hypokinesis. No other diagnostic data is included in his records. He had an implantable cardioverter-defibrillator (ICD) placed 2 years ago and he reports no device firing since device placement, although he has not had his device interrogated in over 12 months. Other past medical history includes systemic hypertension, mixed hyperlipidemia, type 2 diabetes mellitus for the past 4 years on oral medication only, and gout. He has no known allergies, and his current medication list is as follows: carvedilol 25 mg po bid, lisinopril 10 mg po qd, isosorbide mononitrate 30 mg po qd, hydralazine 20 mg po tid, furosemide 40 mg po qd, aspirin 81 mg po qd, simvastatin 40 mg po qhs, and metformin 500 mg po bid. Physical exam reveals a nonacute male that appears older than his stated age. His blood pressure is 112/70, heart rate is 82, and body mass index (BMI) is 25. Pertinent findings include trace rales at his bilateral posterior lung bases and 1+ bilateral lower extremity edema. His cardiac exam is significant for a laterally displaced apical beat with a II/VI holosystolic murmur heard best at the apex and radiating to the back, as well as a third heart sound.

As part of his workup, the following tests are ordered: electrocardiogram (ECG), chest x-ray (CXR), TTE, and a nuclear medicine pharmacologic stress test. ECG reveals normal sinus rhythm, heart rate 98, left bundle branch block (LBBB) with a QRS measuring 142 msec, and nonspecific T-wave changes (**Figure 8-1**). CXR shows bibasilar atelectasis with cardiomegaly (**Figure 8-2**). TTE images and report reviewed severe global hypokinesis of the left ventricle with an estimated LVEF of 20%, left ventricle mildly to moderately dilated, mild to moderate MR, mild left atrial enlargement, and mildly dilated right ventricle with mildly reduced systolic function of the right ventricle (**Figure 8-3**). Nuclear medicine pharmacologic stress test reveals a dilated left ventricle with no evidence of previous infarction or ischemia and LVEF of 23% (**Figure 8-4**). Labs reveal a slightly elevated creatinine of 1.54 but otherwise normal chemistry panel. B-type natriuretic peptide (BNP) is slightly elevated at 196 and hemoglobin A1c is 7.1. Complete blood count (CBC), thyroid-stimulating hormone (TSH), fasting lipids, and liver function tests are all within normal limits.

CASE PRESENTATION: PATIENT B

Patient B presents to a general internal medicine clinic to establish care. Her previous physician from another health care system recently retired and she unfortunately has no medical records available. She is a pleasant 45-year-old white female. On history, she reports some mild chest pain, which occurs a few times a week with a substernal location and no radiation. She says it feels "aching" in quality and is 7/10 at worst with no specific alleviating or aggravating factors and no associated symptoms. It occurs for a few minutes at a time and resolves with no specific intervention. She also reports dyspnea and fatigue with exertion; she says she can climb two flights of stairs without stopping, but due to these symptoms, she would be short of breath and tired once she got to the top. She can complete her activities of daily living without problem. She otherwise denies light-headedness, syncope, nausea/emesis, diaphoresis, PND, orthopnea, palpitations, abdominal distension, lower extremity edema, recent weight changes, or changes in appetite. She further denies anxiety, vision changes, headaches, or any specific gastroenterology or genitourinary

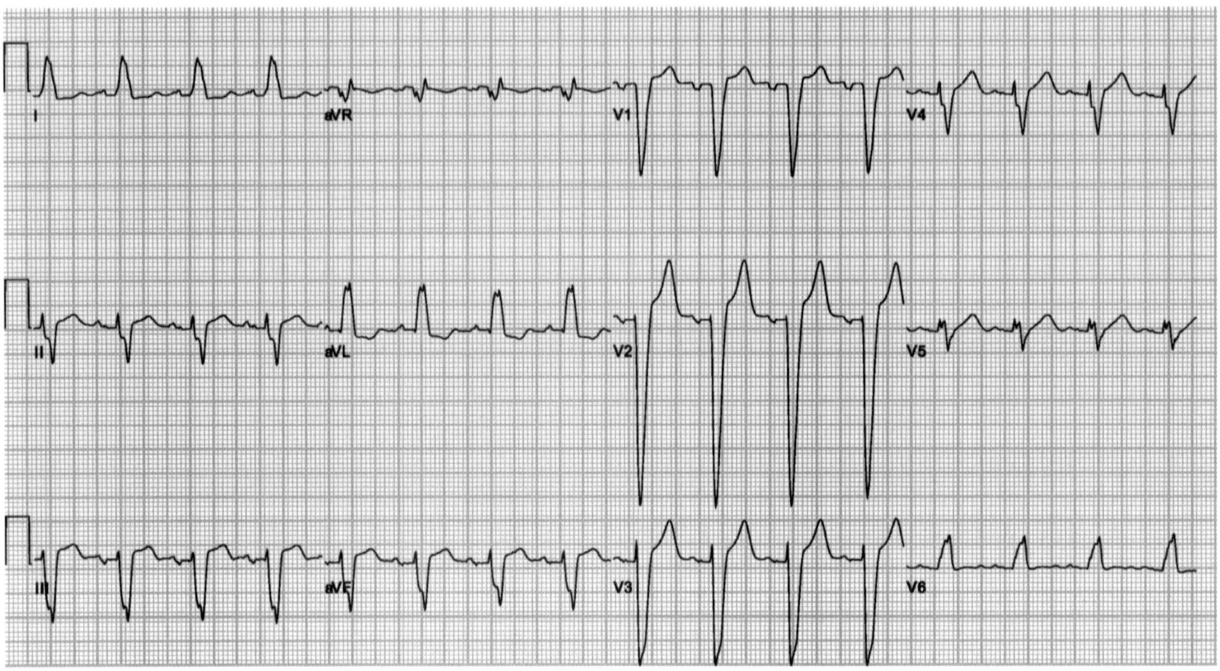

Figure 8-1
Electrocardiogram (ECG) reveals normal sinus rhythm, heart rate 96, left bundle branch block with a QRS interval measuring 142 milliseconds, and nonspecific T-wave changes.

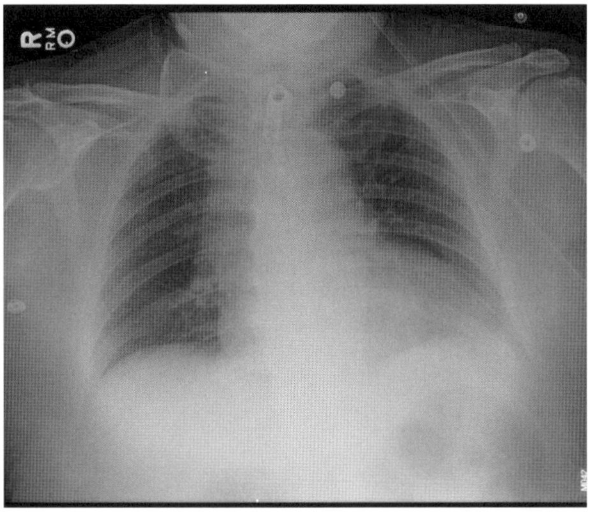

Figure 8-2
Chest x-ray (CXR) shows bibasilar atelectasis with cardiomegaly.

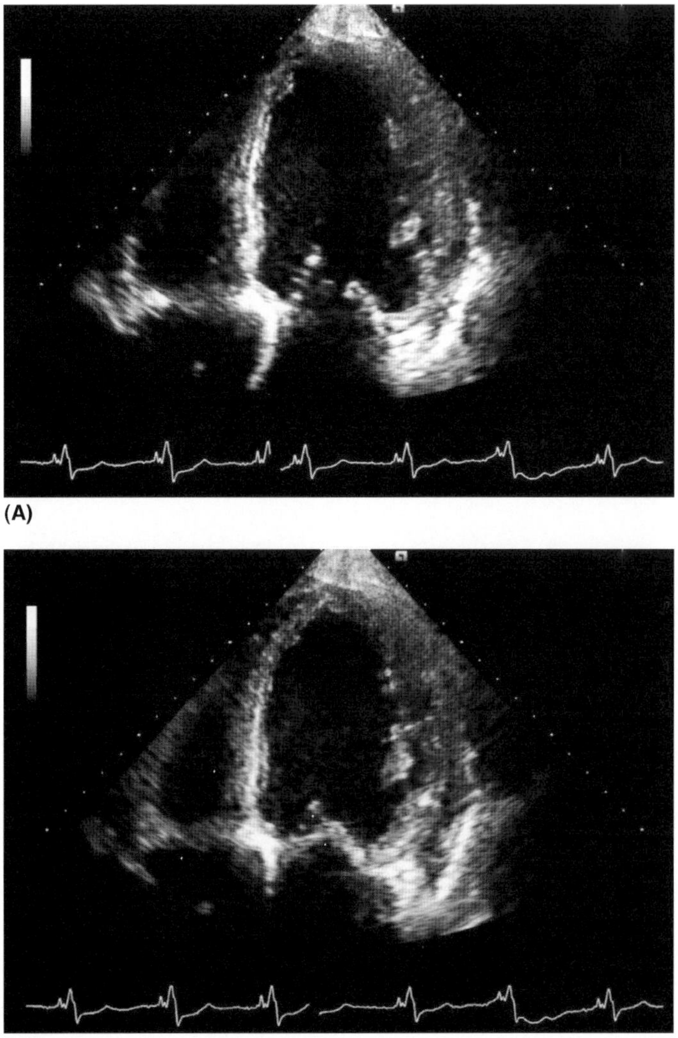

(A)

(B)

Figure 8-3
Transthoracic echocardiogram (TTE) shows severe global hypokinesis of the left ventricle with an estimated left ventricular ejection fraction (LVEF) of 20% (A and B), mild to moderate mitral regurgitation (C), mild left atrial enlargement (A and B), and mildly dilated right ventricle with mildly reduced systolic function of the right ventricle (A and B). *(Continued)*

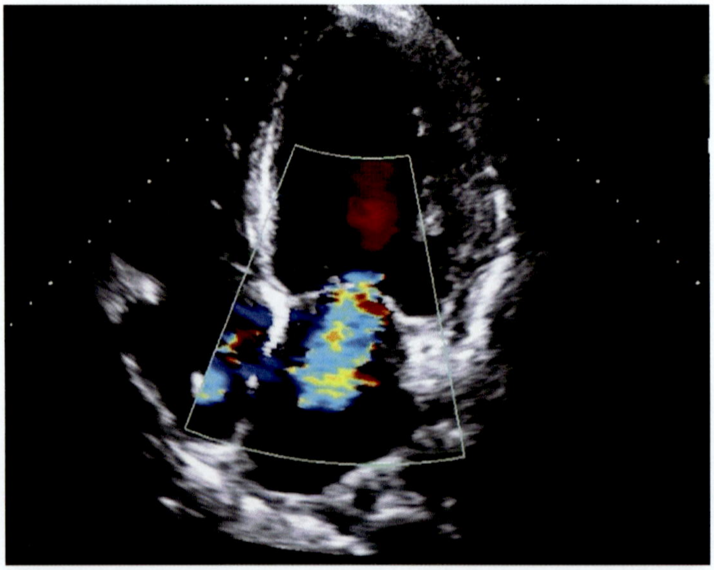

(C)

Figure 8-3 *(Continued)*

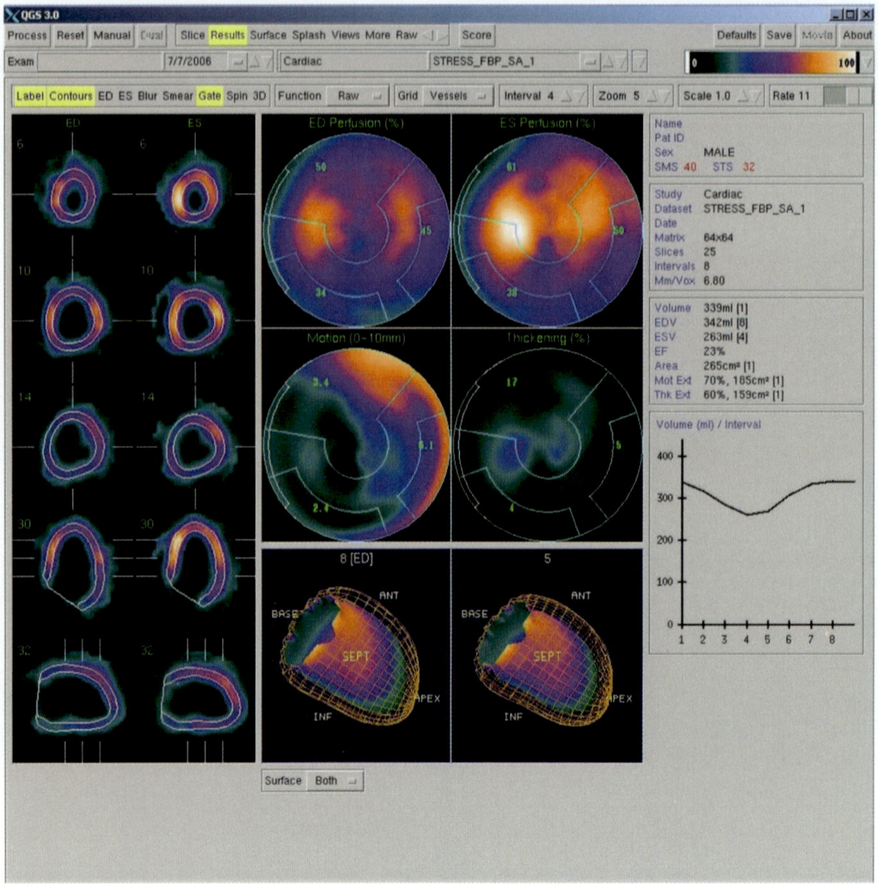

(A)

Figure 8-4
Nuclear medicine pharmacologic stress test reveals a dilated left ventricle with no evidence of previous infarction or ischemia and LVEF of 23%. *(Continued)*

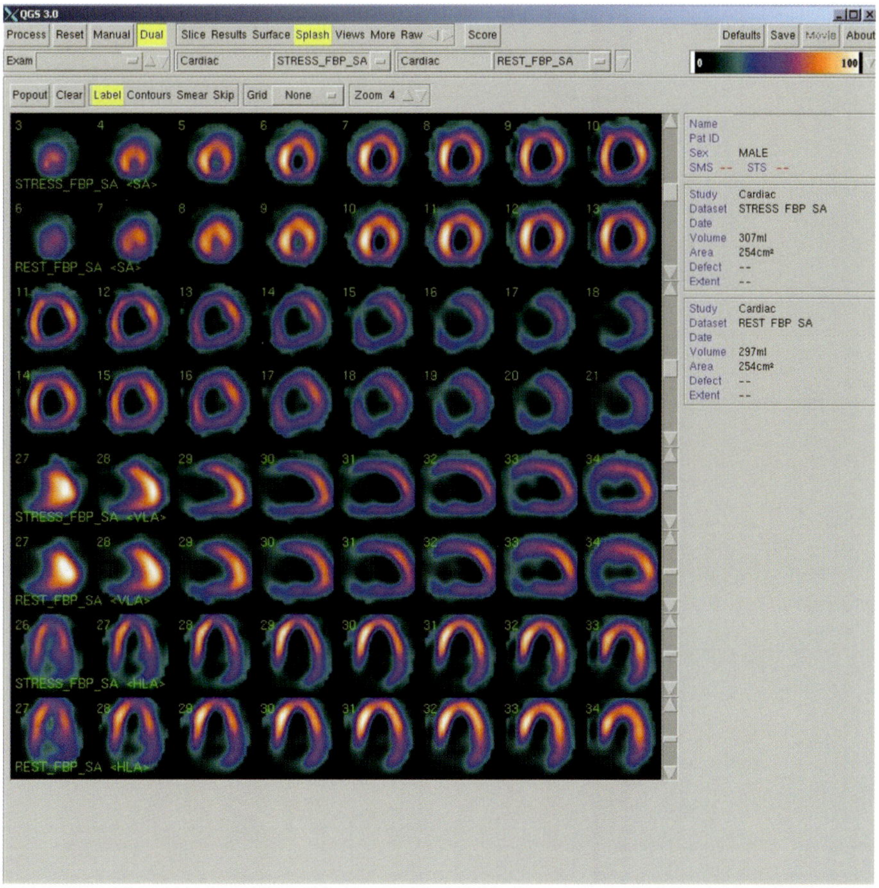

(B)

Figure 8-4 *(Continued)*

symptoms. She reports excellent compliance with her medication regimen and twice-weekly monitoring of her blood pressure and weights. Blood pressure ranges from the 120 to 130s systolic and 80s diastolic at home, and weight is stable at 160 pounds. A complete, 12-point review of symptoms is otherwise unremarkable. She states that she drinks one glass of red wine per week and that she has never smoked tobacco or used illicit drugs. Her family history is significant for a mother who died suddenly at the age of 41 from a myocardial infarction (MI). She has no other known family history of early (before the age of 65) coronary artery disease, heart failure, sudden cardiac death, arrhythmia, or known cardiomyopathy.

With regard to her past medical history, she reports that she had an MI 3 years ago and that she "had a stent placed in the right-sided artery" at that time. She was also told that she had heart failure that "wasn't too bad" per her previous physician. She also endorses a history of systemic hypertension, mixed hyperlipidemia, diet-controlled diabetes mellitus, and depression. She is allergic to sulfa medications. Her medications include carvedilol 37.5 mg po bid, losartan 50 mg po qd, spironolactone 25 mg po qd, aspirin 81 mg po qd, atorvastatin 40 mg po qhs, and citalopram 40 mg po qd.

Physical exam reveals a nonacute, mildly obese female that appears her stated age. Her blood pressure is 126/78, heart rate is 70, and BMI is 31. Pertinent exam findings include clear lung fields and no lower extremity edema. There are no significant positive findings on cardiac or pulmonary examination.

As part of her workup, the following tests are ordered: ECG, CXR, TTE, and a left and right heart catheterization. ECG reveals normal sinus rhythm, heart rate 80, QRS measuring 98 msec, and nonspecific ST and T-wave changes (**Figure 8-5**). CXR is unremarkable (**Figure 8-6**). TTE reveals a normal left ventricular size with mild to moderate systolic dysfunction and estimated LVEF 40% to 45% (**Figure 8-7**). Comparison of Patient A's and Patient B's echocardiogram images is shown in **Figure 8-8**. Left and right heart catheterization reveals no significant coronary stenosis with a patent mid-right coronary artery stent, LVEF 40% on left ventriculogram, and normal left- and right-sided heart pressures (**Figure 8-9**). Labs reveal normal chemistry panel and renal function and normal BNP. Hemoglobin A1c is 6.5. Lipid panel reveals a low density lipoprotein (LDL) of 71 and otherwise normal values. CBC, TSH, and liver function tests are all within normal limits.

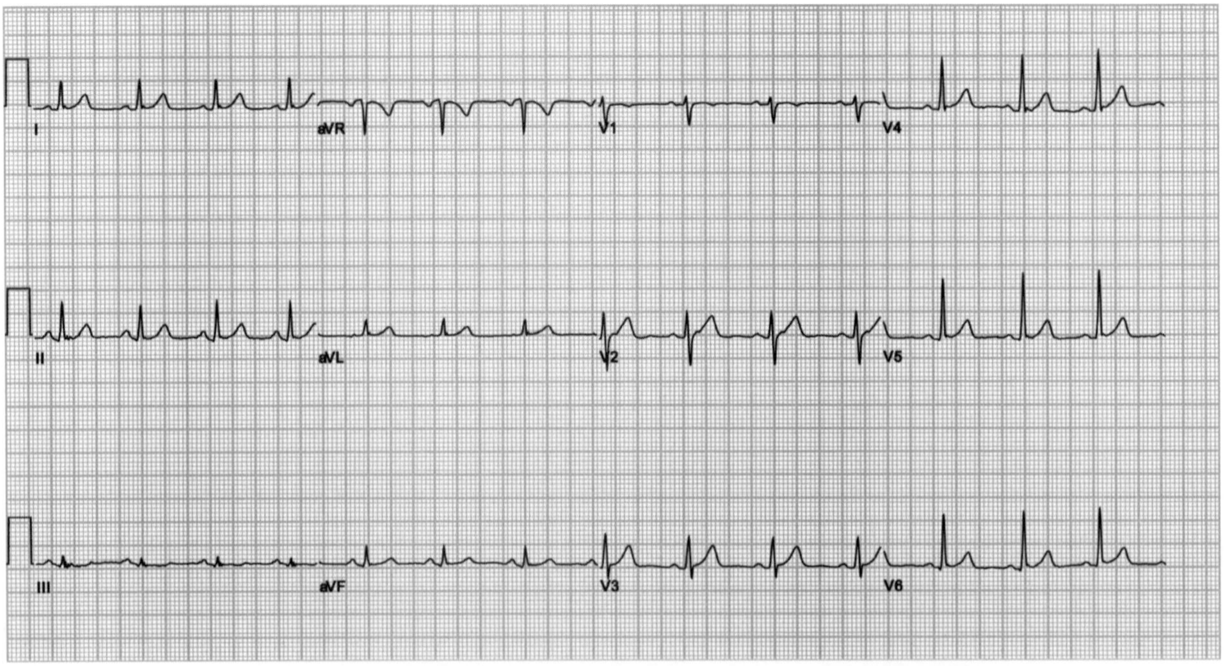

Figure 8-5
ECG reveals normal sinus rhythm, heart rate 80, QRS interval measuring 98 milliseconds, and nonspecific ST and T-wave changes.

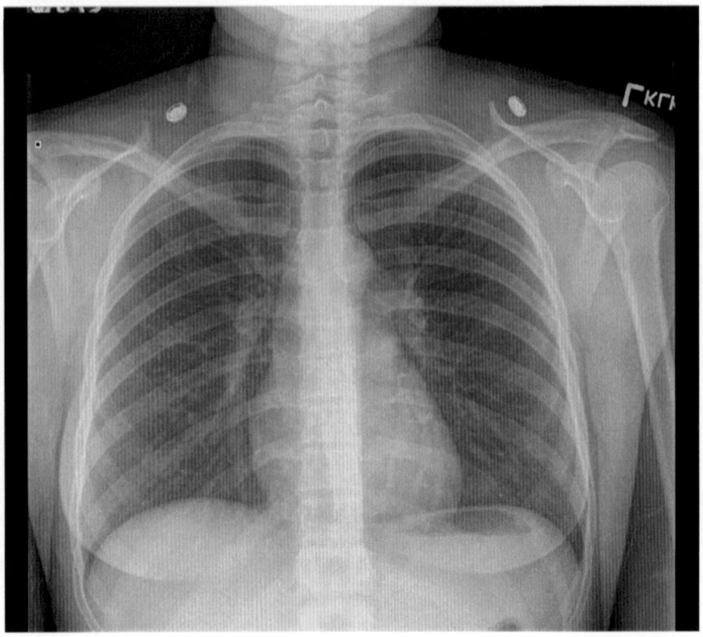

Figure 8-6
CXR is unremarkable.

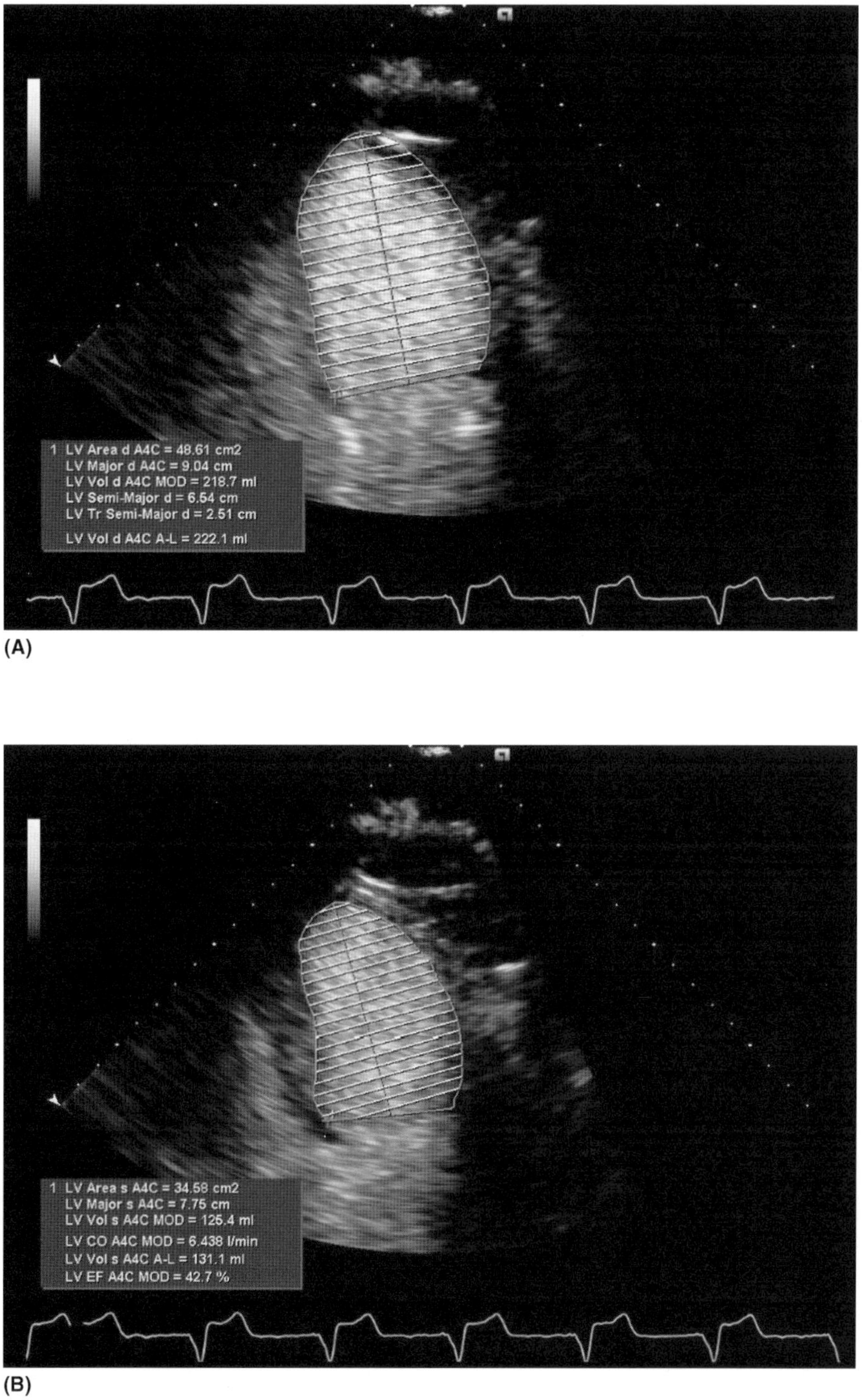

Figure 8-7
TTE reveals a normal left ventricular size with mild to moderate systolic dysfunction and estimated LVEF 40–45% (A and B).

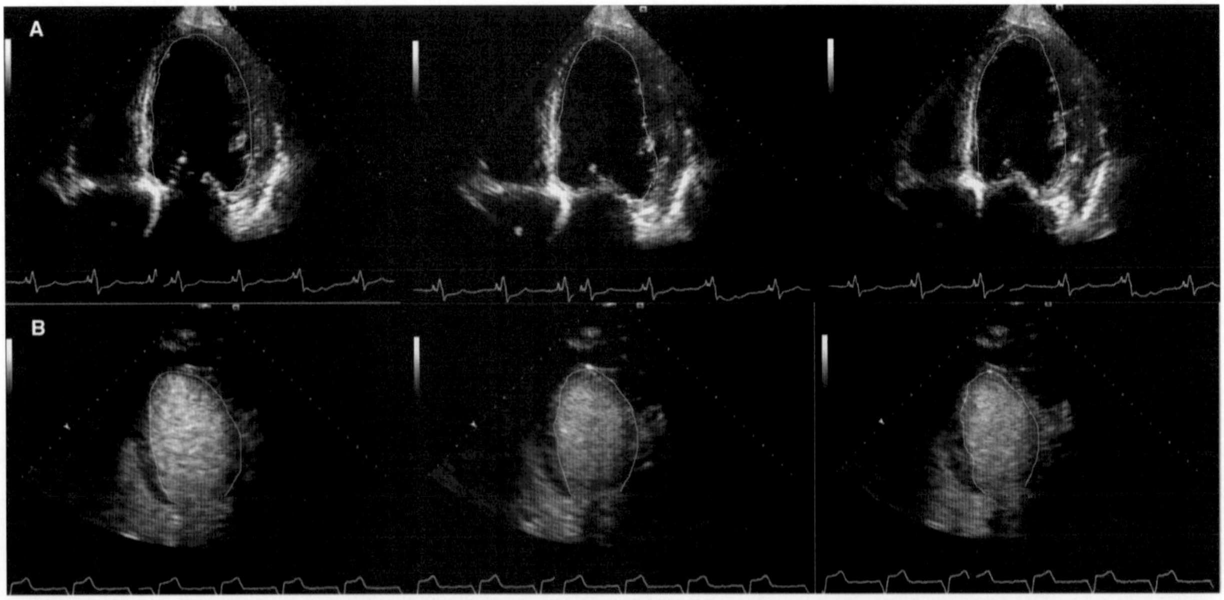

Figure 8-8
TTE images comparing severe systolic dysfunction (Patient A) and mild systolic dysfunction (Patient B).

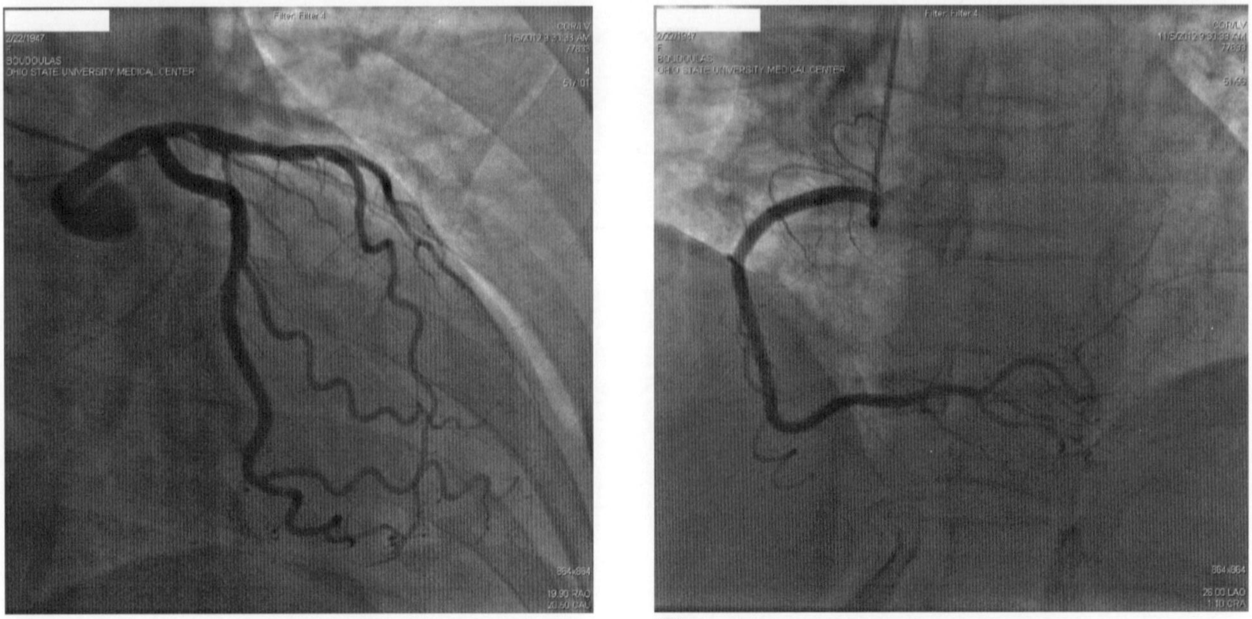

(A) (B)

Figure 8-9
Left and right heart catheterization reveals no significant coronary stenosis with a patent mid-right coronary artery; LVEF of 40% on ventriculogram as well as normal right and left heart pressures were also recorded (not shown).

BACKGROUND

The treatment for heart failure has progressed on several fronts over the past few decades. Medical therapies (including beta-blockers, angiotensin converting enzyme [ACE] inhibitors/angiotensin receptor blockers, spironolactone, and, in specific populations, nitrates and hydrazinophtalazines/hydralazine) have led to marked improvements in both overall symptom management and mortality (1). Device therapy has also led to improved outcomes in heart failure patients. Specifically, implanted cardioverter-defibrillators (ICDs) are now the standard-of-care in appropriate patients with both ischemic and non-ischemic cardiomyopathy for primary and secondary prevention of sudden cardiac death (2). Additionally, pacemakers that coordinate simultaneous pacing of both ventricles have also shown benefit (3–5). This type of pacing requires three pacemaker leads: one each in the right atrium, right ventricle, and left ventricle (as opposed to standard pacemakers and ICDs, which typically have leads only in the right atrium and right ventricle). The three-lead system results in atrial-synchronized, BiV pacing. BiV pacing is also referred to as CRT. CRT devices can act alone or can be used together with an ICD device; the combination is often referred to as CRT-ICD or simply CRT-D. CRT has been shown to improve functional status, quality of life, exercise capacity, ventricular remodeling, morbidity, and mortality in selected heart failure patients. It has become a routine part of our armamentarium for the treatment of heart failure. Recommendations for CRT have expanded over the years to include virtually all New York Heart Association (NYHA) Classes, but they have also contracted based on QRS morphology and, to some extent, QRS duration. Current guideline recommendations for CRT will be discussed later in this chapter.

MECHANISMS

Weak hearts with failing pump function may have a bundle branch block or other intraventricular conduction delay, termed ventricular dyssynchrony. This can cause further worsening of pump function in an already weakened ventricle, resulting in poor contraction efficiency. Therefore, the benefit of CRT lies in the resynchronization of BiV and left ventricular pump function and resulting improvement of pump function with reversal of damaging ventricular remodeling. Additionally, several hemodynamic measurements have been shown to improve with CRT. The theory behind the potential benefit for CRT resulted from several studies, which showed that heart failure patients with a LBBB or intraventricular conduction delay (IVCD) had worse symptoms and outcomes than those without (6–8). Less well established, however, are the molecular pathways by which CRT improves these outcomes. Experimental models suggest that reduction in apoptosis and regulation of kinase activity may result in an improvement in ventricular remodeling (9).

In addition, right ventricular-only pacing may result in deleterious effects similar to that of the dyssynchrony of heart failure. In this case, the paced right ventricle contracts before the left ventricle (referred to as interventricular dyssynchrony). This results in an iatrogenic LBBB; the left ventricular septum contracts before the lateral wall of the left ventricle (referred to as intraventricular dyssynchrony; 10–12). Therefore, standard univentricular, dual-chamber pacemakers (right atrium and right ventricle leads only) are not recommended in the presence of heart failure. Rather, BiV pacing (CRT) with three leads is the treatment of choice in patients with heart failure who require pacemaker therapy.

The physiologic mechanisms of benefit of CRT have been well established in several studies. CRT results in an improved contractile function of the left ventricle. In the Multicenter InSync Randomized Clinical Evaluation (MIRACLE) trial, the LVEF increased 3.6% compared to 0.4% with CRT versus controls, respectively, at 6 months (13). The Cardiac Resynchronization-Heart Failure (CARE-HF) trial showed that in patients with a known LBBB or IVCD and LVEF of 25%, CRT improved LVEF by 3.7% at 3 months and 6.9% at 18 months compared to controls (14). Other improved parameters included a rise in systolic pressure of 6 mmHg, suggesting improved contractile function, and a reduction in BNP of 225 pg/mL at 3 months and 1122 pg/mL at 18 months. Improvements were compared to controls with median initial systolic pressure 110 mmHg and median initial BNP 1800 to 1900 pg/mL.

In addition, CRT is known to reverse the damaging process of (pathological) ventricular remodeling. Both the CARE-HF and MIRACLE trials showed improvements in several markers significant for reverse remodeling, including reduced left ventricular end-systolic and end-diastolic dimensions, reduced mitral regurgitant jet area, and reduced left ventricular mass (15–16). Also, reverse remodeling may be a better predictor of long-term outcomes than clinical improvement. A multivariate analysis of several clinical and echocardiographic measurements was performed in a study of 141 patients defined as responders or nonresponders to CRT (17). This study showed that left ventricular end-systolic volume (LVESV) reduction was the only independent predictor for improved cardiovascular or all-cause mortality.

CLINICAL TRIAL DATA IN MODERATE-SEVERE HEART FAILURE

Several large randomized controlled trials have shown the benefit of CRT in selected heart failure populations. Among these, the CARE-HF trial, the COMPANION trial, the MIRACLE trial, and the MIRACLE ICD trial will be discussed (13–14,18–23).

In the MIRACLE trial, 453 patients were enrolled with LVEF equal to or less than 35%, moderate to severe symptoms of heart failure, and a QRS duration of 130 msec or more. Patients were randomly assigned to

CRT with optimal medical therapy for heart failure or optimal medical therapy alone. The primary endpoints were NYHA heart failure class, standardized quality of life scores, and 6-minute walk distance. Patients in the CRT group were noted to have a significant increase in 6-minute walk versus medical therapy alone (39 minutes vs. 10 minutes). There were also significant improvement in NYHA class, quality of life, and exercise capacity according to time on treadmill. LVEF improved significantly in the CRT group by 4.6% and decreased in the medical therapy alone group by 0.2%. Also noted in the CRT group was a decrease in the rate of hospitalization and the use of intravenous medications for heart failure treatment.

Further analysis in the MIRACLE trial included Doppler echocardiograms at 3 and 6 months. Measurements were made of left ventricular end-diastolic and end-systolic volumes, ejection fraction, left ventricular mass, MR severity, peak transmitral velocities during early and late diastolic fillings (E-wave and A-wave, respectively), and the myocardial performance index. At 6 months, the CRT group showed a significant reduction in left ventricular end-diastolic and end-systolic volumes and left ventricular mass. Additional significant findings included an increase in LVEF, improvement in myocardial performance index, and decrease in MR in the CRT group. Non-ischemic cardiomyopathy patients improved to a greater extent than ischemic cardiomyopathy patients.

The MIRACLE ICD trial was designed to examine the efficacy and safety of combined CRT and ICD devices (CRT-D) in NYHA Class III or IV heart failure patients, who are already receiving optimal medical therapy. This was a randomized, double-blinded, parallel-controlled trial that enrolled 369 patients with LVEF of 35% or less, QRS duration of 130 msec or more, at risk of life-threatening arrhythmias, and NYHA Class III or IV, and who also had an indication for an ICD. Eighty-nine percent of the 369 patients were NYHA Class III. Patients were randomized to CRT plus ICD or ICD only. The primary endpoints were changes at baseline and 6 months in quality of life, NYHA functional class, and 6-minute walk test. Also measured were changes in exercise capacity, certain plasma neurohormones, LVEF, overall heart failure status, survival, ventricular arrhythmia incidence, and rate of hospitalization.

At 6 months, patients with CRT-D showed significant improvement in quality of life score and functional class; however, no significant changes were noted in distance walked in 6 minutes. Peak oxygen consumption increased by 1.1 mL/kg/min in the CRT-D group versus 0.1 mL/kg/min in the ICD only group ($P = .4$), and treadmill exercise duration increased by 56 seconds in the CRT-D group versus an 11 second decreased in the ICD only group ($P < .001$). There were no significant differences in arrhythmia determination capabilities and no proarrhythmias were noted.

The MIRACLE ICD II study (an exploratory component of the MIRACLE ICD trial) analyzed the use of CRT in patients with mildly symptomatic heart failure. This was a randomized, double-blind, parallel-controlled clinical trial in NYHA Class II heart failure already on optimal medical therapy. Patients enrolled had an LVEF of 35% or less, a QRS duration of 130 msec or more, and a Class I indication for an ICD. 186 patients were randomized to either CRT-D or ICD only. Endpoints included peak VO_2, VE/CO_2 (both are measurements obtained during a cardiopulmonary exercise stress test), NYHA class, quality of life scores, 6-minute walk test distance, left ventricular volumes, LVEF, and composite clinical response.

In the CRT-D group at 6 months, there were no significant improvements noted in peak VO_2; however, there were significant improvements in ventricular remodeling indexes (left ventricular diastolic and left ventricular systolic volumes) and LVEF. The CRT group also demonstrated statistically significant improvements in VE/CO_2, NYHA heart failure class, and clinical composite response. No significant differences between groups were noted in 6-minute walk test distance or quality of life scores.

The CARE-HF trial enrolled 813 patients with NYHA Class III or IV heart failure, an LVEF less than or equal to 35%, and QRS prolongation on ECG. Ninety-four percent of patients were NYHA Class III heart failure and 62% were non-ischemic. The mean age was 67 years, the median LVEF was 25%, and the median QRS duration was 160 msec. A QRS duration between 120 and 149 msec required an echocardiogram to prove ventricular dyssynchrony. These patients were randomized to standard heart failure medical therapy or standard heart failure medical therapy plus a CRT device. The primary endpoint was urgent hospitalization for a major cardiovascular condition or death from any cause. The secondary endpoint was death from any cause.

At 29 months, several benefits were noted in the CRT group. Mortality was reduced in the CRT group versus medical therapy alone (20% vs. 30%), primarily in deaths caused by worsening heart failure (8.1% vs. 13.9%) but also in sudden cardiac death (7.1% versus 9.4%). The mortality reduction in the CRT group increased with time. There was a significant reduction in the primary endpoint in the CRT group (39% vs. 55%), which also increased with time. This reduction was independent of medical therapy used, LVEF, QRS duration, age, gender, or NYHA heart failure class at time of enrollment. At 38 months, the reduction in mortality from both heart failure and sudden cardiac death continued and mildly increased. Furthermore, at 90 days, there were beneficial effects noted on NYHA heart failure class and quality of life. The positive effects of reverse remodeling are noted in the previous "Mechanisms" section.

The Comparison of Medical Therapy, Pacing, and Defibrillation in Heart Failure (COMPANION) trial examined the role of combination CRT and ICD devices. This trial enrolled 1,520 patients with NYHA Class III or IV heart failure, a QRS duration of 120 msec or more, and a LVEF less than or equal to 35%. The mean age was 67 years with a median LVEF of 21%. Approximately half of the patients had non-ischemic cardiomyopathy, and about 85% were NYHA Class III. All of the NYHA Class III patients were eligible for ICD placement of primary prevention of sudden cardiac death. All patients had received inpatient care for decompensated heart failure in the previous 12 months. The three random assigned groups were as follows: optimal medical therapy for heart failure, CRT, or CRT-D (the CRT and CRT-D groups were also on optimal medical therapy for heart failure). In this study, optimal medical therapy included angiotensin receptor blockers or ACE inhibitors in 89%, beta-blockers in 66%, and spironolactone in 55%.

Significant reductions in the following were noted at 12 months in the two CRT arms compared to the medical therapy only: primary composite endpoint of all-cause hospitalization and all-cause mortality, cardiovascular causes of hospitalization, and cardiovascular causes of death. The primary composite endpoint occurred in 56% of the CRT only arm, 56% of the CRT-D arm, and 68% of the medical therapy only arm. Similar to CARE-HF, the benefit noted in the primary endpoint was independent of medical therapy used, LVEF, NYHA heart failure class, gender, age, or etiology of cardiomyopathy (ischemic vs. non-ischemic). The CRT-D arm was noted to have a significant decrease in the secondary endpoint of all-cause mortality versus medical therapy alone (12% vs. 19%), while the CRT only arm approached significance (15%). Of note, the mortality benefit was noted at device implantation for the CRT-D group, while the CRT only group did not receive this benefit until eight months after implantation. The likely explanation is the immediate reduction in sudden cardiac death provided by an ICD device, whereas the benefit of BiV pacing and resulting reverse remodeling may take several months to occur. Additionally, those patients receiving either CRT alone or CRT-D were noted to have statistically significant improved six minute walk distance, improved systolic pressure, and improved NYHA class compared to medical therapy alone.

Taken together, these landmark trials showed the benefit of CRT in patients with NYHA class III and IV heart failure with LVEF 35% or less and a QRS duration of 120 to 130 msec or above. Specific benefits include reduction of symptoms within one to three months, reduction in hospitalizations, and improvement of survival.

CLINICAL TRIAL DATA IN MILD TO MODERATE HEART FAILURE

Several studies have addressed the use of CRT in NYHA Class I or II heart failure patients. Randomized trials have demonstrated benefit of CRT or CRT-D in these patients, with BiV pacing resulting in reduced LVEF, improvement in functional status, decreased risk of heart failure events, and decreased risk of composite outcomes. CRT-D also has been shown to decrease mortality in NYHA Class II but not Class I patients.

Published in 2008, the REsynchronization reVErses Remodeling in Systolic left vEntricular dysfunction (REVERSE) trial examined the effect of CRT with previously symptomatic NYHA Class I or NYHA Class II heart failure (24). The 610 enrolled patients had a QRS duration of 120 msec or higher and a LVEF of 40% or below. All patients received a CRT device (with or without ICD) and were randomly assigned to active CRT (CRT-ON, 419 total patients) or control (CRT-OFF, total of 191 patients) for 12 months total. The assigned primary endpoint was the heart failure composite response (patients receive a score of improved, unchanged, or worsened). A secondary endpoint (powered prospectively) was left ventricular end-systolic volume index, and hospitalization for worsening heart failure was examined in a prospective secondary analysis of health care use.

The heart failure clinical composite response endpoint compared only the percentage worsened, and it indicated that 16% of patients in the CRT-ON group worsened compared to 21% of patients in the CRT-OFF group (P = .10). Echocardiographic measurements demonstrated that CRT-ON patients had a significantly greater improvement in left ventricular end-systolic volume index and other echocardiographic indicators of left ventricular remodeling. Additionally, time-to-first heart failure hospitalization was significantly decreased in the CRT-ON group.

A meta-analysis from 2011 combined four large CRT trials in patients with reduced LVEF (40% or below) with NYHA Class I or II heart failure (25). Trials included were MIRACLE ICD II, MADIT-CRT,

REVERSE, and the NYHA Class II patients from RAFT (MIRACLE ICD II and REVERSE were discussed previously, and MADIT-CRT and RAFT will be addressed below). In these patients, CRT provided several benefits: reverse remodeling of the left ventricle, decreased progression of heart failure symptoms (ie, progression of NYHA heart failure class), and decreased heart failure events and mortality.

Furthermore, the benefit of CRT in patients with mild heart failure was examined in the Multicenter Automatic Defibrillator Implantation Trial—Cardiac Resynchronization Therapy (MADIT-CRT) trial (26). The 1,820 enrolled patients had a LVEF of 30% or below, QRS duration of 130 msec or greater, and NYHA Class I or II. Eighty-five percent of patients were NYHA class II while the remaining 15% were NYHA Class I, with 55% classified as ischemic cardiomyopathy and 45% of patients classified as non-ischemic cardiomyopathy. Patients were randomized to CRT-D or ICD alone, with the primary endpoint assigned first occurrence of either nonfatal heart failure event or death from any cause. CRT-D resulted in a decrease in the primary endpoint at an average follow-up of 29 months versus ICD alone (17% vs. 25%). A 41% decrease in heart failure events was noted in the CRT-D group. Echocardiographic measurements were also followed and noted reverse remodeling in the CRT group, with the greatest benefit noted in patients with a QRS duration of 150 msec or greater (ie, those patients with more severe ventricular dyssynchrony).

Further analysis of the MADIT-CRT data showed that patients with LBBB had a benefit over those patients without LBBB, including those with either right bundle branch block (RBBB) or nonspecific intraventricular conduction delays (27). LBBB patients who received CRT-D had a decrease in ventricular dysrhythmias and heart failure progression.

In addition, post hoc analysis of MADIT-CRT data revealed differential benefits in ischemic versus non-ischemic patients. In non-ischemic heart failure patients, CRT-D benefits (compared to ICD alone) were greater in those patients with LBBB, diabetes mellitus, and female gender. In ischemic heart failure patients, CRT-D provided benefit in the setting of LBBB, systolic blood pressure less than 115 mmHg, and QRS duration of 150 ms or greater.

The Resynchronization-Defibrillation for Ambulatory Heart Failure Trial (RAFT) study examined the benefit of CRT in patients with mild or moderate heart failure (28). Of the 1,798 enrolled patients, 81% had NYHA Class II heart failure and 19% had NYHA Class III heart failure. All patients had a QRS of 120 msec or higher and a LVEF of 30% or below. Similar to MADIT-CRT, patients were assigned to either CRT-D or ICD alone. Compared to MADIT-CRT, slightly more patients in RAFT had ischemic versus non-ischemic cardiomyopathy (about two in every three patients were ischemic). The assigned primary endpoint was first occurrence of hospitalization for heart failure or death from any cause. The average follow-up was longer than MADIT-CRT (40 months for RAFT versus 29 months for MADIT-CRT). Versus ICD alone, CRT-D decreased the primary endpoint (33% vs. 40%), had fewer overall deaths (21% vs. 26%), and had fewer heart failure hospitalizations (20% vs. 26%). Again, benefit was more pronounced in patients with QRS duration of 150 msec or greater.

Unfortunately, the CRT-D arm of RAFT had a greater occurrence of adverse events noted within the first 30 days after device placement compared to the ICD only arm (13% versus 7%). These included coronary sinus dissection, lead dislodgement, pneumothorax/hemothorax, and device pocket hematoma or infection.

MAJOR SOCIETY GUIDELINES

As the clinical trial data detailed above demonstrates, CRT is an established device-based therapy for heart failure patients; however, indications for appropriate implantation are continually evolving. CRT is appropriate for selected patients with NYHA Class II, III, and IV heart failure with depressed LVEF and ventricular dyssynchrony. A continued area of investigation is the best determinant of ventricular dyssynchrony; several methods have been proposed, including ECG QRS duration and morphology, tissue Doppler echocardiography, or other forms of advanced cardiac imaging (including three-dimensional echocardiography, cardiac magnetic resonance imaging, and advanced electrophysiology studies).

Several society guidelines offer recommendations for CRT device placement for heart failure patients on optimal medical therapy: the 2012 American College of Cardiology/American Heart Association/Heart Rhythm Society (ACC/AHA/HRS) guidelines for device-based therapy of rhythm abnormalities, the 2009 ACC/AHA heart failure guidelines, the 2010 Heart Failure Society of America guidelines, and the 2010 focused update of the European Society of Cardiology device therapy for heart failure guidelines (29–32). The most recent and extensive of these is the 2012 guidelines from the ACCF/AHA/HRS. While expanding the guideline recommendations to selected NYHA Class I and II patients, this guideline also limits the CRT indication by QRS duration and QRS morphology (**Table 8-1**). The strongest indication for CRT (a Class I

Table 8-1
ACCF/AHA/HRS Recommendations for CRT in Patients With Systolic Heart Failure

2012 DEVICE-BASED THERAPY FOCUSED UPDATE RECOMMENDATIONS	COMMENTS
CLASS I INDICATIONS	
CRT is indicated for patients who have LVEF less than or equal to 35%, sinus rhythm, LBBB with a QRS duration greater than or equal to 150 ms, and NYHA Class II, III, or ambulatory IV symptoms on GDMT. (Level of Evidence: A for NYHA Class III/IV; Level of Evidence: B for NYHA Class II)	Modified recommendation (specifying CRT in patients with LBBB of ≥ 150 ms; expanded to include those with NYHA Class II symptoms).
CLASS IIA	
CRT can be useful for patients who have LVEF less than or equal to 35%, sinus rhythm, LBBB with a QRS duration 120 to 149 ms, and NYHA Class II, III, or ambulatory IV symptoms on GDMT. (Level of Evidence: B)	New recommendation
CRT can be useful for patients who have LVEF less than or equal to 35%, sinus rhythm, a non-LBBB pattern with a QRS duration greater than or equal to 150 ms, and NYHA Class III/ambulatory Class IV symptoms on GDMT. (Level of Evidence: A)	New recommendation
CRT can be useful in patients with atrial fibrillation and LVEF less than or equal to 35% on GDMT if a) the patient requires ventricular pacing or otherwise meets CRT criteria and b) AV nodal ablation or pharmacologic rate control will allow near 100% ventricular pacing with CRT. (Level of Evidence: B)	Modified recommendation (wording changed to indicate benefit based on ejection fraction rather than NYHA Class; level of evidence changed from C to B).
CRT can be useful for patients on GDMT who have LVEF less than or equal to 35% and are undergoing new or replacement device placement with anticipated requirement for significant (> 40%) ventricular pacing. (Level of Evidence: C)	Modified recommendation (wording changed to indicate benefit based on ejection fraction and need for pacing rather than NYHA Class); class changed from IIb to IIa).
CLASS IIB	
CRT may be considered for patients who have LVEF less than or equal to 30%, ischemic etiology of heart failure, sinus rhythm, LBBB with a QRS duration of greater than or equal to 150 ms, and NYHA Class I symptoms on GDMT. (Level of Evidence: C)	New recommendation
CRT may be considered for patients who have LVEF less than or equal to 35%, sinus rhythm, a non-LBBB pattern with QRS duration 120 to 149 ms, and NYHA Class III/ambulatory Class IV on GDMT. (Level of Evidence: B)	New recommendation
CRT may be considered for patients who have LVEF less than or equal to 35%, sinus rhythm, a non-LBBB pattern with a QRS duration greater than or equal to 150 ms, and NYHA Class II symptoms on GDMT. (Level of Evidence: B)	New recommendation
CLASS III: NO BENEFIT	
CRT is not recommended for patients with NYHA Class I or II symptoms and non-LBBB pattern with QRS duration less than 150 ms. (Level of Evidence: B)	New recommendation
CRT is not indicated for patients whose comorbidities and/or frailty limit survival with good functional capacity to less than 1 year. (Level of Evidence: C)	Modified recommendation (wording changed to include cardiac as well as noncardiac comorbidities).

Note: CRT = cardiac resynchronization therapy; DBT = device-based therapy; GDMT = guideline-directed medical therapy; LBBB = left bundle branch block; LVEF = left ventricular ejection fraction; NYHA = New York Heart Association.

indication) is for patients who have an LVEF less than or equal to 35%, sinus rhythm, LBBB with a QRS duration greater than or equal to 150 ms, and NYHA Class II, III, or ambulatory IV symptoms on optimal medical therapy. Several additional but somewhat weaker recommendations follow this one, and a couple of Class III ("is not recommended") indications are included.

RETURN TO CASE PRESENTATIONS

Our case presentations represent two "typical" clinic patients with heart failure with whom appropriate device therapy should be addressed. Patient A has NYHA Class III and American College of Cardiology/American Heart Association (ACC/AHA) Stage C heart failure in the setting of a non-ischemic cardiomyopathy. He has a severely depressed LVEF of 15% to 20% on recent imaging and a QRS of 142 ms on recent ECG. His TTE also indicates BiV failure (although a dyssynchrony study was not performed) and his ECG demonstrates a LBBB. He already has an ICD in place. He is on optimal medical therapy for an African American male with heart failure. His other chronic medical conditions (hypertension, hyperlipidemia, diabetes mellitus, and gout) are under good control and not life threatening.

Based on current major society guidelines and clinical trial data, this patient would likely benefit from an upgrade to a CRT-D device. His LVEF, QRS duration, and functional status all indicate the need for BiV pacing. In addition, he has been on optimal heart failure medications for several months. Although a small risk exists with the device implantation procedure, in the hands of an experienced operator, this risk is no more than 1% for a serious complication. Potential benefits of CRT upgrade include decrease in mortality, improvement in functional status, induction of reverse remodeling, and increase in LVEF. He will need close outpatient follow-up, including enrollment in a device clinic for routine monitoring.

Patient B has NYHA Class II and ACC/AHA Stage C heart failure, due to coronary artery disease and ischemic cardiomyopathy. She has a strong family history of sudden cardiac death at an early age due to myocardial infarction and coronary artery disease. She has a mildly depressed LVEF of 40% to 45% on recent imaging and a QRS of 112 msec on recent ECG. She does not have a permanent pacemaker or ICD in place currently or previously. She is on optimal medical therapy for heart failure and will need continued monitoring of her lipid profile. Her other chronic medical conditions (hypertension, hyperlipidemia, diabetes mellitus, and depression) are under good control and not life threatening. She needs counseling and possible nutrition consult with regard to her obesity and need for "dry" weight loss.

Based on current major society guidelines and clinical trial data, this patient would not currently benefit from CRT, CRT-D, or ICD device therapy. Her LVEF, although mildly depressed, is above 35%. Her QRS does not meet criteria for CRT. Even with the new recommendations for CRT in NYHA Class I and II heart failure patients based on the MADIT-CRT trial data, she does not meet criteria for LVEF (below 30%) or QRS duration (130 msec). In addition, she does not have LBBB on ECG. However, she should be followed closely in the outpatient setting, with at least yearly echocardiograms and clinical evaluation of functional status at least every 6 months. She may benefit from a cardiac magnetic resonance imaging study to evaluate for microvascular disease. Her heart failure may progress in the future to the point where she would benefit from device therapy. Given the evolving nature of appropriate indications for CRT and the continued major society guideline updates based on new clinical trial data, she may benefit from CRT in the future.

REFERENCES

1. Hunt SA, Abraham WT, Chin MH, et al. 2009 focused update incorporated into the ACC/AHA 2005 guidelines for the diagnosis and management of heart failure in adults: a report of the American College of Cardiology Foundation/American Heart Association Task Force on Practice Guidelines: developed in collaboration with the International Society for Heart and Lung Transplantation. *Circulation*. 2009;119(14):e391–479.
2. Aronow WS. Implantable cardioverter-defibrillators. *Am J Ther*. 2010;17(6):e208–220.
3. Abraham WT, Hayes DL. Cardiac resynchronization therapy for heart failure. *Circulation*. 2003;108(21):2596–2603.
4. Auricchio A, Abraham WT. Cardiac resynchronization therapy: current state of the art: cost versus benefit. *Circulation*. 2004;109(3):300–307.
5. Burkhardt JD, Wilkoff BL. Interventional electrophysiology and cardiac resynchronization therapy: delivering electrical therapies for heart failure. *Circulation*. 2007;115(16):2208–2220.
6. Duncan AM, Francis DP, Gibson DG, et al. Limitation of exercise tolerance in chronic heart failure: distinct effects of left bundle-branch block and coronary artery disease. *J Am Coll Cardiol*. 2004;43(9):1524–1531.
7. Shamim W, Francis DP, Yousufuddin M, et al. Intraventricular conduction delay: a prognostic marker in chronic heart failure. *Int J Cardiol*. 1999;70(2):171–178.
8. Baldasseroni S, Opasich C, Gorini M, et al. Left bundle-branch block is associated with increased 1-year sudden and total mortality rate in 5517 outpatients with congestive heart failure: a report from the Italian network on congestive heart failure. *Am Heart J*. 2002;143(3):398–405.
9. Chakir K, Daya SK, Tunin RS, et al. Reversal of global apoptosis and regional stress kinase activation by cardiac resynchronization. *Circulation*. 2008;117(11):1369–1377.
10. Wilkoff BL, Cook JR, Epstein AE, et al. Dual-chamber pacing or ventricular backup pacing in patients with an implantable defibrillator: the Dual Chamber and VVI Implantable Defibrillator (DAVID) Trial. *JAMA*. 2002;288(24):3115–3123.
11. Sweeney MO, Hellkamp AS, Ellenbogen KA, et al. Adverse effect of ventricular pacing on heart failure and atrial fibrillation among patients with normal baseline QRS duration in a clinical trial of pacemaker therapy for sinus node dysfunction. *Circulation*. 2003;107(23):2932–2937.
12. Sweeney MO, Prinzen FW. A new paradigm for physiologic ventricular pacing. *J Am Coll Cardiol*. 2006;47(2):282–288.

13. St John Sutton MG, Plappert T, Abraham WT, et al. Effect of cardiac resynchronization therapy on left ventricular size and function in chronic heart failure. *Circulation.* 2003;107(15):1985–1990.
14. Cleland JG, Daubert JC, Erdmann E, et al. The effect of cardiac resynchronization on morbidity and mortality in heart failure. *N Engl J Med.* 2005;352(15):1539–1549.
15. Zhang Q, Fung JW, Auricchio A, et al. Differential change in left ventricular mass and regional wall thickness after cardiac resynchronization therapy for heart failure. *Eur Heart J.* 2006;27(12):1423–1430.
16. Breithardt OA, Sinha AM, Schwammenthal E, et al. Acute effects of cardiac resynchronization therapy on functional mitral regurgitation in advanced systolic heart failure. *J Am Coll Cardiol.* 2003;41(5):765–770.
17. Yu CM, Bleeker GB, Fung JW, et al. Left ventricular reverse remodeling but not clinical improvement predicts long-term survival after cardiac resynchronization therapy. *Circulation.* 2005;112(11):1580–1586.
18. Cleland JG, Daubert JC, Erdmann E, et al. Longer-term effects of cardiac resynchronization therapy on mortality in heart failure [the CArdiac REsynchronization-Heart Failure (CARE-HF) trial extension phase]. *Eur Heart J.* 2006;27(16):1928–1932.
19. Bristow MR, Saxon LA, Boehmer J, et al. Cardiac-resynchronization therapy with or without an implantable defibrillator in advanced chronic heart failure. *N Engl J Med.* 2004;350(21):2140–2150.
20. Saxon LA, Bristow MR, Boehmer J, et al. Predictors of sudden cardiac death and appropriate shock in the Comparison of Medical Therapy, Pacing, and Defibrillation in Heart Failure (COMPANION) Trial. *Circulation.* 2006;114(25):2766–2772.
21. Abraham WT, Fisher WG, Smith AL, et al. Cardiac resynchronization in chronic heart failure. *N Engl J Med.* 2002;346(24):1845–1853.
22. Young JB, Abraham WT, Smith AL, et al. Combined cardiac resynchronization and implantable cardioversion defibrillation in advanced chronic heart failure: the MIRACLE ICD Trial. *JAMA.* 2003;289(20):2685–2694.
23. Abraham WT, Young JB, León AR, et al. Effects of cardiac resynchronization on disease progression in patients with left ventricular systolic dysfunction, an indication for an implantable cardioverter-defibrillator, and mildly symptomatic chronic heart failure. *Circulation.* 2004;110(18):2864–2868.
24. Linde C, Abraham WT, Gold MR, et al. REVERSE (REsynchronization reVErses Remodeling in Systolic left vEntricular dysfunction) Study Group. Randomized trial of cardiac resynchronization in mildly symptomatic heart failure patients and in asymptomatic patients with left ventricular dysfunction and previous heart failure symptoms. *J Am Coll Cardiol.* 2008;52(23):1834–1843.
25. Santangeli P, Di Biase L, Pelargonio G, et al. Cardiac resynchronization therapy in patients with mild heart failure: a systematic review and meta-analysis. *J Interv Card Electrophysiol.* 2011;32(2):125–135.
26. Moss AJ, Hall WJ, Cannom DS, et al. Cardiac-resynchronization therapy for the prevention of heart-failure events. *N Engl J Med.* 2009;361(14):1329–1338.
27. Zareba W, Klein H, Cygankiewicz I, et al. Effectiveness of cardiac resynchronization therapy by QRS morphology in the Multicenter Automatic Defibrillator Implantation Trial-Cardiac Resynchronization Therapy (MADIT-CRT). *Circulation.* 2011;123(10):1061–1072.
28. Tang AS, Wells GA, Talajic M, et al. Cardiac-resynchronization therapy for mild-to-moderate heart failure. *N Engl J Med.* 2010;363(25):2385–2395.
29. Tracy CM, Epstein AE, Darbar D, et al. 2012 ACCF/AHA/HRS focused update of the 2008 guidelines for device-based therapy of cardiac rhythm abnormalities: a report of the American College of Cardiology Foundation/American Heart Association Task Force on Practice Guidelines and the Heart Rhythm Society [corrected]. *Circulation.* 2012;126:1784–1800.
30. Hunt SA, Abraham WT, Chin MH, et al. 2009 focused update incorporated into the ACC/AHA 2005 Guidelines for the diagnosis and management of heart failure in adults: a report of the American College of Cardiology Foundation/American Heart Association Task Force on Practice Guidelines: developed in collaboration with the International Society for Heart and Lung Transplantation. *Circulation.* 2009;119(14):e391–479.
31. Dickstein K, Vardas PE, Auricchio A, et al. 2010 focused update of ESC Guidelines on device therapy in heart failure: an update of the 2008 ESC guidelines for the diagnosis and treatment of acute and chronic heart failure and the 2007 ESC guidelines for cardiac and resynchronization therapy. Developed with the special contribution of the Heart Failure Association and the European Heart Rhythm Association. *Eur J Heart Fail.* 2010;12(11):1143–1153.
32. Heart Failure Society of America, Lindenfeld J, Albert NM, et al. HFSA 2010 comprehensive heart failure practice guideline. *J Card Fail.* 2010;16(6):e1–194.

9

Hemodynamic Optimization in the Patient With Refractory Systolic Heart Failure

NANCY K. SWEITZER

CASE PRESENTATION

Mr. Smithers is a patient you have followed for more than 10 years. He is a 67-year-old male with ischemic cardiomyopathy. He had his first myocardial infarction just before you met him, and had stenting of the left anterior descendin artery at that time. Eight years ago, he presented with unstable angina, and angiography showed severe three-vessel disease. He underwent coronary artery bypass grafting, but was noted postoperatively to have a reduced ejection fraction of 40%. He was stable medically for about 7 years after his bypass, but during the past year he has had worsening symptoms of heart failure. He complains of increasing shortness of breath at lower levels of exertion, and has stopped working. On noninvasive testing, he has had a decrease in ejection fraction to 25%, and estimates of pulmonary artery pressures are increasing. He has been hospitalized four times in the past 3 months, most recently discharged 1 week ago. While in the hospital at that time, his metoprolol tartrate was temporarily stopped because of his decompensated state, and his lisinopril was halved because of hypotension. He comes to your office for a postdischarge follow-up visit. His weight is down 4 pounds from his admission weight to the hospital. His discharge weight is unknown.

He reports that he feels better than when he went into the hospital, but complains of dyspnea when climbing stairs and showering, not at rest. He has been sedentary since his discharge. He sleeps on four pillows. His appetite has decreased, and he has not been eating well. He is wearing his lower extremity compression hose as directed. He is fatigued and is napping daily, despite sleeping 10 hours per night, up two to three times to urinate. He reports no light-headedness.

On presentation his blood pressure is 117/98, pulse is 88. After crossing the room to the exam table, he is winded with audible expiratory wheezes. He becomes noticeably dyspneic when asked to lie on the exam table. He has venous pulsations noticeable at the angle of the jaw when sitting upright. His abdomen is mildly distended, with hepatomegaly and positive hepatojugular reflux. He has cool extremities with trace edema noted despite the compression hose.

His current medications include: digoxin 0.125 mg daily, lisinopril 5 mg daily, metoprolol tartrate 25 mg bid, spironolactone 25 mg bid, Coumadin, Lasix 80 mg daily, and ASA 81 mg daily.

The above description is typical of a chronic heart failure patient who might present in an ambulatory practice for follow-up after a hospitalization for acute decompensated heart failure (ADHF) with clear ongoing deterioration. He has advanced heart failure and has had multiple hospitalizations. Such a patient is at very high risk for future morbidity and mortality. This situation may arise for a number of reasons:

1. Incomplete therapy for decompensated heart failure, typically the result of incomplete diuresis.
2. Appropriate in-hospital therapy for decompensation, but chronic therapy that is not appropriately aggressive.

3. A patient is prescribed appropriate guidelines-based therapy but has an inadequate hemodynamic response to the therapy.
4. True end-stage, Class IV heart failure requiring therapies targeted at this condition, a situation discussed in Chapter 10.

We will address the first three of these causes of refractoriness to standard therapy in this chapter.

Systolic heart failure is a chronic disease resulting in both neurohormonal and hemodynamic abnormalities that impact patient survival, morbidity, symptoms, and quality of life. In a patient with chronic systolic dysfunction, abnormalities of volume status and perfusion, if not addressed, are harbingers of gradual deterioration and future heart failure events (1–3). Recognition of the patient with suboptimal volume status or perfusion in the ambulatory setting, and appropriate therapeutic response to that situation, can be key factors in reducing heart failure admissions and death (4,5). It also leads to improved patient well-being and symptoms.

As care providers, our responsibility is to both stabilize the patient, reduce symptoms to the extent possible, and to stabilize the disease and keep the patient alive, out of the hospital, and free of disease progression for the longest possible time. While at times deterioration in a heart failure patient is the result of the inevitable progressive nature of the disease, often failure to recognize the patient whose regimen is not optimized contributes to disease worsening. The ability to rapidly recognize a patient whose hemodynamic status is not optimized and respond with an appropriate increase in therapy is arguably one of the most important factors in optimal heart failure treatment and prevention of heart failure hospitalization (6).

The ability to recognize ambulatory patients in whom volume status and perfusion are not optimized involves skillful use of imperfect tools, based primarily on patient history and bedside examination (2,7). To hone these bedside skills, care providers require teaching and practice so that diagnostic skill can be applied successfully to management of advanced heart failure patients. Reliance on symptom history alone is typically inadequate, as patients often report feeling normal or back to baseline early during therapy, while they remain decompensated by other measures (8). Physical examination skills such as assessment of jugular venous pressure (JVP) and auscultation of the third heart sound can be critical to detection of ongoing decompensation, but have been lamented as a dying art (9–11). Investment in improved bedside diagnostic skills pays off with the heart failure patient in improved patient outcomes, quality of life, and well-being, and often leads to a highly therapeutic medical encounter that can reinforce the doctor–patient relationship (12).

Volume overload is the most common presentation of decompensated heart failure patients, present in over two thirds of hospitalized patients with heart failure (7,8,13,14). In the past, it was thought that patients with severe systolic dysfunction required elevated intracardiac filling pressures to maintain cardiac output and, at times, this is still taught. It is now recognized that optimum performance of the dysfunctional left ventricle is achieved at essentially normal left-sided filling pressures, once afterload is optimized (15–17). Achieving this optimized state in an individual patient depends on bedside assessment of filling pressures, a notoriously tricky task.

The most useful bedside procedure for determining that a patient's intracardiac pressures are elevated is examination of the neck for jugular venous pulsations. Elevated right- and left-sided filling pressures are consistently related to heart failure hospitalization rates, and mortality, while the prognostic value of cardiac output is much lower (4). Left atrial pressure is concordant with right atrial pressure (RAP) in approximately 75% of patients with chronic systolic left ventricular dysfunction (18,19). During effective therapy, pressures on both sides of the heart fall in parallel (20,21). This is important because filling pressures on the right side can be readily assessed at the bedside in most patients, and used to guide therapy. The presence of hepatojugular reflux can increase sensitivity for detection of elevated intracardiac pressures to greater than 80% (22–24). Other signs and symptoms are less sensitive and specific for heart failure decompensation, and may be absent despite severe elevation of intracardiac pressures. These include edema and rales. A thorough review of clinical assessment in heart failure is available in Chapter 1 and elsewhere (7,8).

The neck vein examination in a heart failure patient should be conducted differently than is traditionally taught. As patients may present with markedly elevated filling pressures, and engorgement of the jugular veins, examination of patients reclined at 30 degrees may be misleading. If very high pressure is present, the veins may be so engorged that ability to distinguish pulsations is lost. It is more useful to examine a patient with systolic dysfunction in an upright position initially, lowering the angle of examination gradually until jugular venous pulsations can be seen (**Table 9-1**; 25).

Achievement of the lowest possible filling pressures in a heart failure patient has been shown to provide sustained hemodynamic benefit (26) and to

Table 9-1
Tips to Assist the Clinician in the Assessment of the Jugular Venous Pressure

1. Begin with the patient sitting upright at 90°. If no pulsation is visible, lower the patient gradually toward the supine position until a pulsation is seen. If no pulsation is seen whether the patient is upright, supine, or at a reclining angle between upright and supine, it will not be possible to estimate the jugular venous pressure.
2. Examine both sides of the neck.
3. Assess both the internal and external jugular veins. If only the external jugular vein is visible, confirm that there are respirophasic changes in the venous pulsation before using it to estimate right atrial pressure.
4. Compress inferior to an identified pulsation to distinguish the noncompressible arterial pulsation from the compressible venous pulsation.

Source: Reference 25.

result in a reduction in mitral regurgitation (16). This appears to occur due to reduced stretch on the left ventricle and decrease in size in the mitral annulus. When achieved by combining diuresis with a reduction in afterload through increased vasodilator doses, this can result in stable to improved forward cardiac output, reduction in intrapulmonary filling pressures, improvement in renal function, and improvements in symptom burden and quality of life (26,27).

When it has been determined that a patient's heart failure is not optimized due to persistently elevated filling pressures, attempts to lower those pressures to normal should be made. This is typically done most successfully by increasing both diuretics and vasodilators, while simultaneously maximizing guidelines-based therapy with beta-blockers, angiotensin converting enzyme inhibitors (ACEI), aldosterone receptor antagonists, and cardiac resynchronization therapy (7). Diuretic therapy in symptomatic heart failure patients should include loop diuretics, titrated to doses associated with a physical examination consistent with euvolemia, or to a significant increase in renal function. It is important to realize, however, that underdiuresis of a chronic heart failure patient may mask significant chronic kidney disease, which becomes more apparent when a euvolemic state is achieved. At times, optimum management of heart failure patients requires tolerating worsened renal function to minimize symptom burden.

Oral heart failure therapy often includes ACEI—excellent vasodilators. If a particular patient is intolerant to ACEI, angiotensin receptor blocking drugs will serve to provide the necessary neurohormonal blockade of the renin-angiotensin system, but are often hemodynamically less effective vasodilators, in part because of the lack of bradykinin potentiation (28). If a patient is felt to require further vasodilation, hydralazine and nitrates may be hemodynamically beneficial, and have been shown to be important adjuncts to guidelines-based RAS blocking therapy in African American patients with heart failure (29).

Patients hospitalized with heart failure may receive vasodilator therapy using IV drugs available only in the hospital, and thus, rapidly reach a compensated state. Drugs that may accomplish this rapidly include nitroglycerin, nitroprusside, or nesiritide (30). While on these IV drugs, patients often become well compensated, with evidence of improved organ function, such as decreases in blood urea nitrogen, creatinine, and bilirubin levels. It is important, however, to ensure that when the IV therapy is stopped in such a patient, adequate oral vasodilator therapy is substituted to prevent rapid recurrence of vasoconstriction and decompensation. If a patient recently hospitalized for heart failure appears to be sliding back into decompensation, consider further increases of vasodilator therapy (27).

Nearly all hospitalized heart failure patients have evidence of volume overload. In the absence of very aggressive guidelines-based therapy for heart failure, many are also relatively vasoconstricted. In this situation, vasodilation plus diuretics is the optimal therapeutic choice. Often though, when patients are hospitalized and very decompensated, IV inotropic therapy is elected by the treating physician. Interestingly, in an analysis of the factors determining IV drug choice, practice site was the only significant predictor of inotrope use (31). This fact tells us that physicians do not use patients' clinical examination or characteristics when electing therapy, but, rather, use drugs they are accustomed to using, without appropriate rationale. This approach is likely harmful, and the direct result of the lack of data to guide therapy of ADHF. In addition to the data accumulated over the past several decades regarding harmful effects of inotropic therapy (32–36), data from the Evaluation Study of Congestive heart failure And Pulmonary artery catheterization Effectiveness (ESCAPE) trial demonstrate that use of inotropes by the treating team is associated with worse outcomes, despite adjustment for severity of illness (31,37).

Uptitration of vasodilator drugs in heart failure may be limited by blood pressure, although most heart failure hospitalizations are associated with hypertension (13,14). At times, failure to uptitrate to target doses is the result of incorrect assumptions about ideal blood pressure. When the left ventricle is dysfunctional, optimal afterload reduction typically results in a systolic blood pressure below 120 mmHg, ideally between 90 and 110 mmHg. Good intentioned but mistaken efforts to keep systolic blood pressure

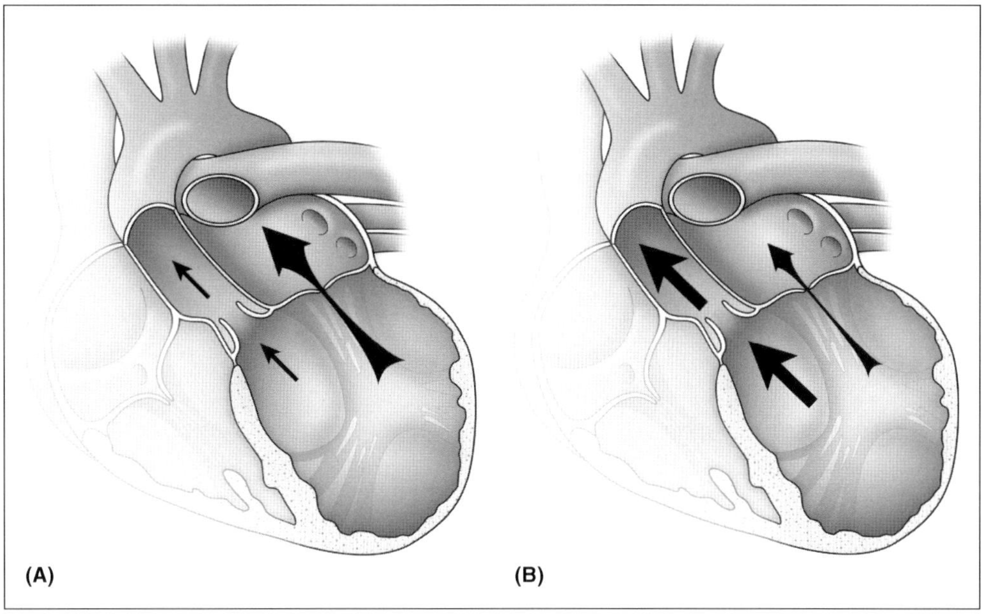

Figure 9-1
(A) Redistribution of blood in the dilated pressure-overloaded heart leads to diminished forward flow and increased backward flow as mitral regurgitation. (B) With aggressive therapy to hemodynamic goals using vasodilators and diuretics, mitral regurgitation is reduced, and forward flow increases.
Source: Adapted from reference 16.

higher in such patients may lead to inadequate vasodilation and contribute to decompensation (13,14). Increasing vasodilator therapy aggressively in a patient with relative hypotension can be disquieting. Efforts to uptitrate guidelines-based therapy may be thwarted by vague patient complaints such as fatigue, light-headedness with position changes that on careful questioning is often transient, or frequent self-monitoring of blood pressure leading to anxiety about outlying values. In addition, other care providers or family members may feel that an appropriate blood pressure is "too low," and advise that medications be reduced. In some cases, right-heart catheterization to measure filling pressures and systemic vascular resistance (SVR) to quantify afterload may be very useful (8). In some patients who appear not to tolerate low dose ACE inhibitor therapy, right-heart catheterization may demonstrate a markedly elevated SVR, suggesting that hypotension is resulting from poor cardiac output in the face of increased afterload. In such cases, significant uptitration of ACE inhibitors or other vasodilators is often possible with no decrease in blood pressure. When afterload is optimally matched to ventricular function, forward cardiac output is maximized, mitral regurgitation is reduced, and blood pressure and renal function often improve and become more stable (**Figure 9-1**). Occasionally, patients appear to have a tremendous drive to vasoconstriction, and require exceedingly high doses of these medications for optimization, as high

Table 9-2
Goals During Hemodynamic Optimization

HEMODYNAMIC PARAMETER	GOAL RANGE
Right atrial pressure	≤ 8 mmHg
Pulmonary capillary wedge pressure	≤ 16 mmHg
Systemic vascular resistance	800–1200 dynes*sec/cm^5
Systolic blood pressure	> 80 mmHg

as captopril 100 mg every 6 hours in combination with high-dose oral nitrate therapy. Carvedilol may be more vasodilating than metoprolol, and may be a reasonable choice in such a circumstance, although whether this is a lasting effect is controversial (38,39).

In particularly difficult cases, a pulmonary artery catheter may be inserted for hemodynamic diagnosis, and then left in place during determination of the optimal regimen of oral medications (8). Routine use of invasive hemodynamic assessment is not warranted in heart failure (21), but such an approach can be useful in select refractory cases. Using hemodynamics, one can ensure that afterload reduction is optimized and filling pressures are as low as achievable with the chosen combination of medications. Such invasively guided determination of an oral medication regimen is termed "tailored therapy" and should result in filling pressures and vasodilation as close to optimal goals as possible (**Table 9-2**). When these optimum values are reached, cardiac output will be maximized in a given patient, and quality of life often improves markedly. If, when optimum SVR and pulmonary capillary wedge pressure (CWP) are reached, a critically low cardiac output is still present, this confirms truly refractory, or Stage IV, heart failure. Such patients have limited treatment options, including palliation, mechanical circulatory support, or transplantation.

CASE PRESENTATION

If we return to our case, Mr. Smithers has clearly presented to your clinic undertreated with regard to both diuretics and vasodilator therapy. He is admitted to the hospital, and treated with IV diuretics and IV vasodilators. Despite initial improvement, he rapidly worsens with withdrawal of these medications. You decide to place a pulmonary artery catheter for hemodynamic guidance.

Invasive hemodynamics are shown in **Table 9-3**, Column A, and are notable for moderately increased filling pressures, markedly elevated vascular resistances, and significantly impaired cardiac output.

You begin IV nitroprusside, and uptitrate it to achieve optimal vasodilation, which occurs at a dose of 0.2 mcg/min. His improved hemodynamics are shown in **Table 9-3**, Column B. Despite use of no inotropic medication, cardiac output (CO) has improved substantially as SVR was reduced, without a significant change in blood pressure. The relationship between cardiac output and SVR is inverse, and also affected by the pressure difference across the systemic arterial bed, as described by the hemodynamic equation CO = MAP-RA/SVR, where SVR is expressed in Wood Units. The fall in RAP that typically occurs with improved heart failure therapy helps increase cardiac output, and decreased right-sided venous pressures are an important component of adequate hemodynamic therapy and improved organ perfusion (4,15).

These new hemodynamics reassure you that when optimally vasodilated, your patient has adequate cardiac output. His filling pressures remain elevated above optimal levels, so you continue diuresing him aggressively to achieve a CWP less than 15 mmHg. You transition him off the IV nitroprusside to oral therapy, keeping the catheter in place to gauge response. He is transitioned from nitroprusside to captopril plus oral nitrates, with doses rapidly uptitrated as tolerated to maintain his SVR of 800 to 1200 dynes*sec/cm^5. When you have uptitrated the doses, he is switched to longer acting medications: enalapril 10 mg po bid and isosorbide mononitrate 120 mg daily. His beta-blocker has been changed to carvedilol to comply with guidelines, and this has been uptitrated to 12.5 mg bid once his volume status was controlled. At this point, his symptoms are vastly improved, his exercise tolerance has increased, he is able to stand without light-headedness, and his hemodynamics remain optimized, as shown in **Table 9-3**, Column C.

When a patient presents with decompensation and the determination is made that they have achieved an optimized volume status, attention should switch to dosing of other oral medications, particularly neurohormonal blocking drugs and vasodilators. These drugs should be uptitrated to guidelines-based doses, or to the highest dose, that does not produce

Table 9-3
Patient's Invasive Hemodynamics Over Time

HEMODYNAMIC PARAMETER	A BASELINE	B ON IV THERAPY	C AFTER IN-HOSPITAL TRANSITION TO ORAL THERAPY	D 8 MONTHS LATER
BP	94/55	92/46	92/46	98/60
RAP (mmHg)	28	18	6	5
PA (S/D/M, mmHg)	52/31/40	40/21/29	43/20/27	28/12/17
CWP (mmHg)	21	23	7	8
Cardiac Output	3.3	5.5	5.0	5.5
Cardiac Index	1.6	2.6	2.4	2.6
SVR (dynes*sec/cm^5)	2,325	994	1,063	1,130
PVR (Wood Units)	6.1	1.1	2.2	1.6

Note: BP = blood pressure; PA = pulmonary artery; S/D/M = systolic/diastolic/mean; CWP = capillary wedge pressure; PVR = pulmonary vascular resistance; RAP = right atrial pressure; SVR = systemic vascular resistance.

intolerable side effects. Aggressiveness in optimizing dose of these medications not only saves lives, but also prevents decompensation and hospitalization in heart failure patients. Guidelines-based dosing of these medications is discussed in Chapter 1.

A few final points deserve mention. When hemodynamic optimization, or tailored therapy, is pursued in a heart failure patient, regular physical examination should continue. Often physicians cease examining a patient when invasive hemodynamic monitoring is present. This, however, is often the most instructive time to examine a patient. Physical examination in the presence of invasive hemodynamic monitoring can help a provider identify jugular venous pulsations in a patient with a more difficult neck examination, for example. One can determine how warm a patient's periphery feels when the SVR is optimized to 1000 dynes*sec/cm^5, and learn the precise degree of concordance between RAP and CWP in a given patient. Knowledge of such factors can be used to maintain optimized status over time as an outpatient, using serial outpatient examination and adjustment of therapy when the examination deviates from what has been shown to be "optimal" in a given patient. Using this approach, optimum hemodynamics can be maintained over months to years, and many patients have further hemodynamic improvement over time with such attentive examination-based therapy (26).

CASE PRESENTATION

In the case of Mr. Smithers, when you have achieved optimized hemodynamics, his skin feels extremely warm to the touch on the forearms and shins. His JVP is visible at 7 cm above the RA lying at 30 degrees, and is not visible when sitting upright. In the first month after discharge, you see him every 1 to 2 weeks, and uptitrate his carvedilol to the goal dose of 25 mg bid. Several times over the next 6 months in clinic you notice that his JVP has crept up above 10 cm H_2O. You increase his diuretics in response, even though he is not complaining of symptoms of volume retention at the time, and his JVP decreases back down below 8 cm H_2O. Once, in clinic, you note that his periphery is significantly cooler than it had been when he was optimized. His blood pressure has also crept up to 125/82. You double his enalapril to 20 mg po bid. Eight months after his initial hospitalization, he presents with atypical chest pain, and because of his significant coronary disease history, the decision is made to pursue angiography. Curious, you ask the interventional team to perform a right-heart catheterization prior to the angiogram. On exam you feel that his heart failure is optimized: His JVP is 6 cm H_2O, his periphery is very warm, his pulse is 66, and his blood pressure is 104/72. You are gratified to get the hemodynamics shown in **Table 9-3**, Column D, demonstrating continued optimal volume status and perfusion with your tailored management approach.

Finally, there are patients in whom physical examination is difficult, unhelpful, or even misleading. If a patient reports severe symptoms, in the absence of discernible physical examination evidence of decompensation, exercise testing for functional capacity and pulmonary artery catheterization can both be very useful in select cases, to determine whether the heart failure is in fact worse than recognized, or, conversely, whether a search for an alternative cause of the symptoms is in order. When the physical examination and the history do not agree, obtaining more objective data can often be a critical first step in improving a patient's well-being and outcomes. Confidence in your physical examination skills is the first, and most important, step in managing the ill heart failure patient.

REFERENCES

1. Nohria A, Tsang SW, Fang JC, et al. Clinical assessment identifies hemodynamic profiles that predict outcomes in patients admitted with heart failure. *J Am Coll Cardiol*. 2003;41: 1797–1804.
2. Drazner MH, Rame JE, Stevenson LW, et al. Prognostic importance of elevated jugular venous pressure and a third heart sound in patients with heart failure. *N Engl J Med*. 2001;345:574–581.
3. Zile MR, Bennett TD, St John Sutton M, et al. Transition from chronic compensated to acute decompensated heart failure: Pathophysiological insights obtained from continuous monitoring of intracardiac pressures. *Circulation*. 2008;118:1433–1441.
4. Stevenson LW, Tillisch JH, Hamilton M, et al. Importance of hemodynamic response to therapy in predicting survival with ejection fraction less than or equal to 20% secondary to ischemic or nonischemic dilated cardiomyopathy. *Am J Cardiol*. 1990;66:1348–1354.
5. Lucas C, Johnson W, Hamilton MA, et al. Freedom from congestion predicts good survival despite previous class iv symptoms of heart failure. *Am Heart J*. 2000;140:840–847.
6. Hunt SA, Abraham WT, Chin MH, et al. 2009 focused update incorporated into the ACC/AHA 2005 guidelines for the diagnosis and management of heart failure in adults: a report of the American College of Cardiology Foundation/American Heart Association task force on practice guidelines: developed in collaboration with the International Society for Heart and Lung Transplantation. *Circulation*. 2009;119:e391–479.
7. Gheorghiade M, Follath F, Ponikowski P, et al. Assessing and grading congestion in acute heart failure: a scientific statement from the acute heart failure committee of the heart failure association of the european society of cardiology and endorsed by the European Society of Intensive Care Medicine. *Eur J Heart Fail*. 2010;12:423–433.

8. Nohria A, Mielniczuk LM, Stevenson LW. Evaluation and monitoring of patients with acute heart failure syndromes. *Am J Cardiol*. 2005;96:32G–40G.
9. Conn RD, O'Keefe JH. Cardiac physical diagnosis in the digital age: An important but increasingly neglected skill (from stethoscopes to microchips). *Am J Cardiol*. 2009;104:590–595.
10. Mangione S, Nieman LZ, Gracely E, et al. The teaching and practice of cardiac auscultation during internal medicine and cardiology training. A nationwide survey. *Ann Intern Med*. 1993; 119:47–54.
11. Vukanovic-Criley JM, Criley S, Warde CM, et al. Competency in cardiac examination skills in medical students, trainees, physicians, and faculty: a multicenter study. *Arch Intern Med*. 2006; 166:610–616.
12. Chomsky DB, Lang CC, Rayos G, et al. Treatment of subclinical fluid retention in patients with symptomatic heart failure: Effect on exercise performance. *J Heart Lung Transplant*. 1997;16: 846–853.
13. Gheorghiade M, Abraham WT, Albert NM, et al. Systolic blood pressure at admission, clinical characteristics, and outcomes in patients hospitalized with acute heart failure. *J Am Med Assoc*. 2006;296:2217–2226.
14. Adams KF Jr, Fonarow GC, Emerman CL, et al. Characteristics and outcomes of patients hospitalized for heart failure in the united states: rationale, design, and preliminary observations from the first 100,000 cases in the Acute Decompensated Heart Failure National Registry (ADHERE). *Am Heart J*. 2005;149:209–216.
15. Stevenson LW, Tillisch JH. Maintenance of cardiac output with normal filling pressures in patients with dilated heart failure. *Circulation*. 1986;74:1303–1308.
16. Rosario LB, Stevenson LW, Solomon SD, et al. The mechanism of decrease in dynamic mitral regurgitation during heart failure treatment: importance of reduction in the regurgitant orifice size. *J Am Coll Cardiol*. 1998;32:1819–1824.
17. Stevenson LW. Theodore e. Woodward award: coming in out of the rain. Relieving congestion in heart failure. *Trans Am Clin Climatol Assoc*. 2009;120:177–187.
18. Chakko S, Woska D, Martinez H, et al. Clinical, radiographic, and hemodynamic correlations in chronic congestive heart failure: conflicting results may lead to inappropriate care. *Am J Med*. 1991;90:353–359.
19. Drazner MH, Brown RN, Kaiser PA, et al. Relationship of right- and left-sided filling pressures in patients with advanced heart failure: a 14-year multi-institutional analysis. *J Heart Lung Transplant*. 2012;31:67–72.
20. Shah MR, Stinnett SS, McNulty SE, et al. Hemodynamics as surrogate end points for survival in advanced heart failure: an analysis from first. *Am Heart J*. 2001;141:908–914.
21. Binanay C, Califf RM, Hasselblad V, et al. Evaluation study of congestive heart failure and pulmonary artery catheterization effectiveness: the escape trial. *J Am Med Assoc*. 2005;294:1625–1633.
22. Butman SM, Ewy GA, Standen JR, et al. Bedside cardiovascular examination in patients with severe chronic heart failure: importance of rest or inducible jugular venous distension. *J Am Coll Cardiol*. 1993;22:968–974.
23. Ewy GA. The abdominojugular test: Technique and hemodynamic correlates. *Ann Intern Med*. 1988;109:456–460.
24. Mueller C, Frana B, Rodriguez D, et al. Emergency diagnosis of congestive heart failure: impact of signs and symptoms. *Can J Cardiol*. 2005;21:921–924.
25. Vader JM, Drazner MH. Clinical assessment of heart failure: utility of symptoms, signs, and daily weights. *Heart Failure Clinics*. 2009; 5:149–160.
26. Hamilton MA, Stevenson LW, Child JS, et al. Sustained reduction in valvular regurgitation and atrial volumes with tailored vasodilator therapy in advanced congestive heart failure secondary to dilated (ischemic or idiopathic) cardiomyopathy. *Am J Cardiol*. 1991;67:259–263.
27. Ritzema J, Troughton R, Melton I, et al. Physician-directed patient self-management of left atrial pressure in advanced chronic heart failure. *Circulation*. 2010;121:1086–1095.
28. Cruden NL, Witherow FN, Webb DJ, et al. Bradykinin contributes to the systemic hemodynamic effects of chronic angiotensin-converting enzyme inhibition in patients with heart failure. *Arterioscler Thromb Vasc Biol*. 2004;24:1043–1048.
29. Taylor AL, Ziesche S, Yancy C, et al. Combination of isosorbide dinitrate and hydralazine in blacks with heart failure. *N Engl J Med*. 2004;351:2049–2057.
30. Intravenous nesiritide vs nitroglycerin for treatment of decompensated congestive heart failure: A randomized controlled trial. *J Am Med Assoc*. 2002;287:1531–1540.
31. Elkayam U, Tasissa G, Binanay C, et al. Use and impact of inotropes and vasodilator therapy in hospitalized patients with severe heart failure. *Am Heart J*. 2007;153:98–104.
32. Elis A, Bental T, Kimchi O, et al. Intermittent dobutamine treatment in patients with chronic refractory congestive heart failure: A randomized, double-blind, placebo-controlled study. *Clin Pharmacol Ther*. 1998;63:682–685.
33. Cuffe MS, Califf RM, Adams KF Jr, et al. Short-term intravenous milrinone for acute exacerbation of chronic heart failure: a randomized controlled trial. *J Am Med Assoc*. 2002;287:1541–1547.
34. Abraham WT, Adams KF, Fonarow GC, et al. In-hospital mortality in patients with acute decompensated heart failure requiring intravenous vasoactive medications: An analysis from the Acute Decompensated Heart Failure National Registry (ADHERE). *J Am Coll Cardiol*. 2005;46:57–64.
35. Cohn JN, Goldstein SO, Greenberg BH, et at. A dose-dependent increase in mortality with vesnarinone among patients with severe heart failure. Vesnarinone trial investigators. *N Engl J Med*. 1998;339;1810–1816.
36. Uretsky BF, Jessup M, Konstam MA, et al. Multicenter trial of oral enoximone in patients with moderate to moderately severe congestive heart failure. Lack of benefit compared with placebo. Enoximone multicenter trial group. *Circulation*. 1990;82:774–780.
37. Allen LA, Rogers JG, Warnica JW, et al. High mortality without escape: the registry of heart failure patients receiving pulmonary artery catheters without randomization. *J Card Fail*. 2008;14:661–669.
38. Sanderson JE, Chan SK, Yip G, et al. Beta-blockade in heart failure: A comparison of carvedilol with metoprolol. *J Am Coll Cardiol*. 1999;34:1522–1528.
39. Gilbert EM, Abraham WT, Olsen S, et al. Comparative hemodynamic, left ventricular functional, and antiadrenergic effects of chronic treatment with metoprolol versus carvedilol in the failing heart. *Circulation*. 1996;94;2817–2825.

III

Heart Failure With Multiple Treatment Issues

10

Evaluation and Management of the Heart Transplant Candidate

MAURICIO VELEZ AND MARYL R. JOHNSON

BACKGROUND

Advanced heart failure therapies, including mechanical circulatory support and cardiac transplantation, remain the best treatment options for individuals with refractory heart failure symptoms in spite of maximally tolerated medical therapy (Stage D heart failure). Among these therapies, cardiac transplantation offers the best long-term survival, with 50% of recipients surviving at least 10 years after transplantation (**Figure 10-1**; 1). That said, recent advances in mechanical circulatory support technology and clinical care have led to consistent improvement in clinical outcomes for patients supported by left ventricular assist devices (LVADs) with expected 12-month survival of approximately 70% for the HeartMate II® (Thoratec Corporation, Pleasanton, CA) device (2), and up to 86% for the Heartware® device (Heartware Incorporated, Framingham, MA), which is still the subject of ongoing clinical trials (3). These survival statistics compare to close to 85% mean 1-year survival for heart transplant recipients (1).

CASE PRESENTATION

XY is a 57-year-old man with chronic heart failure due to non-ischemic cardiomyopathy, who was referred to an advanced heart failure and transplant cardiology center for evaluation for heart transplantation.

The patient was diagnosed with non-ischemic cardiomyopathy 4 years ago after he presented to his primary care physician's office with a history of progressive exercise intolerance due to dyspnea and fatigue for 4 months. His dyspnea had progressed to the point where he was only able to walk one block and climb one flight of stairs before he developed shortness of breath. He used to be an avid golfer who did not like to use a cart, but over the course of the previous year, he found himself using a cart more often to avoid dyspnea until he found himself unable to play anymore. He had also developed decreased appetite and early satiety, yet he noticed a weight gain of 15 pounds over 4 months along with the appearance of lower extremity edema. At that initial visit, his primary care doctor decided to admit him to the hospital for treatment of acutely decompensated heart failure.

XY had a past medical history of hypertension, obesity, and sleep apnea. He was being treated with atenolol and aspirin. He regularly used continuous positive airway pressure (CPAP) at night. He was a former smoker of half a pack of cigarettes daily, but he quit 10 years earlier after his first son was born. He worked as an auto mechanic in his own shop for 15 years. He was married with two adult children. He drank alcohol socially and never used recreational drugs.

At the time of admission to the hospital, his physical exam was notable for a blood pressure of 140/95, with a heart rate of 75 beats per minute, and a weight of 225 lb and height of 5 ft 9 in (body mass index [BMI] 33.2 kg/m^2). His carotid pulses were brisk bilaterally and he had jugular venous distention with an estimated central venous pressure of 14 cm H_2O. His lungs showed crackles at both bases. His cardiac examination showed a diffuse apical impulse located at the intersection of the sixth left intercostal space and the anterior axillary line. His rhythm was regular, with a soft S1 and a paradoxically split S2. He had an S3, but no S4. He also had a

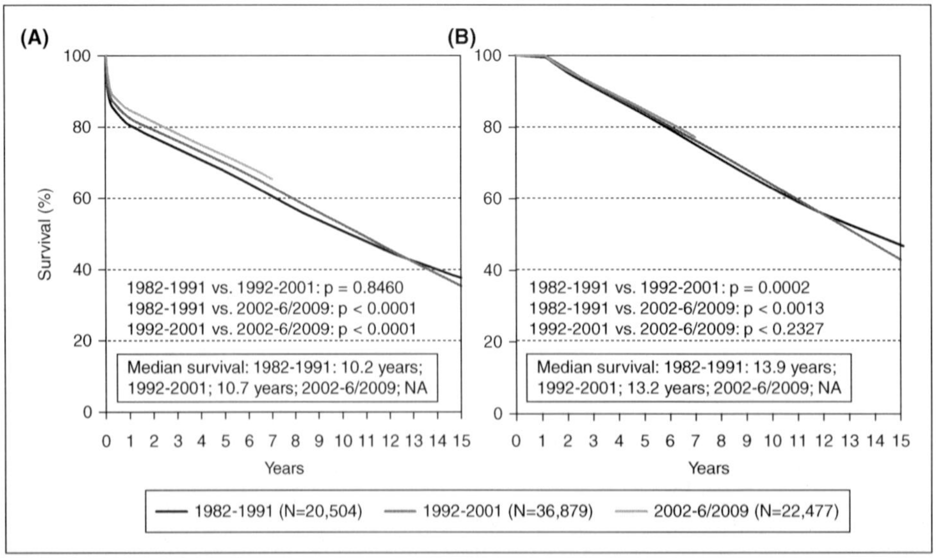

Figure 10-1
Cardiac transplant survival. Panel A. The expected half-life for a cardiac allograft is over 10 years. Panel B. For recipients who survive the first year posttransplant, the expected allograft half-life (conditional half-life) is over 13 years.
Source: With permission from reference 1.

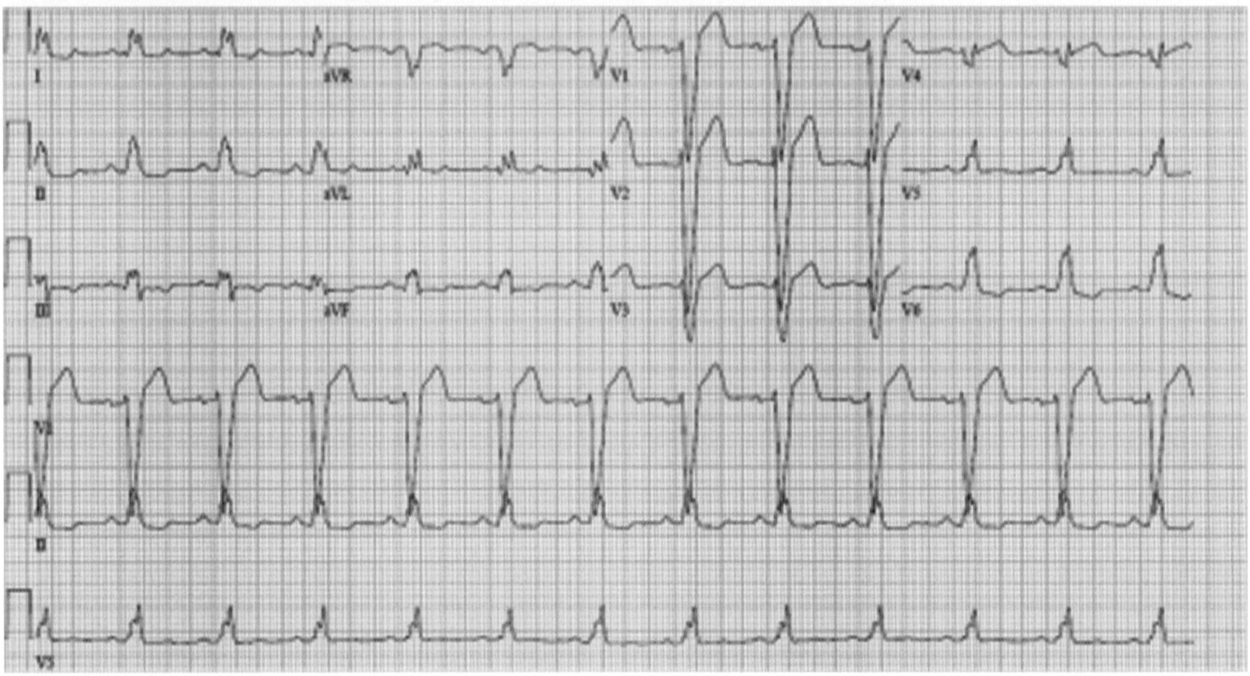

Figure 10-2
Electrocardiogram. XY's electrocardiogram shows normal sinus rhythm at 78 beats per minute. His QRS has a left bundle branch block morphology with a duration of 168 msec.

3/6 systolic murmur heard at the apex that radiated to the axilla. His abdomen was mildly distended and his liver was mildly enlarged. His extremities were warm and dry, with 1+ pitting edema up to the thighs bilaterally. His distal pulses were strong bilaterally.

His electrocardiogram (ECG) showed normal sinus rhythm at 75 bpm with a left bundle branch block with a QRS duration of 168 msec (**Figure 10-2**). His chest x-ray revealed cardiomegaly with a cardiothoracic ratio greater than 0.5, and increased lung vascular markings indicative of pulmonary congestion (**Figure 10-3**). Additional laboratory evaluation included a complete blood count, electrolytes and renal function, liver function tests, thyroid function tests, and iron studies (**Table 10-1**).

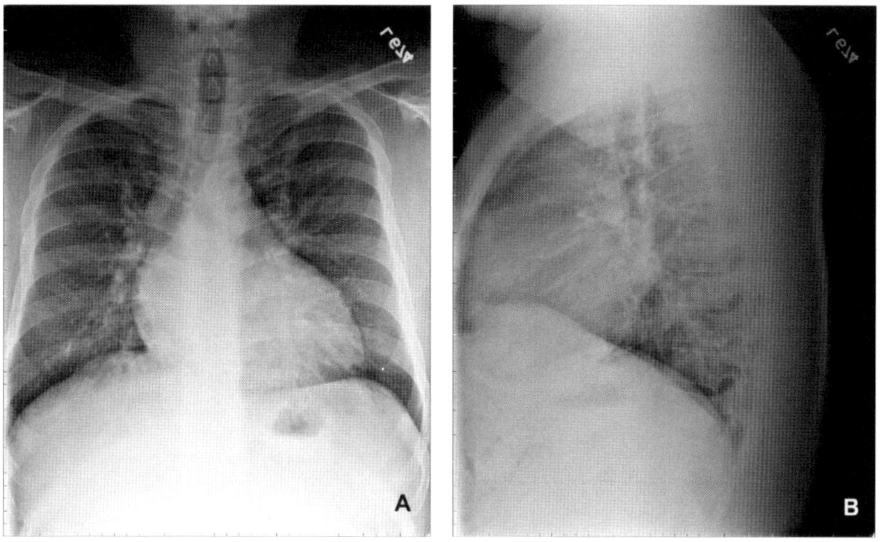

Figure 10-3
Chest x-ray. Panel A shows a postero anterior x-ray view of the chest with evidence of cardiomegaly and prominent lung vascular markings suggestive of pulmonary congestion. Panel B shows a lateral view that again demonstrates cardiomegaly without evidence of pleural effusions.

Table 10-1
Laboratory Evaluation at the Time of Index Hospitalization

PARAMETER	RESULT	PARAMETER	RESULT
WBC	6.9 K/μL	AST	32 IU/L
Hemoglobin	11 g/dL	ALT	51 IU/L
Hematocrit	33%	Total protein	7.1 g/dL
Platelets	222 K/μL	Albumin	3.6 g/dL
Sodium	144 mEq/L	Total bilirubin	0.5 mg/dL
Potassium	4 mEq/L	Direct bilirubin	0.1 mg/dL
Chloride	106 mEq/L	Alkaline phosphatase	58 IU/L
CO_2	29 mEq/L	Total cholesterol	144 mg/dL
Blood urea nitrogen	9 mg/dL	Triglycerides	126 mg/dL
Creatinine	1.2 mg/dL	HDL-C	45 mg/dL
Glucose	107 mg/dL	LDL-C	74 mg/dL
Calcium	8.8 mg/dL	TSH	3.02 μIU/mL
Magnesium	2.2 mg/dL	Ferritin	144 mg/dL
Phosphorus	2.9 mg/dL	Iron saturation	24%

Note: ALT = alanine aminotransferase; AST = aspartate aminotransferase; CO_2 = carbon dioxide; HDL-C = high density lipoprotein cholesterol; LDL-C = low density lipoprotein cholesterol; TSH = thyroid stimulating hormone; WBC = white blood cell count.

During that hospitalization, XY was treated with IV furosemide and he was started on lisinopril and carvedilol. He was evaluated with a transthoracic echocardiogram that revealed a markedly dilated left ventricle with severely reduced left ventricular systolic function with an ejection fraction of 15% and mild mitral regurgitation (**Figure 10-4**). A cardiologist that was consulted for further evaluation recommended coronary angiography. This study showed nonobstructive coronary artery disease. A right-heart catheterization was not done at that time.

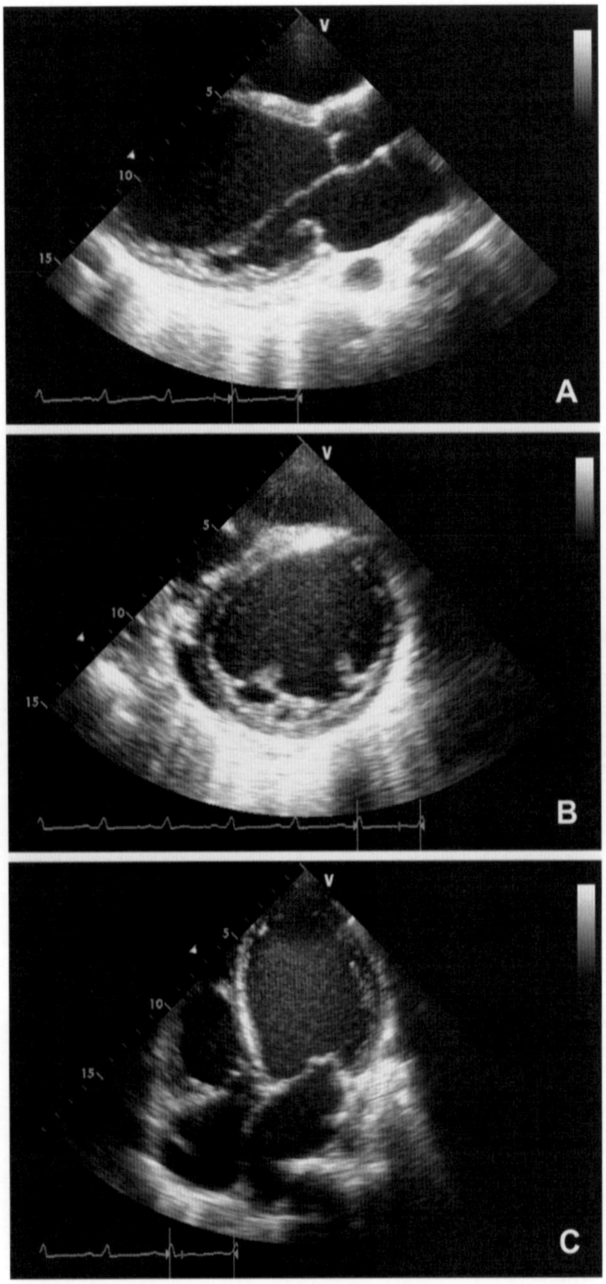

Figure 10-4
Echocardiogram. Panel A shows a still image from the parasternal long axis view demonstrating a severely dilated left ventricle. Panel B shows the parasternal short axis view. Panel C shows the apical four-chamber view, where the left ventricle shows evidence of remodeling as indicated by its globular shape. There is bowing of the interatrial septum from left to right suggesting increased left atrial pressure. Moderate mitral regurgitation was also noted (not shown). The right ventricle was mildly dilated.

XY's symptoms improved with medical treatment and he was discharged from the hospital. He was instructed to follow a 2 gm sodium diet with a 2 L per day fluid restriction and was advised to weigh himself daily and call his physician's office if he gained more than 2 pounds in a day or 5 pounds total. He regained the ability to walk up to a half mile before he developed dyspnea or fatigue and began playing golf again. However, he continued to have mild dyspnea with moderate exertion. He continued to follow with a cardiologist in the outpatient setting. XY's cardiologist optimized his medical regimen for cardiomyopathy over the course of 3 months by achieving goal doses of lisinopril (40 mg p.o. daily) and carvedilol (25 mg p.o. twice daily). He later added spironolactone 25 mg p.o. daily.

After being on optimal medical therapy for 3 months, a repeat echocardiogram revealed that XY's left ventricular systolic function remained severely reduced with a left ventricular ejection fraction of 20%. In view of this, and the fact that he had persistent symptoms and a wide QRS on his ECG, his cardiologist recommended cardiac resynchronization therapy with an implantable cardioverter-defibrillator (CRT-D). A biventricular pacemaker/implantable cardioverter-defibrillator (ICD) was implanted 6 months after the index hospitalization.

XY remained stable with NYHA function Class II exercise tolerance until 1 year ago, when he began noticing that his exercise capacity started to decline again. He was able to walk only a half block and could only climb half a flight of stairs before developing shortness of breath and tiredness. His symptoms gradually progressed to the point where he developed dyspnea at rest with three-pillow orthopnea and paroxysmal nocturnal dyspnea. For this reason, he was admitted to the hospital again and was treated for acute-on-chronic heart failure. After that hospitalization 1 year ago, XY had several other episodes of decompensated heart failure with progressive reduction in his exercise tolerance.

During XY's last hospitalization, his ICD fired twice for ventricular tachycardia, despite the fact that his potassium and magnesium were normal. He was found to be hypotensive with a blood pressure (BP) of 85/65 and in significant respiratory distress, so he was transferred to a tertiary care center with an advanced heart failure program for further evaluation and treatment.

XY was admitted to the ICU at the tertiary center under the care of an advanced heart failure cardiologist. His medical regimen upon transfer included furosemide 120 mg IV every 12 hours. Lisinopril, carvedilol, and spironolactone had been discontinued due to hypotension. His physical examination revealed a BP of 87/58, pulse of 94 per minute and regular, respiratory rate of 20 per minute, oxygen saturation of 93% on room air, and temperature of 36.9°C. He appeared pale, somnolent, and fatigued, but was easy to rouse. His jugular venous pressure was elevated, with the pulsation seen at his earlobe with him sitting at 90° and with hepatojugular reflux present. His lungs showed decreased breath sounds and dullness at both bases. His cardiac exam revealed a diffuse and laterally displaced apical impulse, with a regular rhythm with occasional extrasystoles. He had a soft S1 and S2, with an audible S3 and S4. Again noted was a holosystolic murmur present at the apex, with 3/6 intensity and radiation to the axilla. The abdomen was soft and mildly distended. The liver was enlarged and pulsatile. The extremities were cool and had sluggish capillary refill. There was 1+ dependent edema up to the hips bilaterally.

His chest x-ray revealed cardiomegaly and bilateral pleural effusions. His CRT-D device was noted. His renal function tests were now significant for elevated blood urea nitrogen (BUN) at 54 mg/dL and creatinine at 1.9 mg/dL. His aspartate aminotransferase (AST), alanine aminotransferase (ALT), and total bilirubin were also elevated at 77 IU/L, 84 IU/L, and 2.1 mg/dL, respectively.

XY had a Swan-Ganz catheter placed for hemodynamic guidance in therapy adjustments. As shown in **Table 10-2**, his invasive hemodynamics showed markedly elevated intracardiac filling pressures with a depressed cardiac index and elevated systemic vascular resistance. He was started on IV milrinone at 0.375 mcg/kg/min and his dose of IV furosemide was increased. This resulted in an improvement in his blood pressure, mentation, urine output, and other symptoms. His renal and liver function normalized with intropic support with milrinone.

After starting milrinone, XY developed frequent runs of nonsustained ventricular tachycardia (VT). His potassium and magnesium were noted to be low and were repleted, which led to decreased ventricular ectopy. However, he later received two ICD shocks for sustained VT associated with hypotension and altered mental status, in spite of normalized electrolytes. He was started on IV amiodarone to suppress ventricular ectopy. His mentation and urine output improved and his ventricular arrhythmias did not recur.

Since his renal function normalized after treatment with IV milrinone, XY's preload and afterload reduction therapy with an angiotensin-converting enzyme (ACE) inhibitor was resumed. Carvedilol was not resumed during this hospitalization due to XY's evidence of cardiogenic shock upon presentation. His CRT-D device was interrogated and was found to be operating properly with stable lead impedance and 98.9% biventricular pacing. XY was transferred out of the ICU, the milrinone was weaned off, and the patient was discharged home on lisinopril 20 mg daily and an increased dose of oral furosemide.

After discharge, XY remained quite limited with NYHA functional Class III symptoms. In view of this, his heart failure cardiologist proposed the need to consider advanced therapies including LVAD and heart transplantation. XY expressed interest in proceeding and the evaluation process was started.

EVALUATION FOR VENTRICULAR ASSIST DEVICE AND CARDIAC TRANSPLANT CANDIDACY

The purpose of the evaluation process to determine candidacy for a ventricular assist device (VAD) and cardiac transplantation is to assess whether an individual patient is ill enough to justify the risk of LVAD placement or listing for cardiac transplantation and to rule out any physical, psychological, or social factors that would decrease the likelihood of success should the patient receive an LVAD or transplant. In the physical sphere, factors that will decrease the patient's longevity independent from cardiac disease, and factors that will increase the risk of perioperative or postoperative complications are usually considered contraindications to LVAD implantation and transplantation. In the psychological sphere, uncontrolled psychiatric illness, substance abuse, and behavioral patterns that interfere with compliance with medications and visits constitute significant barriers. Lastly, from a social point of view, lack

Table 10-2
Invasive Hemodynamic Evaluation Pre- and Post-IV Milrinone

HEMODYNAMIC PARAMETER	BASELINE	MILRINONE 0.375 mcg/kg/min
CVP (m), mmHg	22	12
RV (s/d), mmHg	64/22	42/12
PA (s/d/m), mmHg	64/35/45	42/17/25
PCWP (m), mmHg	32	15
CO, L/min	2.3	3.9
CI, L/min/m^2	1.1	1.9
ABP (s/d/m), mmHg	85/65/72	92/60/71
SVR, dyn·s/cm^5	1,739	1,210
PVR, WU	5.7	2.6

Note: ABP = systemic arterial blood pressure (systolic/diastolic/mean); CI = cardiac index; CO = cardiac output; CVP = central venous pressure (mean); PA = pulmonary artery pressure (systolic/diastolic/mean); PCWP = pulmonary capillary wedge pressure (mean); PVR = pulmonary vascular resistance (Wood units); RV = right ventricular pressure (systolic/end-diastolic); SVR = systemic vascular resistance. Baseline invasive hemodynamics show marked volume overload with elevated CVP and PCWP along with elevated SVR and a severe reduction in cardiac index. The introduction of milrinone and treatment with intravenous diuretics resulted in a reduction of intracardiac filling pressures and improvement in cardiac index.

of an adequate circle of support persons that can assist the individual during the initial recovery phase constitutes another contraindication to proceeding.

CARDIOPULMONARY STRESS TESTING

The first step in XY's evaluation was to obtain a cardiopulmonary exercise stress test (CPET). The use of peak oxygen consumption during exercise has been validated as a useful measure to determine which patients are sick enough to derive a survival benefit from cardiac transplantation. It had been generally accepted that a peak oxygen consumption (VO_2) of less than 14 mL/kg/min identifies individuals most likely to have a survival benefit from transplantation (4). However, patients treated with contemporary heart failure therapies, especially beta-blockers, have improved survival despite the achievement of lower peak VO_2 levels, so a threshold of less than 12 mL/kg/min is currently used in patients on beta-blocker therapy (5). Peak VO_2 responses help predict survival benefit with transplant, such that the benefit is greater in individuals with a peak VO_2 less than 10 mL/kg/min with maximal effort, indicated by achievement of an anaerobic threshold and a respiratory exchange ratio (RER) greater than 1.1. Therefore, individuals with a peak VO_2 less than 10 mL/kg/min who reach anaerobic threshold are generally considered transplant candidates.

Individuals with a peak VO_2 between 10 to 14 mL/kg/min and who have significant activity limitations may be considered probable candidates as well. Advanced heart failure patients may not be able to exercise maximally due to physical deconditioning, lack of motivation or other factors, so peak VO_2 often has to be interpreted in the setting of submaximal exercise. In this case, the slope of ventilation to carbon dioxide (VE/VCO_2) and the proportion of peak VO_2 achieved compared to what is expected for age, weight, and gender can add useful prognostic information. A VE/VCO_2 slope greater than 35 or a peak VO_2 that is less than 50% of predicted are indicators of a poor prognosis and reasons cardiac transplantation could be a reasonable consideration.

XY underwent a CPET that revealed a peak VO_2 of 11.6 mL/kg/min (40% of predicted) after reaching anaerobic threshold and with an RER of 1.12.

Given his significant exercise limitations, this level of peak oxygen consumption indicates that XY should be evaluated for cardiac transplantation. If the patient's prognosis from the CPET remains uncertain, composite scores defined to predict the outcomes of patients with ambulatory heart failure, including the Heart Failure Survival Score (6) or the Seattle Heart Failure Model (7), may also be applied to estimate a patient's prognosis; however, it should be realized that both of these scores tend to overestimate survival of patients with heart failure severe enough to consider heart transplantation or LVAD implantation (8).

PULMONARY HYPERTENSION

An important step in the evaluation of patients for cardiac transplantation is to rule out irreversible pulmonary hypertension. Elevated pulmonary artery (PA) pressure increases the likelihood of posttransplant right ventricular failure and decreases long-term survival following heart transplantation. In general, when PA systolic pressure is 50 mmHg or greater, the transpulmonary gradient (TPG) is high (PA mean–pulmonary capillary wedge pressure [PCWP] greater than or equal to 16), or pulmonary vascular resistance (PVR) is high (greater than 3 Wood units), evaluation for the reversibility of pulmonary hypertension should be performed.

In the majority of heart failure patients, pulmonary hypertension is the result of left ventricular systolic dysfunction, so-called pulmonary venous hypertension, therefore afterload and preload reduction are usually enough to reduce PA pressures. However, this may not be the case in patients with underlying valvular and congenital heart disease and those with pulmonary arterial hypertension.

Patients with pulmonary hypertension should be further evaluated with a vasodilator challenge. This involves invasive hemodynamic monitoring while the patient receives IV sodium nitroprusside, nitroglycerin, or nesiritide or breathes inhaled nitric oxide. The goal is to reduce PA pressures and the PVR without causing systemic hypotension or a reduction in cardiac output. Data suggests that individuals with an elevated PVR or transpulmonary gradient in spite of a vasodilator challenge have a high incidence of right heart failure and increased posttransplant mortality, therefore transplantation is usually contraindicated in this setting (9). Frequently, implantation of an LVAD can result in acceptable pulmonary pressures, even if they have not been attained with medical therapy (10). Therefore, in patients ill enough to require LVAD placement, pulmonary pressures should be reassessed after a period of VAD support if pulmonary hypertension is the only factor precluding consideration for heart transplantation.

As noted before, XY's initial invasive hemodynamics revealed moderate pulmonary hypertension with a borderline TPG and PVR. However, treatment with IV diuretics and inotropes lowered his PA pressures along with his TPG and PVR as expected.

Individuals with high PA pressures should be monitored with serial right-heart catheterization every 3 to 6 months to rule out recurrence or progression of pulmonary hypertension that would jeopardize their transplant candidacy.

PHYSICAL FACTORS

In addition to peak VO_2 and PA pressures, multiple other factors play a significant role in determining transplant candidacy. Current International Society for Heart and Lung Transplantation (ISHLT) guidelines for evaluation of transplant candidates (11,12) recommend that individuals should not be transplanted beyond the age of 70, as there is a trend toward increased mortality after transplant with advancing age.

With regard to other physical factors, conditions that increase the risk of perioperative and posttransplant morbidity and mortality must be assessed as part of the evaluation process. Obesity, cancer, diabetes with evidence of end-organ damage, and peripheral arterial disease may constitute contraindications to transplantation when present.

Patients with high BMI have generally been considered to be at higher risk of perioperative morbidity when they undergo cardiac surgery. Early studies suggested that obese cardiac transplant recipients (BMI greater than or equal to 30 kg/m^2) have a near twofold increase in the likelihood of death at 5 years posttransplant compared with recipients who were overweight or who had normal weight. In addition, obese recipients have a higher likelihood of acute rejection during the first year compared to nonobese recipients (13). More recent data have questioned the effect of obesity on outcomes following heart transplantation (14). However, ISHLT guidelines for selection of candidates for heart transplantation still recommend a BMI less than 30 or weight no greater than 140% of ideal body weight as a criteria for transplant listing, with weight loss to these levels recommended prior to listing for potential candidates above these weight thresholds. If obesity is the only factor precluding transplantation, implantation of an LVAD to allow the patient to become more physically active and have a better opportunity to achieve weight loss might be an appropriate bridge to transplant candidacy, even though adequate weight loss is not always achieved.

OTHER SYSTEMIC DISEASE

In addition, other conditions such as diabetes, especially if uncontrolled or with associated end-organ damage, peripheral arterial disease, and advanced chronic kidney disease are associated with poor posttransplant outcomes (15) and are considered relative contraindications. Advanced chronic kidney disease, especially if there is need for pretransplant dialysis, can be addressed with simultaneous heart–kidney transplantation, if the patient is considered a suitable candidate (16).

XY was not a diabetic, as his fasting blood glucose and hemoglobin A1C were within the normal range without the use of insulin or oral hypoglycemic medications. He underwent a carotid and vertebral artery ultrasound and resting ankle-brachial index studies, which revealed no peripheral arterial disease. His renal function was assessed with BUN and creatinine, which were 16 mg/dL and 1.5 mg/dL, respectively. His estimated glomerular filtration rate (GFR) according to the Modified Diet in Renal Disease (MDRD) equation was 62.1 mL/min, consistent with Stage 2 chronic kidney disease (mild impairment in GFR).

TOBACCO USE

Cigarette smoking increases the risk of cardiac allograft vasculopathy and malignancy after transplant; therefore, active tobacco use is a contraindication to transplant. It is general practice to advise potential candidates to quit smoking and avoid exposure to second-hand smoke. Transplant candidates usually must have a tobacco-free period of at least 6 months prior to listing (11,12). Random urine or serum nicotine or cotinine levels can be used once the patient is listed to monitor for relapses or exposure to second-hand smoke. Similarly, recreational drug and alcohol abuse are contraindications to LVAD implantation and transplantation.

PSYCHOLOGICAL FACTORS

In addition to physical factors, psychological and social issues need to be evaluated, as unfavorable behavioral patterns, including a history of noncompliance, or the absence of adequate support during the perioperative and initial recovery period represent common contraindications to transplantation and VAD implantation.

The psychological evaluation should be carried out by an experienced psychologist or other mental health professional who will assess the potential candidate for a history of psychiatric illness, including substance abuse, and treatment appropriateness. In the absence of psychiatric illness, certain behavioral patterns or cognitive deficits may raise red flags, as they may interfere with the patient's ability to comply with treatment or may limit his or her ability to understand instructions and recommendations. When the psychological evaluation raises concerns, the transplant psychologist or the patient's own therapist or psychiatrist can collaborate to optimize treatment or offer psychotherapy to address any concerning issues. If severe enough, psychological factors can be contraindications to transplantation or implantation of an LVAD.

Transplant and LVAD recipients require support from family, friends, or community members in the perioperative period and initial recovery phase to be able to manage the complexities and demands of these life-changing therapies. At least one, and preferably more than one, support person should be identified prior to transplant listing or LVAD implantation.

HEALTH MAINTENANCE

In addition to all the factors mentioned so far, potential cardiac transplant and LVAD candidates are tested to assess other end-organ function including liver and pulmonary function. The patient's health maintenance schedule should be up-to-date as recommended by the United States Preventive Services Taskforce (17). Also, in cardiac transplant candidates, an infectious evaluation is necessary, including HIV, herpes simplex virus, Hepatitis A, B, and C, cytomegalovirus, and Epstein-Barr virus exposure status. Patients should have immunity against common communicable diseases for which a vaccine is available. If immunity is not present, patients should be vaccinated prior to listing. Pneumococcal vaccination and influenza vaccination should be given if appropriate.

HISTOCOMPATIBILITY TESTING

Histocompatibility testing is another important step in the evaluation of cardiac transplant candidates. Screening for the presence of anti-human leucocyte antigen (HLA) antibodies directed to HLA Class I and II antigens allows for the appropriate selection of a donor heart. High levels of anti-HLA antibodies make finding a suitable donor more challenging and prolong the time that a candidate must wait on the list. In addition, a high antibody level is associated with an increased risk of early allograft failure and increased posttransplant mortality. The level of anti-HLA antibodies is commonly expressed as the panel reactive antibody (PRA).

PRA testing has most commonly been performed by exposing the lymphocytes from a pool of random individuals to the recipient's serum to detect the presence of anti-HLA antibodies. PRA is typically expressed as a percentage, which reflects the number of samples that show an immune reaction with the recipient's serum out of all the available random individual samples in the pool. A PRA greater than or equal to 10% is considered a risk factor for poor posttransplant outcomes (18). The recent development of solid phase assays for anti-HLA antibodies using beads or columns has improved the sensitivity of antibody detection and is requiring the transplant community to redefine the level of antibody present that should cause concern and require prospective crossmatching.

PRAs will increase in response to sensitizing events including blood transfusions and implantation of an LVAD (19). Under these circumstances, transplant candidates should be evaluated with serial PRAs to detect the development of new anti-HLA antibodies.

After careful consideration by the multidisciplinary cardiac transplant team, it was determined that XY's mortality risk justified the consideration of cardiac transplantation. After review of his history, test results, and input from the various consultants involved, XY was found to be a candidate for transplantation and was listed.

A summary of all the evaluations discussed is presented in **Table 10-3**. This constitutes the standard, comprehensive cardiac transplant evaluation.

Table 10-3
Elements of the Evaluation for Cardiac Transplant Candidacy for Patient XY

GENERAL STATUS	
Age	Gender
Height	Weight
BMI	ABO blood group and Rh factor
Panel reactive antibody	
CARDIAC STATUS	
Electrocardiogram	Echocardiogram
Coronary angiography	Right heart catheterization
Cardiopulmonary exercise test	
INFECTIOUS DISEASE EVALUATION	
Hepatitis B surface antibody (HBsAb)	Herpes simplex virus-2 IgG
Hepatitis B surface antigen (HBsAg)	Epstein-Barr virus IgG
Hepatitis B core antibody (HBcAb)	Varicella-zoster virus IgG
Hepatitis C antibody (Anti-Hep C)	T. pallidum hemagglutination assay (TPHA)
Hepatitis A antibody (Anti-Hep A)	Rapid plasma reagin (RPR)
Cytomegalovirus IgM	Toxoplasma IgM
Cytomegalovirus IgG	Toxoplasma IgG
Epstein-Barr virus IgM	HIV 1 and 2 antibodies
Herpes simplex virus-1 IgG	Quantiferon-TB gold test
ORGAN FUNCTION, CANCER SCREENING, AND ROUTINE STUDIES	
Liver function tests	Coagulation studies
Electrolytes and renal function	Thyroid function tests
Urinalysis	Prostate specific antigen (PSA)
Chest x-ray (postero-anterior and lateral views)	Pulmonary function tests
Iron studies	Pre-albumin
Abdominal ultrasound	Digital rectal exam
Carotid ultrasound	Ankle-brachial index
Bone density (dual-energy x-ray absorptiometry)	Colonoscopy
Dental evaluation (Panorex)	
SUBSTANCE ABUSE SCREENING	
Urine cotinine	Urine drug screen
CONSULTATIONS	
Cardiothoracic surgery	Social work
Clinical psychology	Financial counselor

BRIDGING TO CARDIAC TRANSPLANTATION WITH A VENTRICULAR ASSIST DEVICE

One month after being listed, XY decompensated once again and was hospitalized for treatment of acute-on-chronic heart failure with NYHA Class IV symptoms including orthopnea and paroxysmal nocturnal dyspnea (PND). He was again found to be hypotensive and markedly volume overloaded. He was admitted to the ICU and received a Swan-Ganz catheter. His invasive hemodynamics showed elevated intracardiac filling pressures and low cardiac index with a PCWP of 28 mmHg and a cardiac index of 1.8 L/min/m^2. He was placed back on milrinone and the dose was increased to 0.5 mcg/kg/min. He was also started on IV furosemide. Plans for implantation of an LVAD were expedited.

Continuous IV infusion of inotropic drugs such as milrinone and dobutamine has been used for treatment of chronic heart failure refractory to medical therapy. However, inotrope use has not been associated with increased survival in advanced heart failure, and may even increase mortality (20,21). Except for some select cases, chronic IV inotrope use is not the ideal strategy as bridge to transplantation. However, inotropes are often used as a bridge to an LVAD while evaluation for candidacy for LVAD implantation and/or heart transplantation is ongoing. Advances in mechanical circulatory support have led to the development of reliable implantable devices that can support ventricular function in patients with refractory heart failure symptoms. Clinical trials have shown that VADs are superior to chronic inotropes as a bridge to transplantation (22) or as destination therapy in carefully selected patients who are not candidates for heart transplantation (23).

The first generation of LVADs consisted of pulsatile pumps that were large and noisy and had several moving parts that deteriorated within 12 to 24 months, usually leading to pump malfunction. The prototype device for this generation was the HeartMate XVE VAD® (Thoratec Corporation, Pleasanton, CA). Second generation VADs provide continuous as opposed to pulsatile flow. This design improved upon pulsatile pumps by offering smaller size and much greater durability with fewer moving parts. Driveline caliber also decreased, which is thought to reduce the likelihood of driveline infection. The prototype device for this generation is the HeartMate II VAD® (Thoratec Corporation, Pleasanton, CA; **Figure 10-5**). This device

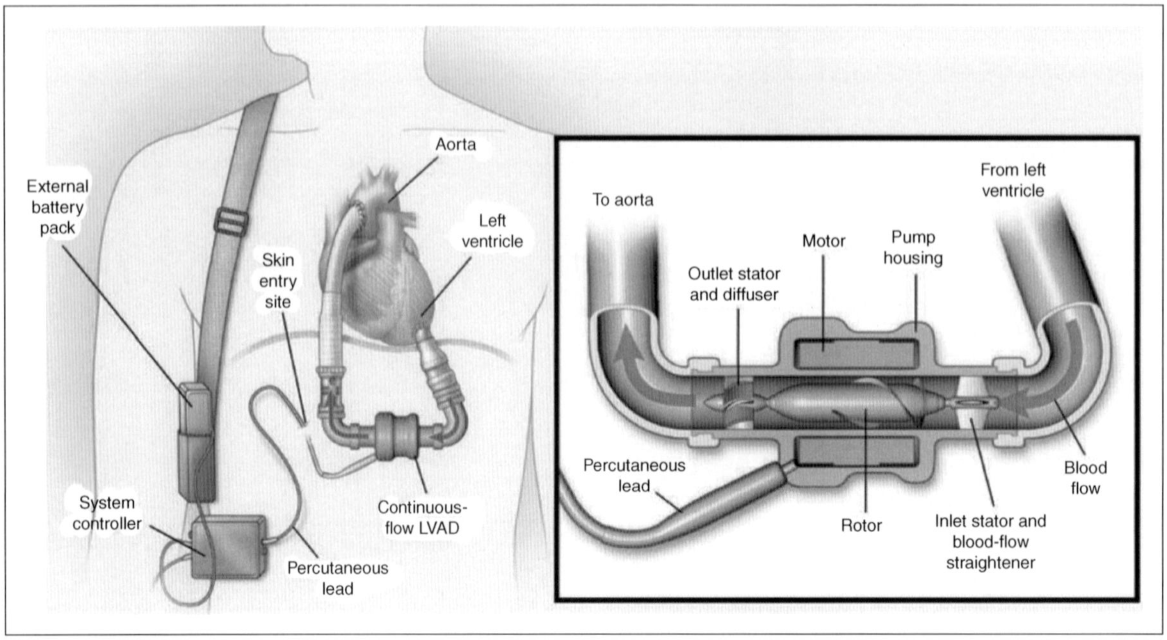

Figure 10-5
Schematic of left ventricular assist device in place with internal and external components. The ventricular assist device is placed in a pre- or intraperitoneal pocket. The device inflow cannula is inserted in the apex of the left ventricle. The device constantly receives blood from the left ventricle and the pump mechanism maintains continuous flow during systole and diastole. Blood is ejected into the ascending aorta through an outflow graft. The only moving part in this device is the pump rotor, which is spun by the pump motor. The percutaneous lead is tunneled under the skin and exits the patient to connect to the system controller and external battery pack.

Source: With permission from reference 24.

demonstrated efficacy for bridging to transplantation in a prospective clinical trial (24). Life expectancy with an LVAD has improved significantly with newer continuous flow devices. Current 12-month survival with the HeartMate II VAD® is estimated at 85%. That represents a significant improvement compared to historical survival rates with previous generation pulsatile devices (**Figure 10-6**).

The evaluation for LVAD candidacy is very similar to that of cardiac transplantation. In addition to the components required for cardiac transplantation, attention is given to clinical factors that can lead to complications in the perioperative period. Among all possible complications, acute right ventricular (RV) failure is particularly serious. Left VADs require adequate RV systolic function to fill the LVAD and in turn maintain adequate LVAD flow. Post-LVAD RV failure leads to multiorgan dysfunction, prolonged intubation, prolonged ICU stays, increased risk of bleeding, renal failure, and higher mortality (25,26). Most cases of post-LVAD RV failure can be managed with temporary use of IV inotropes, inhaled nitric oxide, or short-term mechanical right ventricular support.

Although several risk factors for post-LVAD RV failure have been identified, no particular risk factor or prediction model is specific enough to predict the risk of RV failure with a high level of accuracy (**Table 10-4**; 27).

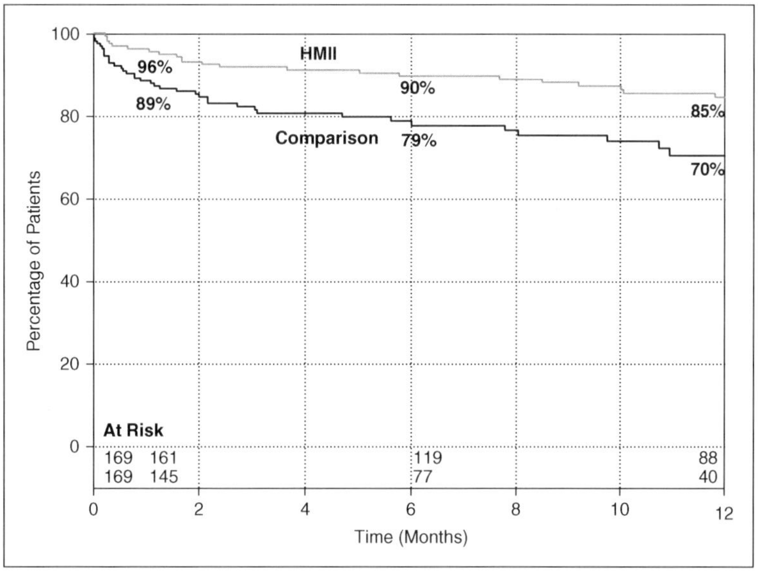

Figure 10-6
Kaplan-Meier survival for HeartMate II® LVAD compared with pulsatile devices. Percentages are the survival rates at 30 days, 6 months, and 12 months. HMII (HeartMate II®). Comparison represents patients implanted with the HeartMate® XVE and Thoratec IVAD®.
Source: With permission from reference 29.

Table 10-4
Risk Factors for Post-LVAD Acute Right Ventricular Failure

General	Smaller BSA, female gender, prior TIA/stroke, prior sternotomy
Pre-op events/interventions	Cardiac arrest within 24 hours of admission or any time prior to surgery, mechanical ventilation, renal replacement therapy
Medications	Intravenous vasopressin or norepinephrine, antiarrhythmics
Echocardiographic/hemodynamic	Severe RV dysfunction by echocardiogram, PASP < 50 mmHg, low cardiac index, RVSWI < 450 mmHg·mL/m^2
Laboratory	BUN ≥ 48 mg/dL, creatinine ≥ 2.3 mg/dL, WBC ≥ 12,200/L, platelets ≤ 120,000/L, albumin ≤ 3 g/dL, AST ≥ 80 IU/L, total bilirubin ≥ 2 mg/dL

Note: AST = aspartate aminotransferase; BUN = blood urea nitrogen; PASP = pulmonary artery systolic pressure; RV = right ventricle; RVSWI = right ventricular stroke work index; TIA = transient ischemic attack; WBC = white blood cell count.
Source: Adapted from reference 27.

Table 10-5
Invasive Hemodynamics Pre- and Post-LVAD

HEMODYNAMIC PARAMETER	MILRINONE 0.375 mcg/kg/min	MILRINONE 0.5 mcg/kg/min + IV FUROSEMIDE 15 mg/hr	POST-LVAD
CVP (m), mmHg	18	8	5
RV (s/d), mmHg	64/16	55/7	30/5
PA (s/d/m), mmHg	64/30/41	55/24/34	30/15/20
PCWP (m), mmHg	28	21	12
CO, L/min	3.0	4.4	5
CI, L/min/m²	1.4	2.1	2.4
ABP (s/d/m), mmHg	82/60/64	94/63/73	78 (MAP)
SVR, dyns/cm⁵	1,333	1,181	1,168
PVR, WU	4.4	3.0	1.6

Note: ABP = systemic arterial blood pressure (systolic/diastolic/mean); CI = cardiac index; CO = cardiac output; CVP = central venous pressure (mean); LVAD = left ventricular assist device; MAP = mean arterial pressure; PA = pulmonary artery pressure (systolic/diastolic/mean); PCWP = pulmonary capillary wedge pressure (mean); PVR = pulmonary vascular resistance (Wood units); RV = right ventricular pressure (systolic/end-diastolic); SVR = systemic vascular resistance.

Invasive hemodynamics revealed recurrence of cardiogenic shock in spite of ongoing milrinone use. Further increase in milrinone dosing and aggressive use of IV furosemide led to improvement in intracardiac filling pressures and cardiac index. Prior to LVAD implantation, invasive hemodynamics can provide supplemental information about right ventricular function. Post-LVAD hemodynamics define the degree of reversibility of pulmonary hypertension with optimal unloading of the left ventricle.

XY's right ventricle was evaluated with echocardiography. It was found to be mildly dilated with moderate systolic dysfunction. He also had moderate tricuspid regurgitation, with an estimated RV systolic pressure of 60 mmHg. His laboratory assessment was significant for WBC 9,000/L, platelets 198,000/L, BUN 24 mg/dL, creatinine 1.1 mg/dL, AST 54 IU/L, albumin 3.4 g/dL, and total bilirubin 1 mg/dL.

A repeat right-heart catheterization showed the findings presented in **Table 10-5**. On the higher dose of milrinone, XY maintained a PA systolic pressure greater than or equal to 50 mmHg and his RV stroke work index (RVSWI) was 598 mmHgxmL/m². Given these findings and the absence of significant end-organ dysfunction, it was felt that XY's right ventricle would have a low likelihood of perioperative RV failure. He was scheduled for LVAD implantation, received the device, and recovered uneventfully.

Mechanical circulatory support with LVADs carries the risk of complications including bleeding, thromboembolism, infection, development of anti-HLA antibodies, and device failure (24). The likelihood of complications has decreased with technological improvements and intensive follow-up. In general, transplant candidates who are supported with VADs must be closely monitored by a multidisciplinary team of health care professionals to ensure the best possible outcomes. Complications that may be observed during mechanical circulatory support with an LVAD are listed in **Table 10-6**.

Table 10-6
LVAD-Related Complications

COMPLICATION	ESTIMATED INCIDENCE
Driveline infection	15–20%
Gastrointestinal bleeding	25–55%
Hemorrhagic stroke	1.1%
Ischemic stroke	4%
Pump thrombosis	1.4–4%

Source: Adapted from reference 28.

Given that XY's PA pressures were mildly elevated prior to LVAD implantation, his post-LVAD pulmonary pressures were carefully evaluated to be certain he was a transplant candidate. With LVAD unloading, PA pressure decreased to 30/15, PCWP was 12, and cardiac output was 5 L/min, giving a PVR of 1.6 Wood units, which is clearly acceptable to be considered a transplant candidate (**Table 10-5**). This decrease in PA systolic pressure after LVAD implantation is commonly seen in candidates whose pulmonary hypertension fails to respond to maximal vasodilator therapy (10), either in the immediate post-LVAD period or upon reassessment after a period of LVAD support. His PRA was tested serially to detect the development of anti-HLA antibodies, but it remained at 0% throughout the wait period. After a wait time of 187 days, a suitable donor was found and XY received a heart transplant without complications.

REFERENCES

1. Stehlik J, Edwards LB, Kucheryavaya AY, et al. The Registry of the International Society for Heart and Lung Transplantation: twenty-eighth adult heart transplant report—2011. *J Heart Lung Transplant*. 2011;30(10):1078–1094.
2. Slaughter MS, Rogers JG, Milano CA, et al. Advanced heart failure treated with continuous-flow left ventricular assist device. *N Engl J Med*. 2009;361(23):2241–2251.
3. Slaughter MS. Evaluation of the HeartWare HVAD Left Ventricular Assist System for the Treatment of Advanced Heart Failure: results of the ADVANCE Bridge to Transplant Trial and Update with Continued Access Patients. Presented at the *International Society for Heart and Lung Transplantation Scientific Meeting. San Diego*, CA, 2011.
4. Mancini DM, Eisen H, Kussmaul W, et al. Value of peak exercise oxygen consumption for optimal timing of cardiac transplantation in ambulatory patients with heart failure. *Circulation*. 1991;83(3):778–786.
5. Peterson LR, Schechtman KB, Ewald GA, et al. The effect of beta-adrenergic blockers on the prognostic value of peak exercise oxygen uptake in patients with heart failure. *J Heart Lung Transplant*. 2003;22(1):70–77.
6. Aaronson KD, Schwartz JS, Chen TM, et al. Development and prospective validation of a clinical index to predict survival in ambulatory patients referred for cardiac transplant evaluation. *Circulation*. 1997;95(12):2660–2667.
7. Levy WC, Mozaffarian D, Linker DT, et al. The Seattle Heart Failure Model: prediction of survival in heart failure. *Circulation*. 2006;113(11):1424–1433.
8. Gorodeski EZ, Chu EC, Chow CH, et al. Application of the Seattle Heart Failure Model in ambulatory patients presented to an advanced heart failure therapeutics committee. *Circ Heart Fail*. 2010;3(6):706–714.
9. Stobierska-Dzierzek B, Awad H, Michler RE. The evolving management of acute right-sided heart failure in cardiac transplant recipients. *J Am Coll Cardiol*. 2001;38(4):923–931.
10. Martin J, Siegenthaler MP, Friesewinkel O, et al. Implantable left ventricular assist device for treatment of pulmonary hypertension in candidates for orthotopic heart transplantation-a preliminary study. *Eur J Cardiothorac Surg*. 2004;25(6):971–977.
11. Mehra MR, Jessup M, Gronda E, et al. Rationale and process: International Society for Heart and Lung Transplantation guidelines for the care of cardiac transplant candidates—2006. *J Heart Lung Transplant*. 2006;25(9):1001–1002.
12. Mehra MR, Kobashigawa J, Starling R, et al. Listing criteria for heart transplantation: International Society for Heart and Lung Transplantation guidelines for the care of cardiac transplant candidates—2006. *J Heart Lung Transplant*. 2006;25(9): 1024–1042.
13. Lietz K, John R, Burke EA, et al. Pretransplant cachexia and morbid obesity are predictors of increased mortality after heart transplantation. *Transplantation*. 2001;72(2):277–283.
14. Kashem MA, Fitzpatrick JT, Nikolaidis L, et al. BMI effects in heart transplant survival: single institution vs. national experience. *J Heart Lung Transplant*. 2009;28(2 Suppl):S116–S117.
15. Taylor DO, Edwards LB, Boucek MM, et al. The Registry of the International Society for Heart and Lung Transplantation: twenty-first official adult heart transplant report—2004. *J Heart Lung Transplant*. 2004;23(7):796–803.
16. Gill J, Shah T, Hristea I, et al. Outcomes of simultaneous heart-kidney transplant in the U.S.: a retrospective analysis using OPTN/UNOS data. *Am J Transplant*. 2009;9(4):844–852.
17. U.S. Preventive Services Task Force. The guide to clinical preventive services 2010–2011: recommendations of the U.S. Preventive Services Task Force. http://www.ahrq.gov/clinic/pocketgd1011/pocketgd1011.pdf. Accessed on October 9, 2011.
18. Lavee J, Kormos RL, Duquesnoy RJ, et al. Influence of panel-reactive antibody and lymphocytotoxic crossmatch on survival after heart transplantation. *J Heart Lung Transplant*. 1991;10(6);921–929.
19. Joyce DL, Southard RE, Torre-Amione G, et al. Impact of left venticular assist device (LVAD)-mediated humoral sensitization on post-transplant outcomes. *J Heart Lung Transplant*. 2005;24(12):2054–2059.
20. Cuffe MS, Califf RM, Adams KF, et al. Short-term intravenous milrinone for acute exacerbation of chronic heart failure. *JAMA*. 2002;287(12):1541–1547.
21. O'Connor CM, Gattis WA, Uretsky BF, et al. Continuous intravenous dobutamine is associated with an increased risk of death in patients with advanced heart failure: insights from the Flolan International Randomized Survival Trial (FIRST). *Am Heart J*. 1999;138(1):78–86.
22. Frazier OH, Rose EA, Oz MC, et al. Multicenter clinical evaluation of the HeartMate vented electric left ventricular assist system in patients awaiting heart transplantation. *J Thorac Cardiovasc Surg*. 2001;122(6):1186–1195.
23. Rose EA, Gelijns AC, Moskowitz AJ, et al. Long-term use of a left ventricular assist device for end-stage heart failure. *N Engl J Med*. 2001;345(20):1435–1443.
24. Miller LW, Pagani FD, Russell SD, et al. Use of a continuous-flow device in patients awaiting heart transplantation. *N Engl J Med*. 2007;357(9):885–896.
25. Dang NC, Topkara VK, Mercando M, et al. Right heart failure after left ventricular assist device implantation in patients with chronic congestive heart failure. *J Heart Lung Transplant*. 2006;25(1): 1–6.
26. Kavarana MN, Pessin-Minsley MS, Urtecho J, et al. Right ventricular dysfunction and organ failure in left ventricular assist device recipients: a continuing problem. *Ann Thorac Surg*. 2002;73(3): 745–750.
27. Matthews JC, Koelling TM, Pagani FD, et al. The Right Ventricular Failure Risk Score: a pre-operative tool for assessing the risk of right ventricular failure in left ventricular assist device candidates. *J Am Coll Cardiol*. 2008;51(22):2163–2172.
28. Milano CA, Simeone AA. Mechanical circulatory support: devices, outcomes and complications. *Heart Fail Rev*. Published online March 7, 2012. 2013;18(1):35–53.
29. Starling RC, Naka Y, Boyle AJ, et al. Results of the post-U.S. Food and Drug Administration-approval study with a continuous flow left ventricular assist device as a bridge to heart transplantation: a prospective study using the INTERMACS (Interagency Registry for Mechanically Assisted Ciculatory Support). *J Am Coll Cardiol*. 2011;57(19):1890–1898.

11

Low Gradient Aortic Stenosis and Significant Left Ventricular Dysfunction

TODD F. DARDAS AND CATHERINE M. OTTO

INTRODUCTION

The clinical presentation and evaluation of severe aortic stenosis (AS) in adults with preserved left ventricular systolic function is relatively straightforward (1). However, management is more challenging in adults with aortic valve calcification and left ventricular systolic dysfunction because the presentation and physical examination findings may be misleading and standard measures of AS severity may not accurately reflect disease severity. It is especially problematic to identify which patients have primary myocardial disease with insignificant valve disease from those with severe AS causing left ventricular systolic dysfunction. The likelihood of meaningful symptomatic improvement following aortic valve replacement (AVR) must be carefully assessed among patients with decreased cardiac output and apparently severe AS. This chapter reviews the approach to the patient with low-gradient, low-flow AS and left ventricular systolic dysfunction, focusing on valve hemodynamics, selection of patients for provocative testing, estimated prognosis following valve replacement, and options for relief of outflow obstruction.

CASE PRESENTATION

An 83-year-old-man presented with a 6-month history of progressive fatigue and dyspnea. He had a prior history of coronary artery bypass grafting, percutaneous coronary intervention, and left ventricular dysfunction with an ejection fraction of 45%. Current medications were aspirin, atorvastatin, clopidogrel, furosemide, and telmisartan. Blood pressure was 120/80 mmHg with a heart rate of 80 beats per minute. On physical examination jugular venous pressure was 15 mmHg, bibasilar rales were present, and there was a 2/6 systolic murmur with radiation to both carotid arteries, and a delayed and diminished carotid upstroke. Given his coronary disease history, the etiology of his heart failure symptoms was thought to be ischemic disease and he was started on an angiotensin receptor blocker (ARB) and diuretics.

CLINICAL PRESENTATION OF SEVERE AS WITH LEFT VENTRICULAR DYSFUNCTION

In patients with a known diagnosis of AS who are followed prospectively prior to symptom onset, left ventricular systolic dysfunction due to the high afterload imposed by the stenotic valve occurs only rarely.

Typical findings in adults with asymptomatic severe AS are left ventricular hypertrophy (occurring in 75%) with preserved systolic function (average ejection fraction of 60%; 2). Heart failure symptoms typically occur only late in the disease course of AS and most patients have the onset of exertional dyspnea or decreased exercise tolerance before there is evidence of overt heart failure. Even when present, early heart failure symptoms are often due to diastolic dysfunction, rather than a low ejection fraction. However, in patients presenting with heart failure, the possibility of AS should be considered as a potential cause of left ventricular dysfunction and symptoms, particularly if a systolic ejection murmur is present, as in this case. The presence of physical findings consistent with AS can be helpful in this situation. The presence of a mid- to late-peaking systolic murmur (sensitivity 95%, specificity 14%) and a single S_2 sound (sensitivity 76%, specificity 33%) are helpful for detection of AS, while the presence of a carotid delay (sensitivity 32%, specificity 99%) and decreased carotid amplitude (sensitivity 32%, specificity 99%) confirms the diagnosis of severe AS (3). However, these findings are not well validated in patients with systolic heart failure where mitral regurgitation and delayed ejection time may decrease diagnostic accuracy.

CASE PRESENTATION

He had only mild clinical improvement with medical therapy for heart failure. Due to concern for ischemia, he was sent for coronary angiography, which showed 100% occlusion at the ostia of the native vessels, filling of the left anterior descending artery via a left internal mammary artery graft, and patent saphenous vein grafts to obtuse marginal branches and the posterior descending artery. Echocardiography was then obtained that showed an ejection fraction of 36% with mild left ventricular hypertrophy. The aortic valve was trileaflet and heavily calcified with limited aortic valve cusp opening. The peak aortic valve velocity was only 3.8 m/s with a mean systolic gradient of 27 mmHg but calculated valve area was 0.7 cm^2 (**Figure 11-1**).

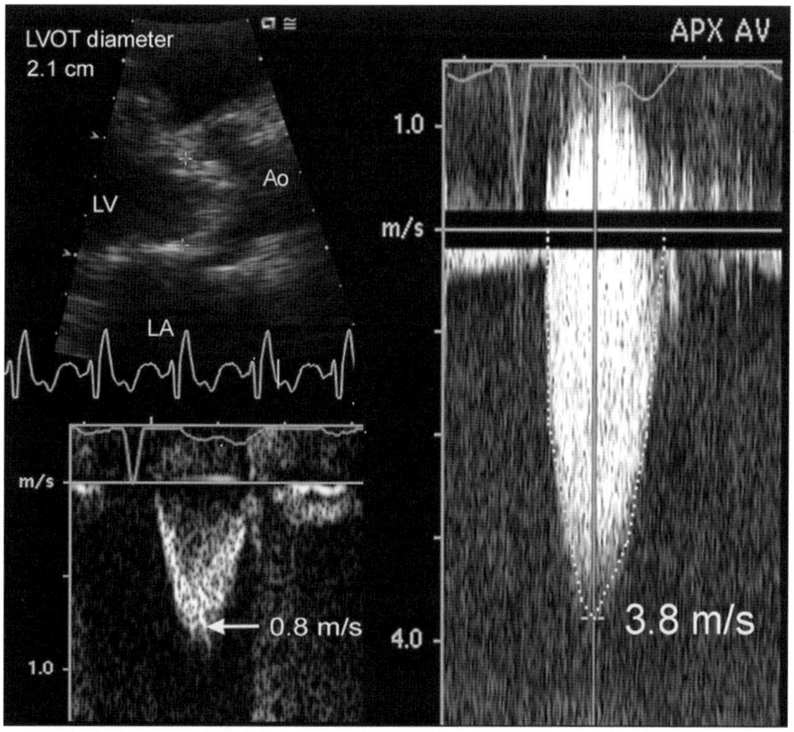

Figure 11-1
Baseline aortic valve appearance and measurements. Severe aortic valve calcification and limited aortic valve opening in a transthoracic parasternal long axis view (upper left). The left ventricular outflow tract (LVOT) diameter is measured at 2.1 cm at the level of the annulus in mid-systole. The velocity in the LVOT of 0.8 m/s is measured using pulsed-wave Doppler from an apical window to obtain a parallel intercept angle with flow. The sample volume should be immediately adjacent to the valve leaflet to ensure that diameter and flow are measured at the same location (bottom left). The maximum aortic valve velocity is recorded using continuous wave Doppler from the window (in this case apical), which yields the highest velocity signal. The velocity of 3.8 m/s is lower than expected for the continuity equation valve area of 0.7 cm^2 in this patient.
Note: Ao = aorta; APX = apex; LA =, left atrium; LV = left ventricle.

DIAGNOSIS OF LOW-GRADIENT AS

Severe AS is defined as an aortic velocity over 4.0 m/s, a mean gradient over 40 mmHg, or a valve area less than 1.0 cm^2 when left ventricular systolic function is normal. However, even when the aortic velocity and mean gradient do not meet severe AS criteria, the findings of heart failure, aortic leaflet calcification with reduced motion, and a valve area less than 1.0 cm^2 suggest the possibility of significant AS. Although there are several proposed definitions of low-gradient AS (LGAS) in the literature, in clinical practice this diagnosis should be considered when velocity or pressure gradient is less than expected for valve area; specifically, a calculated valve area of less than 1.0 cm^2 with a mean gradient less than 40 mmHg or peak aortic velocity less than 4 m/s (4). The dilemma in patients with small valve area with a relatively low velocity and gradient is to determine if these findings reflect true severe AS or only moderate AS with reduced valve opening due to a low transaortic volume flow rate.

The first step in resolving this dilemma is to review the primary data; there are several challenges in recording and measuring Doppler data, so potential sources of error should be excluded. The most common source of underestimation of AS severity is a nonparallel intercept angle between the ultrasound beam and high-velocity aortic jet. Careful attention to technical details, optimal patient positioning, and an experienced sonographer are needed to ensure accurate measurement of aortic jet velocity. Even so, underestimation of velocity (and pressure gradient) can occur because the three-dimensional angle of the transvalvular jet may be eccentric; in some cases, invasive catheter measurement of transaortic pressure gradient may be needed.

Overestimation of stenosis severity occurs if transaortic stroke volume (SV) is underestimated. The left ventricular outflow tract (LVOT), or annulus diameter, is measured adjacent to the valve leaflets, taking care to identify the septal myocardium and anterior mitral leaflet edges. LVOT diameter rarely changes over time in an adult so the same measurement should be used on serial studies. Left ventricular outflow velocity is measured at the same site at the diameter measurement, just on the left ventricular side of the aortic valve, with correct positioning confirmed by the presence of an aortic valve closing click on the Doppler waveform. Left ventricular outflow velocities recorded more apically from the valve plane are lower, resulting in underestimation of SV and an erroneously small calculated valve area. In some cases, valve area is small with a low gradient because the patient is small. Indexing aortic valve area (AVA) to body surface area or using the dimensionless ratio of the left ventricular outflow to transaortic velocity may be helpful. A velocity ratio less than 0.25 or an indexed valve area less than 0.6 cm^2/m^2 suggests severe AS.

Transthoracic Doppler generally provides all the data needed for clinical decision making. However, transesophageal imaging may be helpful when better definition of valve anatomy (bicuspid versus trileaflet), evaluation of valve calcification, or measurement of LVOT diameter is needed.

Once technical issues in stenosis severity measurement have been excluded, the next step is evaluation and treatment for any alternative causes of left ventricular dysfunction. In a contemporary cohort of patients with severe AS and left ventricular dysfunction, 64% had obstructive coronary artery disease (CAD) and 54% had a history of myocardial infarction (5). In the absence of alternate causes for left ventricular systolic dysfunction or when response to the therapy is suboptimal, the presence of a calcified aortic valve, regardless of resting valve hemodynamics, raises the possibility that severe AS may be the cause of left ventricular systolic dysfunction—so-called afterload mismatch.

After evaluation of left ventricular dysfunction, attention is next directed to further evaluation of valve hemodynamics to avoid overestimating the degree of stenosis attributable to irreversible valve calcification. Some patients have "pseudostenosis" due to a weakened ventricle that does not fully open the aortic valve cusps, leading to overestimation of the severity of intrinsic valve disease (6). If only moderate AS is present, valve replacement is unlikely to be beneficial. In contrast, if truly severe stenosis is present, AVR will result in a significant improvement in survival and reduction in symptoms, typically with an accompanying improvement in ejection fraction.

In patients who have symptoms consistent with severe AS and concomitant moderate-to-severe left ventricular dysfunction, the first step in evaluation is to look at the degree of aortic valve calcification. Typically, transthoracic imaging is adequate for assessing leaflet thickness and the severity of calcification. If further assessment is needed, transesophageal imaging, fluoroscopy, or CT imaging may be helpful. If AS severity remains uncertain, additional testing with inotropic stress to determine the true degree of AS may be considered.

CASE PRESENTATION

The patient next underwent low-dose dobutamine stress echocardiography (DSE; **Table 11-1** and **Figure 11-2**).

Table 11-1

Echocardiographic Measurements Over the Course of Aortic Stenosis Diagnosis and Treatment

STUDY	CONDITION	AS V_{max} (m/s)	$LVOT_V$ (m/s)	ΔP_{mean} (mmhg)	$LVOT_D$ (cm)	AVA (cm^2)	EF (%)
1	Rest	3.8	0.8	33	2.1	0.73	36
2	DSE Rest	3.7	0.8	33	2.1	0.74	29
	DSE 10 mcg/kg/min	3.9	0.9	42	2.1	0.80	37
	DSE 20 mcg/kg/min	4.3	1	52	2.1	0.80	43
3	Post TAVI	2.3	1.1	11	2.1	1.65	50

Note: AS = aortic stenosis; AVA = aortic valve area; DSE = dobutamine stress echocardiography; EF = ejection fraction; $LVOT_D$ = left ventricular outflow tract diameter; $LVOT_V$ = left ventricular outflow tract velocity; TAVI = trans-catheter aortic valve implantation; V_{max} = peak velocity.

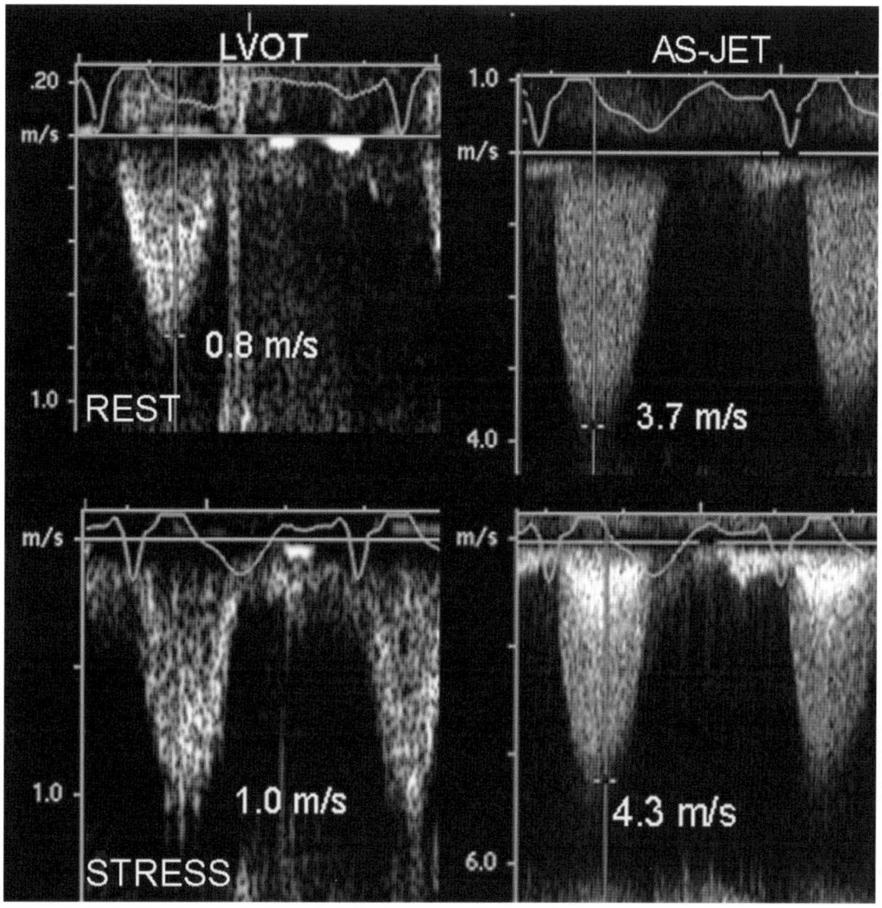

Figure 11-2

Dobutamine stress echocardiography results. Left ventricular outflow tract (LVOT) velocities measured with pulsed-wave Doppler at rest (top left) and with dobutamine 20 mcg/kg/min (bottom left). Peak aortic valve velocities measured at rest (top right) and with dobutamine 20 mcg/kg/min (bottom right). The increase in aortic valve area (AVA) from 0.74 cm^2 to 0.80 cm^2 with a velocity increase from 3.7 m/s to 4.3 m/s confirms the presence of severe aortic stenosis.

LOW-DOSE DOBUTAMINE STRESS TESTING

Dobutamine is used to increase the cardiac contractility and assess changes in valve hemodynamics with either echocardiography or invasive hemodynamics (**Figure 11-3**; 7). Dobutamine increases flow across the aortic valve by increasing myocardial contractility. The additional power of contraction can further open relatively compliant aortic valve cusps that otherwise appear stenotic under resting conditions. As flow increases and opening forces increase, the calculated

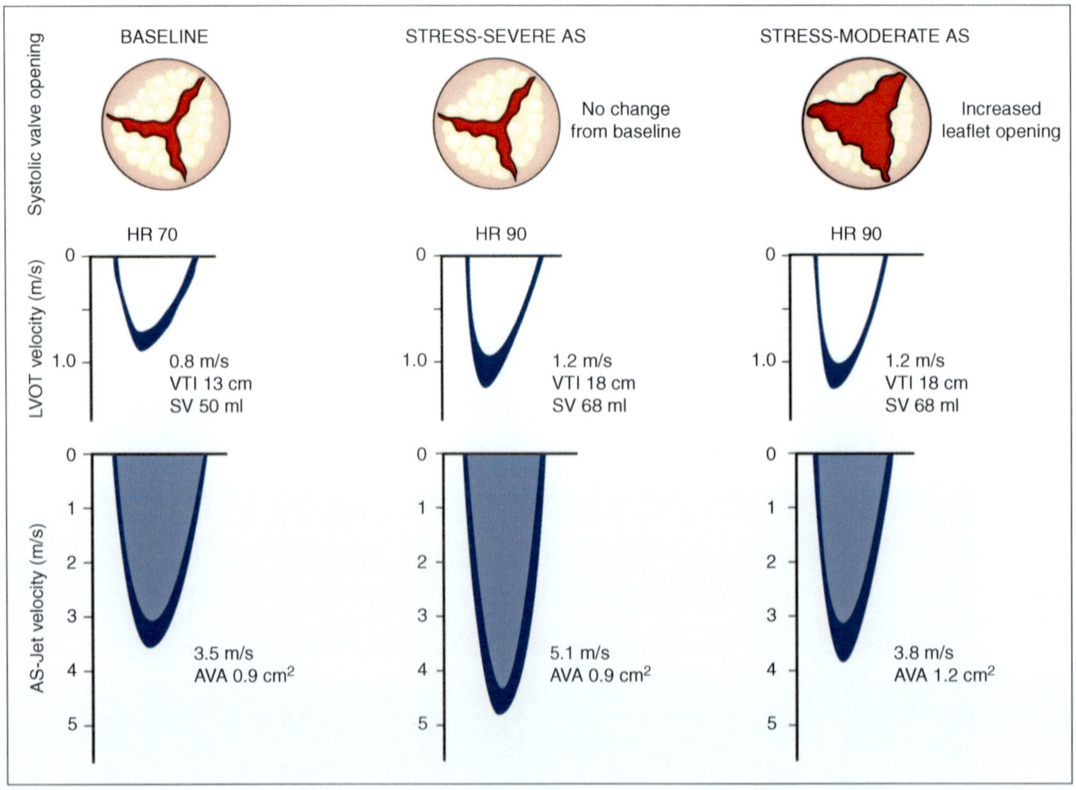

Figure 11-3

Schematic diagram of the changes in aortic valve opening and Doppler flows with dobutamine stress echocardiography (DSE) for low-output, low-gradient aortic stenosis (AS). The baseline data show a hypothetical patient with an EF of 35% and limited leaflet systolic opening, a left ventricular outflow tract (LVOT) velocity of 0.8 m/s, velocity time integral (VTI) of 13 cm, and transaortic stroke volume (SV) of 50 ml. At baseline, aortic jet velocity (AS-jet) is 3.5 m/s, and aortic valve area (AVA) is 0.9 cm^2. If true severe AS is present (middle panel), as ejection fraction (EF) increases from 35% to 45%, transaortic flow rate increases but aortic opening is fixed, resulting in a marked increase in aortic velocity (and pressure gradient) with no change in valve area. In a patient with the same baseline data but "pseudo-severe AS," the increase in EF and transaortic stroke volume (SV) "push" the aortic leaflets to open more so there is a smaller increase in aortic velocity in association with an increase in AVA. Current diagnostic testing relies on Doppler data with dobutamine stress testing because direct imaging of valve anatomy is not adequate for visualization of the exact systolic orifice.

Source: Otto CM, Owens DS. Stress testing for structural heart disease. In: Gillam LD Otto CM (eds.), *Advanced Approaches in Echocardiography*. Philadelphia, PA: Elsevier; 2011. Copyright Elsevier, 2011. Used with permission.

AVA will increase and the mean gradient will increase only modestly or remain unchanged if pseudostenosis is present. In the presence of pseudostenosis, valve area increases by 0.2 cm^2 or greater to a final valve area over 1.0 cm^2. Typically, ejection fraction increases by more than 20%, the aortic valve gradient remains less than 40 mmHg, and aortic velocity remains less than 4.0 m/s (**Figure 11-4**).

When true severe stenosis is present, the calcified noncompliant valve leaflets show no change in motion despite incremental increases in flow rate. Thus, valve area is unchanged while aortic velocity and gradient increase in proportion to the increase in flow rate across the valve. The American Society of Echocardiography and European Association of Echocardiography define severe AS as an aortic velocity over 4.0 m/s or mean gradient greater than 40 mmHg with a valve area that does not exceed 1.0 cm^2 at any point during the study (4). An alternate definition has been suggested by the True Or Pseudo severe Aortic Stenosis (TOPAS) research group, based on calculation of the projected valve area at a normal flow rate, using the change in valve area on DSE. Using this method, AVA is plotted against aortic valve flow (mL/s based on aortic valve volume/ejection time) and the AVA at 250 mL/s is estimated via regression (5). A projected AVA of less than or equal to 1.0 cm^2 was found to have the highest discrimination for severe stenosis. However, this more complex approach to data analysis has not gained wide clinical acceptance.

The last outcome of dobutamine stress testing is "lack of contractile reserve" which is defined as a failure of ejection fraction or transaortic SV or ejection fraction to increase by at least 20% relative to resting values (4). Lack of contractile reserve indicates primary myocardial dysfunction with the inability to augment function

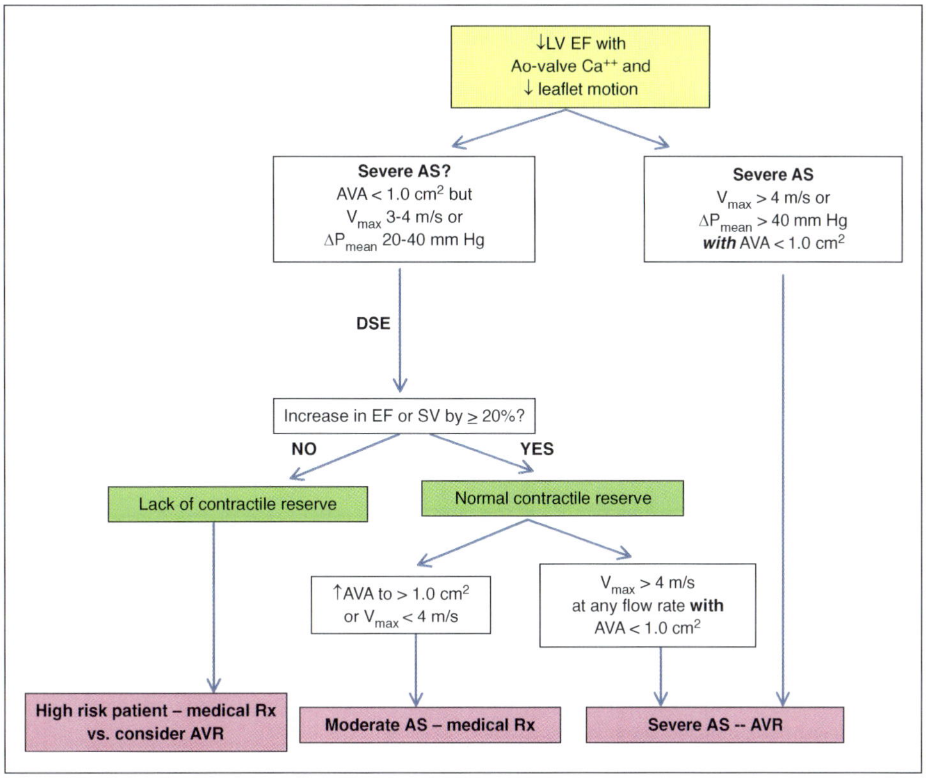

Figure 11-4
Flow chart for suggested approach to identification, evaluation, and surgical candidacy for low-gradient aortic stenosis (AS). An aortic valve area (AVA) <1.0 cm^2 and the presence of a peak velocity (V_{max}) less than 4 m/s or mean gradient (ΔP_{mean}) <40 mmHg identifies those with low gradient AS. Those with a small AVA and V_{max} >4 m/s or ΔP_{mean} >40 mmHg have severe AS regardless of LV ejection fraction (EF). Dobutamine stress echocardiography is a reasonable approach when velocity is lower than expected for valve area in order to assess the change in V_{max} and AVA with changes in transaortic stroke volume (SV). Those who have pseudosevere AS require further observation for progression to severe stenosis but do not require aortic valve replacement (AVR) at this time. Those with severe AS and contractile reserve should undergo AVR. In those without contractile reserve, AS severity is indeterminate; however, selected patients may benefit from high-risk AVR.

during infusion of an inotropic agent. Patients with contractile reserve have a poor prognosis with either medical or surgical therapy and the optimal approach to clinical management is controversial (6,8,9).

Dobutamine stress echocardiography should only be performed with careful physician supervision in cases where the results will change clinical management. The protocol should begin with either 2.5 or 5.0 mcg/kg/min and increase by 5 to 10 mcg/kg/min (**Figure 11-5**). Doses should not be escalated, nor should the protocol continue if the diagnosis of severe stenosis is confirmed or heart rate exceeds 10 to 20 beats per minute greater than resting values. Among unselected patients undergoing DSE, life-threatening complications include ventricular tachycardia (0.1%), ventricular fibrillation (0.03%), and acute myocardial infarction (0.015%; 10). However, most of these patients had coronary disease; the risk of life-threatening complications is likely higher among patients with AS. We recommend close physician supervision, limiting the maximum dose of dobutamine used, and promptly stopping the test for any complications.

LOW GRADIENT AS WITH PRESERVED EJECTION FRACTION

Severe stenosis with low aortic valve gradients can also occur among patients with preserved systolic function. Although ejection fraction is normal, left ventricular hypertrophy due to AS or to hypertension results in diastolic dysfunction and small ventricular volumes. For example, these findings are common in elderly women with AS who have smaller ventricles with more diastolic dysfunction compared to men with a similar degree of valve obstruction. Sometimes, these patients have small ventricular volumes that are appropriate for body size with a reduced valve area in the absence of truly severe AS. In other cases, the low transaortic SV results in a relatively low velocity and gradient even when severe AS is present. Retrospective analysis of the randomized controlled trial of simvastatin and ezetimibe in AS (SEAS) suggested no difference (P = .19) in freedom from cardiovascular death among those with preserved ejection fraction

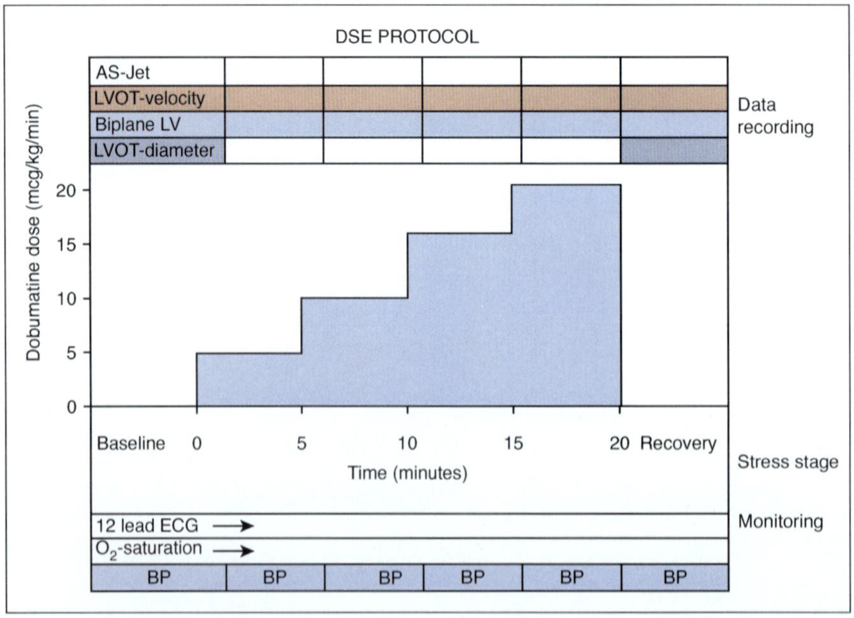

Figure 11-5
Diagram of the dobutamine stress protocol for evaluation of low-output, low-gradient aortic stenosis (AS). The dobutamine dose is increased every 3 to 5 minutes with Doppler-echo data recording (as shown in the bars at the top of the figure) and patient monitoring (as shown in the bars along the bottom). AS-jet, aortic stenosis maximum velocity recorded with continuous wave Doppler; biplane LV, biplane images for calculation of left ventricular ejection fraction.

Note: AS = aortic stenosis

Source: Otto CM, Owens DS. Stress testing for structural heart disease. In: Gillam LD Otto CM (eds.), *Advanced Approaches in Echocardiography*. Philadelphia, PA: Elsevier; 2011. Copyright Elsevier, 2011. Used with permission.

and severe AS with low gradient (AVA less than 1.0 cm^2, mean gradient less than or equal to 40 mmHg) and those with moderate AS (AVA 1.0–1.5 cm^2 and mean gradient 25–40 mmHg; **Figure 11-6**; 11). However, Pibarot et al report a decrease in survival among those with severe AS with preserved SV index compared to those with paradoxically low SV index with normal ejection fraction (P = .006; 12). After adjusting for age and gender this difference was less apparent (P = .045), but the issue of low-gradient severe AS with a normal ejection fraction remains an area of clinical controversy.

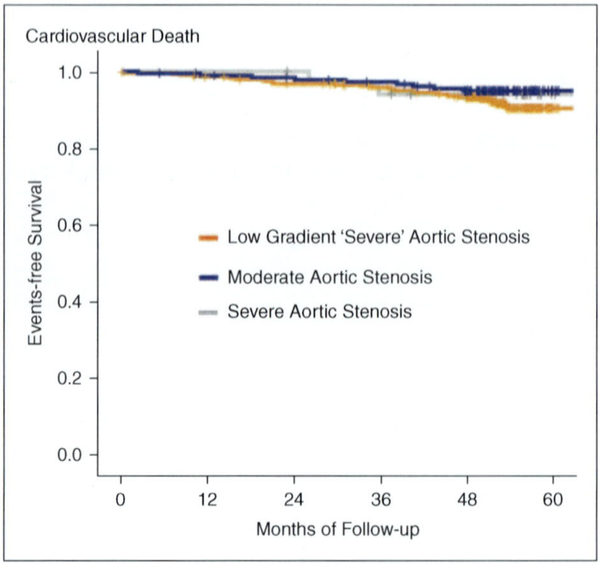

Figure 11-6
Cardiovascular death among patients with preserved LVEF and LGAS, moderate AS, and severe AS. Patients with preserved EF and LGAS have similar outcomes to those with moderate AS, while those with severe AS have markedly worse outcome.

Note: AS = aortic stenosis; LVEF = left venricular ejection fraction; LGAS = low gradient aortic stenosis.

Source: Jander N, Minners J, Holme I, et al. Outcome of patients with low gradient "severe" aortic stenosis and preserved ejection fraction. *Circulation*. 2011;123(3): 887–895. Copyright Wolters Kluwer Health, 2011. Used with permission.

CASE PRESENTATION

Based on the results of the dobutamine stress echocardiogram and the presence of a severely calcified valve, the patient was referred for AVR. Surgical risk was estimated using the Society of Thoracic Surgeons Score, which predicted a 10% mortality largely based on renal insufficiency (estimated glomerular filtration rate [GFR] 53 mL/min) and third-time redo sternotomy. Due to his high surgical risk, he then underwent further evaluation including CT imaging of his ilio-femoral anatomy to determine suitability for a retrograde transcatheter aortic valve implantation.

MEDICAL OPTIONS AND PALLIATION

When valve replacement is not possible due to excessive risk, medical management of patients with AS and left ventricular dysfunction is based on expert-level opinion and observational cohorts of patients. Of course, treatment with vasoactive, negative inotropic, or diuretic agents should be approached with extreme caution in patients with suspected severe AS, as peripheral resistance, chronotropy, inotropy, and volume status are necessary to maintain adequate perfusion. However, treatment with angiotensin converting enzyme inhibitors (ACE-I) or ARBs has now been shown to be safe and may reduce adverse cardiovascular events among patients with severe AS (13). In this series of 2,118 patients with AS, only 25 had left ventricular dysfunction and there was no reduction in all-cause mortality.

Sodium nitroprusside use in those with left ventricular dysfunction and severe AS was historically thought to be deleterious, as it would increase the aortic valve gradient. Khot et al demonstrated the safety and effectiveness of low-dose sodium nitroprusside titrated to a mean arterial pressure of 60 to 70 mmHg in 25 patients with severe AS and cardiac index less than 2.2 L/min/m^2, all of whom had an increase in cardiac index (14). This study suggests that closely monitored nitroprusside may be useful in the acute management of severe AS. In summary, studies of medical therapy suggest that pharmacotherapy can be attempted to treat concomitant diseases, such as systolic dysfunction or hypertension, but must be applied cautiously with careful hemodynamic monitoring.

Balloon valvuloplasty can be used to transiently improve valve hemodynamics and palliate symptoms among patients with severe AS. Among patients not included in the Placement of Aortic Transcatheter Valve (PARTNER) trial, but who underwent screening, balloon aortic valvuloplasty was with a univariate predictor of increased mortality (hazard ratio [HR] 1.6; P = .044), but was not an independent predictor of mortality in a multivariate model including EuroSCORE and other variables associated with operative risk and disease severity. Given the lack of long-term benefit in this study and in previous registries, balloon aortic valvuloplasty can only be considered a temporizing measure to bridge highly selected, critically ill patients to definitive therapy with AVR.

SELECTION FOR AORTIC VALVE SURGERY

Guidelines published by the American College of Cardiology and American Heart Association recommend surgery for confirmed severe AS when left ventricular systolic dysfunction is present, regardless of symptom status (Class I, level of evidence C; 6).

Survival among patients with severe AS and severely decreased ejection fraction has been favorable. Conolly et al. reported on 154 subjects, all of whom had severe AS (15). The mean ejection fraction was 27%. After AVR, 30-day mortality was 9% and preoperative ejection fraction was not associated with differential survival. These findings suggest that among those with decreased left ventricular function, AVR remains beneficial and is associated with improving mortality, compared to medical treatment.

AVR is not recommended for those with moderate AS and left ventricular dysfunction (pseudostenosis). Instead, management is focused on heart failure therapy. A relatively high short-term mortality is seen with left ventricular dysfunction and moderate AS, which may simply reflect advanced heart failure but also suggests some may progress to more severe AS (16–18). Further registry data may be helpful in determining the clinical course and optimal management of these patients.

In patients with severe AS but lack of contractile reserve, decision making is difficult. Although surgical mortality is high and outcomes are suboptimal after valve replacement, survival is even worse with medical therapy (**Figure 11-7**; 18). In a cohort of 136 patients with LGAS, those with contractile reserve had a 3-year survival after AVR of 79% survival compared to less than 25% with medical therapy. Although those without contractile reserve (32% of the group) had a 3-year

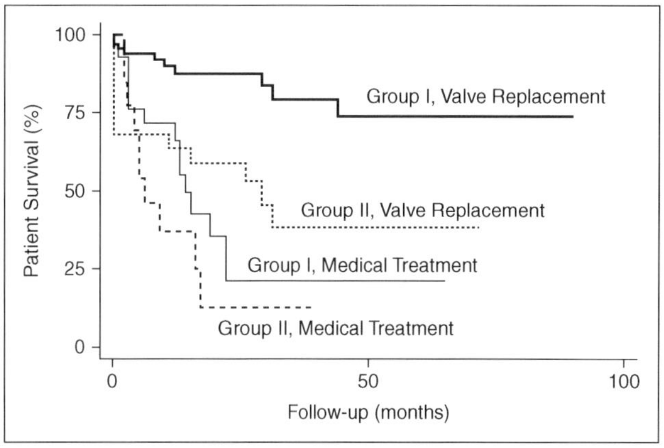

Figure 11-7
Survival from identification of low gradient aortic stenosis (AS) by echo or following aortic valve replacement (AVR) among patients with or without contractile reserve. Survival following AVR was improved for those receiving AVR within groups with or without contractile reserve relative to those not selected for AVR.

Source: Monin JL, Quere JP, Monchi M, et al. Low-gradient aortic stenosis: operative risk stratification and predictors for long-term outcome: a multicenter study using dobutamine stress hemodynamics. *Circulation*. 2003;108(3): 319–324. Copyright Wolters Kluwer Health, 2011. Used with permission.

survival of only about 40% with AVR, survival with medical therapy was only 15% at 2 years (18).

In another study that used propensity score matching to avoid selection bias for or against surgery (19), AVR for LGAS (mean ejection fraction 30%) was associated with improved survival (65±11) versus medical therapy alone (11±7%) at 5 years. However, these results are at odds with data reported by Clavel et al, where AVR was not associated with a survival benefit (HR 1.1, 95% CI 0.76–1.56) after adjusting for age, gender, presence of ischemia, left ventricular ejection fraction, and projected valve area (15).

In aggregate, these studies firmly demonstrate the poor prognosis among patients who have absence of contractile reserve and who are not selected for AVR but leave the issue of optimal therapy unresolved. It is likely that selected patients without contractile reserve will benefit from AVR, although surgical risk is high and outcomes are poor compared to those with contractile reserve. The use of newer valve replacement approaches in this subset of patients has not been studied.

CATHETER-BASED OPTIONS IN LGAS

The development of stented, catheter-implantable valves has resulted in an option for valve replacement that may reduce the high mortality seen among patients with AS and concurrent left ventricular systolic dysfunction. The PARTNER trial randomized patients who were operative candidates to either traditional AVR or transcatheter aortic valve implantation (TAVI; 20). Patients who were deemed too high risk for an operative approach were included in Cohort B. All patients in Cohort A with LGAS had dobutamine stress echo that required the presence of contractile reserve and AVA less than 0.8 cm^2, and either a mean gradient greater than 40 mmHg or peak aortic velocity greater than 4 m/s. The trial demonstrated noninferiority in all-cause mortality between AVR (27%) and TAVI (24%) at 1 year following enrollment (P = .44). Subgroup analysis showed no differential effect between patients with an ejection fraction above or below 55%. Death in the perioperative period was 3.4% with TAVI and 6.5% with AVR (P = .07), suggesting no significant difference between surgical AVR and TAVI.

Clavel et al also reports a modern cohort of nonrandomized patients that underwent either AVR or TAVI with the SAPIEN valve (21). Among the 200 patients described, 83 underwent TAVI. These patients had a mean transvalvular gradient of 37 ± 14 mmHg and left ventricular ejection fraction of 30%. Dobutamine echo was not available in 60% of patients. After adjustment for the propensity of receiving AVR and age, there was no difference in 30-day mortality between the AVR (12%) and TAVI groups (19%, P = .99).

Randomized trials of TAVI in a larger number of subjects with severe AS and contractile reserve are required before the role of TAVI can be determined for patients with LGAS.

CASE PRESENTATION

The patient tolerated TAVI placement without complication. He was seen in follow-up and his symptoms of dyspnea were reduced. He also exhibited an improvement in ejection fraction, increase in AVA, and reduction in mean aortic valve gradient and mean aortic valve gradient (**Figure 11-8**).

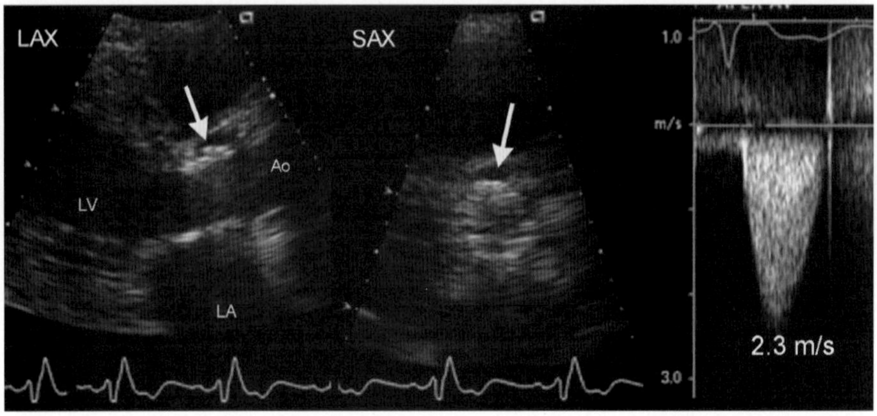

Figure 11-8
Echocardiographic findings following transcatheter aortic valve implantation in our clinical case. The native valve cusps are pushed toward the wall of the aortic root by the implanted aortic valve scaffold as seen in the transthoracic parasternal long axis (arrow, left) and short axis views of the valve (middle). After valve implantation, aortic valve peak velocity now is only 2.3 m/s, which is consistent with a calculated valve area of 1.7 cm^2 (right).

CONCLUSIONS

The finding of severe AS accompanied by a low mean aortic valve gradient and decreased systolic function is associated with worse prognosis, despite the choice of therapy, when compared to patients with severe AS and normal cardiac output. It is important to identify patients with severe AS despite a low gradient as these patients benefit from AVR. Management of those with pseudostenosis and lack of contractile reserve is more challenging and further studies in these patient subgroups are needed.

REFERENCES

1. Otto CM. Valvular aortic stenosis: disease severity and timing of intervention. *J Am Coll Cardiol*. 2006;47(11):2141–2151.
2. Cioffi G, Faggiano P, Vizzardi E, et al. Prognostic effect of inappropriately high left ventricular mass in asymptomatic severe aortic stenosis. *Heart*. 2011;97(4):301–307.
3. Munt B, Legget ME, Kraft CD, et al. Physical examination in valvular aortic stenosis: correlation with stenosis severity and prediction of clinical outcome. *Am Heart J*. 1999;137(2):298–306.
4. Baumgartner H, Hung J, Bermejo J, et al. Echocardiographic assessment of valve stenosis: EAE/ASE recommendations for clinical practice. *J Am Soc Echocardiogr*. 2009;22(1):1–23; quiz 101–102.
5. Clavel MA, Burwash IG, Mundigler G, et al. Validation of conventional and simplified methods to calculate projected valve area at normal flow rate in patients with low flow, low gradient aortic stenosis: the multicenter TOPAS (true or pseudo severe aortic stenosis) study. *J Am Soc Echocardiogr*. 2010;23(4): 380–386.
6. Bonow RO, Carabello BA, Chatterjee K, et al. 2008 focused update incorporated into the ACC/AHA 2006 guidelines for the management of patients with valvular heart disease: a report of the american college of Cardiology/American heart association task force on practice guidelines (writing committee to revise the 1998 guidelines for the management of patients with valvular heart disease): endorsed by the Society of Cardiovascular Anesthesiologists, Society for Cardiovascular Angiography and Interventions, and Society of Thoracic Surgeons. *Circulation*. 2008;118(15):e523–e661.
7. Otto CM, Owens DS. Stress testing for structural heart disease. In: Gillam LD Otto CM (eds.), *Advanced Approaches in Echocardiography*. Philadelphia, PA: Elsevier; 2011.
8. Burwash IG, Hay KM, Chan KL. Hemodynamic stability of valve area, valve resistance, and stroke work loss in aortic stenosis: a comparative analysis. *J Am Soc Echocardiogr*. 2002;15(8):814–822.
9. Nishimura RA, Grantham JA, Connolly HM, et al. Low-output, low-gradient aortic stenosis in patients with depressed left ventricular systolic function: the clinical utility of the dobutamine challenge in the catheterization laboratory. *Circulation*. 2002;106(7):809–813.
10. Sicari R, Nihoyannopoulos P, Evangelista A, et al. Stress echocardiography expert consensus statement: European Association of Echocardiography (EAE) (a registered branch of the ESC). *Eur J Echocardiogr*. 2008;9(4):415–437.
11. Jander N, Minners J, Holme I, et al. Outcome of patients with low-gradient "severe" aortic stenosis and preserved ejection fraction. *Circulation*. 2011;123(3):887–895.
12. Hachicha Z, Dumesnil JG, Bogaty P, et al. Paradoxical low-flow, low-gradient severe aortic stenosis despite preserved ejection fraction is associated with higher afterload and reduced survival. *Circulation*. 2007;115(22):2856–2864.
13. Nadir MA, Wei L, Elder DH, et al. Impact of renin-angiotensin system blockade therapy on outcome in aortic stenosis. *J Am Coll Cardiol*. 2011;58(6):570–576.
14. Khot UN, Novaro GM, Popovic ZB, et al. Nitroprusside in critically ill patients with left ventricular dysfunction and aortic stenosis. *N Engl J Med*. 2003;348(18):1756–1763.
15. Clavel MA, Fuchs C, Burwash IG, et al. Predictors of outcomes in low-flow, low-gradient aortic stenosis: Results of the multicenter TOPAS study. *Circulation*. 2008;118(14 Suppl);S234–S242.
16. Schwammenthal E, Vered Z, Moshkowitz Y, et al. Dobutamine echocardiography in patients with aortic stenosis and left ventricular dysfunction: predicting outcome as a function of management strategy. *Chest*. 2001;119(6):1766–1777.
17. deFilippi CR, Willett DL, Brickner ME, et al. Usefulness of dobutamine echocardiography in distinguishing severe from nonsevere valvular aortic stenosis in patients with depressed left ventricular function and low transvalvular gradients. *Am J Cardiol*. 1995;75(2):191–194.
18. Monin JL, Quere JP, Monchi M, et al. Low-gradient aortic stenosis: operative risk stratification and predictors for long-term outcome: a multicenter study using dobutamine stress hemodynamics. *Circulation*. 2003;108(3):319–324.
19. Tribouilloy C, Levy F, Rusinaru D, et al. Outcome after aortic valve replacement for low-flow/low-gradient aortic stenosis without contractile reserve on dobutamine stress echocardiography. *J Am Coll Cardiol*. 2009;53(20):1865–1873.
20. Smith CR, Leon MB, Mack MJ, et al. Transcatheter versus surgical aortic-valve replacement in high-risk patients. *N Engl J Med*. 2011;364(23):2187–2198.
21. Clavel MA, Webb JG, Rodes-Cabau J, et al. Comparison between transcatheter and surgical prosthetic valve implantation in patients with severe aortic stenosis and reduced left ventricular ejection fraction. *Circulation*. 2010;122(19):1928–1936.

12

Left Ventricular Dysfunction With Mitral Regurgitation

AMANDA R. VEST AND WILLIAM J. STEWART

CASE PRESENTATION

A 64-year-old male, with an 8-year history of systolic heart failure, coronary artery disease (CAD), diabetes mellitus, sleep apnea, peripheral neuropathy, and hyperlipidemia, presents to the cardiology outpatient clinic regarding his leg swelling, fatigue, and reduced exertional capacity. Up until 3 months ago, his exertional capacity was unlimited and he could cut his lawn with a push mower without shortness of breath. Since then, he has noted the onset of lower extremity swelling and orthopnea, and slept upright in a recliner for the past 2 weeks. Significant fatigue and extremity weakness have caused him to be sleeping greater than 18 hours a day. He also noted loss of appetite and a dry cough. He denies any chest pains. He is an ex-smoker, with a 60 pack-year history, but quit 20 years ago. His family history is negative for atherosclerotic disease.

The patient was diagnosed with heart failure when he initially presented with symptoms of exertional dyspnea and fatigue 8 years ago. At that time, he denied orthopnea, lower extremity edema, or chest pains. He had undergone an echocardiogram showing moderate left ventricular dysfunction with regional segmental hypokinesis, a left ventricular ejection fraction of 30%, and moderate concentric left ventricular hypertrophy, but no ventricular dilatation. Aortic sclerosis, a 4.6 cm dilated ascending aorta, mild mitral leaflet thickening, and 1 to 2+ mitral regurgitation (MR) had also been seen at that time. He proceeded to cardiac catheterization, which showed significant stenosis of the circumflex artery, for which he received a stent and recovered well clinically. In the intervening 8 years, he had been started on a statin for hyperlipidemia, but stopped after developing myopathic pains and took no further lipid-lowering agents. His medications at the time of the current presentation included: aspirin 81 mg daily, lisinopril 2.5 mg daily, furosemide 40 mg daily, digoxin 0.25 mg daily, potassium chloride 20 mEq daily, terazosin 5 mg daily, insulin (Humalog mix 75/25) 80 units twice daily, metformin 1000 mg twice daily, and gabapentin 1000 mg twice daily.

His vital signs showed a heart rate of 61, regular rhythm, blood pressure 113/66, weight 180 lbs, and height 172 cm. He appeared older than his stated age, and was lying supine with mild tachypnea. His jugular venous pressure was elevated at 12 cm above the manubriosternal angle. Lung auscultation revealed bibasilar inspiratory crackles. His apical impulse was laterally displaced, without a right ventricular heave. His first and second heart sounds were normal, with a III/VI holosystolic murmur at the apex radiating to the mid-axillary line, and an audible third heart sound. There was moderate lower extremity edema to the knees bilaterally. His skin peripherally was warm, with normal capillary refill. His mentation and neurological exam were normal.

Patient Data During the Current Evaluation

The patient was admitted from clinic to the inpatient setting for IV diuresis. His *laboratory tests* showed: sodium 139, potassium 4.4, chloride 101, bicarbonate 23, BUN 38, creatinine 1.1, glucose 164, WBC 6.4, hemoglobin 11.0, hematocrit 36.5, platelets 225, total cholesterol 83, LDL 51, triglycerides 73, HDL 17, and HbA1c 7.6%. His admission *electrocardiogram* is shown in **Figure 12-1**. The *chest x-ray* is shown in **Figure 12-2**.

A *resting ^{13}N-ammonia positron emission scan (PET) and ^{18}FDG myocardial viability study* showed significantly reduced perfusion in the basal anterolateral segment, the mid-inferolateral segment, and the basal and inferior segments. The ^{18}FDG metabolic images showed no evidence of unmatched ^{18}FDG uptake in the inferolateral segments (24% of the myocardium), which is consistent with scar—not hibernation—in the circumflex territory. The remaining myocardium showed normal perfusion at rest and normal ^{13}N-ammonia uptake.

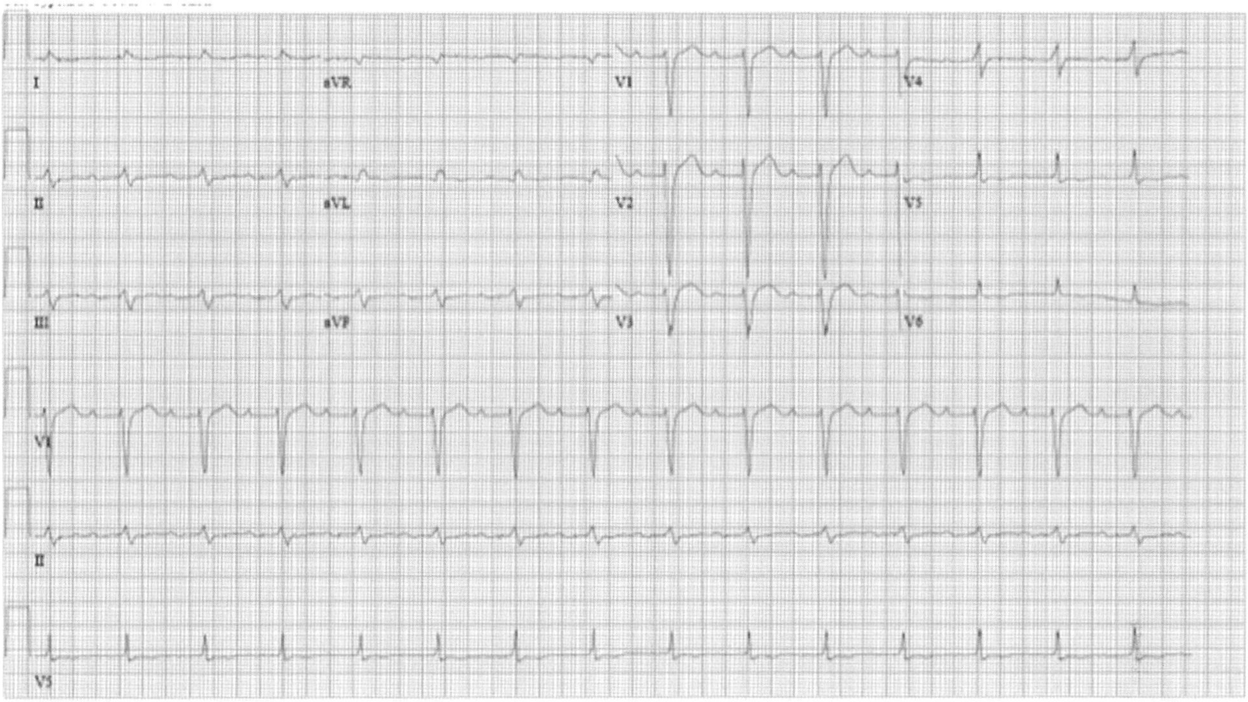

Figure 12-1
Admission electrocardiogram.

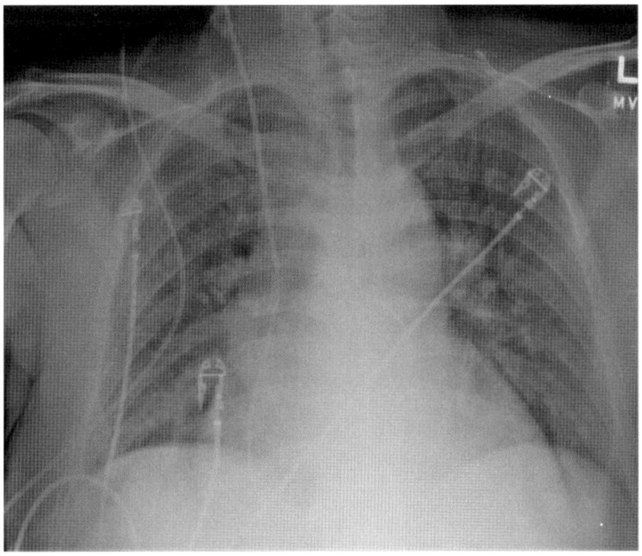

Figure 12-2
Admission chest radiograph.

Gated images at rest showed severely reduced left ventricular wall motion and wall thickening, with a left ventricular ejection fraction of 13% and a dilated left ventricular cavity.

The *transthoracic echocardiogram* (still images in **Figures 12-4–12-7**, **Videos 12-1–12-5** [To view **Videos 12-1–12-5**, please visit the following links: http://www.demosmedpub.com/video/?vid=820; http://www.demosmedpub.com/video/?vid=821; http://www.demosmedpub.com/video/?vid=822; http://www.demosmedpub.com/video/?vid=823; http://www.demosmedpub.com/video/?vid=824]) demonstrated severe left ventricular dilatation, with a ventricular diastolic diameter of 7.0 cm. The left ventricular systolic function was severely decreased, with an ejection fraction of 15% ±5% by three-dimensional assessment. There was global dysfunction with akinesis of the entire inferior wall, posterior wall, and basal inferoseptal segments, and severe hypokinesis of the anterior wall, anterolateral wall, anterior septum, apical lateral segment, mid inferoseptal segment, and apex. The right ventricle was mildly dilated with moderate to severely reduced right ventricular function. There was severe (3–4+) MR with a regurgitant orifice area of 0.4cm^2, mild mitral leaflet thickening, and marked apical tethering of (mostly normal) mitral leaflets **(Figures 12-3, 12-4, 12-5, Videos 12-1, 12-2, 12-3, 12-4, 12-5)**. There was moderate to moderately severe (2–3+) tricuspid regurgitation, with an estimated right ventricular systolic pressure of 64 mmHg, consistent with moderate pulmonary hypertension. The aortic valve was thickened and functionally bicuspid, with no aortic insufficiency. Severe biatrial enlargement was noted.

Cardiac catheterization showed right atrium (RA) mean: 16 mmHg, right ventricle (RV): 65/15 mmHg, pulmonary artery (PA): 70/42 mmHg, pulmonary capillary wedge pressure (PCWP) mean: 28 mmHg, PCWP V wave: 32 mmHg, and a Fick cardiac output of 3.64 l/min, (cardiac index: 1.87 l/min/m^2). The left anterior descending artery was heavily calcified with sequential stenotic lesions of 90% and 80%; the previously stented left circumflex artery showed total occlusion near the origin (**Figure 12-8**, **Video 12-6**; to view the video, please visit http://www.demosmedpub.com/video/?vid=825). The right coronary artery (dominant) was heavily calcified, with 70% stenosis distally (**Figure 12-9**, **Video 12-7**; to view the video, please visit http://www.demosmedpub.com/video/?vid=826).

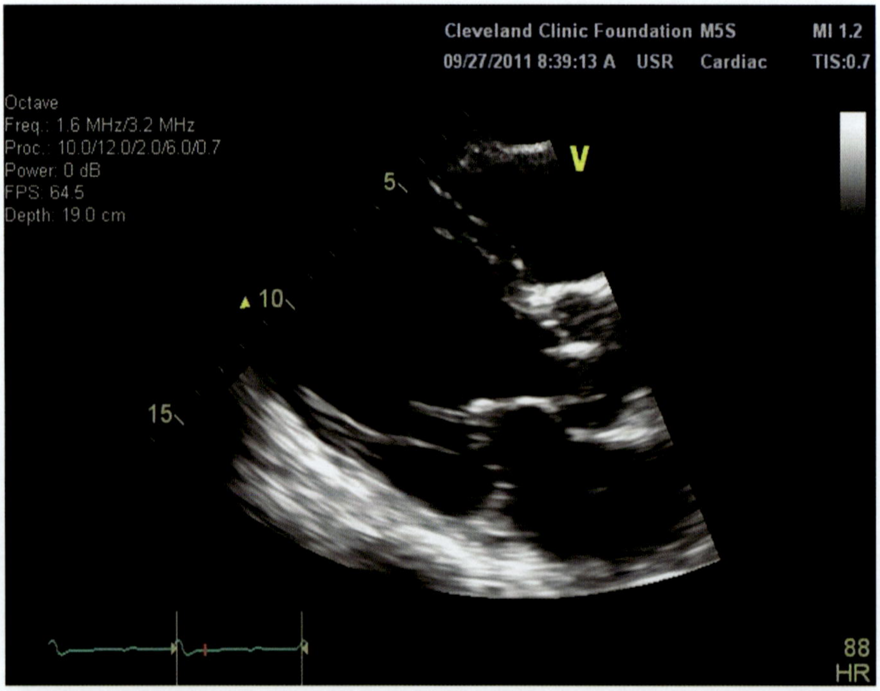

Figure 12-3
Parasternal long axis view of the mitral valve on two-dimensional echocardiogram.

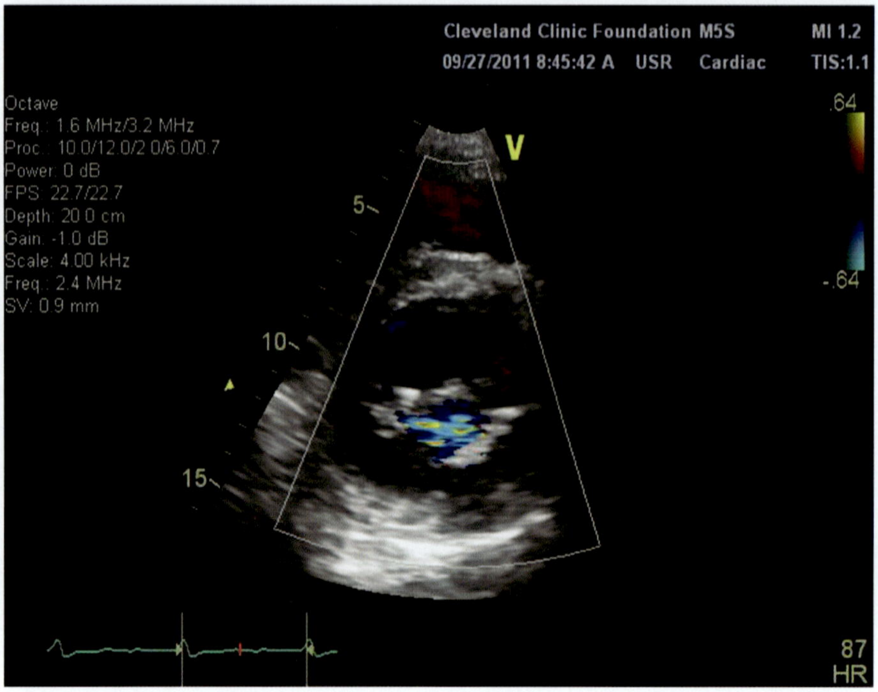

Figure 12-4
Parasternal short axis view of the mitral valve on two-dimensional echocardiogram.

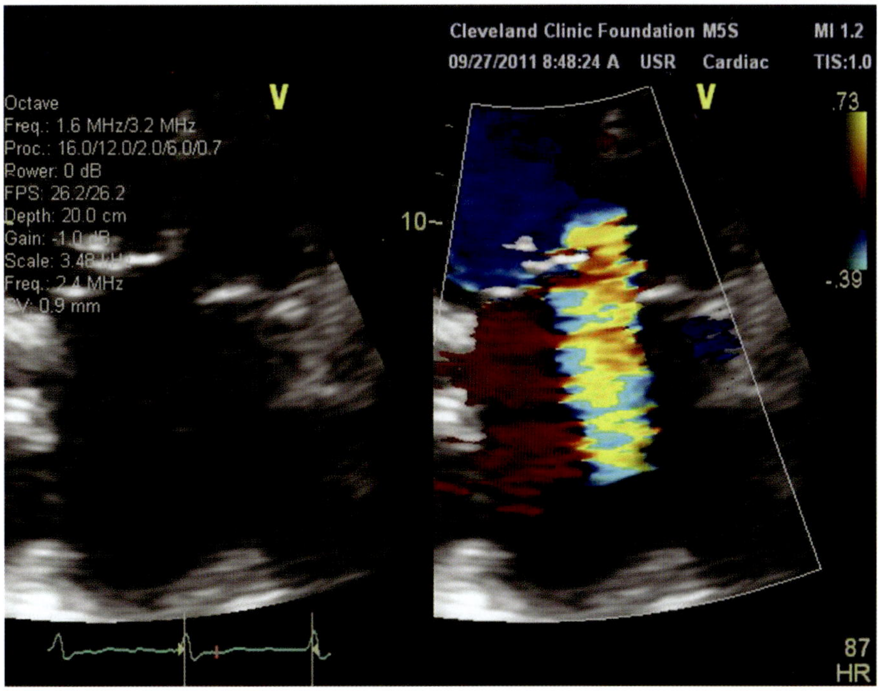

Figure 12-5
Zoomed in apical four-chamber echocardiogram showing the mitral valve on the left panel. The right panel is the same view demonstrating mitral regurgitation (MR) by color Doppler.

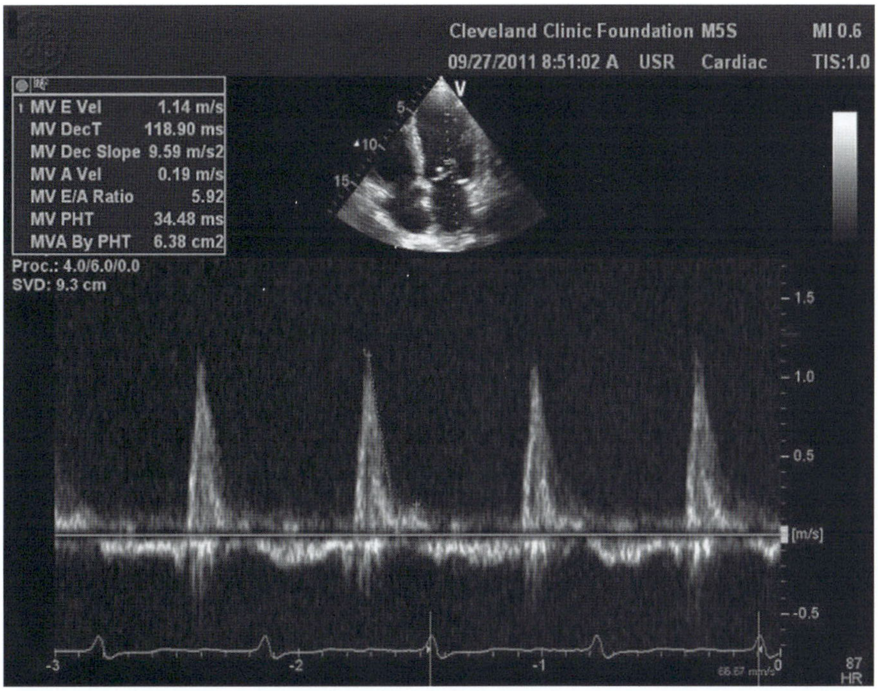

Figure 12-6
Transmitral forward flow across the mitral valve by pulsed Doppler echocardiography.

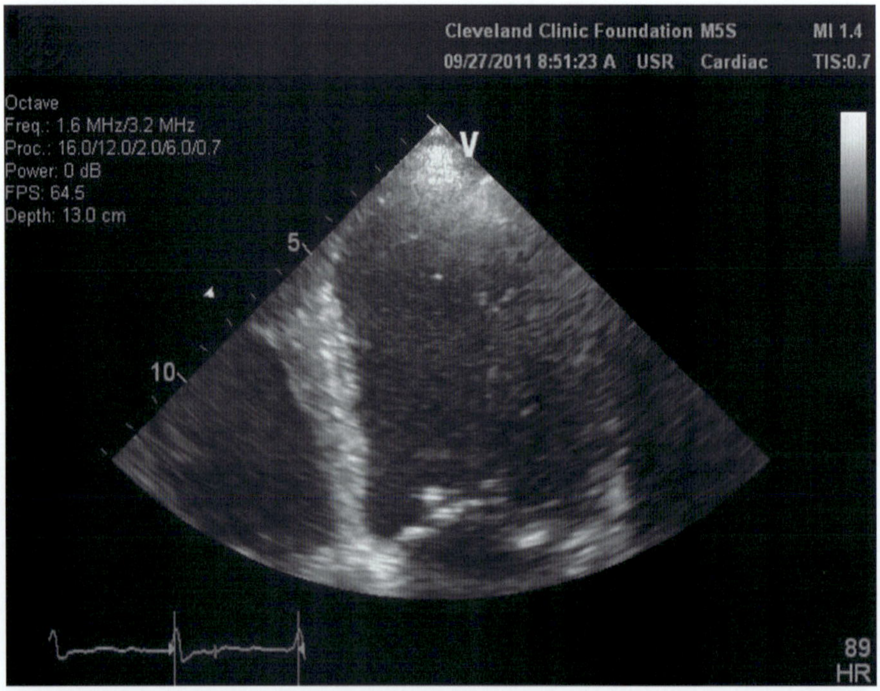

Figure 12-7
Two-dimensional apical four-chamber view of the left ventricle and mitral valve.

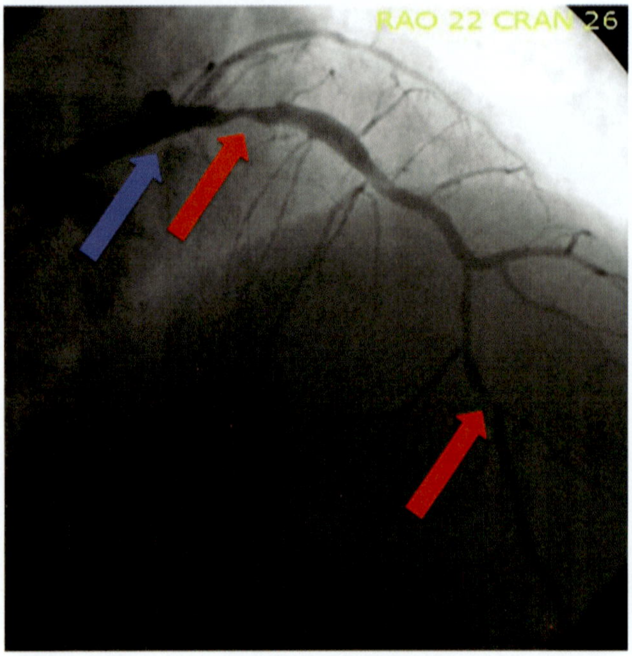

Figure 12-8
Coronary angiogram showing two significant stenoses of the left anterior descending artery (see red arrows). The left circumflex artery is occluded at its origin (blue arrow).

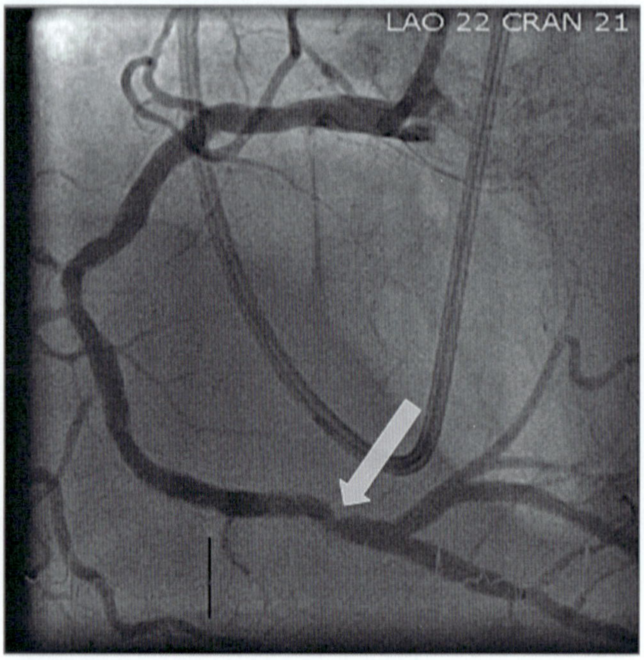

Figure 12-9
Coronary angiogram of the right coronary artery showing distal disease (arrow).

The patient was transferred to the ICU with the pulmonary artery catheter in place, and nitroprusside and nitroglycerin infusions were started. The patient also received IV furosemide, producing good diuresis. The IV afterload reducing agents were titrated and converted to an oral regimen consisting of hydralazine and isosorbide dinitrate over the next few days. Spironolactone was initiated and the lisinopril was uptitrated. By his fifth hospital day, the patient appeared euvolemic and was discharged from the ICU, and was able to ambulate on the ward without symptoms. The patient was then evaluated for several possible additional treatment strategies:

1. Coronary artery bypass grafting with mitral valve repair or replacement.
2. Percutaneous revascularization with coronary stents, and later consideration of mitral surgery or percutaneous mitral valve repair.
3. Cardiac resynchronization therapy and cardiac defibrillator implantation.

There were many uncertainties to be considered, including: What degree of recovery of left ventricular function could be expected with successful revascularization? To what extent is the MR responsible for the symptomatic deterioration of the patient? Is there a primary pathology of the mitral valve, given the mitral valve thickening, in addition to the functional regurgitation? Is the severe MR solely due to geometrical changes within the failing left ventricle? Would surgical mitral valve repair or replacement improve the patient's symptoms? Would biventricular pacing improve the ejection fraction, MR, and/or symptoms?

BACKGROUND

Similar MR cases are often encountered in the heart failure clinic and pose a series of diagnostic and therapeutic dilemmas for the cardiologist. One of the central issues is the "chicken or egg" consideration: Was MR the initial pathology that caused subsequent left ventricular dysfunction, or did left ventricular dilatation affect the mitral annulus and induce "functional" MR (FMR)? A third consideration, which could potentially follow either one of these causative sequences, arises from the presence of severe CAD in the setting of MR. Infarction or transient ischemia can disrupt mitral leaflet coaptation either via changes in ventricular geometry (whereby left ventricular dysfunction is the primary defect) or, less commonly, by causing elongation or rupture of a papillary muscle (making the valve the primary pathology).

This chapter will consider the pathophysiology of these key scenarios: primary valvular MR with secondary left ventricular dysfunction, FMR secondary to left ventricular dysfunction, and MR due to active myocardial ischemia.

The diagnostic approaches and management options available for each condition will be explored. The evidence that guides case selection for the various current surgical and percutaneous approaches will also be reviewed.

MITRAL VALVE ANATOMY

The structure of the mitral valve merits consideration prior to discussion of the various regurgitant pathologies. The normal mitral apparatus consists of the anterior and posterior leaflets, the mitral annulus, the chordae tendineae, and the papillary muscles. When functioning correctly, the apparatus will bring the two mitral leaflets together in systole, creating the coaptation zone at the leaflet tips and so preventing ejection of blood backwards into the left atrium. The annulus is a fibromuscular ring situated in the left atrioventricular groove that serves as the anchoring point for the valve leaflets. During systole, the normal annular circumference may decrease by as much as a fifth, promoting successful coaptation of the leaflets. The anterior portion of the annulus is continuous with the fibrous cardiac skeleton and therefore deters anterior dilatation, whereas the posterior annulus is much more vulnerable to deformation due to changes in left ventricular geometry. If dilatation of the posterior annulus occurs, the shape of the annulus changes from elliptical to a more circular configuration, which compromises leaflet coaptation.

The posterior leaflet comprises three scallops: the middle scallop is designated P2, with the lateral scallop P1, and medial scallop P3. The corresponding areas of the anterior leaflet are designated A1, A2, and A3, although it does not have scallops. The posterior-medial and anterior-lateral commissures define distinct regions at the ends of the line of systolic coaptation of the two leaflets. Systolic apposition of a few millimeters of leaflet tissue all along the coaptation line deters retrograde blood flow in the face of the left ventricular systolic pressure. The posterior leaflet is shorter and broader based than the anterior leaflet, and extends over two thirds of the annular circumference. The shorter height of the posterior leaflet keeps the coaptation line in a more posterior position and well away from the ventricular septum. This helps to prevent movement of the anterior leaflet tips into a position that obstructs left ventricular outflow tract (LVOT) flow (known as systolic anterior motion [SAM] of the mitral valve). The coaptation zones of both leaflets are thicker and rougher with insertion of numerous chordae.

The chordae are fibrous extensions from the heads of the papillary muscles that prevent leaflet prolapse or flail. Primary (marginal) chordae are those attaching to the rough zone of the leaflet margins. Secondary (body) chordae attach to the ventricular side of the mid portions of the leaflets. Tertiary (basal) chordae attach to the base of the posterior leaflet at the hinge points, providing linkage across the ventricle. The papillary muscles are part of the left ventricle, originating between the apical and middle thirds of the left ventricular free wall. Unfortunately, this arrangement increases the mitral valve's sensitivity to ventricular dilatation and remodeling. The papillary muscles are divided into the anterior and posterior groups. The anterior papillary muscle blood supply usually originates from both the left anterior descending and circumflex arteries, whereas the posterior papillary muscle is primarily supplied by the right coronary in patients with right coronary dominance and is therefore more vulnerable to ischemia or infarction from disease of a single vessel.

LEFT VENTRICULAR DYSFUNCTION IN PATIENTS WITH MR DUE TO PRIMARY VALVULAR ETIOLOGY

Primary MR can result from malfunction of any component of the mitral valve apparatus. The most common MR etiology is myxomatous degeneration of the valve leaflets. This encompasses a spectrum of pathologies, including chordal elongation and rupture, annular dilatation, and leaflet redundancy. There may be prolapse of a single segment (P2 is especially vulnerable), or a multisegmented bileaflet prolapse. Prolapse describes extension of a leaflet more than 2 mm beyond the plane of the annulus into the left atrium during systole; flail is present when the leaflet tip is unsupported by chordae and extends freely into the left atrium in systole. There are multiple other potential etiologies for primary valvular MR, including rheumatic heart disease, endocarditis, congenital deformities such as a cleft mitral valve, and mitral annular calcification.

Due to the insidious onset of clinical symptoms and signs, the valvular insufficiency can already be severe and may be accompanied by left ventricular changes by the time the patient becomes symptomatic and presents for evaluation. Exertional dyspnea and limitation of exercise capacity are the usual first symptoms, which may progress to frank heart failure. MR may already be accompanied by pulmonary hypertension and right heart failure in advanced cases. Atrial fibrillation commonly results from valvular MR, due to left atrial dilation and atrial myocardial dysfunction.

On examination of the patient with MR, the apical impulse may be laterally displaced if left ventricular dilation is present. An apical holosystolic murmur is usually audible, enveloping the second heart sound, and best heard with the patient in the left lateral decubitus position during exhalation. The murmur often radiates into the mid-axillary line, and in severe MR to the left paravertebral area. The murmur augments during increases in afterload, such as isometric handgrip exercises, or IV alpha-adrenergic agonists. As a result of the volume overload state associated with valvular MR, a third heart sound is commonly audible at the apex. When decompensated systolic heart failure is present, elevated jugular venous pressure and fine inspiratory pulmonary crackles may be evident. Findings of pulmonary hypertension such as a right ventricular heave and a loud P2 are commonly found. Hepatomegaly, ascites, and peripheral edema suggest right ventricular failure secondary to left ventricular failure.

Echocardiography with color Doppler is pivotal both in diagnosing MR and determining the severity and mechanism of the valve lesion. Multiple parameters should be interrogated, as listed in **Table 12-1**, rather than relying on a single value for quantification of the regurgitation. Severity is graded as 1+ for mild, 2+ for moderate, 3+ for moderately severe, and 4+ for severe regurgitation. Echocardiography also permits assessment of the size of the left atrium and ventricle, measurement of left ventricular systolic function, and estimation of pulmonary artery pressure. Regurgitation caused by prolapse or flail results in a jet directed to the opposite side of the left atrium to the affected leaflet (ie, posterior jet with anterior leaflet prolapse). MR caused by leaflet restriction (rheumatic, ischemic) is directed toward same side of the left atrium as the most fibrotic and restricted leaflet.

MR is associated with increased preload and normal or decreased afterload, because a proportion of left ventricular stroke volume is ejected retrogradely into the lower pressure left atrium. The regurgitant flow fills the ventricle again in the next cardiac cycle, thereby increasing the total left ventricular stroke volume. The left ventricular dilates, mediated by Starling forces. Based partly on sympathetic and other compensatory responses, forward cardiac output is maintained at a normal level in most patients well into the chronic phase of the disease. The total left ventricular stroke volume and ejection fraction are usually increased in severe MR, even though the regurgitant volume ejected back into the left atrium does not contribute to forward stroke volume. Therefore, the ejection fraction may be an overrepresentation of true ventricular function in patients with severe MR.

With time, left atrial dilation helps to accommodate the increased volume to maintain lower left

Table 12-1
Qualitative and Quantitative Parameters Useful in Grading Mitral Regurgitation Severity

	MILD	MODERATE		SEVERE
Numeric grade	1+	2+	3+	4+
LA and left ventricular sizes	Usually normal	Normal or dilated		Dilated
Color Doppler flow jet area	Small, central jet (usually < 4 cm^2 or < 20% LA area)	Signs of MR greater than mild, but no severe MR criteria		Large central jet (usually > 10 cm^2 or > 40% LA area) or wall-impinging jet of any size
Vena contracta width (cm)	< 0.3	0.3–0.69		≥ 0.7
Regurgitant volume (ml)	< 30	30–44	40–59	≥ 60
Regurgitant fraction (%)	< 30	30–39	40–49	≥ 50
Regurgitant orifice area (cm^2)	< 0.20	0.20–0.29	0.30–0.39	≥ 0.40

Note: Proposed thresholds for the severity of MR may be lower in the ischemic FMR (effective regurgitant orifice area > 0.2 cm^2, regurgitant volume > 30 ml) than for valvular MR

Source: Adapted from reference 31.

ventricular filling pressures. Ventricular remodeling also occurs, resulting in left ventricular dilation with eccentric hypertrophy. This cardiac compensation may enable patients with significant MR to remain minimally symptomatic, or even asymptomatic, for many years. However, subclinical development of contractile dysfunction can proceed undetected, especially because it is hidden by the increased total left ventricular stroke volume. Unfortunately, left ventricular dilatation and dysfunction may have become irreversible by the time the patient presents for evaluation. The presence of any drop in resting ejection fraction or a significant increase in left ventricular systolic volume accompanying severe MR are poor prognostic factors that will confer a higher risk of postoperative decompensated heart failure even if successful surgery is accomplished.

FMR SECONDARY TO LEFT VENTRICULAR DYSFUNCTION

In contrast to primary MR with subsequent left ventricular dysfunction, the mitral leaflets are structurally normal in FMR, but they are tethered apically by the left ventricular enlargement. In one series of 2,057 cardiomyopathy patients with a left ventricular ejection fraction of less than 40% and heart failure symptoms, 56% had MR. The 5-year survival of cardiomyopathy patients with moderately severe or severe MR was 40%, lower than the 54% rate seen in cardiomyopathy patients without MR (1).

The processes that link left ventricular remodeling to poor mitral leaflet coaptation are still an area of active research. The relationship is complicated by the fact that "MR begets MR," with the valvular insufficiency inducing further ventricular dilatation. The presenting symptoms of FMR are usually indistinguishable from other individuals with heart failure. However, atrial fibrillation is more likely to be a feature of left ventricular dysfunction with MR, due to more severe left atrial enlargement. As in primary MR, the physical exam should be directed toward signs of decompensated heart failure and appreciation of a displaced apical impulse, a holosystolic murmur, S3 gallop, or features of pulmonary hypertension and right heart failure.

Initial evaluation with transthoracic echocardiography (TTE) allows characterization of both the valve and ventricle. Beyond interrogation of the MR (with particular reference to any PM rupture, leaflet restriction, or MV tethering), echocardiography defines abnormalities of left ventricular structure and function. As illustrated in **Figure 12-10**, ventricular dilatation results in apical displacement of the insertion point of the papillary muscles, because of the fixed length of the papillary muscles and chords in the face of a dilated left ventricle. Apical tethering of the intrinsically normal leaflets toward the left ventricular apex hinders proper leaflet coaptation. Regionality of left ventricular dysfunction may suggest ischemia or infarction as an etiology, although it is not a reliable indicator of coronary disease. Importantly, the severity of MR is not necessarily related to the overall degree of left ventricular dysfunction. Instead, the presence of FMR is far more reflective of the regional geometric disturbances, such as an inferolateral infarction coexisting with an anterior infarction, producing severe regurgitation independent of ventricular volume (2).

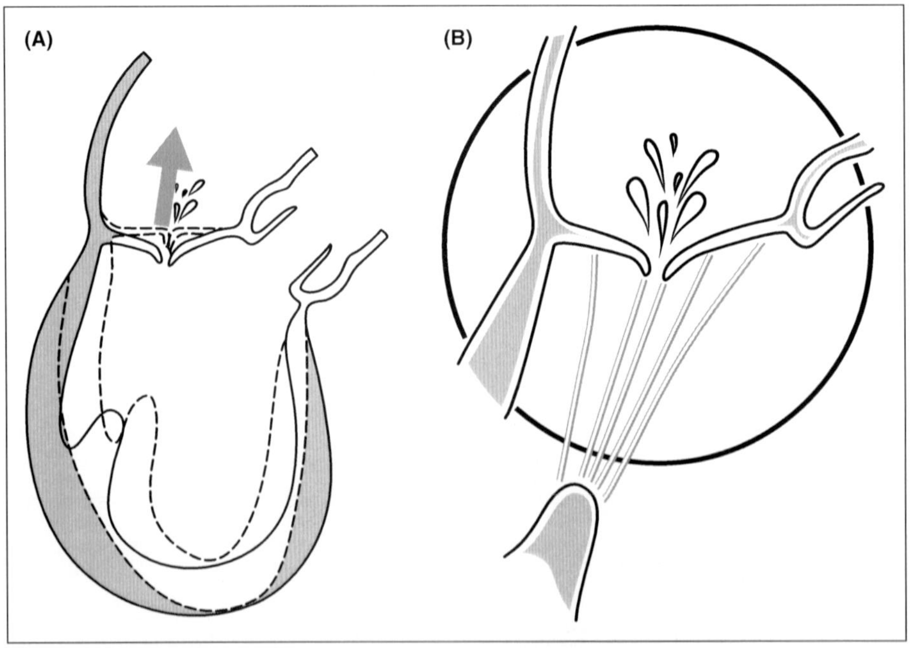

Figure 12-10
(A) Normal anatomy of the ventricle and leaflets in broken lines. Dilated left ventricle in solid lines, demonstrating change in position of the papillary muscle and apical tethering of the leaflets. (B) Zoomed in illustration of the leaflets and chordae causing functional mitral regurgitation by the apical tethering mechanism.

In addition to the resting TTE, an exercise echocardiogram can add particularly useful information in the FMR setting. The most common parameters evaluated in such studies are inducible ischemia and inducible increases in right ventricular systolic pressure, each of which aid understanding of the mechanism of the patient's condition. Several investigators have also highlighted the dynamic nature of FMR and the value of exercising a patient with mild or moderate MR on resting echocardiograms. With exertion, there may be significant changes in loading conditions that modulate ventricular geometry and shift the balance between valvular tethering and closing forces. Exercise-induced changes in the severity of MR may be predictive of morbidity and mortality (3). Although calculation of effective regurgitant orifice area (ROA) is difficult in postexercise imaging when the heart rate is high, Lancellotti and colleagues described the relationship between changes with stress in ROA and tenting area, which was particularly useful in post-myocardial infarction patients with left ventricular ejection fraction less than 45%, at least mild MR, and no exercise-induced ischemia (4). A series of 60 patients with idiopathic dilated cardiomyopathy also highlighted the correlation between exertional ventricular dysynchrony and MR severity (5).

Most patients with left ventricular dysfunction and MR of uncertain etiology should proceed to cardiac catheterization. Coronary angiography defines the presence of CAD, as well as the location, extent, and revascularization options for the patient. Evaluation by right heart catheterization may also be useful if uncertainty remains after echocardiography about the hemodynamics or the severity of the MR. The utility of diagnostic testing in determining between the etiologies of MR with associated left ventricular dysfunction is summarized in **Table 12-2**.

It remains unclear why certain patients with left ventricular dysfunction develop mild, moderate, or severe MR and yet others do not, and so clinical and anatomic predictors of FMR development continue to be sought. Studies do not show a correlation between the degree of left ventricular ejection fraction reduction and the presence of FMR (6), even though distortion of left ventricular anatomy does appear to be the root cause. In vivo studies have supported left ventricular "sphericalization" as a mechanism, with apical and radial displacement of the papillary muscles and lateral tethering forces creating extra tension on the chordae. However, a more spherical left ventricular geometry is a common finding in heart failure patients and exists without MR in some patients. The mitral annular circumference has traditionally been described as enlarged in FMR, although that presumption has been questioned recently. Left ventricular dilation and regional wall motion abnormalities, especially of the wall underlying the posterior papillary muscle, are frequently implicated, and there may be decreased

Table 12-2
Summary of Diagnostic Tests in Mitral Regurgitation With Associated Left Ventricular Dysfunction

	PRIMARY VALVULAR MR	FUNCTIONAL MR, INCLUDING ISCHEMIC ETIOLOGIES
Transthoracic echocardiogram	Shows leaflet motion and structural abnormalities of the MV (flail, prolapse, restriction), severity of MR and left ventricular dysfunction, and pulmonary artery pressure	Demonstrates apical tethering secondary to left ventricular dilatation, quantifies left ventricular volumes and dysfunction
Exercise echocardiogram	Provides objective assessment of exercise capacity, symptom severity, rest and exercise left ventricular size and function, and pulmonary pressure, adding to clinical data on need for valve repair/replacement	Detects exercise-induced ischemia, data on symptom severity, left ventricular size and function, the clinical need for valve repair/replacement; also has a prognostic role in ischemic MR
Transesophageal echocardiogram	Superior delineation of regurgitant mechanisms, detail on feasibility of repair	Superior delineation of regurgitant mechanisms, degree and symmetry of apical tethering
Coronary angiography	Useful for excluding CAD prior to operative mitral valve repair/replacement	Often required to exclude/confirm an ischemic cause for left ventricular dysfunction, and may permit percutaneous revascularization as an attempt to lessen MR from acute ischemia and infarction
Invasive hemodynamics	Occasionally useful in quantifying the hemodynamic significance of the MR (PA and wedge pressure) when non-invasive means are insufficient	May have a role in determining the degree of heart failure decompensation, and optimizing medical treatment, in critically ill patients

mitral valve closing forces, or focally increased tethering forces resulting from the segmental left ventricular dysfunction. The valve leaflets have generally been considered passive in these structural changes.

However, recent evidence using three-dimensional echocardiography has challenged some of these assumptions. Chaput and colleagues presented a new method of measuring diastolic leaflet area and compared leaflet size in normal subjects, individuals with dilated cardiomyopathy, and individuals with inferior wall dyskinesis (7). They found an increase in leaflet size by more than 30% in both of the left ventricular dysfunction groups, with and without MR, compared to those with normal hearts, at a single evaluation time point. This cast the mitral leaflets in a more active role in heart failure, implying the potential for a compensatory increase in leaflet surface area apparently to compensate for structural abnormalities of the left ventricular and mitral annulus. The authors postulated that FMR results when the compensatory increase in leaflet size is insufficient.

MR DUE TO ACTIVE MYOCARDIAL ISCHEMIA

MR may present acutely with active myocardial ischemia or acute infarction. It is often associated with pulmonary edema and/or cardiogenic shock, which carries a very poor prognosis. Other patients with long-standing CAD may have significant chronic MR, which develops insidiously with the onset of global or regional abnormalities of left ventricular function. The typical scenario is an older patient with regional wall motion abnormalities and reduced systolic function, with moderate to severe MR and a CAD history of acute or chronic angina. However, it may not be possible to distinguish the ischemic etiology of MR and left ventricular dysfunction from the other etiologies already described by the patient's history and exam alone. Among patients with CAD, the presence of MR clearly portends a worse prognosis, and significant uncertainty remains as to the best management strategy.

Ischemic MR may arise via one of several mechanisms, as summarized in **Table 12-3**. Alterations in left ventricular geometry are a much more common etiology than actual infarction of the papillary muscles.

The presence of MR after myocardial infarction carries a poorer prognosis post-revascularization when compared to patients without MR. In one 5-year study of asymptomatic individuals with a recent myocardial infection, the adjusted relative risk of heart failure or cardiac death was 2.97 for the presence of MR, and 4.4 for an effective ROA exceeding 0.20 cm^2 (8). Even mild regurgitation has been

Table 12-3
Ischemia or Infarction May Give Rise to One or More of the Following Mechanisms of MR

Mechanisms for MR due to active myocardial ischemia:
Altered left ventricular geometry, causing acute left ventricular dilation and apical displacement of mitral leaflets
Papillary muscle (PM) rupture or chordal elongation
Mechanisms for chronic ischemic MR:
PM necrosis causing leaflet tethering and poor coaptation
Decreased MV closing forces because of left ventricular systolic dysfunction
Left ventricular cavity dilation causing apical tethering of mitral leaflets

demonstrated as a risk factor for 3-year mortality (hazard ratio [HR] 2.0, 95% CI 1.4–3.0; 9). Lancellotti and colleagues have also demonstrated the value of exercise echo in patients with an ischemic etiology for their MR and left ventricular dysfunction, confirming that large exercise-induced increases in ROA, and transtricuspid pressure gradient (inducible pulmonary hypertension), are predictors of mortality within this subset of patients (10).

NONSURGICAL MANAGEMENT OF MR WITH ASSOCIATED LEFT VENTRICULAR DYSFUNCTION

All patients with MR and left ventricular dysfunction, regardless of whether the MR is a primary valve problem or secondary to a cardiomyopathic process, should be titrated onto the standard heart failure medical regimen to deter deleterious remodeling. This includes an angiotensin-converting enzyme (ACE) inhibitor or angiotensin receptor blocker, a beta-blocker, and spironolactone, as tolerated by blood pressure, potassium, and renal function. Loop diuretics are also often required for control of congestive symptoms, and angina (or silent ischemia when present) should also be managed with appropriate medications. However, it should be noted that the administration of afterload-reducing medications is not an established management strategy for MR per se, and is not recommended by the major society guidelines in the absence of left ventricular dysfunction. Although IV afterload reducers such as nitroprusside and nitroglycerin are commonly used to manage acute MR, existing small studies of oral afterload reduction in chronic MR with preserved left ventricular systolic function have been largely negative. There is some limited evidence for the use of beta-blockers in the absence of reduced left ventricular ejection fraction. The mechanism of benefit has been proposed as a reduction in left ventricular mass and ventricular sphericity; favorable geometrics were associated with decreased MR during carvedilol treatment in a small group of patients with MR and left ventricular systolic dysfunction (11).

Atrial fibrillation occurs in many patients with MR and left ventricular dysfunction of any cause; rate control or restoration of sinus rhythm may considerably improve symptoms. Beta-blockers are the mainstay of ventricular rate-controlling therapy, and strategies such as antiarrhythmic drugs, electrical cardioversion, and pulmonary vein isolation may be selectively employed to restore and maintain sinus rhythm. However, if severe MR remains uncorrected, successful maintenance of sinus rhythm is less likely because the left atrium is dilated and left atrial pressure is high. In accordance with current American Heart Association (AHA) guidelines, endocarditis prophylaxis is not routinely indicated in patients with native MR, but prophylaxis is still recommended after implantation of a prosthetic valve replacement.

Cardiac resynchronization therapy (CRT) should also be considered for NYHA Classes II to IV patients who are already on an optimal medication schedule, provided they meet criteria for biventricular pacing. In some carefully selected patients with prolongation of the QRS interval (especially a left bundle branch block [LBBB]) and left ventricular ejection fraction less than or equal to 35%, significant improvements in the degree of MR and exertional capacity can be achieved with CRT. These benefits may be the result of improved synchronicity between the anterior and posterior papillary muscles, improved contractility of the mitral annulus, favorable remodeling, or improvement in mitral closing forces due to stronger left ventricular pump function (12).

SURGERY IN PATIENTS WITH MR AND LEFT VENTRICULAR DYSFUNCTION

Table 12-4 lists the variables that are generally taken into consideration when determining the appropriateness of mitral valve surgery in primary MR. Elective mitral surgery is indicated for symptomatic patients with moderately severe to severe primary MR and left ventricular dysfunction. In addition, the presence of left ventricular dysfunction is a Class IB indication for surgery even in asymptomatic patients per current guidelines (13). Therefore, asymptomatic individuals who have primary MR, which is truly severe, and who are already showing adverse changes in left ventricular dimensions and function, should be considered for surgery to limit further ventricular deterioration. The American College of Cardiology (ACC)/AHA guidelines specify a left ventricular ejection fraction less than or equal to 60% and/or left ventricular end-systolic dimension greater than or equal to 40 mm as indications for surgical evaluation. Management is less clear for individuals who have mild to moderate MR, in whom it is harder to determine if the MR is actually the cause of the left ventricular dysfunction (the "chicken or egg" problem). The final decision on whether or not to operate should also be tailored to the age and comorbidities of the patient, the potential for successful valve repair, and the likelihood that surgical intervention will improve outcomes.

The decision regarding the utility of surgery is particularly complex in patients with very significant left ventricular systolic impairment (eg, LVEF less than 20%–30%), as postoperative outcomes are known to be poorer in this group, especially when left ventricular dilation is extreme. For these patients, the ACC/AHA guidelines suggest that if mitral valve repair seems likely to be achievable, surgery should still be contemplated. Even though the left ventricular dysfunction may persist postoperatively, symptomatic benefit and limitation of future deterioration in left ventricular function may be achieved if the MR severity is reduced.

The question of likelihood of repair is always an important consideration, because mitral valve repair carries a much more favorable long-term prognosis in terms of periperative mortality, preservation of left ventricular function, thromboembolism, endocarditis, and postoperative survival than mitral valve replacement. However, freedom from reoperation is no greater with repair than replacement. The feasibility of valve repair depends on the etiology and mechanism of MR. Uncomplicated mitral valve prolapse or flail can be repaired at experienced centers in 90% or more of cases, in the absence of extensive leaflet calcification, moderate or more rheumatic fibrosis, or severe damage from endocarditis. A cleft valve or FMR is less likely to be successfully repaired with durable results.

Repair techniques almost always involve insertion of an annuloplasty ring to reduce annular diameter. In patients with primary valvular dysfunction, repair may also include resection or plication of leaflets, a patch to repair a perforation, insertion of artificial chordae, or chordal shortening or transposition.

In patients whose MR is known to be functional in origin, consideration of surgery is a more complex decision because the literature offers far less clear evidence supporting a role for surgery in FMR, compared to primary mitral valve disease. Studies have been distorted by the heterogeneity of mechanisms for both left ventricular and mitral valve dysfunction

Table 12-4
Variables in Determining the Appropriateness of Mitral Valve Surgery in Primary Mitral Regurgitation

Left ventricular size and function
Exercise capacity
Repairability of the valve
Mechanism of MR, including presence of flail leaflet
Severity of MR
Pulmonary artery pressures > 50 mmHg at rest or > 60 mmHg at peak exercise
Atrial fibrillation
Age and other comorbidities (worse post-op outcomes if > 75 years, CAD or renal impairment)
Left ventricular size and function at peak exercise

in FMR, as well as the heterogeneity of surgical interventions that have been performed. However, there is good evidence that mitral valve repair is feasible in patients with FMR and advanced heart failure, is usually well hemodynamically tolerated, and is associated with acceptable short-term mortality outcomes (14). Of 48 patients with NYHA Classes III to IV heart failure and refractory 4+ FMR, who underwent surgical placement of undersized flexible annuloplasty rings with or without bypass grafting, 12- and 24-month survival rates were 82% and 71% respectively, with reduced hospitalizations, left ventricular volumes, and sphericity (15).

Mitral valve replacement is indicated when repair is not technically possible; the modern standard employs chordal preservation techniques that leave the subvalvular structures mostly intact, and hence reduce the incidence of postoperative left ventricular dysfunction resulting from disruption of the internal skeleton of the heart. The choice of a mechanical versus bioprosthetic valve is a balance between the risks of thrombosis and chronic anticoagulation with a mechanical valve, versus the risks of leaflet degeneration with a bioprosthetic valve. Primary mitral bioprosthetic valve failure affects approximately 30% of patients at 10 years and around 44% by 15 years, with less structural failure in the mechanical valve patients (16).

One of the limitations of the surgical approach in FMR is the failure of standard mitral annuloplasty to address the underlying problem, which is the left ventricle. Some innovative solutions to modify the left ventricular size and shape have been devised, though none has gained widespread acceptance. This includes the Batista operation, in which a portion of the left ventricular free wall was resected (17); this procedure is no longer practiced. The Acorn trial tested a sock-like external restraint device termed the CorCap (Acorn Cardiovascular, St Paul, MN) to inhibit left ventricular enlargement, combined with mitral valve repair/replacement (mitral annuloplasty ring in 84%). That trial showed fairly positive results with surgery for 91 NYHA Classes II to IV patients with greater than or equal to 3+ FMR (18). The 30-day operative mortality was 1.6%. At 5 years, total mortality was 30%, MR recurrence was 19% (compared to 30%–40% with mitral repair alone), and there was a progressive reduction in the left ventricular end-systolic and end-diastolic volumes postoperatively (28% reduction from baseline). There was a trend toward a greater decrease in left ventricular end-diastolic volume in patients who received the external restraint device, compared to subjects receiving mitral valve surgery alone (average difference of 16.5 mL, $P = .05$).

It should be highlighted that although improvements in MR, symptoms, and functional capacity have been demonstrated from mitral valve repair or replacement in FMR (19), there is no data to suggest a mortality benefit (20). The failure to affect survival in these reasonably small trials may reflect the poor prognosis of the underlying cardiomyopathy having more of a negative impact than the surgical strategy. The European Society of Cardiology (ESC) does recommend mitral valve surgery in patients with severe MR, a low ejection fraction, and ongoing symptoms despite optimal non-surgical management of the heart failure (21); the AHA/ACC 2008 guideline update does not give recommendations specific to FMR.

In FMR patients, the aim of mitral valve repair or replacement is often to improve symptoms. In selected patients, it may postpone, or even avoid, the need for advanced mechanical therapy or transplantation for highly symptomatic heart failure. However, surgery should not be attempted in patients who have already deteriorated into the terminal stages of heart failure and have little chance of recovering fully from the operation. For symptomatic advanced heart failure patients with mild or moderate degrees of FMR, mitral valve surgery is unlikely to result in symptomatic benefit and should therefore be avoided. Although some patients report significantly improved symptoms after annuloplasty surgery, most patients with MR and left ventricular dysfunction do not gain complete symptom relief.

Severe FMR from an ischemic etiology with left ventricular dysfunction poses another distinct problem for the clinician. It is clear that the presence of any degree of MR in the setting of CAD has a significant negative impact on survival, with MR emerging as the foremost predictor of survival in a large cohort of elective percutaneous coronary intervention (PCI) patients (22). In 711 patients with a range of left ventricular functions who underwent PCI for revascularization, moderate to severe MR at the time of intervention was an independent predictor of mortality, with a 57% survival rate at 5 years in the presence of MR, compared to 97% for individuals without regurgitation (23). Patients with moderate to severe MR differed from patients with mild or no MR in that they were older, more frequently female, and more likely to have a coronary artery bypass graft, myocardial infarction, and lower ejection fraction.

There is no robust evidence to support a long-term survival benefit from the addition of mitral valve repair or replacement to coronary artery bypass grafting (CABG) in the setting of chronic FMR of ischemic etiology. Mihalijevic et al found that annuloplasty (for MR) with CABG reduced postoperative

MR and did improve early symptoms, compared to CABG alone, but surgery did not benefit long-term functional status or survival (24). In addition, the durability of valve repair in ischemic MR is significantly lower than that of degenerative mitral valve disease. In some studies, the frequency of recurrence of MR was alarmingly high. The severity of posterior papillary muscle displacement appeared to be a predictor of MR recurrence after ring annuloplasty (25).

Some surgical authorities argue that the current standard of care for ischemic MR should be valve repair with a restrictive annuloplasty using a complete rigid or semi-rigid ring, with coronary artery bypass grafting (26). Their argument is that the absence of a mortality benefit in studies thus far is due to use of incomplete rings that do not deter postoperative dilation of the anterior annulus and further ventricular remodeling. Using that strategy in 100 consecutive ischemic MR patients, the degree of preoperative left ventricular dilation was found to be pivotal in predicting surgical outcomes (27). A left ventricular end-diastolic diameter exceeding 65 mm decreased the likelihood of successful reverse remodeling, and correlated with poor midterm survival. The ACC/AHA guidelines (**Table 12-5**) do not state specific recommendations to guide decision making in patients with symptomatic chronic FMR from ischemia with left ventricular dysfunction. The European Society of Cardiology (ESC) guidelines are somewhat more prescriptive, and state indications for mitral valve surgery (**Table 12-6**), although the level of evidence for patients with a depressed ejection fraction is IIaC.

Table 12-5
ACC/AHA Guideline Indications for Mitral Valve Surgery in Mitral Regurgitation

CLASS I
(a) Mitral valve (MV) surgery is recommended for the symptomatic patient with acute severe mitral regurgitation (MR).
(b) MV surgery is of benefit for patients with chronic severe MR and New York Heart Association (NYHA) functional class II, III, or IV symptoms in the absence of severe left ventricular dysfunction (severe left ventricular dysfunction is defined as ejection fraction < 0.30) and/or severe left ventricular dilation (defined as end-systolic dimension > 55 mm).
(c) MV surgery is of benefit for asymptomatic patients with chronic severe MR and mild to moderate left ventricular dysfunction, ejection fraction 0.30 to 0.60, or end-systolic dimension ≥40 mm.
(d) MV repair is preferred over MV replacement in most patients with severe chronic MR who require surgery, and patients should be referred to surgical centers experienced in MV repair.
CLASS IIA
(a) MV repair is reasonable in experienced surgical centers for asymptomatic patients with chronic severe MR with preserved left ventricular function (ejection fraction > 0.60 and end-systolic dimension < 40 mm) in whom the likelihood of successful repair without residual MR is > 90%, and expected perioperative morbidities are low.
(b) MV surgery is reasonable for asymptomatic patients with chronic severe MR, preserved left ventricular function, and new-onset atrial fibrillation.
(c) MV surgery is reasonable for asymptomatic patients with chronic severe MR, preserved left ventricular function, and pulmonary hypertension (pulmonary artery, PA, systolic pressure > 50 mm Hg at rest or > 60 mm Hg with exercise).
(d) MV surgery is reasonable for patients with chronic severe MR due to a primary abnormality of the mitral apparatus and NYHA functional class III–IV symptoms and severe left ventricular dysfunction (ejection fraction < 0.30 and/or end-systolic dimension > 55 mm) in whom MV repair is highly likely.
CLASS IIB
MV repair may be considered for patients with chronic severe secondary MR due to severe left ventricular dysfunction (ejection fraction < 0.30) who have persistent NYHA functional class III–IV symptoms despite optimal therapy for heart failure, including biventricular pacing.
CLASS III
(a) MV surgery is not indicated for asymptomatic patients with MR and preserved left ventricular function (ejection fraction > 0.60 and end-systolic dimension < 40 mm) in whom significant doubt about the feasibility of repair exists.
(b) Isolated MV surgery is not indicated for patients with mild or moderate MR.

Source: From the 2008 Update to the ACC/AHA Valve Disease Guidelines.

Table 12-6
Indications for Mitral Surgery in Chronic Ischemic Mitral Regurgitation

- Severe MR, LVEF > 30%, patient scheduled for CABG-IC
- Moderate MR, patient scheduled for CABG if mitral repair is feasible - IIaC
- Severe MR, symptomatic patients, LVEF < 30%, candidate for revascularization - IIaC
- Severe MR, LVEF > 30%, no option for revascularization, recurrent symptoms on optimal medical therapy, low comorbidity – IIbC
Proposed thresholds for the severity of MR are lower in the ischemic type (effective regurgitant orifice area > 0.2 cm^2, regurgitant volume > 30 ml) than the general thresholds for MR

Source: From reference 30.

EMERGING MINIMALLY INVASIVE AND TRANSCATHETER OPTIONS TO TREAT MR

Traditional open-heart surgery through a full sternotomy is no longer the only option for MR correction. Given the additional postoperative risk conferred by a depressed left ventricular ejection fraction for a patient undergoing open heart surgery, there is strong interest in developing less invasive options for patients with MR and left ventricular dysfunction. Minimally invasive video-assisted approaches to mitral valve repair via hemi-lower sternotomy or right thoracotomy incisions may be options in some experienced centers and selected patients, offering smaller incisions and more rapid postoperative recovery. However, they require considerable expertise, and have not yet shown superior mortality outcomes, probably because the mitral repair itself is unchanged.

Transcatheter mitral valve repair is an emerging treatment option in which an implantable device is delivered via catheter to reduce MR. Current techniques emulate existing surgical procedures. The devices currently under investigation utilize one of two approaches: structural modification of the leaflets themselves or annular remodeling.

The clip approach is currently the best-studied percutaneous option. The Endovascular Valve Edge-to-Edge Repair Study (EVEREST) II group recently reported 12-month results for 279 patients with 3 to 4+ MR randomized to MitraClip (Abbott Vascular, Menlo Park, CA) versus surgical mitral valve repair or replacement (28). This clip is positioned to bring the tips of the middle portion of the anterior and posterior leaflets together. This creates a double-orifice valve, and has been used extensively in highly selected patients with myxomatous mitral valve disease and FMR. In the EVEREST II trial, 55% of subjects in the percutaneous repair group met the primary composite end point of freedom from death, mitral valve (MV) surgery as a second procedure, or 3 or 4+ MR at 1 year, compared to 73% in the surgery group (P = .007). There was no difference between the groups in all-cause mortality. A significantly lower adverse event rate in the percutaneous group disappeared when blood transfusion was excluded as a complication. The MitraClip is currently being implanted in the United States as part of a continued access registry, and has been used in FMR patients extensively in Europe.

The alternate devices that aim to reduce the mitral annular diameter are in earlier stages of development at this time. The proximity of the coronary sinus (CS) to the mitral valve has been exploited in some experimental designs to achieve this structural modification. However, the variability of the proximity of the mitral annulus to the CS and to the left circumflex artery may limit achievement of the desired goals. Percutaneous annuloplasty devices under investigation include a fixed length, double-anchor CS device called the Carillon Mitral Contour System (Cardiac Dimensions, Kirkland, WA). The recent TITAN trial (Transcatheter Implantation of Carillon Mitral Annuloplasty Device) demonstrated significant reductions in regurgitant volume (34.5 ±11.5 mL to 17.4 ±12.4 mL, P < .001), left ventricular end-diastolic volume (208.5 ±62.0 mL to 178.9 ±48.0 mL, P < .001), end-systolic volume (151.8 ±57.1 mL to 120.7 ±43.2 mL, P = .015), and increased 6-minute walk distance at 12 months among 36 implanted patients (29). Seventeen patients who had the device recaptured at the time of attempted implantation served as controls, and showed progressive left ventricular dilatation. Thirty-day mortality was 1.9%.

Additional inventions include the Monarc device (Edwards Lifesciences, Irvine, CA), which deploys two stents into the CS with the connecting coil bridge being tightened over time, and a CS anchor that connects to the interatrial septum via a cord under tension called the Percutaneous Septal Shortening System (Ample Medical, Foster City, CA). It remains unclear at the current time whether such devices will have a significant future impact on symptom relief and/or improved survival for individuals with MR and left ventricular dysfunction.

FOLLOW-UP OF PATIENTS WITH MR RECEIVING SURGERY, TRANSCATHETER INTERVENTIONS, OR MEDICAL TREATMENT

Patients with severe MR who do not undergo a valvular intervention or surgery should be evaluated semi-annually with echocardiography, and sometimes with stress echocardiography. Patients with moderate MR should be evaluated annually. In those who do undergo surgical repair/replacement or transcatheter procedures, baseline postprocedure echocardiography should be performed ideally at 4 to 6 weeks after the intervention, although this is often performed before hospital discharge for practical purposes. MR can recur because of failure of the repair or due to progression of the underlying disease. Therefore, annual clinical evaluations are recommended, and yearly echocardiography is also a reasonable choice.

CASE OUTCOME

The 64-year-old male with coronary disease and MR, presented above, was judged to have advanced decompensated left ventricular systolic dysfunction of ischemic etiology. The left anterior descending (LAD) and right coronary artery (RCA) territories included some viable myocardium, so it was hoped that revascularization might improve the systolic function. However, it was also recognized that the progression in MR over the past 8 years was likely contributing to the degree of left ventricular dilatation and dysfunction. Therefore, it was unclear whether revascularization alone would significantly improve the patient's ejection fraction or his symptomatology. Given this uncertainty, the significant risk of an open-heart procedure with severe left ventricular dilation and dysfunction, and the lack of evidence to support a survival benefit of mitral valve repair or replacement in this setting, the patient was advised to undergo percutaneous coronary intervention as the first therapeutic procedure. This was successfully accomplished with a 4.0 x 15 mm bare metal stent to the proximal LAD, and a 3.5 x 12 mm bare metal stent to the distal RCA. Clopidogrel was added to the existing aspirin therapy.

Although coronary artery disease is the major underlying etiology of this patient's left ventricular dysfunction and MR, it was considered unlikely that post-revascularization improvements in ventricular function would fully reverse the apical tethering of the mitral valve. Indeed, the severe MR persisted in the immediate post-PCI period. Therefore, CRT was recommended to the patient, particularly in view of his prolonged QRS interval of 130 ms with a LBBB morphology on the electrocardiogram. His LVEF below 35% also met criteria to receive an implantable cardiac defibrillator (CRT-D) for prevention of sudden cardiac death. On discharge from the hospital, the patient was fitted with an external LifeVest® defibrillator. He then returned in 3 months for dysynchony evaluation by echocardiography and underwent placement of a CRT-D device. In early follow-up, he was doing fairly well, though still moderately symptomatic.

REFERENCES

1. Trichon BH, Felker GM, Shaw LK, et al. Relation of frequency and severity of mitral regurgitation to survival among patients with left ventricular systolic dysfunction and heart failure. *Am J Cardiol*. 2003;91(5):538–543.
2. Song JM, Qin JX, Kongsaerepong V, et al. Determinants of ischemic mitral regurgitation in patients with chronic anterior wall myocardial infarction: a real time three-dimensional echocardiography study. *Echocardiography*. 2006;23(8):650–657.
3. Cieślikowski D, Baron T, Grodzicki T. Exercise echocardiography in the evaluation of functional mitral regurgitation: a systematic review of the literature. *Cardiology Journal*. 2007;14(5):436–446.
4. Lancellotti P, Lebrun F, Pierard LA. Determinants of exercise-induced changes in mitral regurgitation in patients with coronary artery disease and left ventricular dysfunction. *J Am Coll Cardiol*. 2003;42(11):1921–1928.
5. D'Andrea A, Caso P, Cuomo S, et al. Effect of dynamic myocardial dysynchrony on mitral regurgitation during supine bicycle exercise stress echocardiography in patients with idiopathic dilated cardiomyopathy and "narrow" QRS. *Eur Heart J*. 2007;28(8):1004–1011.
6. Yiu SF, Enriquez-Sarano, M, et al. Determinants of the Degree of Functional Mitral Regurgitation in Patients With Systolic Left Ventricular Dysfunction A Quantitative Clinical Study. *Circulation*. 2000;102(12):1400–1406.
7. Chaput M, Handschumacher MD, Tournoux F, et al. Mitral leaflet adaptation to ventricular remodeling occurrence and adequacy in patients with functional mitral regurgitation. *Circulation*. 2008;118(8):845–852.
8. Grigioni F, Detaint D, Avierinos J, et al. Contribution of ischemic mitral regurgitation to congestive heart failure after myocardial infarction. *J Am Coll Cardiol*. 2005;45(2):260–267.

9. Aronson D, Goldsher N, Zukermann R, et al. Ischemic mitral regurgitation and risk of heart failure after myocardial infarction. *Arch Intern Med*. 2006;166(21):2362–2368.
10. Lancellotti P, Gerard PL, Pierard LA. Long-term outcomes of patients with heart failure and dynamic function mitral regurgitation. *Eur Heart J*. 2005;26(15):1528–1532.
11. Lowes BD, Gill EA, Abraham WT, et al. Effects of carvedilol on left ventricular mass, chamber geometry, and mitral regurgitation in chronic heart failure. *Am J Cardiol*. 1999;83(8):1201–1205.
12. Breithardt OA, Sinha AM, Schwammenthal E, et al. Acute effects of cardiac resynchronization therapy on functional mitral regurgitation in advanced systolic heart failure. *J Am Coll Cardiol*. 2003;41(5):765–770.
13. Bonow RO, Carabello BA, Chatterjee K, et al. 2008 Focused Update Incorporated Into the ACC/AHA 2006 Guidelines for the Management of Patients With Valvular Heart Disease. *J Am Coll Cardiol*. 2008;52(13):e1-e142.
14. Bolling SF, Deeb GM, Brunsting LA, et al. Early outcomes of mitral valve reconstruction in patients with end-stage cardiomyopathy. *J Thorac Cardiovasc Surg*. 1995;109(4):676–682.
15. Bolling SF, Pagani FD, Deeb GM, et al. Intermediate-term outcome of mitral reconstruction in cardiomyopathy. *Thorac Cardiovasc Surg*. 1998;115(2):381–388.
16. Hammermeister K, Sethi GK, Henderson WG, et al. Outcomes 15 years after valve replacement with a mechanical versus a bioprosthetic valve: final report of the Veterans Affairs randomized trial. *J Am Coll Cardiol*. 2000;36(4):1152–1158.
17. Batista RJV, Verde J, Nery P, et al. Partial left ventriculectomy to treat end-stage heart disease. *Ann Thorac Surg*. 1997;64(3):634–638.
18. Acker MA, Jessup M, Bolling SF, et al. Mitral valve repair in heart failure: five-year follow-up from the mitral valve replacement stratum of the Acorn randomized trial. *J Thoarc and Cardiovasc Surgery*. 2011;142(3):569–574.
19. Bishay ES, McCarthy PM, Cosgrove DM, et al. Mitral valve surgery in patients with severe left ventricular dysfunction. *Eur Cardiothroac Surg*. 2000;17(3):213–221.
20. Wu AH, Aaronson KD, Bolling SF, et al. Impact of mitral valve annuloplasty on mortality risk in patients with mitral regurgitation and left ventricular systolic dysfunction. *J Am Coll Cardiol*. 2005;45(3):381–387.
21. Vahanian A, Baumgartner H, Bax J, et al. Guidelines on the management of valvular heart disease. The Task Force on the Management of Valvular Heart Disease of the European Society of Cardiology. *Eur Heart J*. 2007;28(2):230–268.
22. Ellis SG, Whitlow PL, Raymond RE, et al. Impact of mitral regurgitation on long-term survival after percutaneous coronary intervention. *Am J Cardiol*. 2002;89(3):315–318.
23. Pastorius CA, Henry TD, Harris KM. Long-term outcomes of patients with mitral regurgitation undergoing percutaneous coronary intervention. *Am J Cardiol*. 2002;100(8):1218–1223.
24. Mihaljevic T, Lam BK, Rajeswaran J, et al. Impact of mitral valve annuloplasty combined with revascularization in patients with functional ischemic mitral regurgitation. *J Am Coll Cardiol*. 2007;49(22):2191–2201.
25. Matsunaga A, Tahta SA, Duran CMG. Failure of reduction annuloplasty for functional ischemic mitral regurgitation. *J Heart Valve Dis*. 2004;13(3):390–398.
26. Anyanwu AC, Adams DH. Ischemic mitral regurgitation: recent advances. *Curr Treat Options Cardiovasc Med*. 2008;10(6):529–537.
27. Braun J, van de Veire NR, Klautz RJ, et al. Restrictive mitral annuloplasty cures ischemic mitral regurgitation and heart failure. *Ann Thoarc Surg*. 2008;85(2):430–437.
28. Feldman T, Foster E, Glower DD, et al. for the EVEREST II Investigators. Percutaneous Repair or Surgery for Mitral Regurgitation. *N Engl J Med*. 2011;364(15):1395–406.
29. Siminiak T, Wu JC, Haude M, et al. Treatment of functional mitral regurgitation by percutaneous annuloplasty: results of the TITAN trial. *Eur J Heart Fail*. May 21, 2012 [Epub ahead of print].
30. Vahanian A, Baumgartner H, Bax J, et al. Guidelines on the management of valvular heart disease. *Eur Heart J*. 2007;28(2): 230–268.
31. Zoghbi WA, Enriquez-Sarano M, Foster E, et al. American Society of Echocardiography Report. Recommendations for evaluation of the severity of native valvular regurgitation with two-dimensional and Doppler echocardiography. *J Am Soc Echocardiogr*. 2003;16(7):777–802.

RESOURCES

Landmark Articles

Bargiggia GS, et al. A new method for quantification of mitral regurgitation based on color flow Doppler imaging of flow convergence proximal to regurgitant orifice. *Circulation* 1991;84: 1481–1489.

Bonow RO, et al. 2008 Focused update incorporated into the 2006 American College of Cardiology/American Heart Association Task Force on Practice Guidelines for the Management of Patients With Valvular Heart Disease. *J Am Coll Cardiol*. 2008;52;e1–e142.

Duran CG, Pomar JL, Revuelta JM. Conservative operation for mitral insufficiency: critical analysis supported by postoperative hemodynamic studies of 72 patients. *J Thorac Cardiovasc Surg*. 1980;79: 326–337.

Enriquez-Sarano M, Schaff HV, Orszulak TA, et al. Valve repair improves the outcome of surgery for mitral regurgitation: a multivariate analysis. *Circulation*. 1995;91:1022–1028.

Enriquez-Sarano M, Tajik AJ, Schaff HV, et al. Echocardiographic prediction of left ventricular function after correction of mitral regurgitation: results and clinical implications. *J Am Coll Cardiol*. 1994;24:1536–1543.

Feldman T, Foster E, Glower D, et al. Percutaneous repair or surgery for mitral regurgitation. *N Engl J Med*. 2011;364:1395–1406.

Freed LA, et al. Prevalence and clinical outcome of mitral-valve prolapse. *N Engl J Med*. 1999;341:1–7.

Leung DY, Griffin BP, Stewart WJ, et al. Left ventricular function after valve repair for chronic mitral regurgitation: predictive value of preoperative assessment of contractile reserve by exercise echocardiography. *J Am Coll Cardiol*. 1996;28:1198–1205.

Milano CA, Daneshmand MA, Rankin JS, et al. Survival prognosis and surgical management of ischemic mitral regurgitation. *Ann Thorac Surg*. 2008; 86:735–744.

Schofer J, Siminiak T, Haude M, et al. Percutaneous mitral annuloplasty for functional mitral regurgitation: results of the CARILLON Mitral Annuloplasty Device European Union Study. *Circulation*. 2009;120:326–333.

Key Reviews

Block PC. Percutaneous transcatheter repair for mitral regurgitation. *J Interv Cardiol.* 2006;19:547–551.

Carabello BA. The current therapy for mitral regurgitation. *J Am Coll Cardiol.* 2008;52:319–326.

Ciarka A, Van de Veire N. Secondary mitral regurgitation: pathophysiology, diagnosis, and treatment. *Heart.* 2011;97:1012–1023.

Irvine T. Assessment of mitral regurgitation. *Heart.* 2002;88:iv11–iv19.

Krishnaswamy A, Gillinov AM, Griffin BP. Ischemic mitral regurgitation: pathophysiology, diagnosis, and treatment. *Coron Artery Dis.* 2011;22:359–370.

Mihaljevic T, Gillinov AM, Jarrett C et al. Endoscopic robotically-assisted mitral valve repair. Multimedia Manual of Cardiothoracic Surgery; 2009.

Stewart WJ. Choosing the golden moment for mitral valve repair. *J Am Coll Cardiol.* 1994;24:1544–1546.

Thomas JD. Doppler echocardiographic assessment of valvular regurgitation. *Heart.* 2002;88:651–657.

Relevant Book Chapters

Alpert JS, Sabik J, Cosgrove DM. Mitral valve disease. In: Topol EJ, ed. *Textbook of Cardiovascular Medicine*, 2nd ed. Philadelphia. PA: Lippincott, Williams & Wilkins; 2002:483–509.

Griffin BP, Stewart WJ. Echocardiography in patient selection, operative planning, and intraoperative evaluation of mitral valve repair. In: Otto CM, ed. *The Practice of Clinical Echocardiography*, 2nd ed. Philadelphia, PA: WB Saunders; 2002:417–434.

Meier DJ, Landolfo CK, Starling MR. Role of echocardiography in the timing of surgical intervention for chronic mitral and aortic regurgitation. In: Otto CM, ed. The Practice of Clinical Echocardiography, 2nd ed. Philadelphia, PA: WB Saunders; 2002: 389–416.

Otto CM, Bonow RO. Valvular heart disease. In: Bonow RO, Mann DL, Zipes DP, Libby P, eds. *Heart Disease: A Textbook of Cardiovascular Medicine*, 9th ed. Philadelphia, PA: Elsevier Saunders; 2012:1468–1539.

13

Symptomatic Obstructive Hypertrophic Cardiomyopathy

RACHEL STECKELBERG AND PAUL SORAJJA

INTRODUCTION

Hypertrophic cardiomyopathy (HCM) is a common, inheritable cardiac disorder with a prevalence of 1 in 500 persons (1). Although the vast majority of afflicted individuals have minimal or no cardiac symptoms, there is a subset of patients who suffer from dyspnea, angina, or syncope. The pathophysiology underlying these symptoms is complex, arising from an interplay of diastolic dysfunction, myocardial ischemia, and, in many patients, the presence of dynamic left ventricular outflow tract (LVOT) obstruction. Delineation of these contributing factors is important in the management of patients with HCM, as definitive therapies for relief of heart failure symptoms are available for appropriate candidates (2). This chapter discusses the comprehensive evaluation and management of patients with symptomatic HCM.

CASE PRESENTATION

Clinical History

A 62-year-old man presents for evaluation of exertional dyspnea. Six years ago, he was diagnosed with HCM after an abnormal resting electrocardiogram (ECG) was discovered during a routine general medical examination. At the time of his diagnosis, the patient was asymptomatic. However, over the past year, he has developed dyspnea and angina, both of which now occur with mild levels of activity, such as climbing less than a flight of stairs and ambulating short distances (less than 50 yards). His symptoms are exacerbated in the postprandial state and during hot weather. There is no history of presyncope or syncope. The patient works as a building contractor, and his symptoms have been interfering with his occupation. His medical history is significant for hypertension and hyperlipidemia. Current medications are metoprolol (100 mg twice daily), diltiazem (120 mg twice daily), and atorvastatin (20 mg daily). There is no family history of HCM.

Physical Examination

The patient appears healthy, but is notably overweight (height, 160 cm; weight 90 kg). Vital signs are normal (blood pressure, 115/72 mmHg; heart rate, 62 bpm). Lungs are clear. Carotid upstroke is brisk and not bifid; jugular venous pulse is normal. The precordium demonstrates a sustained, nondisplaced apical impulse. The first and second heart sounds are normal with physiological splitting, and no murmurs, gallops, or rubs are present. During squat-to-stand maneuver, there is a dynamic, 2/6 systolic ejection murmur heard best at the left lower sternal border. The remainder of the physical examination is unremarkable. His ECG shows sinus rhythm, left ventricular hypertrophy, and secondary repolarization abnormalities.

Imaging and Noninvasive Testing

Transthoracic echocardiography demonstrates findings of HCM (**Figure 13-1**). The ventricular septum measures 24 mm in maximal thickness, with less severe hypertrophy involving the posterior wall (15 mm). There is no dynamic LVOT obstruction at rest or during Valsalva strain. Trivial mitral regurgitation

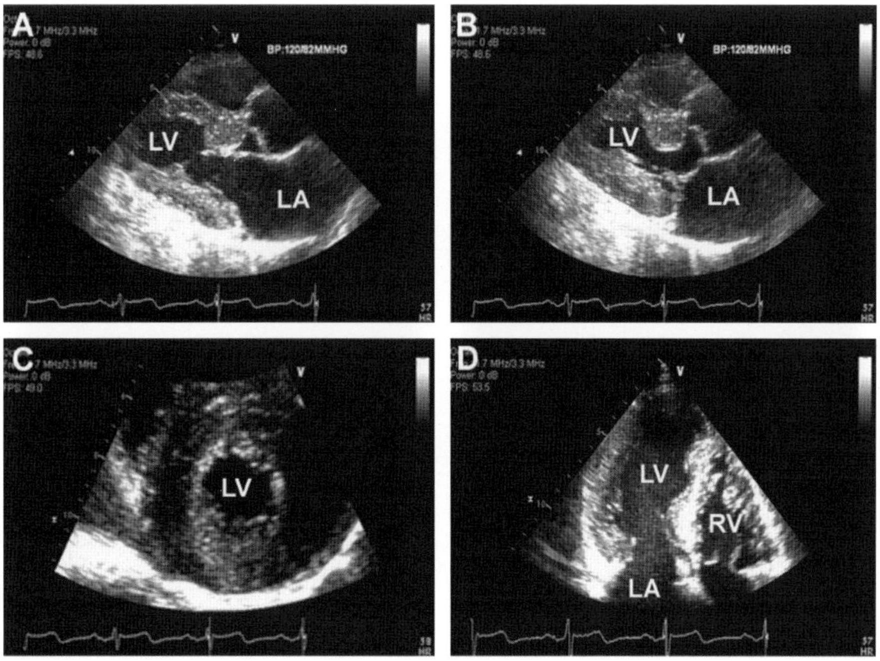

Figure 13-1
Echocardiography of a 62-year-old man with HCM. (A) End-diastolic frame showing severe asymmetric ventricular septal hypertrophy. (B) End-systolic frame showing no systolic anterior motion of the mitral valve and no left ventricular outflow tract (LVOT) obstruction. (C) Short-axis and apical four-chamber. (D) Views showing severe myocardial hypertrophy.

(MR) is present. Left ventricular size and function are normal (ejection fraction, 65%). A cardiac MRI study shows minimal delayed gadolinium hyperenhancement in the ventricular septum at the insertion of the right ventricle; remainder of findings are similar to those of echocardiography. A 24-hour ambulatory ECG demonstrates less than 10 premature atrial contractions; no ventricular ectopics or ventricular tachycardia is observed.

The patient undergoes a maximum oxygen consumption treadmill study, where he exercises for 9 minutes. His systolic blood pressure augments from 110 to 170 mmHg, with a normal increase in the heart rate. Mild chest pain occurs at peak exercise that is nonlimiting and spontaneously dissipates during recovery. The exercise ECG is not interpretable due to pre-existing ST-segment abnormalities in the setting of left ventricular hypertrophy. Metabolic gas exchange measurement demonstrates a peak myocardial oxygen consumption (VO_2) of 22.0 ml/kg/min (70% predicted), a respiratory exchange ratio of 1.2 liters, and significant plateau in the O_2 pulse, consistent with cardiac output limitation.

Cardiac Catheterization

The patient undergoes invasive hemodynamic assessment with transseptal catheterization. The right-sided pressures were normal; mild elevation in left atrial pressure (mean, 15 mmHg) and no significant LVOT obstruction is present (**Figure 13-2**). During isoproterenol administration (1–3 mg/min), there is a dynamic LVOT gradient of 55 to 75 mmHg with a characteristic Brockenbrough response in the aortic pressure on the postectopic

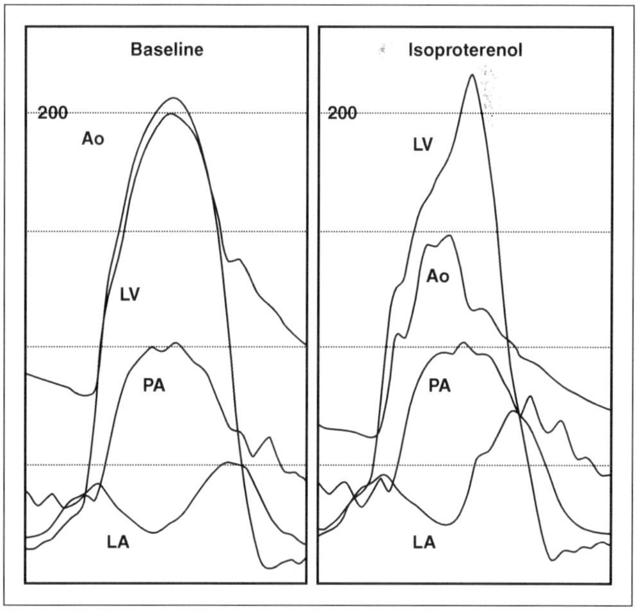

Figure 13-2
Invasive hemodynamics. At baseline, there was no significant left ventricular outflow tract gradient. With infusion of isoproterenol, there is a 74 mmHg gradient across the left ventricular outflow tract. Simultaneous echocardiography demonstrated systolic anterior motion of the mitral valve.

Note: Ao = ascending aortic pressure; LA = left atrial pressure; LV = left ventricular pressure; PA = pulmonary artery pressure.

ventricular beat. Simultaneous echocardiography demonstrates systolic anterior motion (SAM) of the mitral valve. There is no significant atherosclerosis on coronary angiography.

Septal Reduction Therapy

Given the evidence of dynamic LVOT obstruction and the presence of drug-refractory, limiting symptoms, the patient undergoes counseling for septal reduction therapy. The significant functional limitation observed on his treadmill exercise study also is noted. The options of both surgical myectomy and alcohol septal ablation are discussed in detail. The patient chooses surgical myectomy, which is successfully performed and leads to a residual LVOT gradient of less than 5 mmHg at rest and after provocation. His hospital course is uncomplicated, and the patient has complete relief of his cardiac symptoms in follow-up.

HCM is a common disorder, the complexities of which have fascinated and challenged clinicians for over 50 years. The case described herein illustrates many of the challenges germane to the evaluation and management of patients with HCM.

CLINICAL SYMPTOMS AND PHYSICAL SIGNS

While many patients with HCM have minimal or no symptoms, others can be significantly debilitated. Multiple pathological mechanisms lead to the development of symptoms in these patients, including diastolic dysfunction, myocardial ischemia, atrial or ventricular arrhythmias, and LVOT obstruction with or without dynamic MR. Sudden cardiac death may be the initial manifestation of the disorder. Notably, HCM accounts for approximately 35% of sudden deaths among all persons under 35 years of age, and is the leading cause of sudden death in this age group (1,2).

Several physical signs suggest the presence of HCM in suspected patients. The carotid upstroke is rapid due to the hyperdynamic nature of the disease, and may be bifid in those with LVOT obstruction. The atrial wave of the jugular venous pulse may be heightened if there is significant infundibular hypertrophy. The apical impulse is nearly always sustained, localized, and may be bifid or trifid. A fourth heart sound is frequently present, especially in younger patients. Paradoxical splitting of the second heart sound also may occur with significant LVOT obstruction.

Dynamic LVOT obstruction conventionally has been defined as a gradient of greater than 30 mmHg. Importantly, LVOT obstruction in HCM is exquisitely sensitive to changes in ventricular load and contractility (**Figure 13-3**). Overall, dynamic LVOT obstruction is present in 25% of patients at rest, while another 30% to 40% of patients have evidence of obstruction only after provocative maneuvers (3–5). Thus, physical examination maneuvers should be performed routinely to illicit the presence of dynamic LVOT obstruction and to differentiate it from other causes of systolic murmurs. Increases in inotropy and

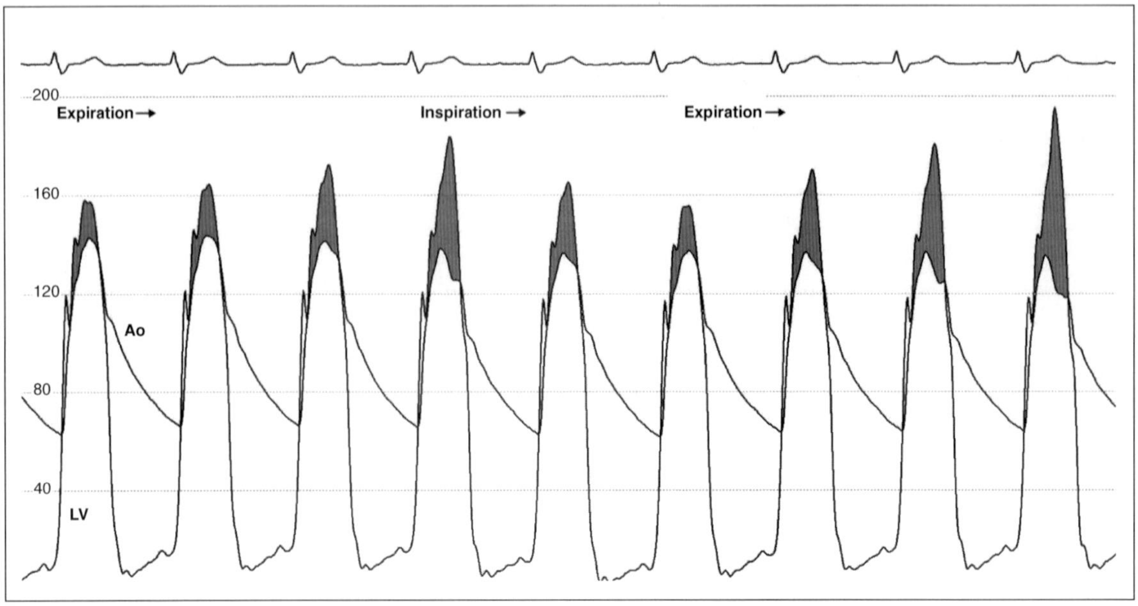

Figure 13-3
Dynamic respiratory change in the left ventricular outflow tract gradient in HCM. These changes in gradient were observed in normal respiration, resulting from only mild respiratory changes in ventricular afterload.

decreases in either preload or afterload will lead to worsening of dynamic LVOT obstruction. Thus, the systolic ejection murmur due to obstructive HCM augments during Valsalva strain, after squat-to-stand maneuver, following amyl nitrate inhalation, during physical exercise, and on the postventricular ectopic beat. The murmur of MR secondary to LVOT obstruction and decreased mitral leaflet coaptation also may exhibit some of these dynamic qualities. These physical examination maneuvers are an important part of the clinical evaluation due to the known variability of the LVOT gradient. Evidence of latent LVOT obstruction should be sought in symptomatic patients, in whom appropriate medical and surgical therapies can provide definitive relief of symptoms.

TWO-DIMENSIONAL AND DOPPLER ECHOCARDIOGRAPHY

Echocardiography is the most common imaging method for diagnosing HCM due to its noninvasive nature and widespread availability. Cardiac MRI also may be utilized, and provides incremental diagnostic utility when echocardiography is inconclusive (eg, apical or eccentric hypertrophy; 6). With either imaging modality, it is important to correlate the morphologic abnormalities with the clinical findings, including electrocardiography, as infiltrative cardiomyopathies can mimic the findings of HCM. The diagnosis of HCM is made on the basis of a nondilated ventricle and myocardial hypertrophy (typically greater than or equal to 15 mm) that cannot be attributed to another cardiac or systemic etiology (2).

The common patterns of myocardial hypertrophy in patients with HCM are asymmetric septal, concentric, and apical, but eccentric or lateral wall hypertrophy also has been observed (**Figure 13-4**; 6,7). Asymmetric septal hypertrophy refers to hypertrophy that predominantly involves the ventricular septum (septal: posterior wall thickness greater than 1.5). Asymmetric septal hypertrophy is the most frequent pattern of myocardial hypertrophy (60%), and gave rise to the early nomenclature of the disease (eg, idiopathic hypertrophic subaortic stenosis). Conversely,

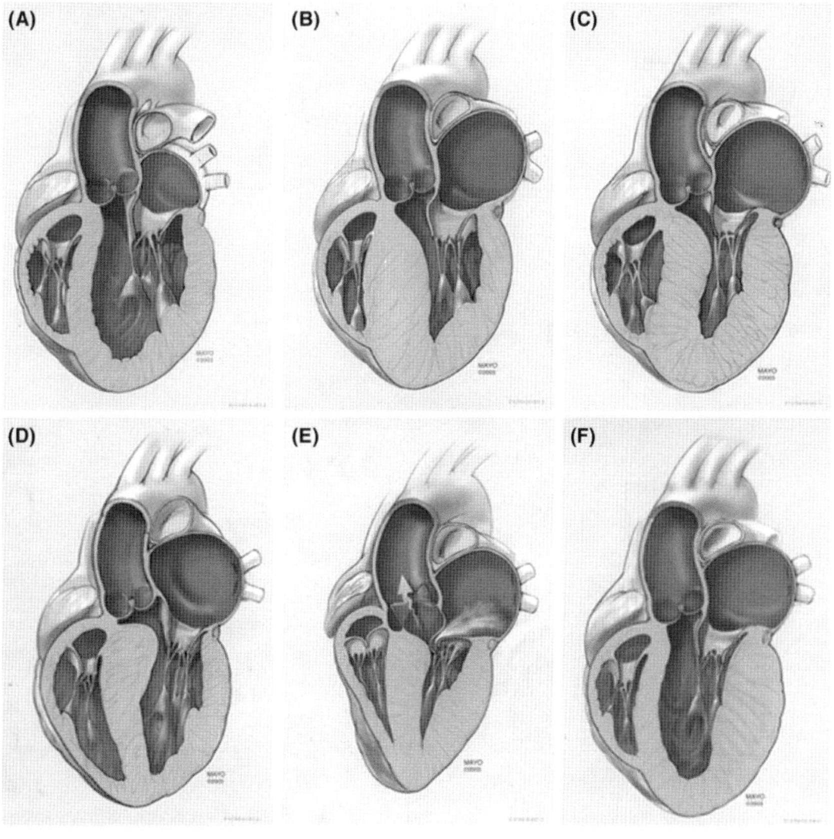

Figure 13-4
Patterns of hypertrophy in patients with HCM. (A) normal; (B) asymmetric ventricular septal hypertrophy; (C) concentric hypertrophy; (D) basal septal hypertrophy; (E) apical hypertrophy; (F) eccentric or lateral hypertrophy.

Source: Reprinted with permission. Copyright, Mayo Clinic Foundation.

concentric hypertrophy involves the entire left ventricle in a relatively symmetrical manner. Apical hypertrophy is confined to segments distal to the origin of the papillary muscles.

Echocardiography is fundamental to the detection and characterization of dynamic LVOT obstruction at rest and after provocative maneuvers. In patients with obstructive HCM, there is a dynamic LVOT gradient and SAM of either the anterior and/or posterior leaflet of the mitral valve. The onset, severity, and duration of SAM correlate with the severity of the LVOT gradient. It is important to distinguish the Doppler signal of the LVOT gradient ("dagger-shaped") from that due to MR (symmetrical shape; **Figure 13-5**). Other important goals of the echocardiographic examination are to evaluate for the presence of concomitant aortic disease, intrinsic MR, and anomalous papillary muscles; these abnormalities have implications for the choice of septal reduction therapy in symptomatic patients.

INVASIVE CARDIAC CATHETERIZATION

Hemodynamic evaluation with cardiac catheterization is indicated in HCM patients with symptoms that are not readily explained by the results of noninvasive imaging. The principal advantage of invasive hemodynamic catheterization is the direct measurement of absolute intracardiac pressures, which cannot be accurately assessed with current echocardiographic methods in patients with HCM. Invasive hemodynamic catheterization also is required when the gradient cannot be determined by echocardiography in symptomatic patients who are suspected of having latent LVOT obstruction (eg, contamination with MR signal, poor body habitus for imaging; 8).

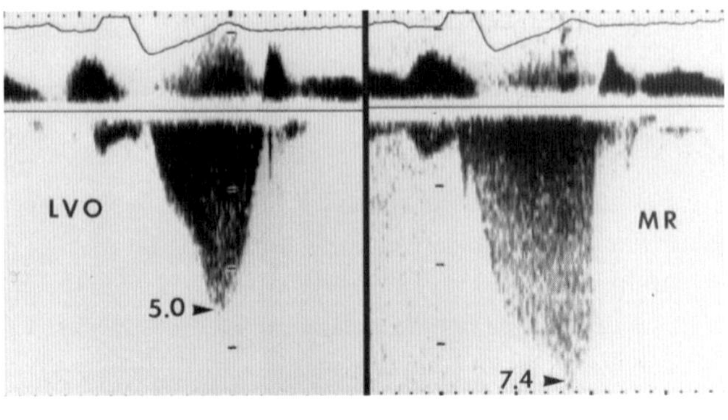

Figure 13-5
Differentiation of the signal of mitral regurgitation (MR) versus that of left ventricular outflow (LVO) obstruction. Care must taken to differentiate these two Doppler signals as contamination with MR with lead to a significant overestimation of the left ventricular outflow tract (LVOT) gradient.

The optimal method for assessing the LVOT gradient is a transseptal approach with placement of a balloon-tipped catheter (eg, 7 Fr Berman catheter, Arrow International Inc., Reading, PA) at the left ventricular inflow region and a pigtail catheter placed retrograde in the ascending aorta for simultaneous measurement of the LVOT gradient. The transseptal approach helps to avoid catheter entrapment, which can be difficult to distinguish from changes in left ventricular pressure that occur due to the dynamic nature of LVOT obstruction (6–8). Use of an 8 Fr Mullins sheath for transseptal access also enables recording of left atrial pressure via the sidearm for assessment for concomitant diastolic dysfunction. Alternatively, left ventricular pressure can be assessed with a 5 or 6 Fr catheter placed retrograde across the aortic valve. Absence of catheter entrapment should be confirmed with hand contrast injections or demonstration of pulsatile flow from the catheter with disconnection from the extenders used for pressure transduction.

The diagnosis of dynamic obstruction is made through detection of a significant LVOT gradient with the characteristic "spike-and-dome" configuration in the aortic pressure contour. Dynamic LVOT obstruction can be observed at rest or with provocation using physical or pharmacologic exercise (**Figure 13-6**). The Brockenbrough response refers to the decrease in aortic pulse pressure on the post-ventricular ectopic beat. This phenomenon occurs due to the marked increase in contractility, worsening of LVOT obstruction, and consequential decrease in left ventricular forward stroke volume. Amyl nitrate or isoproterenol (1 to 10 mg/min) can be administered for determining the presence of latent LVOT obstruction (9). Simultaneous echocardiography should also be used to document systolic anterior motion of the mitral valve.

GENERAL MANAGEMENT GUIDELINES

The major goals in managing patients with HCM include symptom relief, identification of those at an increased risk of sudden death, and intervening in patients who are considered high risk. As a significant proportion of sudden deaths occur during or following exercise, it is generally recommended that these patients abstain from competitive sports or

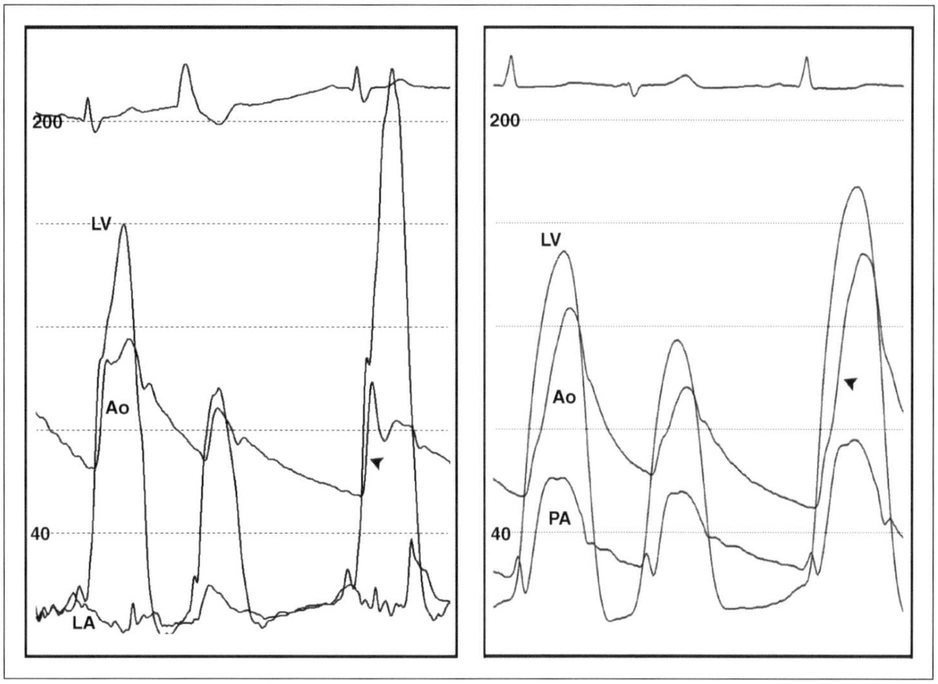

Figure 13-6
Pressure tracings after a premature ventricular beat in a patient with dynamic left ventricular outflow tract (LVOT) obstruction due to hypertrophic cardiomyopathy (left) and in a patient with fixed obstruction due to aortic stenosis (right). Note the decrease in aortic pulse pressure (arrowheads) following the premature ventricular beat in the patient with hypertrophic cardiomyopathy (ie, Brockenborough response) that does not occur in the patient with aortic stenosis.

other strenuous physical activities. Patients should also be counseled to remain well hydrated and avoid situations that may put them at increased risk of vasodilation (eg, hot tubs, saunas, etc.). Counseling on the genetic nature of HCM should be offered, in addition to recommendations of screening of first-degree relatives for the condition. Of note, the presence of concomitant coronary artery disease is associated with an adverse prognosis in patients with HCM (10). Thus, for patients with symptoms of angina, evaluation for epicardial coronary atherosclerosis should be performed in those at risk, and lead to appropriate therapies for both primary and secondary prevention.

MEDICAL THERAPY

Negative inotropic agents are the mainstay of pharmacologic therapy in symptomatic patients with HCM. The most commonly used drugs are beta-adrenergic antagonists, which improve diastolic filling time and the imbalance between myocardial oxygen demand and ischemia (2). These agents also reduce intraventricular flow velocities by depressing contractility, thereby alleviating LVOT obstruction and high-intracavitary pressures in susceptible patients. Other frequently prescribed drug agents are calcium-channel blockers and disopyramide, both of which operate through mechanisms similar to beta-adrenergic antagonists (11). Of note, calcium-channel blockers should be used cautiously in patients with LVOT obstruction, as these drugs potentially can lead to worsening of the LVOT gradient and result in pulmonary edema. Also, disopyramide may lead to anticholinergic side effects and is known to accelerate atrioventricular nodal conduction. Disopyramide should be initiated under cardiac monitoring to exclude proarrhythmic effects. In all patients with dynamic LVOT obstruction, peripheral vasodilators and diuretics should be avoided due to their adverse effects on ventricular load.

SEPTAL REDUCTION THERAPY

For patients with significant LVOT obstruction and severe symptoms refractory to appropriate medical treatment, definitive means of septal reduction therapy should be considered. Of note, several studies have demonstrated impaired survival of patients with obstructive HCM, even in the absence of significant symptoms (12,13). However, septal reduction therapy is indicated only for relief of symptoms, and there currently is no role for these therapies as prophylaxis for improvement in survival.

Surgical Myectomy

Surgical myectomy has evolved over the past five decades to become the gold standard therapy for the relief of drug-refractory symptoms due to LVOT obstruction in patients with HCM (2,14). In this procedure, a surgeon uses a transaortic approach to widen the LVOT by debulking the thickened ventricular septum under direct visualization. Not uncommonly, the resection is carried deep into the mid-ventricular septum (ie, extended myectomy), leading to full reconstruction of the outflow tract (**Figures 13-7** and **13-8**). Surgical myectomy leads to a greater than 90% reduction in the LVOT gradient

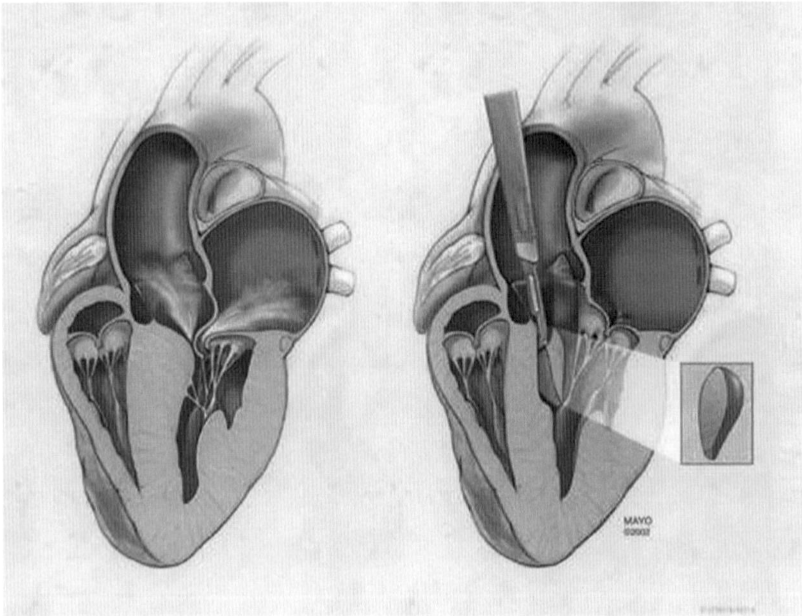

Figure 13-7
Surgical myectomy. The surgeon uses a transaortic approach to resect myocardial hypertrophy from the ventricular septum, often extending down to the base of the papillary muscles.
Source: Reprinted with permission. Copyright, Mayo Clinic Foundation.

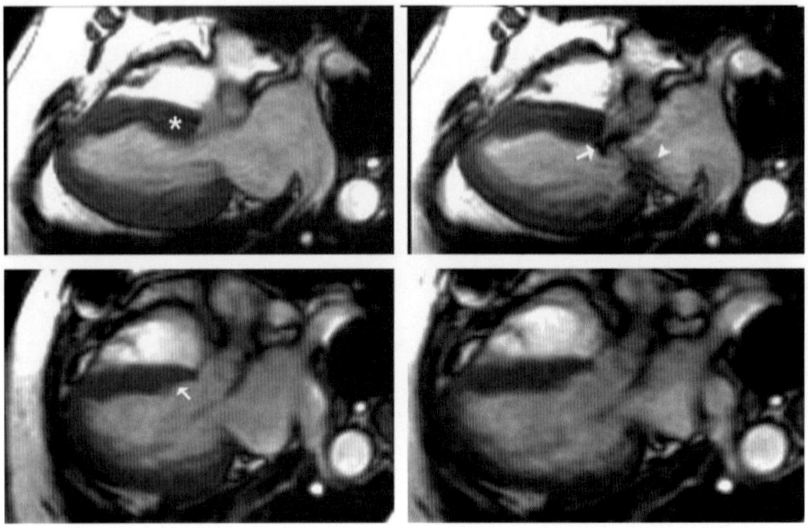

Figure 13-8
Cardiac MRI before and after surgical myectomy. Top, end-diastolic (left) and end-systolic (right) frames demonstrating ventricular septal myocardial hypertrophy (asterisk), systolic anterior motion of the mitral valve (arrow), and posteriorly directed mitral regurgitation (arrowhead). Bottom, end-diastolic (left) and end-systolic (right) frames demonstrating resection of the ventricular septum (arrow) with resolution of left ventricular outflow tract (LVOT) obstruction and mitral regurgitation.

with residual gradients typically less than 5 mmHg. While historical studies reported significant hazards with the procedure, the evolution of operative techniques and cardiac anesthesia had led to a current operative mortality of less than 1% when performed in experienced surgical centers (14).

Surgical myectomy leads to durable symptom relief in more than 90% of patients with HCM. The benefits of surgical myectomy have been attributed to elimination of LVOT obstruction, reduction in myocardial ischemia, improvement in diastolic function, and alleviation of MR. In addition, several studies have demonstrated highly favorable long-term survival after the procedure with follow-up ranging from 10 to 25 years. Notably, in one study from the Mayo Clinic, the survival of the myectomy patients ($n = 289$) was no different from the expected survival of a similar general U.S. population of individuals (83% vs. 88% at 10 years, $P = .20$; **Figure 13-9**; 14). Survival of these myectomy patients also was superior to patients with LVOT obstruction who did not have surgery. Although treatment was not randomized in this study, these data support the notion that appropriately selected patients may have normal life expectancy following surgical myectomy.

Alcohol Septal Ablation

In 1995, alcohol septal ablation was introduced as an alternative to surgical myectomy for the relief of LVOT obstruction (15). The aim of this procedure is to induce a localized myocardial infarction of the proximal ventricular septum, thereby leading to a reduction in systolic septal thickening and excursion into the LVOT. During alcohol septal ablation, an angioplasty balloon is placed in a septal perforator artery using standard coronary catheters and flexible guidewires (**Figure 13-10**). Contrast echocardiography is used to delineate the area supplied by the septal artery, with targeting of only the myocardial area that is intimately involved with the development of LVOT obstruction. Following this confirmation, 1 to 3 ml of desiccated alcohol is infused slowly through the balloon catheter into the septal artery. The use of alcohol is preferred because this agent immediately results in a discrete myocardial infarction. In other percutaneous methods (eg, vascular coiling, covered stent placement), a therapeutic infarction may not result due to septal collateralization. Alcohol septal ablation typically results in an infraction size of 8% to 10% of the left ventricular mass.

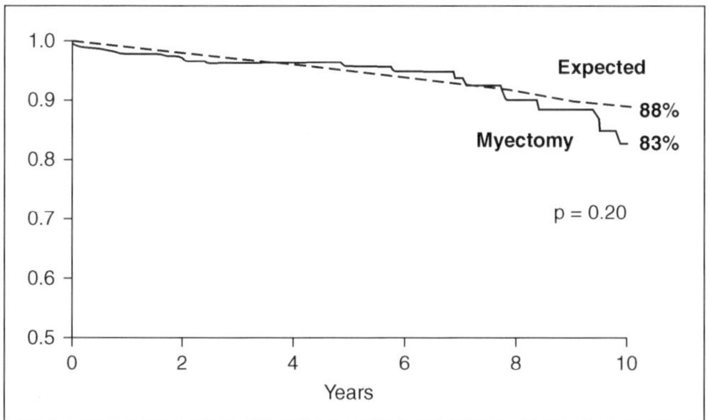

Figure 13-9
Expected versus observed survival after surgical myectomy. Expected survival was calculated using published U.S. population mortality rates.
Source: Reprinted with permission (14).

Acute hemodynamic success with relief of the LVOT gradient occurs in 80% to 85% of patients who undergo alcohol septal ablation (16). This success rate is lower than open surgery due to the dependency of the procedure on septal artery anatomy. Of note, the most common reason for procedural failure is the lack of an appropriate septal artery, which may be either too small or tortuous for successful cannulation with the angioplasty catheter in 10% to 20% of patients. Further reduction in the LVOT gradient over 3 to 6 months after the procedure can occur due to ventricular remodeling and basal septal thinning.

The published procedural mortality of alcohol septal ablation is 1% to 2% (2,17,18). The major complication is pacemaker dependency from complete atrioventricular block, the occurrence of which is related to the presence of underlying conduction system disease. Alcohol septal ablation results in a right bundle branch block (RBBB) in approximately 50% of cases. Thus, patients with pre-existing left bundle branch block (LBBB), severe left axis deviation, or wide QRS are at the highest risk of permanent pacemaker dependency (19). However, the risk of complete atrioventricular block remains approximately 10% even if the baseline ECG is normal. Thus, all patients without a prior pacemaker undergo placement of a temporary device followed by monitoring in an ICU with the device in place for 3 to 4 days after ablation. Other procedural complications of alcohol septal ablation that have been reported include dissection of the left anterior descending artery, free wall infarction from collateralization or untoward extravasation of alcohol, and cardiac perforation due to temporary pacemaker placement.

Overall, in comparison to surgical myectomy, alcohol septal ablation has been associated with comparable early survival and similar significant improvements in New York Heart Association (NYHA)

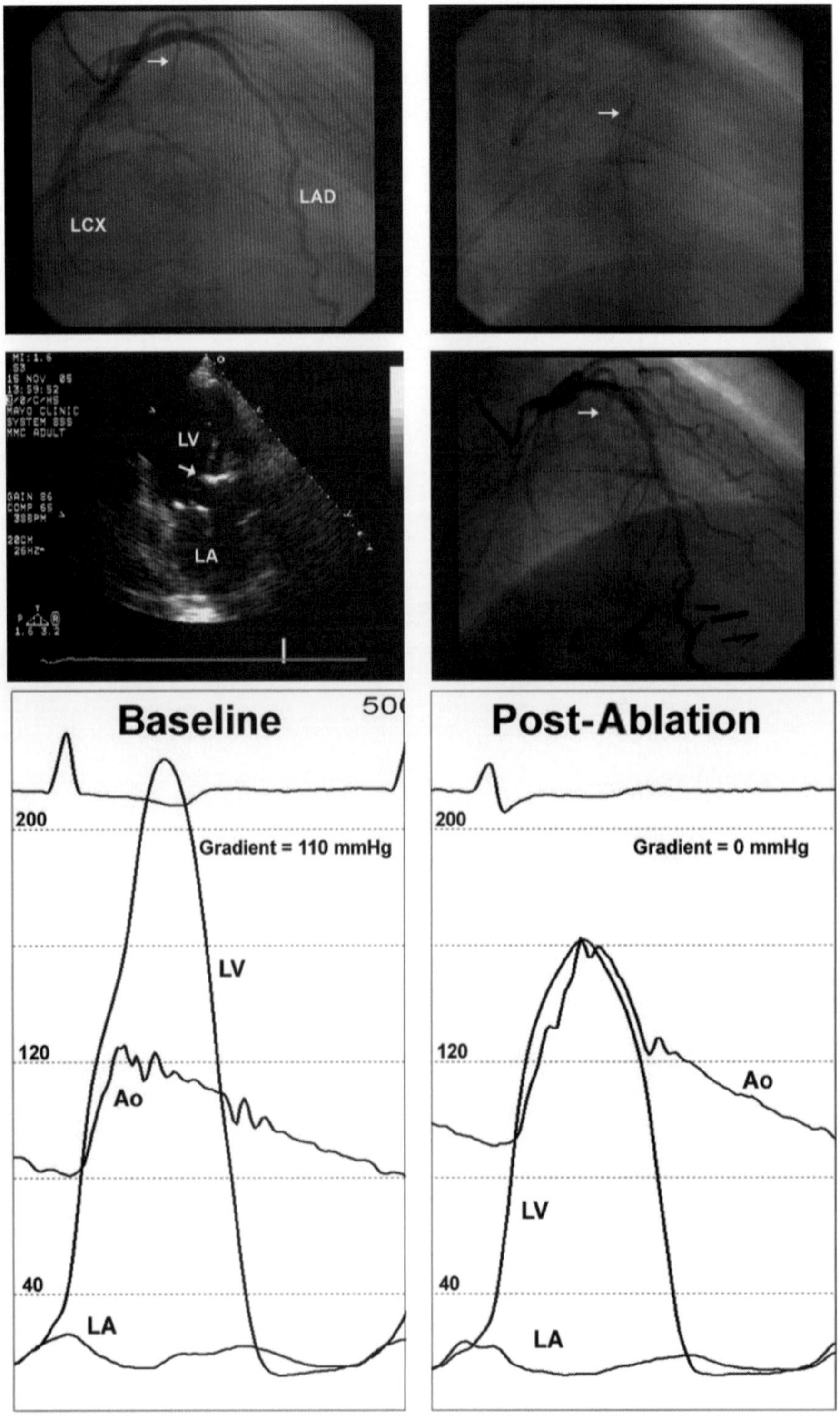

Figure 13-10
Percutaneous alcohol septal ablation. Top left: Baseline angiogram of the left coronary artery showing the septal perforator artery (arrow) to be used for ablation. Top right: An over-the-wire balloon (arrow) is inflated in the perforator artery followed by contrast injection through the balloon. Middle left: Echocardiographic contrast is injected through the balloon and visualized with simultaneous echocardiography. Middle right: Following injection of alcohol, the septal artery (arrow) is obliterated. Bottom left: Before septal ablation, the left ventricular outflow tract (LVOT) gradient is 110 mmHg. Bottom right: Following septal ablation, there is no LVOT gradient.

Note: Ao = ascending aorta; LA = left atrium; LAD = left anterior descending; LCX = left circumflex; LV = left ventricle.

functional class and objective measures of exercise tolerance, such as treadmill time and peak myocardial oxygen consumption (**Figure 13-11**; 20–27). One notable exception is the difference in outcome for younger patients (less than 65 years of age), in whom surgical myectomy has been shown to be superior in terms of survival free of severe symptoms (**Figure 13-12**; 16). The reasons for this discrepancy are not clear, but may be related to the relatively higher residual gradients after alcohol septal ablation (approximately 10 to 15 mmHg). These residual gradients may be tolerated as well by younger or more active individuals.

The vast majority of studies on alcohol septal ablation have a follow-up duration of less than 5 years, leading to remaining questions regarding the long-term effects of the septal infarction (2,28–30). Given the complexity of decision making in the management of HCM, it is important that the evaluation and counseling for septal reduction therapy be performed in a multidisciplinary setting devoted to the comprehensive, longitudinal care of these patients. For alcohol septal ablation, proper selection is critical to the success of the procedure. Appropriate criteria include: (a) severe, drug-refractory cardiac symptoms (NYHA functional Class III/IV or Canadian Cardiac Society angina Class III/IV) due to obstructive HCM; (b) dynamic LVOT obstruction due to systolic anterior motion of the mitral valve (gradient greater than or equal to 30 mmHg); (c) ventricular septal thickness greater than or equal to 15 mm; (d) absence of significant intrinsic mitral valve disease; (e) absence of need for concomitant cardiac surgical procedure (eg, bypass grafting, valve replacement); and (f) informed patient consent. Informed patient consent requires full understanding of the paucity of long-term data on survival after septal ablation, the relatively lower success rate due to its dependence on coronary anatomy, risk of pacemaker dependency, and potential complications related to instrumentation of the coronary arteries. Although younger age has not been an absolute contraindication to the procedure, alcohol septal ablation generally has been reserved for older adult patients due to the limited data on long-term survival and better outcomes observed with surgical myectomy in those patients less than 65 years of age.

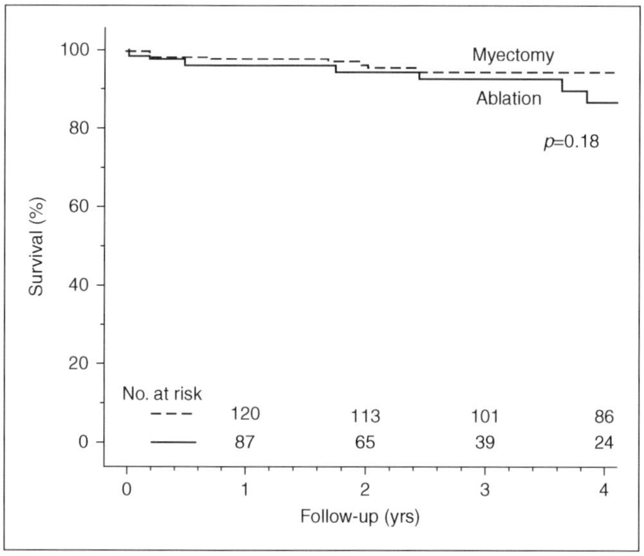

Figure 13-11
Survival free of all-cause mortality after surgical myectomy versus alcohol septal ablation.
Source: Reprinted with permission (16).

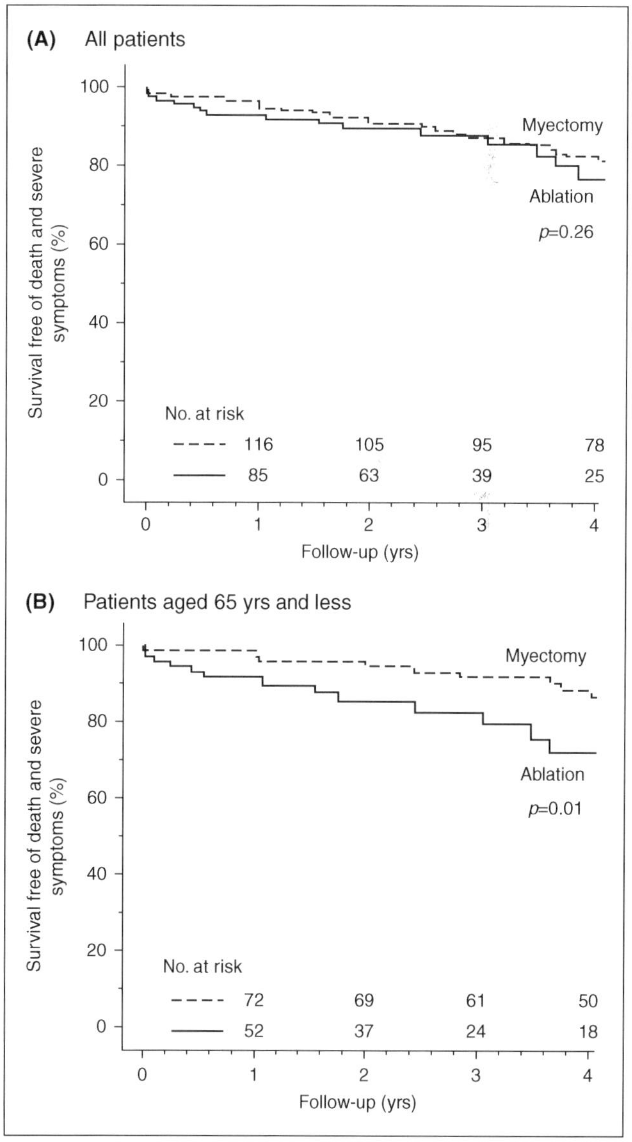

Figure 13-12
Survival free of death and severe symptoms after surgical myectomy versus alcohol septal ablation for (A) all patients and (B) those aged 65 years or less.
Source: Reprinted with permission (16).

NONOBSTRUCTIVE HCM

For patients with symptoms and no evidence of LVOT obstruction, the primary pathophysiologic process is that of diastolic dysfunction. As previously described, drugs with negative inotropic and chronotropic effects are the predominant therapy in these patients. Reducing myocardial ischemia is also beneficial, but may be more difficult to achieve as there are no overt structural lesions that can be corrected. For patients with HCM who have impaired systolic function (ie, "burnt-out" variant), vasodilators, diuretics, beta-receptor antagonists, and other conventional pharmacologic or device therapies should be employed.

For patients with apical HCM, a novel procedure of surgical myectomy of the left ventricular apex has been developed at Mayo Clinic (31). In this procedure, the surgeon uses a transapical approach to directly debulk myocardial hypertrophy of the left ventricular apex, distal septum, and papillary muscles with the goal of enlarging the left ventricular cavity and improving stroke volume. In a report of 44 patients who underwent apical myectomy, there were significant improvements in left ventricular diastolic pressure (28 ±9 to 24 ±7 mmHg), end-diastolic volume (55 ±17 to 68 ±18 mL), and stroke volume (56 ±17 to 63 ±19 mL). After a follow-up of 2.6 years, 74% were NYHA functional Class I or II. Of note, for patients with severe symptoms who otherwise are not operative candidates, cardiac transplantation is the only therapeutic option.

RISK STRATIFICATION FOR SUDDEN CARDIAC DEATH

Sudden cardiac death is a devastating complication of HCM. While historical reports previously suggested a high incidence, studies of unselected populations of patients with HCM have demonstrated an annual occurrence of approximately 1% (2,32). Identification and treatment of HCM patients at increased risk of sudden cardiac death poses unique challenges. These include considerable disease heterogeneity, different patient (or family) tolerance of risk, the relatively low incidence of sudden cardiac death, variable definitions of the risk factors, and the potential complications of device implantation.

Risk stratification for sudden cardiac death in HCM is recommended as part of the routine initial evaluation of patients who are eligible for therapy with an implantable cardioverter-defibrillator (ICD), with repeat evaluations performed at regular intervals in follow-up (every 12 to 24 months). It is important to note the low positive predictive value of each risk factor (approximately 10% to 20%). Thus, the vast majority of patients with risk factor(s) will not experience sudden cardiac death. Decision making with regard to the need for ICD implantation in HCM should be individualized according to patient preference, age, the type, and number of risk factors present, as well as the risks of lifelong ICD implantation.

Patients with a history of prior cardiac arrest, ventricular fibrillation, or sustained ventricular tachycardia have a high risk of recurrence (approximately 10% per year) and should receive an ICD as part of a secondary prevention strategy (33). Other established risk factors for sudden cardiac death are massive myocardial hypertrophy (greater than or equal to 30 mm thickness), family history of sudden death due to HCM, unexplained syncope, abnormal blood pressure response to exercise, and nonsustained ventricular tachycardia.

Of note, LVOT obstruction also has been associated with increased risk of sudden cardiac death in some, but not all, studies (12). Possible explanations for the lack of strong association between LVOT obstruction and risk of sudden cardiac death include the dynamic variability of obstruction, its modifiable nature via medical therapy and surgery, and the relatively small size of patient cohorts studied. Notably, one study examined HCM patients with a history of ICD who underwent surgical myectomy for symptomatic LVOT obstruction (34). In this study, the incidence of ICD discharge after surgery was only 0.2%. Severe dynamic LVOT obstruction currently is not utilized as an independent risk factor, but may be considered in the context of other risk factors for sudden cardiac death when weighing the risks and benefits of ICD implantation. In instances where septal reduction therapy may be performed, the modifiable nature of LVOT obstruction should be taken into account.

CONCLUSION AND KEY POINTS

1. Dynamic LVOT obstruction in HCM is exquisitely sensitive to ventricular load and contractility.
2. In symptomatic patients with HCM, provocative maneuvers should be performed to assess for the presence of dynamic LVOT obstruction to identify candidates for septal reduction therapy.

3. Surgical myectomy is the gold standard therapy for symptomatic obstructive HCM, with symptom relief and procedure success occurring in more than 90% of the patients and a surgical mortality of less than 1% when performed in experienced centers.
4. Alcohol septal ablation is an effective alternative therapy for symptomatic obstructive HCM. Patient selection and operator experience are critical to the success of the procedure. The main complication of alcohol septal ablation is permanent pacemaker dependency.

REFERENCES

1. Maron BJ. Hypertrophic cardiomyopathy: A systematic review. *JAMA*. 2002;287(10):1308–1320.
2. Gersh BJ, Maron BJ, Bonow RO, et al. 2011 ACCF/AHA guideline forthe diagnosis and treatment of hypertrophic cardiomyopathy: a report of the American College of Cardiology Foundation/American Heart AssociationTask Force on Practice Guidelines.*J Am Coll Cardiol*. November 2, 2011. [Epub].
3. Maron MS, Olivotto I, Zenovich AG, et al. Hypertrophic cardiomyopathy is predominantly a disease of left ventricular outflow tract obstruction. *Circulation*. 2006;114(21):2232–2239.
4. Kizilbash AM, Heinle SK, Grayburn PA. Spontaneous variability of left ventricular outflow tract gradient in hypertrophic obstructive cardiomyopathy. *Circulation*. 1998;97(5):461–466.
5. Geske J, Sorajja P, Nishimura RA, et al. Left ventricular outflow tract gradient variability in patients with hypertrophic cardiomyopathy. *Clin Cardiol*. 2009;32(7):397–402.
6. Maron MS, Maron BJ, Harrigan C, et al. Hypertrophic cardiomyopathy phenotype revisited after 50 years with cardiovascular magnetic resonance. *J Am Coll Cardiol*. 2009;54(3):220–228.
7. Klues HG, Schiffers A, Maron BJ. Phenotypic spectrum and patterns of left ventricular hypertrophy in hypertrophic cardiomyopathy: morphologic observations and significance as assessed by two-dimensional echocardiography in 600 patients. *J Am Coll Cardiol*. 1995;26(7):1699–1708.
8. Geske JB, Sorajja P, Nishimura RA, et al.Evaluation of left ventricular filling pressures by Doppler echocardiography in patients with hypertrophic cardiomyopathy: correlation with direct left atrial pressure measurement at cardiac catheterization. *Circulation*. 2007;116(23):2702–2708.
9. Elesber A, Nishimura RA, Rihal CS, et al. Utility of isoproterenol to provoke outflow tract gradients in patients with hypertrophic cardiomyopathy. *Am J Cardiol*. 2008;101(4):516–520.
10. Sorajja P, Ommen SR, Nishimura RA, et al. Adverse prognosis of patients with hypertrophic cardiomyopathy and epicardial coronary artery disease. *Circulation*. 2003;108(19):2342–2348.
11. Matsubara H, Nakatani S, Nagata S, et al. Salutary effect of disopyramide on left ventricular diastolic function in hypertrophic obstructive cardiomyopathy. *J Am Coll Cardiol*. 1995;26(3): 768–775.
12. Maron MS, Olivotto I, Zenovich AG, et al. Effect of left ventricular outflow tract obstruction on clinical outcome in hypertrophic cardiomyopathy. *N Engl J Med*. 2003;348(4):295–303.
13. Sorajja P, Nishimura RA, Gersh BJ, et al. Outcome of mildly symptomatic or asymptomatic obstructive hypertrophic cardiomyopathy: a long-term follow-up study. *J Am Coll Cardiol*. 2009;54(3):234–241.
14. Ommen SR, Maron BJ, Olivotto I, et al. Long-term effects of surgical septal myectomy on survival in patients with obstructive hypertrophic cardiomyopathy. *J Am Coll Cardiol*. 2005;46(3): 470–476
15. Sigwart U. Non-surgical myocardial reduction for hypertrophic obstructive cardiomyopathy. *Lancet*. 1995;346(8969):211–214.
16. Sorajja P, Valeti U, Nishimura RA, et al. Outcome of alcohol septal ablation for obstructive hypertrophic cardiomyopathy. *Circulation*. 2008;118(2):131–139.
17. Leonardi RA, Kransdorf EP, Simel DL, et al. Meta-analyses of septal reduction therapies for obstructive hypertrophic cardiomyopathy: comparative rates of overall mortality and sudden cardiac death after treatment. *Circ Cardiovasc Interv*. 2010;3(2):97–104.
18. Agarwal S, Tuzcu EM, Desai MY, et al. Updated meta-analysis of septal alcohol ablation versus myectomy for hypertrophic cardiomyopathy. *J Am Coll Cardiol*. 2010;55(8):823–834.
19. Talreja DR, Nishimura RA, Edwards WD, et al. Alcohol septal ablation versus surgical septal myectomy: comparison of effects on atrioventricular conduction tissue. *J Am Coll Cardiol*. 2004;44(12):2329–2332.
20. Firoozi S, Elliott PM, Sharma S, et al. Septal myotomy-myectomy and transcoronary septal alcohol ablation in hypertrophic obstructive cardiomyopathy: a comparison of clinical, haemodynamic and exercise outcomes. *Eur Heart J*. 2002;23(20):1617–1624.
21. Ralph-Edwards A, Woo A, McCrindle BW, et al. Hypertrophic obstructive cardiomyopathy: comparison of outcomes after myectomy or alcohol ablation adjusted by propensity score. *J Thorac Cardiovasc Surg*. 2005;129(2):351–358.
22. Firoozi S, Elliott PM, Sharma S, et al. Septal myotomy-myectomy and transcoronary septal alcohol ablation in hypertrophic obstructive cardiomyopathy: a comparison of clinical, hemodynamic and exercise outcomes. *Eur Heart J*. 2002;23(20):1617–1624.
23. Qin JX, Shiota T, Lever HM, et al. Outcome of patients with hypertrophic obstructive cardiomyopathy after percutaneous transluminal septal myocardial ablation and septal myectomy surgery. *J Am Coll Cardiol*. 2001;38(7):1994–2000.
24. Van der Lee C, ten Cate FJ, Geleijnse ML, et al. Percutaneous versus surgical treatment for patients with hypertrophic obstructive cardiomyopathy and enlarged anterior mitral valve leaflets. *Circulation*. 2005;112(4):482–488.
25. Ralph-Edwards A, Woo A, McCrindle BW, et al. Hypertrophic obstructive cardiomyopathy: comparison of outcomes after myectomy or alcohol ablation adjusted by propensity score. *J Thor Cardiovasc Surg*. 2005;129(2):351–358.
26. Nagueh S, Ommen SR, Lakkis NM, et al. Comparison of ethanol septal reduction therapy with surgical myectomy for the treatment of hypertrophic obstructive cardiomyopathy. *J Am Coll Cardiol*. 2001;38(6):1701–1706.
27. Faber L, Welge D, Fassbender D, et al. One-year follow-up of percutaenous septal ablation for symptomatic hypertrophic obstructive cardiomyopathy in 312 patients: predictors of hemodynamic and clinical response. *Clin Res Cardiol*. 2007;96(12):864–873.
28. Fernandes VL, Nielsen C, Nagueh SF, et al. Follow-up of alcohol septal ablation for symptomatic hypertrophic obstructive cardiomyopathy: the Baylor and Medical University of South Carolina experience 1996 to 2007. *J Am Coll Cardiol Intv*. 2008;1(5):561–570.

29. Jensen MK, Almaas VM, Jaobsson L, et al. Long-term outcome of percutaneous transluminal septal myocardial ablation in hypertrophic obstructive cardiomyopathy: a Scandinavian multicenter study. *Circ Cardiovasc Interv*. 2011;4(3):256–265.

30. ten Cate FJ, Soliman OII, Michels M, et al. Long-term outcome of alcohol septal ablation in patients with obstructive hypertrophic cardiomyopathy: a word of caution. *Circulation*. 2010;3(3):362–369.

31. Schaff HV, Brown ML, Dearani JA, et al. Apical myectomy: a new surgical technique for management of severely symptomatic patients with apical hypertrophic cardiomyopathy. *J Thorac Cardiovasc Surg*. 2010;139(3):634–640.

32. Spirito P, Chiarella F, Carratino L, et al. Clinical course and prognosis of hypertrophic cardiomyopathy in an outpatient population. *N Engl J Med*. 1989;320(12):749–755.

33. Maron BJ, Spirito P, Shen WK, et al. Implantable cardioverter-defibrillators and prevention of sudden cardiac death in hypertrophic cardiomyopathy. *JAMA*. 2007;298(4):405–412.

34. McLeod CJ, Ommen SR, Ackerman MJ, et al.Surgical septal myectomy decreases the risk for appropriate implantable cardioverter defibrillator discharge in obstructive hypertrophic cardiomyopathy. *Eur Heart J*. 2007;28(21):2583–2588.

IV

Heart Failure Associated With Other Systemic Disease

14

Heart Failure in Patients With Chronic Obstructive Pulmonary Disease

SALMAN ALLANA AND WALTER KAO

CASE PRESENTATION

Mr. K is a 70-year-old man, with previously diagnosed severe left ventricular systolic dysfunction due to ischemic cardiomyopathy, who presents with worsening dyspnea on exertion and fatigue over the previous 2 weeks. He denies fever, chills, chest discomfort, palpitations, or syncope, although he notes new lower extremity edema beginning about 1 week ago. He experiences occasional light-headedness, especially with rapid positional change, but this is self-limited. He has an occasional dry cough. He sleeps on two pillows chronically but has taken to using three pillows over the past 3 weeks for "comfort." He denies paroxysmal nocturnal dyspnea (PND).

His past medical history is notable for chronic hypertension and a previous acute anterior myocardial infarction (MI) 8 years ago followed by late percutaneous revascularization. He was implanted with a dual-chamber cardioverter-defibrillator following recovery from his MI. He has had intermittent episodes of atrial fibrillation since then, which are sometimes symptomatic. At the time of his infarction he had been smoking one pack of cigarettes per day since his early 20s. He was advised to quit smoking at that time and has reduced his consumption to 5 to 10 cigarettes/day but has been unable to entirely discontinue this practice. He does not drink alcohol. Pulmonary evaluation following cardiac stabilization included chest radiographic evidence of mild lung hyperinflation and scarring and pulmonary function testing which demonstrated evidence of obstructive lung disease and impaired oxygen diffusion. He does his best to adhere to a low-sodium, low-cholesterol diet.

Current medications include: carvedilol 25 mg BID, enalapril 10 mg BID, spironolactone 25 mg daily, furosemide 20 mg daily, aspirin 325 mg daily, pravastatin 40 mg daily, inhaled salmeterol-fluticasone one puff BID, and inhaled ipratroprium two puffs QID. In addition to the scheduled medications noted, he also uses an albuterol inhaler as needed for dyspnea, typically once every 1 to 2 days (although he has used it more frequently during the last 2 weeks) and home oxygen via nasal prongs at 2 L/minute, also as needed for dyspnea and occasionally to help him sleep.

Examination revealed that he was in mild respiratory distress, although he was able to speak in full sentences. Blood pressure was 122/79, heart rate was 88/minute with occasional extrasystoles, and respiratory rate was 20/minute. He was 5′10″ tall and weighed 185 pounds, which was eight pounds higher than his previous weight 6 months ago. Transcutaneous oxygen saturation was 90% on room air. The sclerae were white and oral mucosa was moist. Tidal volume was decreased bilaterally. There were no wheezes, rhonchi, or rales. Jugular venous pulsations were seen just below the angle of the jaw at 45° inclination. Carotids were decreased in volume without bruits. PMI was not palpable. S1 and S2 were soft, although P2 was relatively prominent. There was a 2/6 moderate pitched holosystolic murmur at the lower left sternal border that became higher pitched at the apex and axilla. The liver edge was palpable 5 cm below the right costal margin and was smooth, firm, slightly tender, and moved with the pulse. There was mild pitting lower extremity edema that was soft and extended to the shins bilaterally. There was no skin discoloration. Pedal pulses were palpable but diminished in amplitude bilaterally. The skin was warm and dry.

A PA and lateral chest x-ray demonstrated moderate cardiomegaly, prominent pulmonary arteries, and evidence of lung hyperinflation but no infiltrates or pleural effusion. A 12-lead electrocardiogram revealed sinus rhythm with occasional ventricular premature beats. Screening laboratory studies demonstrate normal electrolytes, renal function, white blood cell count, and hemoglobin/hematocrit.

CLINICAL EVALUATION

Patients with concomitant chronic obstructive pulmonary disease (COPD) and heart failure represent a growing population in whom diagnosis and treatment is particularly challenging for the cardiologist. This is particularly the case in terms of hemodynamic assessment as symptoms and examination findings in COPD can often mimic or mask those classically seen in a patient with heart failure, particularly when the cardiac condition is longstanding.

Management of a patient with chronic heart failure, particularly in the setting of acute symptomatic deterioration, is often predicated on accurate hemodynamic assessment. This is usually without the benefit of direct invasive measurement, except in the critical care setting. Since the more common scenario is that of left ventricular systolic dysfunction, determination of left ventricular preload (typically left atrial or pulmonary venous pressure) is an important guide to medical management. Absent direct invasive measurement, clinicians typically attempt to determine this quantity using surrogates such as symptoms reflective of impaired pulmonary venous drainage (dyspnea, orthopnea, PND), physical signs (left ventricular filling sounds or rales), or radiographic evidence of pulmonary edema/congestion. Unfortunately, most of these findings can be affected by the presence of concomitant COPD. As is often the case with chronic heart failure, the cardinal symptoms of COPD are typically dyspnea and fatigue, often associated with coughing. In patients with ventilatory impairment, orthopnea and PND can also occur. When the emphysematous component of COPD is prominent, the destruction of lung tissue (and related pulmonary vasculature) may result in increased pulmonary vascular resistance and impairment of right ventricular cardiac output. Other factors that may also increase pulmonary vascular resistance in COPD include endothelial dysfunction, hypoxia mediated pulmonary vasoconstriction, ongoing inflammatory changes, and hyperinflation (1). The resultant increase in right ventricular afterload impairs right ventricular cardiac output, thereby trapping the blood flow on the right side of the heart. This, in turn, decreases the tendency of right ventricular output to overwhelm the pulmonary capillaries and the impaired left ventricle of chronic heart failure patients, thereby preventing the development of many of the common findings seen in isolated left ventricular failure. Due to this dependence of typical left ventricular overload and pulmonary congestion/edema findings on intact right ventricular cardiac output, the more easily detectable clinical findings in patients with COPD and left ventricular systolic dysfunction are frequently related to right ventricular pressure and/or volume overload such as symptoms of systemic edema, elevated jugular venous pressure, a palpable right ventricle, or pulmonary artery and tricuspid regurgitation. This last finding is particularly relevant, since the geometry (and thus function) of the tricuspid valve is dependent on right ventricular size, which can change rapidly based on filling pressure. Changes in tricuspid valve function can, in turn, result in abrupt changes in forward right ventricular output with attendant changes in clinical status.

In the patient discussed above, the central venous pressure as judged on physical examination is increased (elevated jugular venous pulsations and hepatic congestion), which has resulted in probable right ventricular enlargement and tricuspid regurgitation. Right ventricular contractility, however, is probably intact, as the prominent pulmonary valve closure sound (P2) suggests that the right ventricle is still able to generate an elevated pressure head resulting in pulmonary diastolic hypertension, a reassuring finding in this case. Whether this translates to elevated *left* ventricular filling remains uncertain, the patient's known chronic left ventricular systolic dysfunction notwithstanding. As is the case with many patients with chronic left ventricular systolic dysfunction, with or without chronic lung disease, the physical examination and chest radiograph findings may be relatively benign in spite of markedly elevated left ventricular filling pressure. Rales on lung auscultation, as a physical sign, are often relied upon for diagnosis of congestive heart failure (CHF) exacerbation, specifically the presence of (presumed cardiogenic) pulmonary edema. With acute rises in pulmonary capillary pressure, the pulmonary lymphatics cannot rapidly increase the rate of fluid removal; as a result, pulmonary edema occurs at pulmonary capillary pressures as low as 18 mmHg. In contrast, patients with chronic heart failure, in whom the pulmonary capillary wedge pressure is persistently elevated, have increased lymphatic capacity and do not develop pulmonary edema until significantly higher pulmonary capillary pressures are reached. Therefore, it is important to note that patients with heart failure (especially chronic heart failure) may not manifest rales even when they are in a decompensated state. Consequently, the absence of pulmonary congestive findings in this patient does not rule out the need for intensified left ventricular afterload reduction therapy, particularly with well-preserved blood pressure. However, due to the uncertainty that the left-sided filling pressure is elevated, an increase in vasodilator medications should be done with caution since this maneuver may result in systemic hypotension if the left-sided filling pressure is low, a finding masked by the presence of pulmonary vascular disease.

Acute exacerbations of heart failure and COPD both typically present with acute dyspnea. To complicate matters, one condition can also precipitate the other. In most circumstances, history and physical examination should suffice for the diagnosis. In instances when diagnosis is difficult, serum levels of B-type natriuretic peptide (BNP) can be used (2). Additional BNP is released in response to high ventricular filling pressures. Most dyspneic patients with heart failure have values above 400 pg/mL. However, in patients with moderate to severe chronic left ventricular systolic dysfunction or in patients with concomitant kidney disease, a BNP levels may be chronically greater than 400 pg/mL, reducing the utility of BNP measurement for assessing the contribution of hemodynamic decompensation in acute changes in dyspnea. Nevertheless, a BNP value less than 100 pg/mL has a high negative predictive value for ruling out heart failure, that is, cardiogenic pulmonary congestion, as the cause of dyspnea (3).

Due to the frequent uncertainty in the clinical assessment of left ventricular hemodynamics in patients with chronic lung disease, direct measurement of central hemodynamics with right-heart catheterization is often necessary to accurately and precisely guide management. The use of balloon-tipped pulmonary artery catheters has been controversial in the critical care and cardiology literature, and insertion of these devices should not be undertaken lightly (4). However, in selected cases where precise and accurate assessment of left ventricular filling and cardiac output will guide management, this tool can be an extremely important adjunct to standard assessment methods. In experienced hands, the risk and discomfort of pulmonary artery catheterization to the patient is low. Once hemodynamic measures are obtained and medical intervention is initiated, the duration of invasive monitoring can often be brief, sometimes minutes to hours rather than days, thereby minimizing the risks for infection, bleeding, and vascular injury. Unfortunately, because of the controversies surrounding risk-benefit, the use of pulmonary artery catheters has decreased in the current era. This has led to fewer opportunities for trainees to acquire the requisite technical skills for safe deployment of these devices and facility in hemodynamic assessment. However, most invasive cardiology programs and critical care/anesthesia services are still able to provide this service when requested.

Of note, COPD can result in chronic pulmonary hypertension by increasing pulmonary vascular resistance via multiple mechanisms including hypoxic vasoconstriction of pulmonary arterioles, inflammation, endothelial dysfunction, and pulmonary vascular remodeling (1). Evaluation of the etiology of pulmonary hypertension with right-heart catheterization in COPD patients with heart failure may be necessary. This should be undertaken with great care since obtaining accurate and helpful measurements is more challenging in these patients who are likely to have large caliber pulmonary arteries. This may render thermodilution cardiac output measurement inaccurate since the proximal port of the pulmonary artery catheter may be advanced into the right ventricle or even into the proximal pulmonary artery during attempts to obtain an accurate pulmonary artery occlusive or wedge pressure. Also, central venous cannulation via internal jugular or subclavian approach may be more challenging due to hyperinflation of the lungs, which would render the patients at higher risk for pneumothorax.

THERAPY

The standard principals governing care of the patient with heart failure remain operative for patients who have chronic lung disease. However, the maintenance medical therapy of patients with systolic heart failure is predominantly neurohormonally based, with cornerstones of beta-blockers and anti–renin-angiotensin-aldosterone agents. This is in contrast to the hospital management of heart failure patients with acute decompensation that involves hemodynamically based therapies while also continuing and/or optimizing maintenance therapies. Each approach presents different challenges when applied to patients with COPD.

MAINTENANCE THERAPY

In the case of patients with left ventricular systolic dysfunction, interventions that improve cardiac function typically result in decreased left ventricular filling pressure and therefore reduced pulmonary congestion, thereby optimizing ventilation, and oxygenation function, particularly important in patients with COPD. Most heart failure therapies in current use have been extensively studied in large-scale clinical trials. Unfortunately, patients with COPD have typically been excluded from or constitute a very small percentage of the study populations. However, it is reasonable to suggest that most of these agents still exert their beneficial effects on heart failure outcome in the presence of lung disease. Angiotensin converting enzyme (ACE) inhibitors and angiotensin receptor blockers (ARBs) typically result in rapid cardiac unloading and hemodynamic benefit, although these effects can become attenuated over time (5,6). Direct vasodilating agents such as hydralazine and nitrates can exhibit even more potent beneficial hemodynamic effects, although they confer a lesser, but still significant, mortality advantage (7). Digoxin and diuretics, previously the cornerstone of chronic heart failure therapy, play a less prominent role in the current era, but still provide symptomatic, hemodynamic, and morbidity benefits (8). Their hemodynamic effects of preload reduction (and modest inotropy in the case of digoxin) are also likely to benefit pulmonary function, as they would also serve to decrease the tendency to pulmonary congestion. Antialdosterone agents such as spironolactone and eplerenone demonstrate substantial mortality benefits in patients with chronic heart failure and ischemic cardiomyopathy respectively but are generally associated with little hemodynamic change (9,10).

BETA-BLOCKADE

Beta-blockers, in particular bisoprolol, metoprolol succinate, and carvedilol, are known to be beneficial in patients with chronic heart failure with well-documented salutary effects on cardiac function, symptoms, and mortality (11–13). These agents have traditionally been avoided in patients with COPD, particularly those with a prominent component of reactive airways disease, due to a concern that unopposed α-1 sympathetic stimulation could exacerbate airway compromise. Indeed, in almost all of the larger scale placebo controlled clinical trials examining the effect of beta-blockers in heart failure, the diagnosis of COPD/asthma was sufficient to exclude the subject from enrollment. Only the MERIT-HF trial included a small (5.3% of the study population) number of patients with the diagnosis of COPD, and the effects of the study drug (metoprolol succinate) on this subgroup are not known. However, the study as a whole demonstrated marked mortality benefit associated with the β-1 selective metoprolol succinate without any difference in pulmonary complications between the treatment and control populations. Patients with COPD enrolled in other heart failure clinical trials who were taking beta-blockers as incidental background therapy have also done well (6). An element of selection bias may have prevented enrollment of more clinically advanced COPD patients in these trials. However, these observations suggest that heart failure patients with COPD, at least to a moderate degree, should not be denied the benefits of beta-blocker therapy. Whether β-1 selectivity affects the pulmonary tolerance in heart failure patients is also uncertain, although it is important to note that the differing affinities for the β-1 compared to the β-2 receptors that comprise "cardioselectivity" are relative and not absolute. Thus, a heart failure beneficial dose of even a cardioselective beta-blocker, for example, metoprolol succinate 200 mg/day, will likely possess a robust degree of β-2 antagonism, thereby blurring the lines somewhat between "cardioselective" and "noncardioselective" beta-blockers.

PULMONARY THERAPY

With respect to the use of long-acting β-agonist for chronic management of COPD, oral β-agonists have consistently been shown to increase incidence of heart failure (14–17). Inhaled β-agonists are preferred. A pooled analysis of seven randomized controlled trials demonstrated no increased cardiovascular adverse events with inhaled salmeterol over a median duration of 24 weeks (18). Another case-control study observed no significant relationship with inhaled β-agonist with development of ischemic cardiomyopathy (19). The Ambulatory Care Quality Improvement (ACQUIP) study demonstrated increased 1-year adjusted heart failure hospitalizations in patients with COPD and asthma who were prescribed inhaled β-agonist (20). Long-term randomized controlled data of inhaled β-agonist in heart failure population are lacking. Therefore, whether inhaled β-agonists are implicated in the development of heart failure remains uncertain. By contrast, long-acting anticholinergic bronchodilator, tiotropium, has proved effective in COPD and asthma management with reassuring cardiovascular safety data (21,22). These should, therefore, be considered over long-acting β-agonists in patients with COPD with concomitant heart failure.

THERAPY FOR ACUTE EXACERBATIONS

Treatment of acute decompensated heart failure, whether systolic or diastolic, is hemodynamically oriented, typically involving optimization of cardiac filling pressures and cardiac output as well as management of the end-organ manifestations of hemodynamic embarrassment. It is treated the same way in patients with COPD as it is in patients without it, typically employing parenteral diuretics to optimize intravascular volume and oral or parenteral vasodilators (and inotropic agents in more extreme instances) to achieve optimal (un)loading conditions. If a coexistent COPD exacerbation is present or there is evidence of reactive airway disease, it is important to assess the roles of β-2 agonists and corticosteroids that form the cornerstone of the management of the disorder. Acute steroid use may exacerbate intravascular volume by cross reactivity with mineralocorticoid receptors. Therefore, it is extremely important to closely monitor volume status in patients with heart failure who are receiving systemic steroids. β-2–agonists mediate their therapeutic effects in COPD via bronchodilation. However, they also exert numerous unfavorable cardiovascular effects, including tachycardia, hypokalemia, QTc prolongation, and disturbed autonomic modulation and may also precipitate myocardial ischemia and arrhythmias. Inhaled β-agonists have never been prospectively studied in patients with decompensated heart failure. They have short-term favorable hemodynamic effects including enhanced cardiac output and reduced peripheral vascular resistance (23). However, acute improvement may belie myocardial injury leading to increased mortality. Nebulized dosing preparations provide markedly greater exposure than standard inhalers. As the systemic effects of the β-agonists are dose related, these agents must be used with caution in acute situations. Also, it is important to not discontinue or dramatically decrease the beta-blocker dose in acute COPD exacerbation as this will result in abrupt myocardial catecholamine exposure with attendant risks of myocardial ischemia and arrhythmias.

In more severe exacerbations of COPD, temporary mechanical ventilatory support may be required. This intervention may carry profound hemodynamic consequences in individuals with underlying cardiac dysfunction, particularly those with right ventricular dysfunction. The right ventricle, more than the left ventricle, is especially sensitive to acute changes in loading conditions and the increased right ventricular afterload associated with an abrupt transition from negative to positive pressure ventilation may markedly impair right ventricular cardiac output. This may lead, in turn, to decreased left ventricular filling. In scenarios of excessive left ventricular preload, typically associated with cardiogenic pulmonary edema, mechanical ventilator support is extremely beneficial, increasing oxygenation while decreasing left atrial and left ventricular distending pressure. However, in patients with biventricular dysfunction, the deleterious effect of increased right ventricular afterload can effectively trap blood in the right side of the heart, leading to worsening systemic congestion with resultant end-organ dysfunction. Consequently, careful hemodynamic assessment must be undertaken when deciding whether to employ mechanical ventilator support in COPD patients with concomitant cardiac dysfunction, especially right ventricular systolic dysfunction.

SUMMARY

Patients with concomitant lung disease and heart failure constitute a particular challenge for cardiologists. The importance of considering the lung as a circulatory organ cannot be overstated, and care must be taken in the diagnostic phase of care to carefully discriminate between symptoms and signs that are caused by primary pulmonary disease rather than cardiac/hemodynamic decompensation. Even careful physical examination may be inconclusive and more advanced measures such as invasive hemodynamic monitoring may be required to accurately guide therapy.

Once cardiac decompensation is confirmed, standard therapeutic measures should be employed. In the event of coexisting pulmonary decompensation, special caution should be exercised when treating patients with underlying heart failure as interventions with pulmonary benefits may have untoward cardiac effects.

REFERENCES

1. Wrobel JP, Thompson BR, Williams TJ. Mechanisms of pulmonary hypertension in chronic obstructive pulmonary disease: a pathophysiologic review. *J Heart Lung Transplant*. 2012;31(6):557–564.
2. Mueller C, Scholer A, Laule-Kilian K, et al. Use of B-type natriuretic peptide in the evaluation and management of acute dyspnea. *N Engl J Med*. 2004;350(7):647–654.
3. Maisel AS, Krishnaswamy P, Nowak RM, et al.; Breathing Not Properly Multinational Study Investigators. Rapid measurement of B-type natriuretic peptide in the emergency diagnosis of heart failure. *N Engl J Med*. 2002;347(3):161–167.
4. Binanay C, Califf RM, Hasselblad V, et al.; ESCAPE Investigators and ESCAPE Study Coordinators. Evaluation study of congestive heart failure and pulmonary artery catheterization effectiveness: the ESCAPE trial. *JAMA*. 2005;294(13):1625–1633.

5. Cohn JN, Johnson G, Ziesche S, et al. A comparison of enalapril with hydralazine-isosorbide dinitrate in the treatment of chronic congestive heart failure. *N Engl J Med*. 1991;325(5):303–310.

6. Cohn JN, Tognoni G; Valsartan Heart Failure Trial Investigators. A randomized trial of the angiotensin-receptor blocker valsartan in chronic heart failure. *N Engl J Med*. 2001;345(23):1667–1675.

7. Cohn JN, Archibald DG, Ziesche S, et al. Effect of vasodilator therapy on mortality in chronic congestive heart failure. Results of a Veterans Administration Cooperative Study. *N Engl J Med*. 1986;314(24):1547–1552.

8. The DIG Investigation Group. The effect of digoxin on mortality and morbidity in patients with heart failure. *N Eng J Med*. 1997;336:525–533.

9. Pitt B, Zannad F, Remme WJ, et al. The effect of spironolactone on morbidity and mortality in patients with severe heart failure. Randomized Aldactone Evaluation Study Investigators. *N Engl J Med*. 1999;341(10):709–717.

10. Pitt B, Remme W, Zannad F, et al.; Eplerenone Post-Acute Myocardial Infarction Heart Failure Efficacy and Survival Study Investigators. Eplerenone, a selective aldosterone blocker, in patients with left ventricular dysfunction after myocardial infarction. *N Engl J Med*. 2003;348(14):1309–1321.

11. Packer M, Bristow MR, Cohn JN, et al. The effect of carvedilol on morbidity and mortality in patients with chronic heart failure. U.S. Carvedilol Heart Failure Study Group. *N Engl J Med*. 1996;334(21):1349–1355.

12. MERIT-HF Study Group. Effect of metoprolol CR/XL in chronic heart failure: Metoprolol CR/XL Randomised Intervention Trial in Congestive Heart Failure (MERIT-HF). *Lancet*. 1999;353:2001–2007.

13. CIBIS-II Investigators and Committees. The Cardiac Insufficiency Bisoprolol Study II (CIBIS-II): a randomised trial. *Lancet*. 1999;353:9–13.

14. Mettauer B, Rouleau JL, Burgess JH. Detrimental arrhythmogenic and sustained beneficial hemodynamic effects of oral salbutamol in patients with chronic congestive heart failure. *Am Heart J*. 1985;109(4):840–847.

15. Martin RM, Dunn NR, Freemantle SN, Mann RD. Risk of non-fatal cardiac failure and ischaemic heart disease with long acting beta 2 agonists. *Thorax*. 1998;53(7):558–562.

16. Coughlin SS, Metayer C, McCarthy EP, et al. Respiratory illness, beta-agonists, and risk of idiopathic dilated cardiomyopathy. The Washington, DC, Dilated Cardiomyopathy Study. *Am J Epidemiol*. 1995;142(4):395–403.

17. The Xamoterol in Severe Heart Failure Study Group. Xamoterol in severe heart failure. *Lancet*. 1990;336:1–6.

18. Ferguson GT, Funck-Brentano C, Fischer T, Darken P, Reisner C. Cardiovascular safety of salmeterol in COPD. *Chest*. 2003;123(6):1817–1824.

19. Sengstock DM, Obeidat O, Pasnoori V, Mehra P, Sandberg KR, McCullough PA. Asthma, beta-agonists, and development of congestive heart failure: results of the ABCHF study. *J Card Fail*. 2002;8(4):232–238.

20. Au DH, Udris EM, Curtis JR, McDonell MB, Fihn SD; ACQUIP Investigators. Association between chronic heart failure and inhaled beta-2-adrenoceptor agonists. *Am Heart J*. 2004;148(5):915–920.

21. Michele TM, Pinheiro S, Iyasu S. The safety of tiotropium–the FDA's conclusions. *N Engl J Med*. 2010;363(12):1097–1099.

22. Vogelmeier C, Hederer B, Glaab T, et al.; POET-COPD Investigators. Tiotropium versus salmeterol for the prevention of exacerbations of COPD. *N Engl J Med*. 2011;364(12):1093–1103.

23. Maak CA, Tabas JA, McClintock DE. Should acute treatment with inhaled beta agonists be withheld from patients with dyspnea who may have heart failure? *J Emerg Med*. 2011;40(2):135–145.

15

Cardiotoxicity of Anticancer Treatment

STEVEN M. EWER AND KARI B. WISINSKI

INTRODUCTION

Cancer and cardiovascular disease are increasing among an overlapping demographic that shares risk factors such as advanced age and tobacco use. When present together, treatment of one disease often complicates management of the other. Traditional chemotherapy necessarily carries a narrow therapeutic window, and off-target effects are frequently encountered, including potentially serious cardiotoxicity. Several chemotherapeutic agents have been well documented to cause left ventricular dysfunction and heart failure, which can limit cancer treatment and lead to additional morbidity and mortality. This is especially important when chemotherapy is used with curative intent or in the adjuvant setting, where many patients can expect a long survival after their cancer diagnoses. Anthracycline cardiomyopathy is the prototypical example, and a large part of this chapter will be devoted to this topic. Other agents that cause cardiomyopathy can have substantially different clinical features, which are just beginning to be understood, and these will be discussed as well. Lastly, a broad range of other cardiovascular effects that can be seen in the course of cancer treatment will be briefly discussed, including those related to newer targeted agents, radiation therapy, and the underlying malignancy itself.

CASE PRESENTATION: PART 1

A 45-year-old premenopausal woman with a history of hypertension and mild obesity (body mass index [BMI] 32 kg/m^2) is found to have a palpable mass in the left breast during a routine physical exam. A mobile, enlarged axillary lymph node is also appreciated. Diagnostic mammography and ultrasound reveal findings suspicious for carcinoma. Biopsy demonstrates Grade 2 infiltrating ductal carcinoma in the breast and lymph node, which is positive for the expression of estrogen receptor, progesterone receptor, and human epidermal growth factor receptor-2 (HER2). Evaluation for distant metastatic disease is unremarkable. She undergoes left mastectomy with axillary lymph node dissection. Four of 15 lymph nodes are positive, and her oncologist recommends four cycles of adjuvant chemotherapy with doxorubicin and cyclophosphamide, followed by four cycles of paclitaxel with trastuzumab and then completion of 1-year total of trastuzumab. Planned total doxorubicin dose is 240 mg/m^2. Postmastectomy radiation therapy to the left chest wall and draining lymphatics as well as 5 years of adjuvant endocrine therapy with tamoxifen are also recommended. Cardiovascular evaluation prior to chemotherapy reveals a blood pressure of 150/94 mmHg, heart rate 72 beats/minute, normal cardiac auscultation, and no evidence for volume overload. Echocardiogram reveals an ejection fraction of 60%, borderline left ventricular hypertrophy, and mild diastolic dysfunction. She is on amlodipine and hydrochlorothiazide for her hypertension.

ANTHRACYCLINE CARDIOMYOPATHY

Anthracycline cardiomyopathy is one of the most important and best-studied cancer treatment-related cardiac effects. The case presentation brings up many considerations for the clinician, including the unique clinical features of anthracycline cardiomyopathy, risk factors, cardiac monitoring, prevention, and treatment. Anthracyclines are a widely used class of chemotherapeutic agents including doxorubicin, idarubicin, daunorubicin, and epirubicin, which are currently used in the treatment of breast cancer, leukemia, lymphoma, and sarcomas among other malignancies. The structurally related agent mitoxantrone, an anthracenedione, can be considered along with anthracyclines for discussions of cardiotoxicity. The oncologic mechanism involves intercalation into DNA, inhibition of topoisomerase II, and disruption of DNA and RNA synthesis (1).

Therapeutic use of anthracyclines has been limited by a dose-dependent cardiomyopathy that is generally irreversible and can lead to profound heart failure and death or need for heart transplantation. The predominant mechanism of cardiotoxicity is distinct from that of oncologic efficacy, and involves iron-dependent generation of reactive oxygen species and cell membrane disruption, leading to myocyte death (2). Other mechanisms have also been proposed. Electron microscopy of endomyocardial biopsy specimens from patients with anthracycline cardiomyopathy demonstrates the presence of vacuole formation, myofibrillar disarray, and frank necrosis (3). Compared with other organs, the heart is particularly susceptible to oxidative damage due to relative lack of free radical scavengers and minimal regenerative capability.

The risk of clinical heart failure has been found to increase exponentially with cumulative anthracycline dose, which is one of the key features of this toxicity (**Figure 15-1**; 4). A cumulative doxorubicin dose of 450 mg/m^2, roughly associated with a 5% risk of heart failure, has been a traditionally accepted lifetime limit, although this can certainly be adjusted according to individual patient features such as underlying risk for cardiomyopathy, risk of death from the malignancy, alternative therapeutic options for the malignancy, and potential for cure with anthracycline-based treatment. For our patient, a cumulative dose of 240 mg/m^2 would typically be associated with negligible cardiac risk (approximately 1% risk of heart failure) unless additional risk factors were present (4). In addition to prior anthracycline exposure, risk factors for anthracycline-related cardiomyopathy include older age, hypertension, coronary artery disease (CAD), cardiac radiation exposure, and pre-existing structural heart disease (**Table 15-1**; 5). Pre-existing cardiomyopathy would represent a strong contraindication to treatment with anthracyclines, even if compensated. Hypertension alone carries a hazard ratio of 1.6 for the development of anthracycline cardiomyopathy, so our patient's risk is still reasonably low.

Other anthracyclines behave similarly to doxorubicin with respect to cardiotoxicity, but with different cumulative dose limits. There is some data to suggest that epirubicin is less cardiotoxic than doxorubicin for an equivalent level of myelosuppression; a meta-analysis of this topic found a strong trend in this direction, but it did not reach statistical

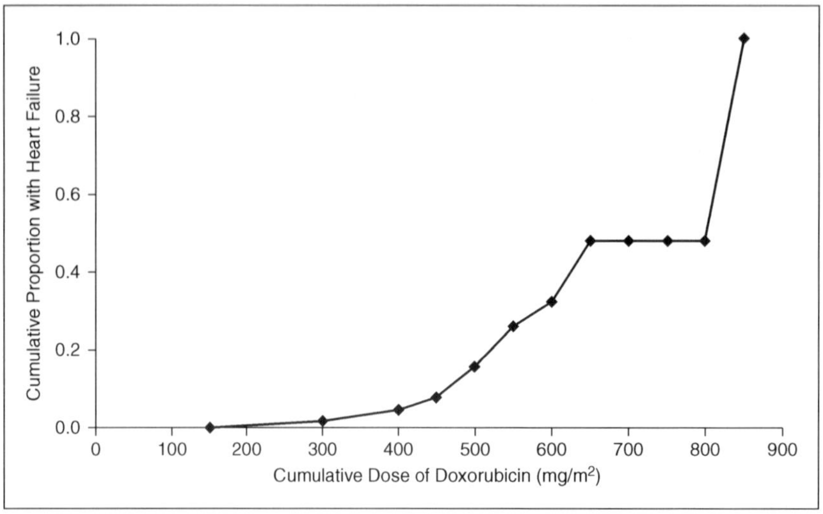

Figure 15-1
Cumulative doxorubicin dose at onset of doxorubicin-related heart failure (4).

Table 15-1
Risk Factors for Anthracycline Cardiomyopathy

RISK FACTOR	HAZARD RATIO	REFERENCE
Prior anthracycline use (cumulative dose)	NA	Von Hoff et al (51)
Age > 65 years	2.25	Swain et al (4)
Hypertension	1.58	Hershman et al (5)
Coronary artery disease	2.21	Hershman et al (5)
Other heart disease	1.53	Hershman et al (5)
Cardiac irradiation	NA	Steinherz et al (52)

Note: NA = not available.

Source: Adapted from reference (10).

significance (6). Liposomal formulations of doxorubicin can significantly reduce cardiotoxicity by altering the pharmacokinetics (reducing peak plasma concentration) and favoring delivery to tissues with immature vasculature (7). However, these agents are not considered interchangeable due to potential differences in spectrum of activity and oncologic efficacy.

Some clinical features of anthracycline cardiotoxicity may be present at the time of administration, including chest discomfort, dyspnea, arrhythmias, and troponin elevation. These findings are likely to represent acute anthracycline injury of the myocardium, although left ventricular function remains preserved at this stage. Emerging data suggests that early troponin elevation in particular has been found to predict future left ventricular dysfunction (8), but is not yet recommended as a standard evaluation. Although not practical for routine screening, endomyocardial biopsy changes generally precede the onset of left ventricular dysfunction, which is detectable by echocardiogram or radionuclide angiography (MUGA scan) at a median onset of 4 months after the completion of anthracycline therapy (9). Classic symptoms and physical exam findings of decompensated heart failure are late findings.

Given the risk for cardiotoxicity, monitoring schedules have been utilized to assess for left ventricular dysfunction during anthracycline administration, particularly when higher cumulative doses are anticipated. Continued exposure to additional cycles of anthracycline after the development of left ventricular dysfunction can result in significant morbidity and mortality, and monitoring serves to minimize this occurrence. Also, earlier diagnosis and rapid initiation of treatment is desirable. Formal monitoring guidelines have not yet been adopted, but many reasonable monitoring strategies have been proposed (10). Left ventricular ejection fraction (LVEF) is measured either by echocardiography or by MUGA scan at baseline. Additional imaging may be appropriate during and after anthracycline therapy depending on individual risk factors and the total anticipated cumulative dose. The two imaging modalities are not completely interchangeable, and for an individual patient a consistent imaging technique should generally be employed. The decision to use echocardiography or MUGA scan is based on cost, local practice patterns, relative strengths of the individual imaging laboratories, and desire to avoid the ionizing radiation associated with MUGA scans.

In the absence of risk factors, LVEF is usually measured at baseline and at a cumulative doxorubicin dose (or equivalent) of 300 mg/m^2 if additional anthracycline is to be given. Thereafter, LVEF is measured more frequently (every 1–2 cycles). One definition of significant LVEF decline is an absolute decrease of 15% or greater, or a decrease of 10% that results in values below the lower limit of normal. It is important to remember that LVEF is an imperfect measure of cardiotoxicity, which can be influenced by variations inherent in the imaging modality, volume status, anemia, levels of circulating catecholamines, afterload, and so on. Care must be taken not to overinterpret small changes in LVEF, as this can lead to unnecessary withdrawal of needed therapy.

Cardiac biomarkers, particularly troponin and B-type natriuretic peptide (BNP), have been investigated in the risk-stratification and monitoring of anthracycline-related cardiotoxicity. Wide availability, low risk, and low cost make biomarkers an attractive supplement to cardiac imaging. In one study, elevation of troponin-I within 72 hours of anthracycline administration and at 1 month was found to predict later LVEF decline and a composite of cardiac endpoints (8). Although BNP levels generally correlate with left ventricular systolic and diastolic function and clinical heart failure, significant interindividual variability makes it difficult to establish clinically useful cutoff values. Further study is required before use of biomarkers is recommended routinely in this setting.

Several strategies can be employed to minimize anthracycline cardiotoxicity. Hemodynamic parameters such as systemic blood pressure, volume status, and, in the setting of atrial arrhythmia, heart rate should be optimized prior to exposure, as increased left ventricular wall stress is likely to exacerbate the cytotoxic injury. Given the cumulative dose relationship demonstrated in **Figure 15-1**, limiting the cumulative anthracycline exposure is one of the most straightforward ways of minimizing risk. Occasionally, a less toxic anthracycline (potentially epirubicin) or a liposomal formulation may be appropriate. Prolonged infusion (up to 72 hours) has been shown to be significantly cardioprotective compared with rapid infusion due to reduced peak plasma concentrations (11). Although infrequently utilized for reasons of cost, convenience, and anticancer efficacy, this can be considered for higher risk individuals when the anthracycline is a necessary component of disease management.

Dexrazoxane, an iron chelator, has been shown to significantly reduce the risk of anthracycline cardiotoxicity, but concerns regarding effects on oncologic efficacy have limited its widespread use (12,13). Current Food and Drug Administration (FDA) indications allow use in metastatic breast cancer patients who have already received 300 mg/m^2 of doxorubicin. Lastly, early data suggest beneficial effects of enalapril (14) and carvedilol (15) use throughout anthracycline administration in preventing left ventricular dysfunction in patients with normal baseline left ventricular function. Confirmation in Phase III studies is required prior to widespread dissemination of this approach.

Treatment of anthracycline-related cardiomyopathy is similar to that of any other cause (16). Although not specifically validated in this population, accumulated evidence supports a final common pathway in the pathophysiology of systolic heart failure. Although one study suggests that treatment within the first 6 months following the completion of anthracycline treatment can reverse some of the left ventricular dysfunction (9), myocardial damage is generally considered permanent, and the data regarding this optimal time frame for treatment are limited. Treatment goals are aimed at preventing progressive left ventricular remodeling and alleviating symptoms of heart failure. Further anthracycline exposure is contraindicated once significant left ventricular dysfunction is encountered.

For our patient, her only risk factor for anthracycline cardiomyopathy is hypertension. Since her planned cumulative doxorubicin dose is 240 mg/m^2, we would still anticipate a very low risk of clinical heart failure. Her baseline LVEF is normal at 60%. It would be appropriate to repeat her imaging at the completion of her four cycles of doxorubicin and cyclophosphamide, since treatment with trastuzumab is also planned. It will be important to control her hypertension prior to and throughout anthracycline treatment. There is some rationale for preferential use angiotensin converting enzyme (ACE) inhibitors and/or carvedilol over amlodipine and hydrochlorothiazide, due to possible protective effects on left ventricular systolic function.

CASE PRESENTATION: PART 2

After four cycles of doxorubicin and cyclophosphamide, the patient describes nonspecific fatigue, but denies symptoms of heart failure. Ejection fraction is measured again by echocardiography prior to initiation of trastuzumab and is found to be low-normal at 55%. After 3 months of treatment with paclitaxel and trastuzumab, she begins to notice exertional dyspnea. Her blood pressure is 142/88 mmHg and heart rate 96 beats/minute. Echocardiogram is repeated with findings of mild left ventricular enlargement, severe systolic dysfunction, LVEF 30%, and moderate diastolic dysfunction. Trastuzumab is held, and her amlodipine and hydrochlorothiazide are discontinued in favor of carvedilol and lisinopril. One month later, she is asymptomatic with ejection fraction improved to 50%. She is now undergoing left chest wall radiation. Trastuzumab is resumed, and is tolerated for the remainder of planned therapy with no further decline in left ventricular systolic function by echocardiography. Additionally, she is started on adjuvant tamoxifen with a planned 5-year course.

In addition to anthracyclines and mitoxantrone, other antineoplastic agents have been found to be associated with left ventricular dysfunction and heart failure, including traditional chemotherapy agents (eg, cyclophosphamide), and targeted agents (eg, trastuzumab, sunitinib, imatinib, and lapatinib). In general, these agents differ from anthracyclines in their mechanism of cardiotoxicity and their associated clinical features. Trastuzumab will be highlighted here as one of the better studied drugs with distinct characteristics.

Trastuzumab is a monoclonal antibody directed against the HER2, and is highly effective in the treatment of breast cancers that overexpress this receptor. Approximately 20% of breast cancers are classified as HER2 positive. Adjuvant trastuzumab therapy has demonstrated nearly a 35% reduction in mortality in this group (17,18). HER2 is also expressed in the heart, and preclinical studies suggested that perturbation of downstream pathways that are important for cardiomyocyte survival and adaptation to stress could result in trastuzumab cardiotoxicity (19,20). Indeed, an early study of patients with metastatic breast cancer found very high incidence of heart failure when trastuzumab and anthracyclines were used concurrently (21). This led to careful characterization of trastuzumab-related cardiac effects in several subsequent large trials.

Among the findings that emerged from the adjuvant trastuzumab trials in women with nonmetastatic breast cancer was that although left ventricular dysfunction was a relatively frequent occurrence, patients fared far better compared to those with anthracycline cardiomyopathy. The incidence of trastuzumab-related New York Heart Association (NYHA) Class III or IV heart failure is estimated at 2.5%, and LVEF decline more than 10% is estimated at 11% (22). Despite left ventricular dysfunction being a relatively frequent occurrence, no significant increase in risk of cardiac mortality or progression to end-stage heart failure was observed. Cardiac function often improved or even normalized after withdrawal of trastuzumab and appropriate medical treatment of left ventricular dysfunction. Patients with trastuzumab-related left ventricular dysfunction sometimes tolerate long-term administration of trastuzumab after recovery from their initial insult. Unlike anthracycline cardiotoxicity, there did not appear to be a cumulative dose phenomenon. Myocardial biopsy specimens from patients with trastuzumab-related left ventricular dysfunction showed a benign appearance (23). These observations led to the concept of distinguishing Type I (anthracycline-like) from Type II (trastuzumab-like) chemotherapy-related cardiac dysfunction (**Table 15-2**; 24).

One of the difficulties in studying trastuzumab-related heart disease is that quite often HER2 and breast cancer patients are also first treated with an anthracycline, similar to the case presented. As clinically apparent anthracycline toxicity can often be delayed by months, it can be difficult to tease apart the offending agent. Furthermore, there is a likely synergistic effect between anthracyclines and trastuzumab, explained perhaps by trastuzumab's interference in the heart's adaptive response to anthracycline injury. The incidence of heart failure seems to be higher when trastuzumab is given concurrently with or shortly after anthracycline, suggesting that the timing of these two agents is important. Interestingly, when trastuzumab is administered prior to anthracycline or in the absence of anthracycline, the incidence of cardiotoxicity is markedly reduced (25,26).

Risk factors for the development of trastuzumab-related left ventricular dysfunction include older age, obesity, antihypertensive therapy, lower pre-trastuzumab LVEF, concurrent anthracycline use (which is contraindicated with doxorubicin, but may be safe with epirubicin), and cumulative anthracycline dose (27–29). Evidence-based guidelines for cardiac monitoring while on trastuzumab have not been developed, but in the adjuvant trials, assessment of LVEF was generally performed at baseline and every 3 months during trastuzumab treatment. For more prolonged administration (ie, in the metastatic breast cancer setting), monitoring is debated and typically is less frequent given the palliative goals of treatment. Symptoms of heart failure should warrant thorough evaluation at the time of presentation. Decisions regarding when to withhold trastuzumab

Table 15-2
Type I versus Type II Chemotherapy-Related Cardiac Dysfunction

TYPE OF DRUG	PROTOTYPE	FINDINGS ON ENDOMYOCARDIAL BIOPSY (ELECTRON MICROSCOPY)	CUMULATIVE DOSE RELATIONSHIP	REVERSIBILITY	ASSOCIATED WITH INCREASED CARDIOVASCULAR MORTALITY
Type I	Doxorubicin	Vacuoles Sarcomere disruption Necrosis	Yes	No (might respond to very early treatment)	Yes
Type II	Trastuzumab	Benign ultrastructural appearance	No	Yes, in most cases	No

Source: Adapted from reference (10).

therapy are based on an individualized assessment of risks and benefits.

Other agents with features compatible with Type II cardiac dysfunction are sunitinib and lapatinib. Sunitinib, a multityrosine kinase inhibitor used in renal cell carcinoma and gastrointestinal stromal tumors, was associated with an 8% risk of heart failure and a 28% risk of LVEF decrease greater than 10% in one study (30). Substantial reversibility was documented, and there was no cumulative dose relationship. Lapatinib, a tyrosine kinase inhibitor with a high specificity for HER2 and the epidermal growth factor receptor (EGFR), has been associated with infrequent left ventricular dysfunction and heart failure, which likewise demonstrated reversibility and lack of cumulative dose relationship (31). Cyclophosphamide can cause a unique hemorrhagic myocardial necrosis, particularly at higher doses (32). As permanent injury can result, cyclophosphamide is best categorized as a Type I agent.

Our patient experienced a mild decrease in LVEF after doxorubicin exposure, which we expect represents real and permanent damage. Her significant further decline after starting trastuzumab was associated with symptoms compatible with heart failure. Her incompletely treated hypertension was likely a contributing factor. Withholding trastuzumab, starting appropriate treatment for left ventricular dysfunction, and normalizing blood pressure resulted in nearly full recovery of LVEF compared to pretrastuzumab levels. Due to the significant reduction in breast cancer mortality expected from trastuzumab, a cautious rechallenge is appropriate. In the majority of patients, rechallenging is successful.

CASE PRESENTATION: PART 3

Five years after initial diagnosis, after presenting with persistent cough, the patient is found to have metastatic disease to the lungs and liver. Liver biopsy reveals adenocarcinoma positive for estrogen receptor, progesterone receptor and HER2. She is started on a regimen of paclitaxel and trastuzumab, but demonstrates disease progression after 6 months, and is then switched to capecitabine and lapatinib. Two weeks later, she presents to the emergency department with chest pain suggesting unstable angina and anterolateral ST depressions on electrocardiogram (ECG). Coronary angiography reveals nonocclusive CAD. The presumptive diagnosis of coronary vasospasm is made, and long-acting nitrates are prescribed. Cautious rechallenge of capecitabine is tolerated thereafter, with no recurrence of angina. She does well for 1 year, until returning to the emergency department with rapidly progressive dyspnea. She is found to be hypotensive and in atrial fibrillation with rapid ventricular response. Chest CT is negative for pulmonary embolus, but reveals a large pericardial effusion. Echocardiogram reveals hemodynamic features of cardiac tamponade, and a pericardial drain is placed. Cytology is positive for metastatic adenocarcinoma.

In addition to the potential for left ventricular dysfunction and systolic heart failure, cancer treatment and the underlying malignant process can affect the cardiovascular system in a variety of other ways. These will be reviewed briefly here.

CARDIAC ISCHEMIA

As illustrated by our case, 5-fluorouracil and its oral prodrug, capecitabine, can be associated with coronary artery vasospasm. The incidence is approximately 4%, and underlying CAD is an important risk factor (33). Presentation typically includes angina and ST changes on ECG, although frank myocardial infarction and ventricular arrhythmias are possible. Treatment of vasospasm with nitrates and/or calcium channel blockers usually allows continued cancer treatment. By a different mechanism, bevacizumab, a monoclonal antibody to the vascular endothelial growth factor-A (VEGF-A), a key factor in cancer angiogenesis, has been associated with arterial thrombotic events, including in the coronary vasculature in approximately 1% of patients (34). Bevacizumab is commonly used in the treatment of advanced lung, colorectal, and renal cell carcinomas.

Aromatase inhibitors, including anastrozole, letrozole, and exemestane, are alternative endocrine therapies to tamoxifen for postmenopausal patients with hormone receptor-positive breast cancer (such as the patient in our case). These agents have been associated with potential lipid abnormalities and several studies have suggested an approximately 30% relative increase in the risk of composite cardiovascular events (35,36). Although the absolute increase in cardiac risk is small, it is worth considering when choosing endocrine therapy for an individual patient, especially when traditional CAD risk factors are present. In contrast, tamoxifen has been associated with a decreased risk of CAD (37).

HYPERTENSION

Significant hypertension has been seen with the antiangiogenesis agents sunitinib, sorafenib, and bevacizumab. The mechanism of oncologic activity involves inhibition of the VEGF pathway, which results in decreased nitric oxide production in the vascular endothelium and subsequent hypertension. Incidence may be as high as 45%, and can be severe enough to cause hypertensive urgency and intracranial hemorrhage (38). Pre-existing hypertension is a risk factor. Strict control of blood pressure before and during treatment with VEGF pathway inhibitors is required, and interruptions in cancer treatment may be necessary in refractory cases. In the case of drugs such as sunitinib, which can also cause left ventricular dysfunction, there may be rationale for preferential use of ACE inhibitors and beta-blockers to control hypertension, although this has not yet been investigated.

THROMBOEMBOLIC DISEASE

Malignancy already predisposes patients to hypercoagulability, which is heightened in such settings as the postoperative state or in the presence of a chronic indwelling venous catheter. An increased risk of venous thromboembolic disease has been noted with several anticancer agents, including tamoxifen, raloxifene, l-asparaginase, and cisplatin. Although little data exist, mechanism has been hypothesized to include contributions from a decrease in the synthesis of proteins C and S and antithrombin, as well as acquired abnormalities of von Willebrand factor. In several studies, the use of tamoxifen was associated with a two- to threefold increase in thromboembolic events, with a substantially higher incidence when tamoxifen was given concurrently with chemotherapy. For breast cancer patients with a prior history of thromboembolic disease, aromatase inhibitors are often preferred to tamoxifen. Our patient received a 5-year course of adjuvant tamoxifen after chemotherapy, and thus accepted a modest increase in thromboembolic risk.

In the setting of multiple myeloma, thalidomide and lenalidomide are particularly thrombogenic when used in combination with corticosteroids or doxorubicin, with an incidence thromboembolism in the range of 20% to 25%. Due to the very high risk of events in this population, prophylaxis with either aspirin or low-molecular weight heparin, depending of level of risk, has been deemed appropriate (39). In addition, in venous thrombotic events, tamoxifen and raloxifene have been associated with a small increase in stroke (40). As mentioned above, bevacizumab has also been associated with arterial thrombotic events (34).

ARRHYTHMIA

As cancer patients are often on multiple medications, acquired long QT syndrome is an important consideration. Drug-induced prolongation of the QT interval increases the risk for Torsades de pointes, a polymorphic ventricular tachycardia that can cause syncope or sudden death. Timely recognition of this phenomenon can help avoid unnecessary mortality. Specific anticancer drugs that have the potential to prolong the QT interval include arsenic trioxide, vandetanib, eribulin, lapatinib, nilotinib, sunitinib, and tamoxifen (41). Other common offenders include methadone, antiemetics, antibiotics (particularly macrolides and fluoroquinolones), and several antidepressant and antipsychotic agents. Monitoring of the QT interval, corrected for heart rate, should be considered in patients receiving these agents, especially if taking multiple QT-prolonging drugs.

RADIATION HEART DISEASE

Our patient received radiation for the left chest wall as part of her treatment. To what extent was the heart involved, and what are her cardiac risks going forward?

Therapeutic radiation that includes the heart in the treatment field can lead to a spectrum of cardiac manifestations, including pericardial disease, restrictive cardiomyopathy, CAD, valvular heart disease, conduction system disease, and even (rarely) secondary cardiac tumors. Treatment of thoracic malignancies such as lymphoma, lung and esophageal cancer, and left-sided breast cancer can result in cardiac radiation exposure. Risk of radiation heart disease depends on total dose (increased risk begins around 15 Gy), volume of the heart involved, and patient age (younger patients assume higher risk; 42). Administration of cardiotoxic chemotherapy can further increase risk. The mechanism of radiation toxicity involves microvascular destruction, direct cellular injury and ultimately, fibrosis (43).

The epidemiology of radiation heart disease is challenging to study, as clinical manifestations often develop years or decades after exposure. Furthermore, substantial improvements in radiation therapy planning and delivery techniques have been made over the years, making older studies obsolete. Patients with breast cancer and Hodgkin's lymphoma are more likely to be affected given their better chance at long-term survival and younger median age compared to those with lung or esophageal cancer. Breast cancer allows the unique opportunity to compare right- versus left-sided disease, since the cardiac radiation exposure is minimal in right-sided disease. Studies analyzing data from the Surveillance, Epidemiology, and End Results (SEER) database revealed a significant increase in cardiac events for left- versus right-sided breast cancer treated with radiation prior to 1980, but no significant differences in patients treated since then (44,45). Whether this temporal difference is due to improved radiation techniques over time or shorter duration of follow-up is difficult to determine.

Pericardial manifestations of radiation include acute and chronic pericarditis, pericardial effusion, and constriction. Unlike other causes of constriction, radiation-related disease is typically noncalcific (46). Treatment of constriction is challenging, as surgical pericardiectomy in an irradiated field carries a high risk of mortality (46). Myocardial irradiation can lead to diastolic dysfunction, heart failure, and a restrictive cardiomyopathy, which can be difficult to distinguish from pericardial constriction, especially when both are present in the same patient, as is often the case. Valvular heart disease related to radiation usually consists of regurgitant lesions, with aortic regurgitation being the most common (47). Aortic stenosis has also been reported. Pathologically, there is endocardial thickening and fibroelastosis. CAD can be caused by both acceleration of the typical atherosclerotic process and a more radiation-specific endovascular proliferation (48). Traditional coronary risk factors play an important role and deserve special attention in cancer survivors with a history of cardiac radiation exposure. Due to its location, the left anterior descending artery is more often involved (49).

METASTATIC DISEASE AND THE HEART

At the later stages of the case presentation, our patient developed additional cardiac problems (arrhythmia and symptomatic pericardial effusion) not as a result of her treatment, but rather from progression of her malignancy. Cardiac metastases can be endocardial or myocardial, but pericardial locations are the most frequently encountered (50). Routes of invasion include direct extension (more common in lung and esophageal cancers), retrograde lymphatic spread (breast and lung cancers), and hematologic seeding (leukemia, lymphoma, and melanoma). The entire spectrum of pericardial syndromes can be seen with malignant pericardial disease. In addition, pericardial effusions can arise from obstruction of lymphatic vessels that drain the heart. Cardiac metastases can be associated with atrial arrhythmias, ventricular arrhythmias, or conduction system disease, depending on location of the tumors. Local inflammation from primary tumors adjacent to the heart such as lung and esophageal cancer can also often lead to atrial arrhythmias. It is important to keep these complications from cancer itself in the differential diagnosis of treatment-related cardiotoxicity, as recognition will often alter the prognosis and treatment strategy.

SUMMARY

Table 15-3 summarizes the major cardiovascular toxicities that have been associated with anticancer therapy. Our patient developed some of these complications from her breast cancer treatment, including cardiomyopathy related to doxorubicin

Table 15-3
Anticancer Agents Associated With Cardiovascular Toxicity

Anticancer Agents
Cardiomyopathy
Type I
Doxorubicin
Daunorubicin
Epirubicin
Idarubicin
Mitoxantrone
Cyclophosphamide
Type II
Trastuzumab
Sunitinib
Lapatinib
Coronary vasospasm
5-Fluorouracil
Capecitabine
Thromboembolic disease
Bevacizumab
Cisplatin
Thalidomide
Lenalidomide
Tamoxifen
Raloxifene
L-Aspariginase
Hypertension
Sunitinib
Sorafenib
Bevacizumab
Long QT
Arsenic trioxide
Nilotinib

and trastuzumab, and angina due to capecitabine-induced coronary vasospasm. She also accepted additional modest increase in cardiovascular risk throughout her course of treatment, which included cyclophosphamide, lapatinib, tamoxifen, and chest wall irradiation. Although her cardiac complications resulted in one episode of systolic heart failure, a brief interruption in her trastuzumab therapy, and a presentation for unstable angina leading to coronary angiography, they did not impact her overall cancer treatment strategy in a major way. If she were to achieve long-term survival, she might be left with mild left ventricular dysfunction that could make her more vulnerable to subsequent cardiac insults in the future. This was probably a reasonable price to pay, since her initial cancer treatment was performed with curative intent. A careful balance of risks and benefits is required prior to embarking on potentially cardiotoxic treatment regimens, and this sometimes requires the help of the cardiology consultant. Good communication between specialists is critically important in optimizing the treatment strategy for these patients. Specialized oncology–cardiology programs are being developed throughout Europe and the United States to address this increasingly complex set of issues.

REFERENCES

1. Chaires JB. Biophysical chemistry of the daunomycin-DNA interaction. *Biophys Chem*. 1990;35(2–3):191–202.
2. Doroshow JH. Effect of anthracycline antibiotics on oxygen radical formation in rat heart. *Cancer Res*. 1983;43(2):460–472.
3. Billingham ME, Mason JW, Bristow MR, Daniels JR. Anthracycline cardiomyopathy monitored by morphologic changes. *Cancer Treat Rep*. 1978;62(6):865–872.
4. Swain SM, Whaley FS, Ewer MS. Congestive heart failure in patients treated with doxorubicin: a retrospective analysis of three trials. *Cancer*. 2003;97(11):2869–2879.
5. Hershman DL, McBride RB, Eisenberger A, Tsai WY, Grann VR, Jacobson JS. Doxorubicin, cardiac risk factors, and cardiac toxicity in elderly patients with diffuse B-cell non-Hodgkin's lymphoma. *J Clin Oncol*. 2008;26(19):3159–3165.
6. van Dalen EC, Michiels EM, Caron HN, Kremer LC. Different anthracycline derivates for reducing cardiotoxicity in cancer patients. *Cochrane Database Syst Rev*. 2006;4:CD005006.
7. Balazsovits JA, Mayer LD, Bally MB, et al. Analysis of the effect of liposome encapsulation on the vesicant properties, acute and cardiac toxicities, and antitumor efficacy of doxorubicin. *Cancer Chemother Pharmacol*. 1989;23(2):81–86.
8. Cardinale D, Sandri MT, Colombo A, et al. Prognostic value of troponin I in cardiac risk stratification of cancer patients undergoing high-dose chemotherapy. *Circulation*. 2004;109(22):2749–2754.
9. Cardinale D, Colombo A, Lamantia G, et al. Anthracycline-induced cardiomyopathy: clinical relevance and response to pharmacologic therapy. *J Am Coll Cardiol*. 2010;55(3):213–220.
10. Ewer MS, Ewer SM. Cardiotoxicity of anticancer treatments: what the cardiologist needs to know. *Nat Rev Cardiol*. 2010;7(10):564–575.
11. Legha SS, Benjamin RS, Mackay B, et al. Reduction of doxorubicin cardiotoxicity by prolonged continuous intravenous infusion. *Ann Intern Med*. 1982;96(2):133–139.
12. Swain SM, Whaley FS, Gerber MC, Ewer MS, Bianchine JR, Gams RA. Delayed administration of dexrazoxane provides cardioprotection for patients with advanced breast cancer treated with doxorubicin-containing therapy. *J Clin Oncol*. 1997;15(4):1333–1340.
13. Swain SM, Whaley FS, Gerber MC, et al. Cardioprotection with dexrazoxane for doxorubicin-containing therapy in advanced breast cancer. *J Clin Oncol*. 1997;15(4):1318–1332.
14. Cardinale D, Colombo A, Sandri MT, et al. Prevention of high-dose chemotherapy-induced cardiotoxicity in high-risk patients by angiotensin-converting enzyme inhibition. *Circulation*. 2006;114(23):2474–2481.
15. Kalay N, Basar E, Ozdogru I, et al. Protective effects of carvedilol against anthracycline-induced cardiomyopathy. *J Am Coll Cardiol*. 2006;48(11):2258–2262.
16. Hunt SA, Abraham WT, Chin MH, et al.; American College of Cardiology Foundation; American Heart Association. 2009 Focused update incorporated into the ACC/AHA 2005 Guidelines for the Diagnosis and Management of Heart Failure in Adults A Report of the American College of Cardiology Foundation/American Heart Association Task Force on Practice Guidelines Developed in Collaboration With the International Society for Heart and Lung Transplantation. *J Am Coll Cardiol*. 2009;53(15):e1–e90.
17. Piccart-Gebhart MJ, Procter M, Leyland-Jones B, et al.; Herceptin Adjuvant (HERA) Trial Study Team. Trastuzumab after adjuvant chemotherapy in HER2-positive breast cancer. *N Engl J Med*. 2005;353(16):1659–1672.
18. Romond EH, Perez EA, Bryant J, et al. Trastuzumab plus adjuvant chemotherapy for operable HER2-positive breast cancer. *N Engl J Med*. 2005;353(16):1673–1684.
19. Zhao YY, Sawyer DR, Baliga RR, et al. Neuregulins promote survival and growth of cardiac myocytes. Persistence of ErbB2 and ErbB4 expression in neonatal and adult ventricular myocytes. *J Biol Chem*. 1998;273(17):10261–10269.
20. Crone SA, Zhao YY, Fan L, et al. ErbB2 is essential in the prevention of dilated cardiomyopathy. *Nat Med*. 2002;8(5):459–465.
21. Slamon DJ, Leyland-Jones B, Shak S, et al. Use of chemotherapy plus a monoclonal antibody against HER2 for metastatic breast cancer that overexpresses HER2. *N Engl J Med*. 2001;344(11):783–792.
22. Moja L, Tagliabue L, Balduzzi S, et al. Trastuzumab containing regimens for early breast cancer. *Cochrane Database Syst Rev*. 2012;4:CD006243.
23. Ewer MS, Vooletich MT, Durand JB, et al. Reversibility of trastuzumab-related cardiotoxicity: new insights based on clinical course and response to medical treatment. *J Clin Oncol*. 2005;23(31):7820–7826.
24. Ewer MS, Lippman SM. Type II chemotherapy-related cardiac dysfunction: time to recognize a new entity. *J Clin Oncol*. 2005;23(13):2900–2902.
25. Slamon D, Eiermann W, Robert N, et al.; Breast Cancer International Research Group. Adjuvant trastuzumab in HER2-positive breast cancer. *N Engl J Med*. 2011;365(14):1273–1283.
26. Joensuu H, Bono P, Kataja V, et al. Fluorouracil, epirubicin, and cyclophosphamide with either docetaxel or vinorelbine,

with or without trastuzumab, as adjuvant treatments of breast cancer: final results of the FinHer Trial. *J Clin Oncol*. 2009;27(34): 5685–5692.

27. Slamon DJ, Leyland-Jones B, Shak S, et al. Use of chemotherapy plus a monoclonal antibody against HER2 for metastatic breast cancer that overexpresses HER2. *N Engl J Med*. 2001;344(11): 783–792.
28. Romond EH, Jeong JH, Rastogi P, et al. Seven-year follow-up assessment of cardiac function in NSABP B-31, a randomized trial comparing doxorubicin and cyclophosphamide followed by paclitaxel (ACP) with ACP plus trastuzumab as adjuvant therapy for patients with node-positive, human epidermal growth factor receptor 2-positive breast cancer. *J Clin Oncol*. 2012;30(31):3792–3799.
29. Suter TM, Procter M, van Veldhuisen DJ, et al. Trastuzumab-associated cardiac adverse effects in the herceptin adjuvant trial. *J Clin Oncol*. 2007;25(25):3859–3865.
30. Chu TF, Rupnick MA, Kerkela R, et al. Cardiotoxicity associated with tyrosine kinase inhibitor sunitinib. *Lancet*. 2007;370(9604):2011–2019.
31. Perez EA, Koehler M, Byrne J, Preston AJ, Rappold E, Ewer MS. Cardiac safety of lapatinib: pooled analysis of 3689 patients enrolled in clinical trials. *Mayo Clin Proc*. 2008;83(6):679–686.
32. Braverman AC, Antin JH, Plappert MT, Cook EF, Lee RT. Cyclophosphamide cardiotoxicity in bone marrow transplantation: a prospective evaluation of new dosing regimens. *J Clin Oncol*. 1991;9(7):1215–1223.
33. Kosmas C, Kallistratos MS, Kopterides P, et al. Cardiotoxicity of fluoropyrimidines in different schedules of administration: a prospective study. *J Cancer Res Clin Oncol*. 2008;134(1):75–82.
34. Sugrue MM, Yi J, Purdie D, et al. Serious arterial thromboembolic events (sATE) in patients (pts) with metastatic colorectal cancer (mCRC) treated with bevacizumab (BV): results from the BRiTE registry [Abstract 4136]. *J Clin Oncol*. 2007;25(Suppl. 18): 4136.
35. Cuppone F, Bria E, Verma S, et al. Do adjuvant aromatase inhibitors increase the cardiovascular risk in postmenopausal women with early breast cancer? Meta-analysis of randomized trials. *Cancer*. 2008;112(2):260–267.
36. Amir E, Seruga B, Niraula S, Carlsson L, Ocaña A. Toxicity of adjuvant endocrine therapy in postmenopausal breast cancer patients: a systematic review and meta-analysis. *J Natl Cancer Inst*. 2011;103(17):1299–1309.
37. Davies C, Pan H, Godwin J. Long-term effects of continuing adjuvant tamoxifen to 10 years versus stopping at 5 years after diagnosis of oestrogen receptor-positive breast cancer: ATLAS, a randomised trial. *Lancet*. 2013;381(9869):805–816.
38. Shord SS, Bressler LR, Tierney LA, Cuellar S, George A. Understanding and managing the possible adverse effects associated with bevacizumab. *Am J Health Syst Pharm*. 2009;66(11): 999–1013.
39. Palumbo A, Rajkumar SV, Dimopoulos MA, et al.; International Myeloma Working Group. Prevention of thalidomide- and lenalidomide-associated thrombosis in myeloma. *Leukemia*. 2008;22(2):414–423.
40. Bushnell CD, Goldstein LB. Risk of ischemic stroke with tamoxifen treatment for breast cancer: a meta-analysis. *Neurology*. 2004;63(7):1230–1233.
41. University of Arizona Center for Education and Research on Therapeutics. Available at: www.azcert.org. Accessed September 7, 2012.
42. Tukenova M, Guibout C, Oberlin O, et al. Role of cancer treatment in long-term overall and cardiovascular mortality after childhood cancer. *J Clin Oncol*. 2010;28(8):1308–1315.
43. Schultz-Hector S. Radiation-induced heart disease: review of experimental data on dose response and pathogenesis. *Int J Radiat Biol*. 1992;61(2):149–160.
44. Darby SC, McGale P, Taylor CW, Peto R. Long-term mortality from heart disease and lung cancer after radiotherapy for early breast cancer: prospective cohort study of about 300,000 women in US SEER cancer registries. *Lancet Oncol*. 2005;6(8):557–565.
45. Giordano SH, Kuo YF, Freeman JL, Buchholz TA, Hortobagyi GN, Goodwin JS. Risk of cardiac death after adjuvant radiotherapy for breast cancer. *J Natl Cancer Inst*. 2005;97(6):419–424.
46. Maisch B, Seferovic PM, Ristic AD, et al.; Task Force on the Diagnosis and Management of Pricardial Diseases of the European Society of Cardiology. Guidelines on the diagnosis and management of pericardial diseases executive summary; The Task force on the diagnosis and management of pericardial diseases of the European society of cardiology. *Eur Heart J*. 2004;25(7):587–610.
47. Adams MJ, Lipsitz SR, Colan SD, et al. Cardiovascular status in long-term survivors of Hodgkin's disease treated with chest radiotherapy. *J Clin Oncol*. 2004;22(15):3139–3148.
48. Brosius FC 3rd, Waller BF, Roberts WC. Radiation heart disease. Analysis of 16 young (aged 15 to 33 years) necropsy patients who received over 3,500 rads to the heart. *Am J Med*. 1981;70(3):519–530.
49. McEniery PT, Dorosti K, Schiavone WA, Pedrick TJ, Sheldon WC. Clinical and angiographic features of coronary artery disease after chest irradiation. *Am J Cardiol*. 1987;60(13):1020–1024.
50. Kralstein J, Frishman W. Malignant pericardial diseases: diagnosis and treatment. *Am Heart J*. 1987;113(3):785–790.
51. Von Hoff DD, Layard MW, Basa P, et al. Risk factors for doxorubicin-induced congestive heart failure. *Ann Intern Med*. 1979;91(5):710–717.
52. Steinherz LJ, Steinherz PG, Tan CT, Heller G, Murphy ML. Cardiac toxicity 4 to 20 years after completing anthracycline therapy. *JAMA*. 1991;266(12):1672–1677.

16

Cardiac Amyloidosis

RYAN KIPP AND PETER S. RAHKO

CASE PRESENTATION

A 55-year-old male with a past medical history significant for coronary artery disease (CAD) and three-vessel coronary artery bypass graft surgery, hypertension, and dyslipidemia presents to his general internist with complaints of increasing fatigue. Six months ago, he was able to run five miles, five times a week without difficulty. He initially noticed that he was having difficulty completing his runs, but recently stopped running because of worsening exercise tolerance. He denies having any angina symptoms. The patient kept a diary of his resting pulse, which shows a gradual increase from the mid-40s 6 months ago to the low-70s currently. He now has difficulty walking up a flight of stairs.

He has also noticed swelling of his legs, particularly over the last month, but denies orthopnea. He admits to a cough waking him in the middle of the night, which improves after 30 minutes of sitting upright at the edge of his bed. He has lost 10 pounds over the last year, but attributes it to a healthier diet. However, he has noticed early satiety. He admits to orthostasis, but denies any episodes of syncope. When asked about bleeding or bruising, he reports having occasional "black eyes" over the last year, but does not remember any trauma prior to these events.

On physical exam, the patient appears well, but slightly pale. His pulse is 82 and regular. His blood pressure is 105/70. He has a nearly resolved ecchymosis near his right eye. Jugular venous distension is about 14 cm of water. On inspiration, the venous distension increases. Carotid pulses have reduced amplitude without bruits. On cardiac examination, there is a regular rhythm with a single S1 and S2, no S3 or S4. There is a II/VI holosystolic murmur best auscultated at the left lower sternal border, no right ventricular heave, and the point of maximal impulse (PMI) is located in the fifth intercostal space in the mid-clavicular line. The lungs have decreased breath sounds in the bases, right greater than left with dullness to percussion and egophony. There are no rales. The abdomen is slightly distended with shifting dullness. The liver edge is firm and pulsatile, and is palpated 2 cm below the costal margin. Hepatojugular reflux is present. His extremities are warm and there is 2+ pitting edema in the lower extremities bilaterally. His neurologic exam is unremarkable.

HISTORY AND PHYSICAL EXAM

This patient presents with numerous clinical features suggestive of progressive heart failure. The important historical features include the short time frame over which his symptoms have developed, as well as the degree of physical limitation he is experiencing. He has developed exercise intolerance and his resting pulse has increased substantially, suggesting decreased stroke volume, requiring an increased heart rate to maintain his cardiac output. His orthostasis may be consistent with poor cardiac output and an inability to augment his output rapidly or impaired autonomic function. His low blood pressure, despite a history of hypertension, also lends support for possible autonomic dysfunction. He also reports having a nocturnal cough, which improves with sitting on the edge of the bed. The cough is likely due to pulmonary congestion resulting from redistribution of his excess systemic fluid.

On physical exam, there are numerous features suggesting myocardial dysfunction. The patient has an elevated jugular venous pressure at approximately 14 cm and lower extremity edema consistent with venous congestion that may indicate right ventricular failure. There is also shifting dullness (ascites) and an enlarged, tender, pulsatile liver suggesting hepatic congestion, supporting a diagnosis of heart failure. His early satiety and weight loss are particularly concerning because they suggest edema of the small bowel and poor nutrient absorption. The resulting protein malnutrition (cardiac cachexia) may result in low albumin levels, contributing further to his edema from low intravascular oncotic pressure.

Absent breath sounds in the lung bases suggest pleural effusions. There is an absence of rales, which could be due to a lack of pulmonary venous congestion. However, patients with long-standing pulmonary venous congestion may develop increased lymphatic clearance of interstitial pulmonary fluid resulting in clear lungs despite elevated pulmonary venous pressures. Therefore, this physical exam finding does not reliably exclude left ventricular failure. Low albumin from cardiac cachexia may also contribute to pleural effusion development.

Together, the patient's history and physical exam are consistent with heart failure. The most common cause of heart failure in the United States is ischemic heart disease. Our patient has a history of obstructive CAD, increasing the possibility that he has developed an ischemic cardiomyopathy. However, there are several subtle, but important, clinical features that suggest another cause.

First, Kussmaul's sign (increased jugular venous distension with inspiration) is present. Kussmaul's sign occurs when there is an inability of the right ventricle to dilate and accommodate the increased venous return from inspiration. Several cardiac diseases can result in this finding, including constrictive pericarditis, restrictive cardiomyopathy, right ventricular infarction or failure, and tricuspid stenosis. Severe tricuspid regurgitation may cause similar findings, but can be distinguished by timing the waveforms of venous distension (in Kussmaul's sign the venous distension increases with inspiration, whereas with severe tricuspid regurgitation the venous distension increases with every systole from a pronounced V-wave). This is an important distinguishing feature, since Kussmaul's sign is not present in a typical ischemic cardiomyopathy. A second physical exam finding suggesting a nondilated cardiomyopathy is the nondisplaced apical impulse, indicating a lack of left ventricular dilation.

The history of periorbital purpura without a history of trauma is suspicious, and suggests amyloidosis, a cause of restrictive cardiomyopathy.

In summary, the patient's history and physical exam is consistent with subacute decompensated heart failure with findings suggestive of constrictive pericarditis or restrictive cardiomyopathy (positive Kussmaul's sign, normal PMI), and one physical exam finding suggesting amyloidosis.

CASE PRESENTATION

The 12-lead electrocardiogram (ECG) shows sinus rhythm with low voltage throughout the limb and precordial leads. There are Q-waves present in the anteroseptal and inferior leads. Compared to his ECG obtained three years ago, there has been a significant loss of electrical voltage in both the limb and precordial leads (**Figure 16-1**).

The transthoracic echocardiogram (TTE) reveals a normal-sized left ventricle with a thickened interventricular septum measuring 20 mm and a thick left ventricular posterior wall measuring 20 mm. The right ventricular wall also appears thickened. There is a sparkling and granular appearance to the myocardium (**Figure 16-2A–C**). The left ventricular ejection fraction (LVEF) is slightly reduced at 50% without regional ventricular wall motion abnormalities. The left and right atria are moderately dilated with thickened walls (**Figure 16-2D**). There is only mild tricuspid regurgitation and no mitral valve or aortic valve dysfunction. Compared to a prior echocardiogram done after his bypass surgery, left ventricular wall thickness has markedly increased.

Pulsed Doppler across the mitral valve shows an elevated E-velocity and short deceleration time. There is still an A-wave, but the E/A ratio is elevated to 2.22 (**Figure 16-2E**). Tissue Doppler shows a reduced absolute e′ and an E/e′ ratio of 11.3 (**Figure 16-2F**). The pulmonary vein inflow shows systolic blunting, consistent with elevated left atrial pressures and loss of A-wave reversal (**Figure 16-2G**). Together, these findings suggest severe (Grade 4) diastolic dysfunction and increased left atrial pressure.

The pericardium is slightly thickened, and a small pericardial effusion is present. There is no exaggerated interventricular septal shift with respiration phases and no exaggerated respiratory variation in Doppler velocity (less than 18%) through the mitral or aortic valves.

ELECTROCARDIOGRAM AND ECHOCARDIOGRAM

The electrocardiogram (ECG) and echocardiogram are instrumental in determining the potential cause of a cardiomyopathy. Our patient's TTE has only slightly reduced left ventricular systolic function without regional wall motion abnormalities and no primary valve disease. However, severe diastolic dysfunction

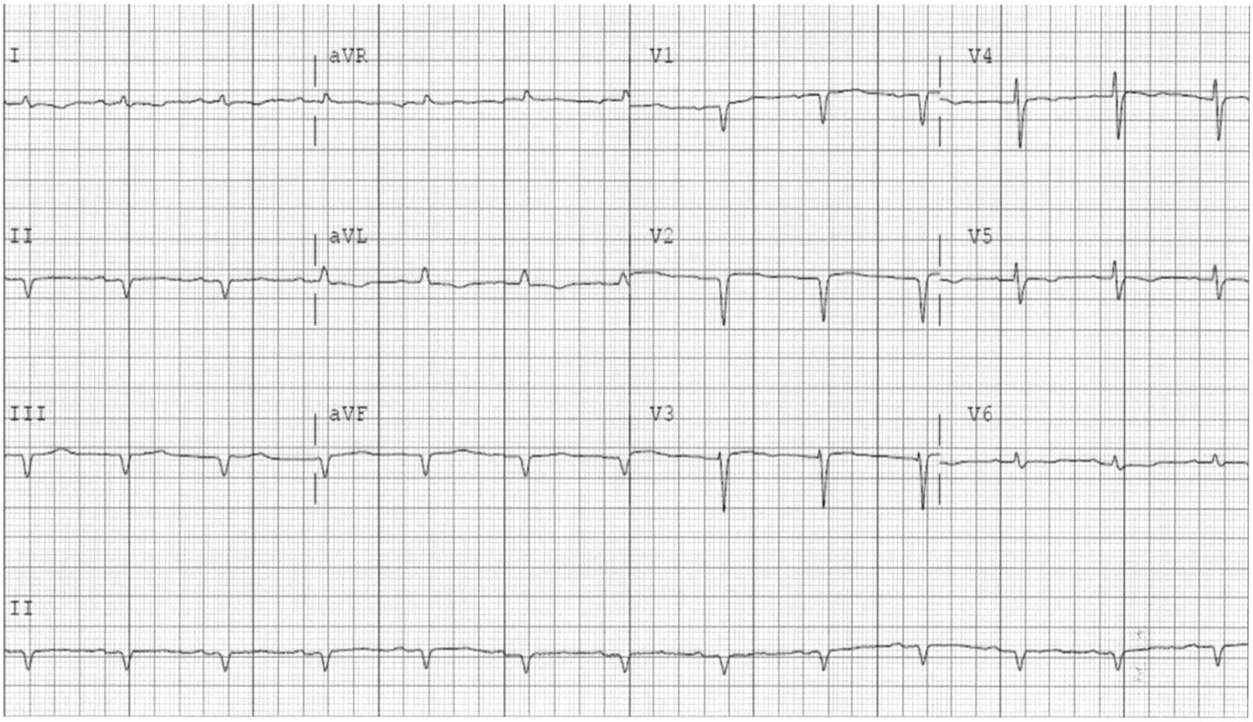

(A)

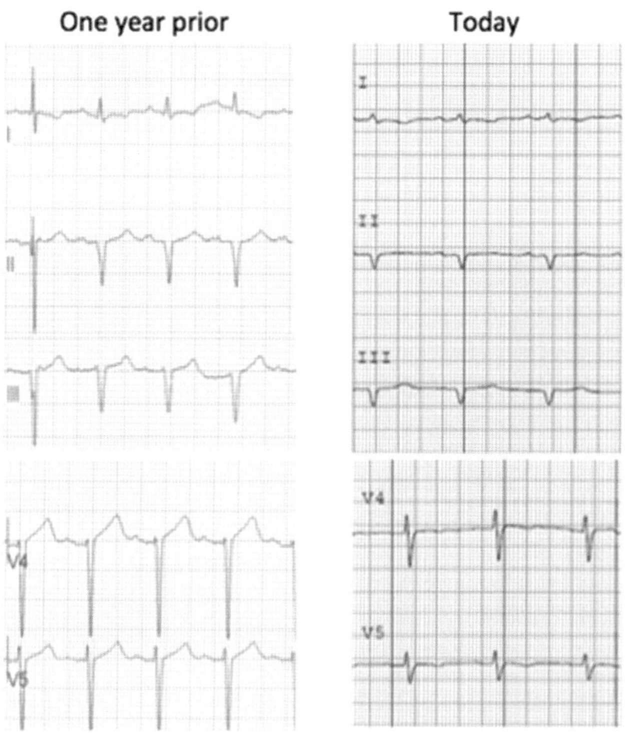

(B)

Figure 16-1

(A) Twelve-lead ECG obtained at this visit shows regular sinus rhythm with normal AV-conduction. There are Q-waves in the anteroseptal and inferior leads with low QRS voltage in the both the precordial (QRS voltage less than 10 mm) and limb (QRS voltage less than 5 mm) leads. (B) Compared to an ECG obtained 1 year ago, the QRS voltage is significantly reduced.

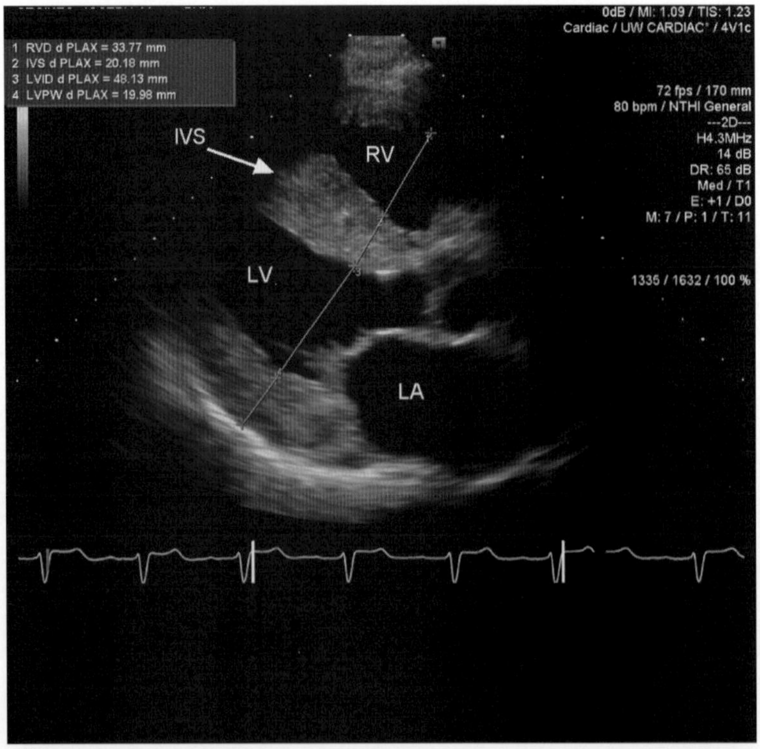

(A)

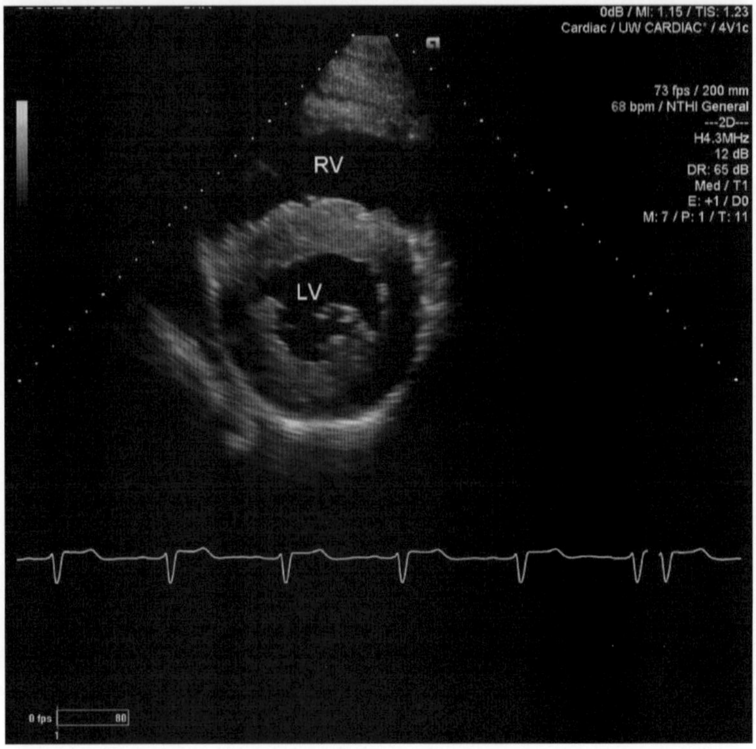

(B)

Figure 16-2

Transthoracic echocardiogram. (A) Parasternal long axis view of the left ventricle with thickening of the interventricular septum and posterior left ventricular wall indicating infiltration. The granular appearance of the thickened myocardium is characteristic of amyloid infiltration. The mitral valve leaflets are also thickened, which can be seen with amyloidosis. (B) Parasternal short axis view of the left ventricle at the level of the mitral valve demonstrates hypertrophy of the left ventricle with granular appearance of the myocardium characteristic of amyloid infiltration. See also **Video 16-1A** and **Video 16-1B** by visiting the following links; http://www.demosmedpub.com/video/?vid=827 and http://www.demosmedpub.com/video/?vid=828 *(Continued)*

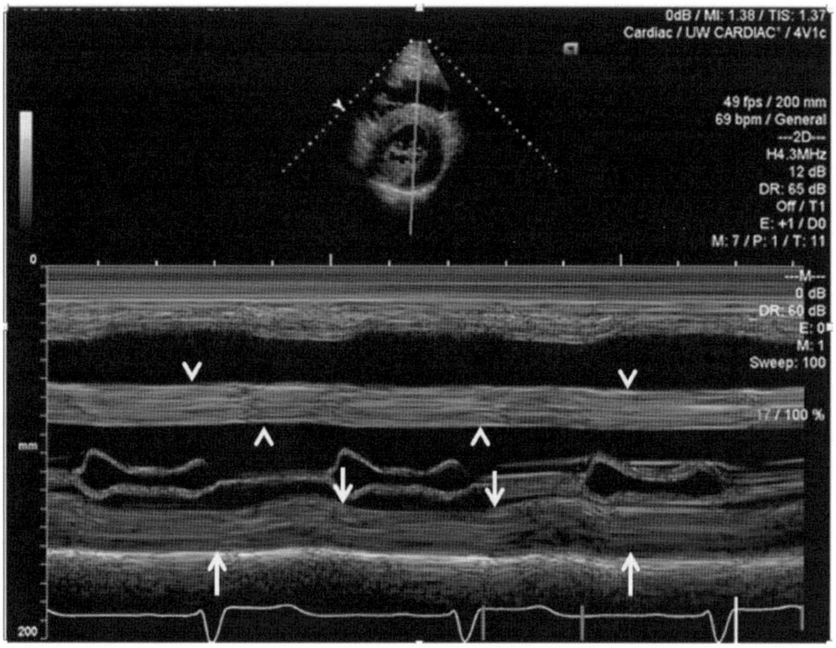

(C)

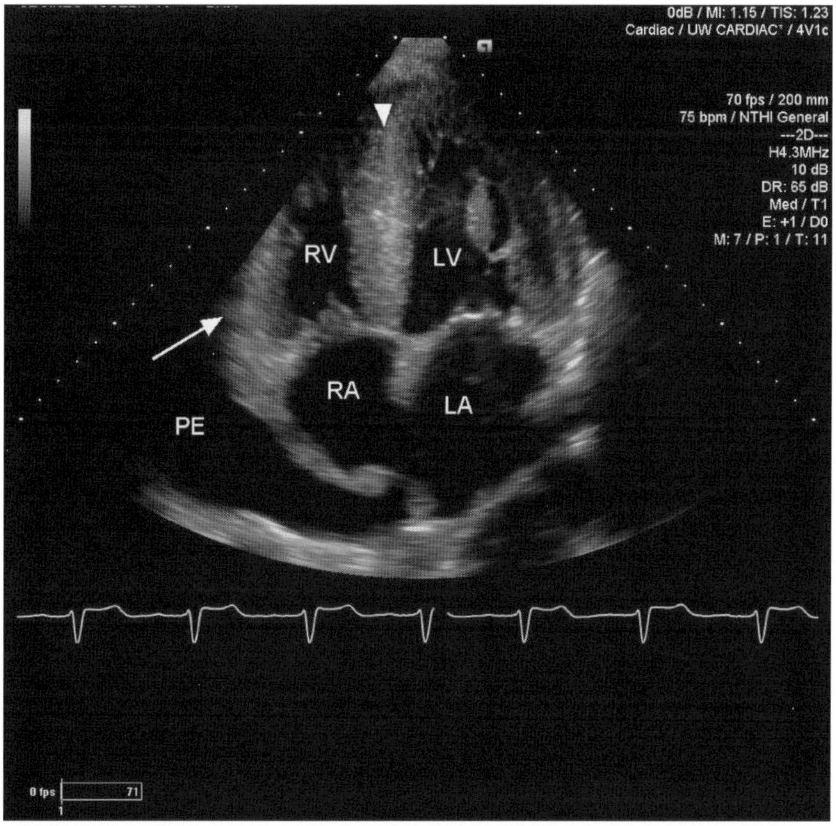

(D)

Figure 16-2 *(Continued)*
(C) M-mode of the parasternal short axis at the level of the mitral valve exemplifies the thickened interventricular septum (arrow head) and posterior wall (arrow). (D) An apical four-chamber view shows thickening of the right ventricular free wall (arrow) suggesting right ventricular infiltration. The left atrium has a diameter of 5.2 cm consistent with moderate atrial dilation. This suggests high left ventricular filling pressures. Thickening of the atrial walls indicates atrial infiltration with amyloid. The arrowhead indicates the thickened interventricular septum. *(Continued)*

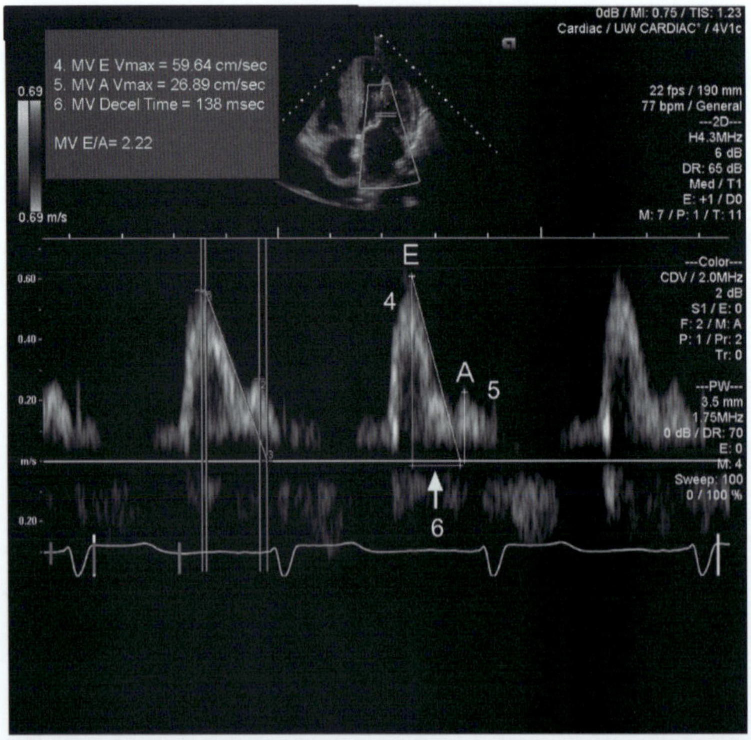

(E)

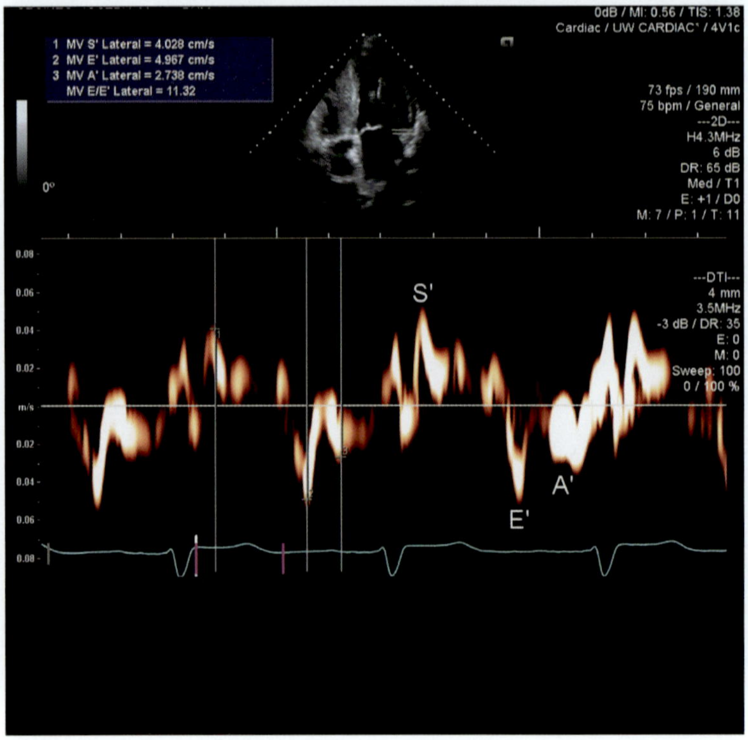

(F)

Figure 16-2 *(Continued)*

(E) The mitral inflow pulse Doppler has a short E-wave deceleration time and an increased E/A ratio. (F) The e′ from the tissue Doppler of the lateral mitral valve annulus is significantly blunted. The E/e′ ratio is also increased. *(Continued)*

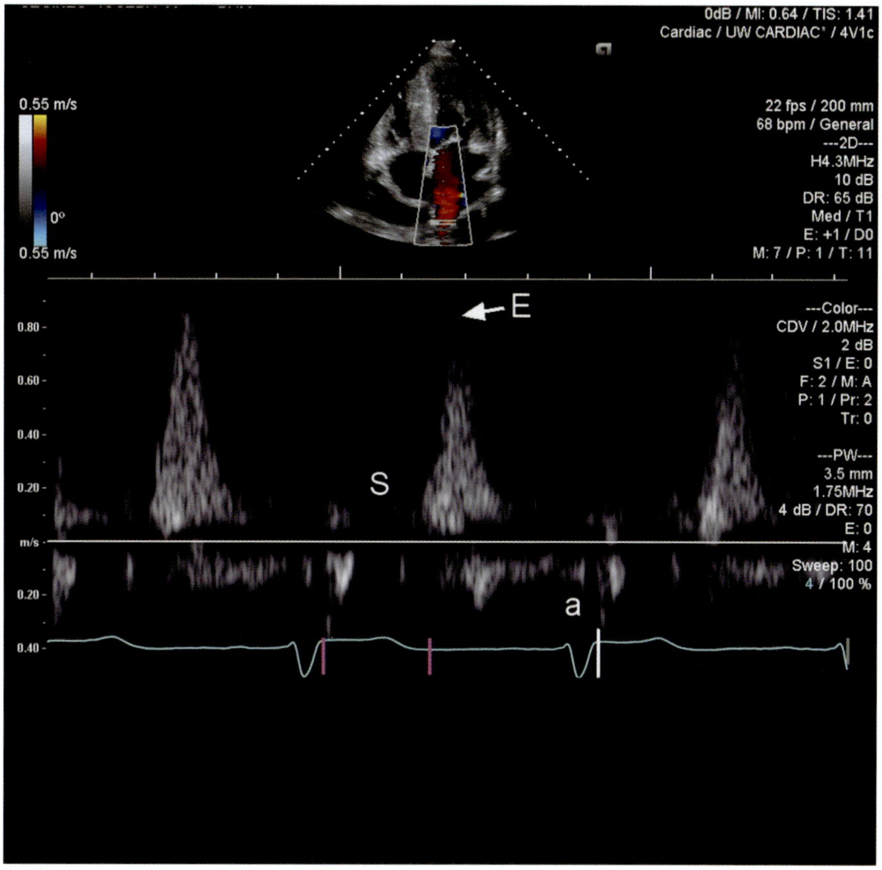

(G)

Figure 16-2 *(Continued)*
(G) Pulse Doppler at the ostium of the right upper pulmonary vein shows severe S-wave blunting with forward flow occurring almost exclusively during diastole (E-wave). A-wave reversal is nearly absent indicating loss of atrial systolic function, possibly from atrial amyloid infiltration. These findings are consistent with severe, irreversible left ventricular diastolic dysfunction and increased left atrial pressure.

Note: IVS = interventricular septum; LA = left atrium; LV = left ventricle; PE = pleural effusion; RA = right atrium; RV = right ventricle.

and signs of elevated left atrial pressure are present. Therefore, this patient has heart failure with preserved systolic function, or diastolic heart failure. To proceed with treatment, the etiology of the diastolic dysfunction needs to be determined. Two general categories of isolated diastolic dysfunction may be considered: constriction or restriction. Constriction is usually caused by a noncompliant pericardium impairing normal myocardial diastolic function, whereas restriction is a primary failure of myocardial relaxation. Restriction is usually caused by a process related to thickened left ventricular walls, such as primary cardiomyopathy (hypertrophic cardiomyopathy) or hypertensive disease (both having a combination of cardiac myocyte hypertrophy and fibroblasts), or an infiltrative process within the myocardium.

There are several findings on our patient's TTE consistent with restrictive cardiomyopathy and no features consistent with constrictive pericarditis. First, there is thickening of the right and left ventricular walls, and the interventricular septum. There is also a sparkling and granular appearance of the myocardium. These findings are most consistent with an infiltrative cardiomyopathy, specifically amyloidosis, which when severe can result in a restrictive cardiomyopathy. It should be noted that the granular backscatter pattern of amyloid disease is less reliable with current generation ultrasound systems that utilize second harmonic imaging than it was with earlier generation fundamental (first harmonic) systems. Additionally, there are numerous signs of severe left ventricular diastolic dysfunction that indicate high filling pressures both on the left and right sides of the heart. These include an elevated E/e′ ratio, a high E-wave velocity with short E-wave deceleration time (indicating rapid but short-lived filling of the left ventricle driven by high left atrial pressure), pulmonary vein systolic inflow blunting (also consistent with elevated left atrial pressures), and an increased E/A ratio. Two important distinctions must be made that further help differentiate restriction from constriction. First, the absolute e′ velocity is low, highly consistent with slowed muscle relaxation and not constriction. It is important to differentiate e′ velocity at the septum to the lateral wall. In a restrictive cardiomyopathy, both locations have reduced velocity. In constriction, septal e′ velocity is usually normal or high and typically of higher velocity than the lateral wall. Second, while reduced, the A-wave velocity is still at least partially preserved (**Figures 16-2F, 16-2G**). This would be less likely in constrictive pericarditis. Taken together, these findings are most consistent with a restrictive cardiomyopathy.

To help further differentiate the type of cardiomyopathy, the echocardiogram and ECG should be evaluated together. Patients with thickened ventricular myocardium from myocyte hypertrophy secondary to hypertensive or hypertrophic cardiomyopathy usually meet the criteria for ventricular hypertrophy on their ECG. Our patient has thickened ventricular myocardium with low voltage, indicating a significant mismatch between the amount of ventricular myocardium present on echocardiography and the electrical signal it is generating on ECG. Additionally, this loss of electrical voltage has developed over the last year. Indeed, while his walls have thickened, his voltage has gone down. There are also Q-waves present without evidence of prior infarction on the echocardiogram. This combination of findings is suggestive of an infiltrating cardiomyopathy, such as:

- Sarcoidosis (systemic deposition of noncaseating granulomas)
- Hemochromatosis (excessive iron absorption with systemic deposition)
- Amyloidosis (deposition of extracellular fibrils of low molecular weight protein subunits derived from normal serum protein. The fibrils form antiparallel β-pleated sheets with systemic deposition and end-organ disruption).

Infiltrating diseases result in low ECG voltage despite increased myocardial mass on TTE due to poor electrical conduction through the infiltrating material. Therefore, despite the appearance of left ventricular hypertrophy (LVH) on TTE, electrical criteria for LVH may not be met. Q-waves develop as a result of electrically silent infiltrating material creating an area of myocardium with poor electrical activity, similar to infarcted myocardium, resulting in preferential electrical conduction away from that area and Q-waves (called pseudo-infarction).

Comparing the degree of myocardial thickening with the QRS voltage assists with distinguishing amyloidosis from other causes of restrictive cardiomyopathy or hypertensive heart disease. An interventricular septum measuring greater than 1.98 cm and low QRS voltage in the limb (QRS voltage less than 5 mm) or precordial (QRS voltage less than 10 mm) leads has a sensitivity and specificity of 72% and 91%, respectively, for the diagnosis of amyloidosis (1).

Therefore, our patient has numerous echocardiographic findings consistent with a restrictive cardiomyopathy, which when combined with ECG and physical exam findings is most likely due to cardiac amyloidosis. These findings are contrasted to typical findings of hypertensive heart disease and constriction in **Table 16-1**.

CARDIAC CT AND CARDIAC MAGNETIC RESONANCE

Cardiac CT can assist with the diagnosis of pericardial constriction through imaging the thickness of the pericardium and allowing the detection of even small amounts of pericardial calcium. However, these findings are neither sensitive nor specific. Cine acquisition can assist with evaluation of septal wall motion, but again this is not a sensitive finding in the diagnosis of constrictive pericarditis.

Cardiac magnetic resonance (CMR) is currently being evaluated for its ability to assist in the work-up of restrictive cardiomyopathy and constrictive pericarditis. As with echocardiography, amyloid deposits result in thickening of the left and right ventricular walls that are imaged well with MR (**Figure 16-3A**). Cardiac amyloidosis also results in a diffuse subendocardial delayed enhancement pattern with gadolinium (**Figure 16-3B**; 2). Delayed gadolinium enhancement on CMR appears to precede left ventricular thickening and may allow earlier diagnosis of cardiac amyloidosis than echocardiography (3). Similarly, patients with pericarditis may also have late gadolinium enhancement confined to the pericardium due to pericardial inflammation, which may assist in distinguishing constrictive pericarditis from restrictive cardiomyopathy. Finally, as with cardiac CT, cine acquisition may allow evaluation of diastolic septal wall motion for distinction of constrictive pericarditis.

Table 16-1
Distinguishing Features of Cardiac Amyloidosis, Cardiac Hypertrophy Secondary to Hypertension, and Constrictive Pericarditis

	RESTRICTIVE CARDIOMYOPATHY		CONSTRICTIVE PERICARDITIS
	Amyloidosis	**Hypertension**	
Macroglossia or periorbital purpura	May be present	Absent	Absent
Orthostatic hypotension	Often present	Absent	May be present
History of carpel tunnel syndrome	Often present	Absent	Absent
Kussmaul's sign	May be present	Absent	Present
Signs of right ventricular heart failure	Present	Absent	Present
ECG findings	Low QRS voltage, particularly in limb leads Pseudo-infarct pattern	Increased QRS voltage with criteria for LVH	Normal QRS voltage
Left ventricular myocardial wall thickness on TTE	Increased	Increased	Normal
Myocardial mass to QRS voltage mismatch	Present	Absent	Absent
Granular appearance of myocardium on TTE	Present	Absent	Absent
Pericardial appearance on TTE	Normal with possible small effusion	Normal	Thickened, calcified
Marked reduction in mitral A-wave velocity on Doppler inflow	Progresses with severity of infiltration	Absent except in end stage disease	Present
Reduced diastolic annular velocities on TTE tissue Doppler imaging	Present and progresses with severity of infiltration	Present in more severe disease	Absent
Mitral annular diastolic velocity ≥8 cm/second on TTE	Absent	Absent	Present (95% sensitivity, 96% specificity for diagnosing constrictive pericarditis; 31)
Respiratory variation of E-wave velocity across mitral valve on TTE	Absent	Absent	Present (>18% variation has a sensitivity and specificity of 79% and 91%, respectively, for the diagnosis of constrictive pericarditis; 32)
"Dip-and-plateau" on right heart catheterization	Present	May be present in severe cases	Present
Equalization of end-diastolic RA, RVEDP, PCWP, and LVEDP	Absent	Absent	Present
Discordance of ventricular pressure tracings (systolic area index > 1.1)	Absent	Absent	Present
MR late gadolinium enhancement	Subendocardium	None	Pericardium, particularly with residual inflammation

Note: LVEDP = left ventricular end diastolic pressure; MR = magnetic resonance; PCWP = pulmonary capillary wedge pressure; RA = right atrial; RVEDP = right ventricular end diastolic pressure; TTE = transthoracic echocardiogram.

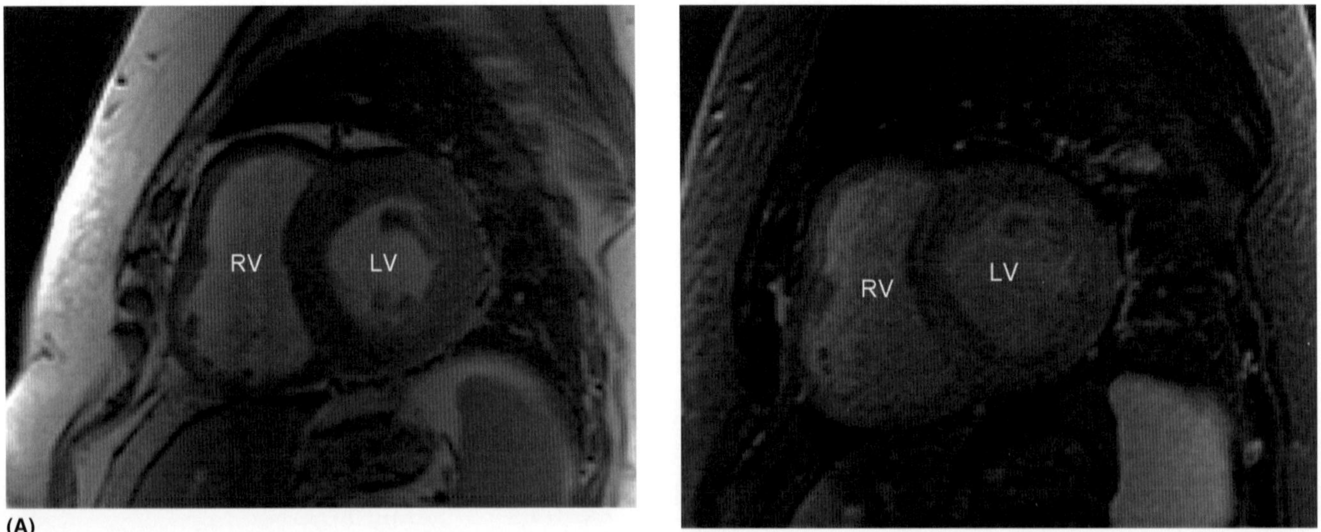

(A) (B)

Figure 16-3
Cardiac MR from a patient with cardiac amyloidosis viewed from the short axis. (A) There is thickening of the right and left ventricular walls. (B) Diffuse delayed gadolinium enhancement of the subendocardium in the right and left ventricles suggests amyloid infiltration.

Note: LV = left ventricle; MR = magnetic resonance; RV = right ventricle.

Source: Images courtesy of Drs. Scott Reader and Christopher Francois.

While cardiac CT and CMR may assist with making the diagnosis of restrictive cardiomyopathy, the clinical utility of these studies in the treatment or prognosis of cardiac amyloidosis has not yet been determined.

CASE PRESENTATION

The most common cause of cardiomyopathy in the United States is CAD. Despite evidence suggesting an infiltrating cardiomyopathy, due to the presence of reduced LVEF and history of obstructive CAD, a cardiac catheterization is performed to exclude progressive coronary disease. A coronary angiogram finds that the three previously placed vein grafts remain patent and he is without significant progression of disease in his native vessels. To provide additional data to assist with distinguishing constrictive pericarditis from restrictive cardiomyopathy, simultaneous right- and left-heart catheterization is also performed.

The catheterization reveals:

Right Atrial Pressure	19 mmHg
Right Ventricular Pressure	42/15 mmHg
Pulmonary Capillary Wedge Pressure	23 mmHg
Left Ventricular Pressure	120/22 mmHg

There is elevated pressure within the right atrium, as well as increased right ventricular pressure. The pressure tracing in the right ventricle has an elevated end-diastolic pressure with a "square-root sign" (**Figure 16-4A**). The pulmonary capillary wedge pressure (PCWP) and left ventricular end-diastolic pressures are also increased. There is no pressure equalization at end-diastole. During normal respiratory cycles, there is concordance between the systolic area ratios (**Figure 16-4B**).

HEMODYNAMICS

Echocardiographic findings can help distinguish constrictive pericarditis from restrictive cardiomyopathy; however, there are patients who may still have a mixed picture. Historical features that increase the likelihood of either condition being present include radiation to the chest, sarcoidosis, or systemic inflammatory conditions. Our patient has one historical feature that predisposes him to the development of constrictive pericarditis: prior coronary artery bypass surgery. Simultaneous left- and right-heart catheterization helps to distinguish between restrictive cardiomyopathy and constrictive pericarditis. It is not sufficient to only evaluate for elevated filling pressures with right heart catheterization, as filling pressures may be normal in up to 20% of patients with amyloid (restrictive) heart disease (4). Additionally, both restrictive and constrictive disease may result in pressure tracings showing the classic right

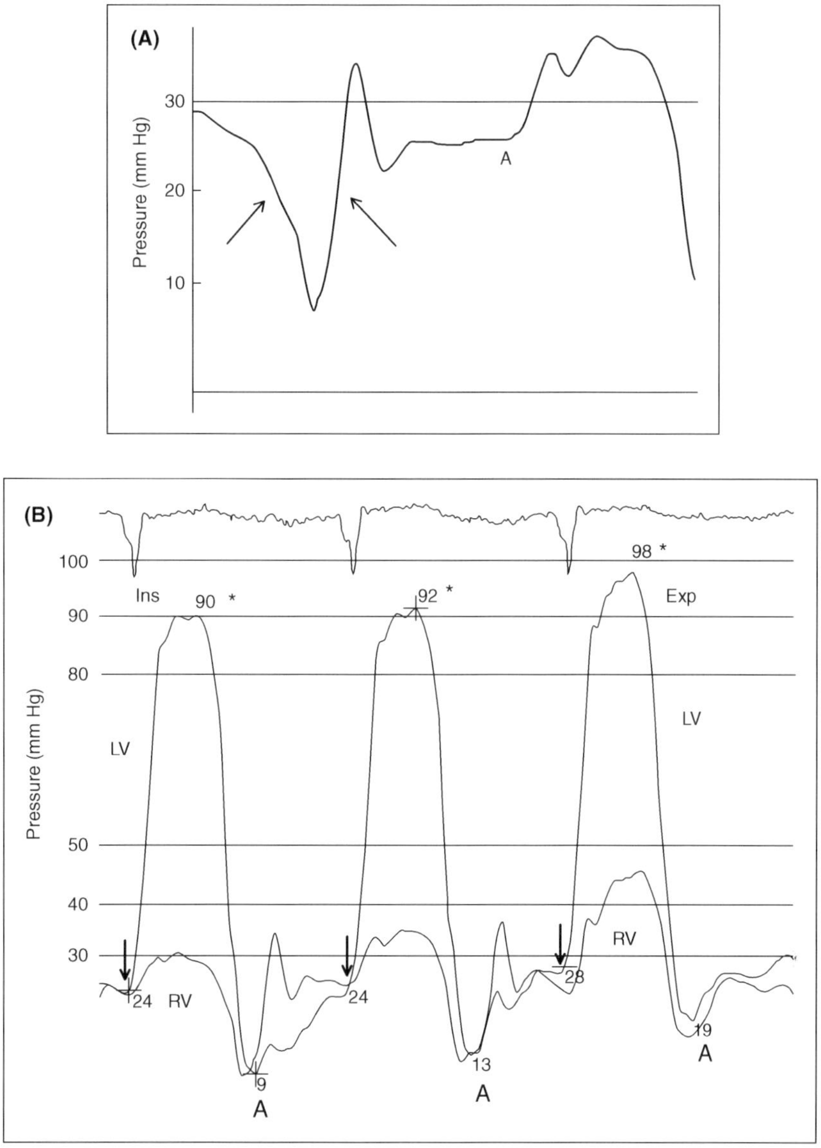

Figure 16-4

(A) Right ventricular pressure tracing with a "square-root sign" (arrows) (also termed "dip-and-plateau") during diastole consistent with restrictive cardiomyopathy or constrictive pericarditis. Elevated end-diastolic pressure is also present (at location A). (B) Simultaneous right and left ventricular pressure tracing. The systolic area index ([RV_{area}/LV_{area} ins]/[RV_{area}/LV_{area} exp]) is less than 1.1, indicating concordance. Concordance can be visualized on this tracing by the simultaneous increase in the LV and RV systolic pressures throughout the course of inspiration. Identification of concordance is consistent with restrictive cardiomyopathy. The left ventricular systolic (*), diastolic (A), and end-diastolic (arrow) pressures are marked. The left and right ventricular end-diastolic pressures are elevated.

Note: Exp = expiration; Ins = inspiration; LV = left ventricle; RV = right ventricle.

ventricle "dip-and-plateau" or "square root sign" (**Figure 16-4A**), which is caused by rapid early filling of the right ventricle during early diastole and early pressure equalization between the right atrium and right ventricle as a result of impaired myocardial relaxation.

In restrictive cardiomyopathies, such as amyloidosis, the right and left ventricles are limited in the amount of blood they can receive due to impaired relaxation. Since the pericardium is not constricting the heart, there is no interventricular dependence for volume within the pericardial sac. Additionally, the normal pericardial sac allows transmission of intrathoracic pressure to the heart. Therefore, the volume and pressure of the right and left ventricles will increase and decrease to similar degrees during inspiration and expiration. This is termed *concordance*. This is in contrast to the pressure tracing seen in constrictive pericarditis, which demonstrates *discordance*. Pressure changes in the right and left ventricle during inspiration and expiration move in opposite directions due to the constricting pericardial sac creating a fixed intrapericardial volume, which in turn raises interventricular dependence for volumes (5).

To assess for discordance and concordance, simultaneous pressure curves from the right and left ventricles are generated. The area under the curve (AUC) for each ventricle during one cardiac cycle can then be calculated (mmHg × second), allowing the calculation of a systolic area ratio: RV_{area}/LV_{area} during end-inspiration and end-expiration (**Figure 16-4B**). The ratio of systolic area during inspiration (RV_{area}/LV_{area} inspiration) divided by the systolic area ratio during expiration (RV_{area}/LV_{area} expiration) is termed the systolic area index. A systolic area index greater than 1.1 indicates discordance and has a 97% sensitivity and 100% specificity at distinguishing constrictive pericarditis from restrictive cardiomyopathy (6). Calculating the systolic area index is the hemodynamic gold standard for distinguishing these two disease processes.

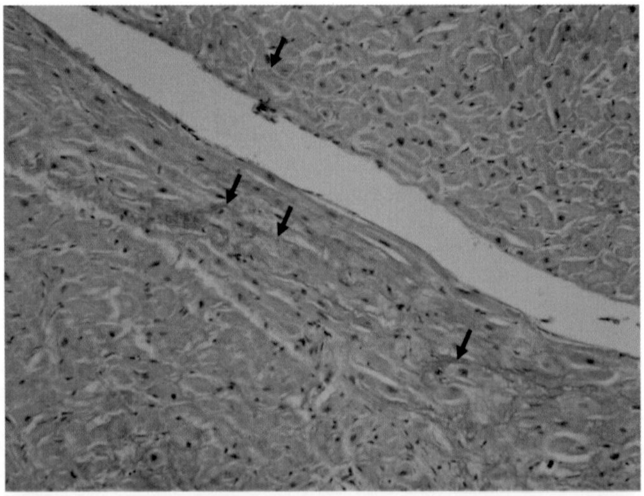

(A)

(B)

Figure 16-5
Endomyocardial biopsy viewed with light microscopy. (A) Staining with standard H and E reveals deposition of eosinophilic material between cardiac myocytes (arrows). (B) Congo red stained tissue viewed under polarized light reveals green birefringence of the extracellular material, consistent with cardiac amyloidosis.
Source: Images courtesy of Drs. Jose Torrealba and Ryan Gertz.

CASE PRESENTATION

Concordance between the right and left ventricular pressures is present, consistent with a restrictive cardiomyopathy. Therefore, a right ventricular endomyocardial biopsy is performed at the conclusion of the cardiac catheterization. Staining of the biopsy with hematoxylin and eosin (H&E) stain demonstrates disruption of the normal myofibril structure with eosinophilic staining of extracellular protein deposits. When stained with Congo red and viewed under polarized light, the extracellular protein has a green birefringence consistent with cardiac amyloidosis (**Figure 16-5**). Transmission electron microscopy demonstrates randomly arranged thin fibrils with an average diameter of 9.17 nm, also consistent with cardiac amyloidosis (**Figure 16-6**).

CLASSIFICATION OF AMYLOID HEART DISEASE

Conclusively establishing the diagnosis of amyloidosis requires documentation of the presence of systemic amyloid deposition. This can be diagnosed through biopsy of affected organs and documentation of amyloid deposits, usually through staining with Congo red and visualization under polarized light where amyloid depositions have a green birefringence. Transmission electron microscopy also allows direct visualization of the amyloid deposits.

In patients with suspected cardiac amyloidosis, an endomyocardial biopsy has the highest yield in making the diagnosis due to the diffuse infiltration of the myocardium with a sensitivity of 90% to 100% (7,8). Other possible biopsy sites include the abdominal fat pad, rectum, or bone marrow biopsy, though the sensitivity at these sites is considerably lower (9). Patients with a previous diagnosis of amyloidosis and hemodynamic findings suggestive of cardiac amyloid infiltration do not require an endomyocardial biopsy to confirm the diagnosis, but rather should be treated as though cardiac involvement is present.

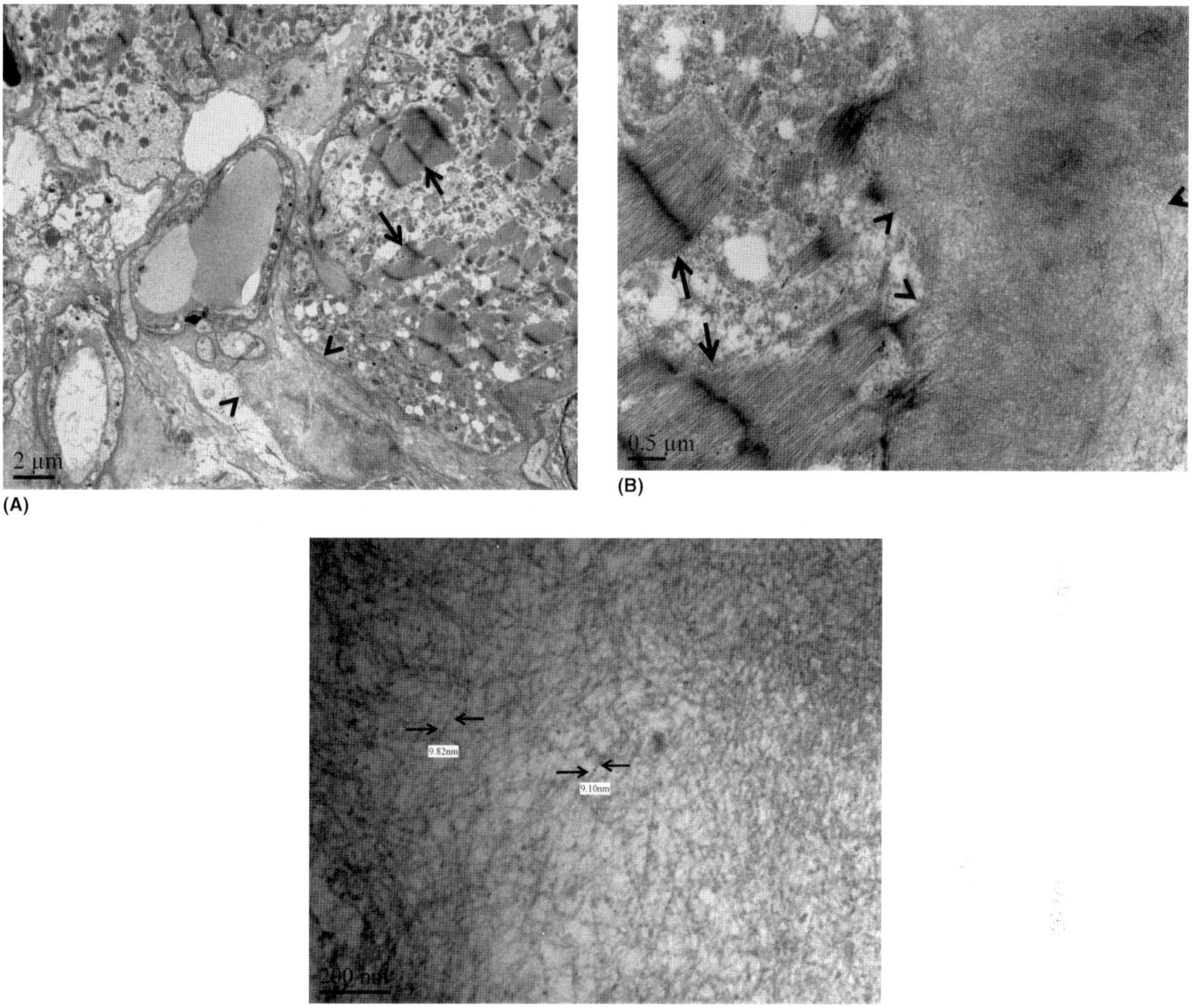

Figure 16-6
Endomyocardial biopsy viewed with transmission electron microscopy. The low (A) and medium (B) powered scans demonstrate extracellular protein deposition (arrowheads) resulting in cardiac myofibril (arrows) disruption characteristic of cardiac amyloidosis. The high power scan (C) shows randomly arranged thin fibrils. The nonbranching fibers (marked by arrows) have a diameter of 9.17 nm and are characteristic of amyloidosis. Amyloid fibers normally have a diameter between 7.5 and 10 nm.

Source: Images courtesy of Dr Jose Torrealba.

Amyloidosis refers to multiorgan infiltration by insoluble fibrillar protein deposits. The severity and type of symptoms present at the time of diagnosis is dependent upon which organs are involved in the disease. It is unusual for patients to present with only cardiac involvement (particularly with light chain amyloidosis [AL]), necessitating thorough work-up for other end-organ involvement once the diagnosis of cardiac amyloidosis has been made. The degree of other end-organ involvement, prognosis, and treatment options are dependent upon the type of amyloidosis present. There are generally four classes of amyloidosis that may manifest with cardiac involvement:

1. AL. Cardiac involvement in up to 50% of patients (10). Most commonly recognized cause of cardiac amyloidosis.
2. Hereditary amyloidosis. Variable cardiac involvement dependent upon the protein type and mutation present.
3. Senile amyloidosis. Nearly every patient over the age of 80 has cardiac senile amyloid

deposition. It is a generally a silent condition until extensive deposition results in clinical heart failure.

4. Secondary amyloidosis (AA). Cardiac involvement in less than 5% of cases (11).

Determining the type of amyloidosis can be accomplished through use of:

1. A thorough physical exam and lab examination to assess for organ involvement and damage (**Table 16-2**).
2. Family history to establish whether a heritable condition is present.
3. Performing immunofluorescence stains of the biopsied tissue to assess for monoclonal light chains.
4. Performing serum and urine protein immunofixation or serum-free light-chain-assay to assess for monoclonal protein bands, specifically assessing the kappa:lambda light-chain ratio. A ratio greater than 1.65 or less than 0.26 is diagnostic of excessive kappa and lambda light chain.
5. Performing bone marrow biopsy to assess for percentage clonal plasma cells, and evaluate for myeloma.
6. Performing DNA studies to assess for heritable amyloidosis mutations.

Systematic application of these tests allows determination of the type of amyloidosis present (**Figure 16-7**).

Table 16-2
Physical Exam and Laboratory Findings in Amyloidosis

Finding
Anasarca[a]
Hepatomegaly[a]
Macroglossia[a]
Diarrhea
Weight loss
Protein malnutrition[a]
Nausea
Gastroesophageal reflux disease
Abdominal pain
Peripheral neuropathy including carpel tunnel syndrome[a]
Autonomic dysfunction including urinary retention or incontinence (due to neuropathy), orthostatic hypotension (due to adrenal infiltration and neuropathy)[a]
Coagulopathy with periorbital purpura[a]
Proteinuria with nephrotic syndrome[a]

Note: The presence of any one symptom is dependent upon the type of amyloid present and end-organ involvement. It is not possible to determine the type of amyloidosis present through physical exam findings alone.
[a]Indicates findings frequently found in AL amyloidosis.

CASE PRESENTATION

Immunohistologic staining of the endomyocardial biopsy supports the diagnosis of AL amyloidosis. The serum-free light-chain assay has a kappa:lambda ratio of 1.9 confirming the diagnosis of AL amyloidosis. Subsequent bone marrow biopsy is positive for clonal plasma cells producing kappa light chains. Troponin I and N-terminal pro-B-type natriuretic peptide (NT-proBNP) levels are at 0.05 μg/L and 550 ng/L, respectively.

BIOMARKERS

Markers of myocardial damage and strain may be positive in patients with cardiac amyloidosis and can support whether cardiac amyloidosis is present (12). Additionally, these markers assist in prognostication on patient outcome. Troponin I levels greater than or equal to 0.1 μg/L and NT-proBNP levels greater than or equal to 332 ng/L are both associated with worse outcomes. Based on these biomarkers, a staging system has been established to assist in determining prognosis for patients who subsequently undergo peripheral blood stem cell transplantation (**Table 16-3**; 13). However, this staging system should not be used alone in determining treatment possibilities.

CASE PRESENTATION

For control of the patient's symptoms of heart failure, his diuretics are continued and the fluid and salt restriction recommendations are re-enforced. Despite the previous diagnosis of hypertension, the patient's blood pressure is now controlled off his angiotensin receptor blocker (ARB). Due to the aggressive nature and poor prognosis associated with cardiac amyloidosis, particularly when presenting with congestive heart failure (CHF), the patient is immediately referred to a hematologist for initiation of chemotherapy.

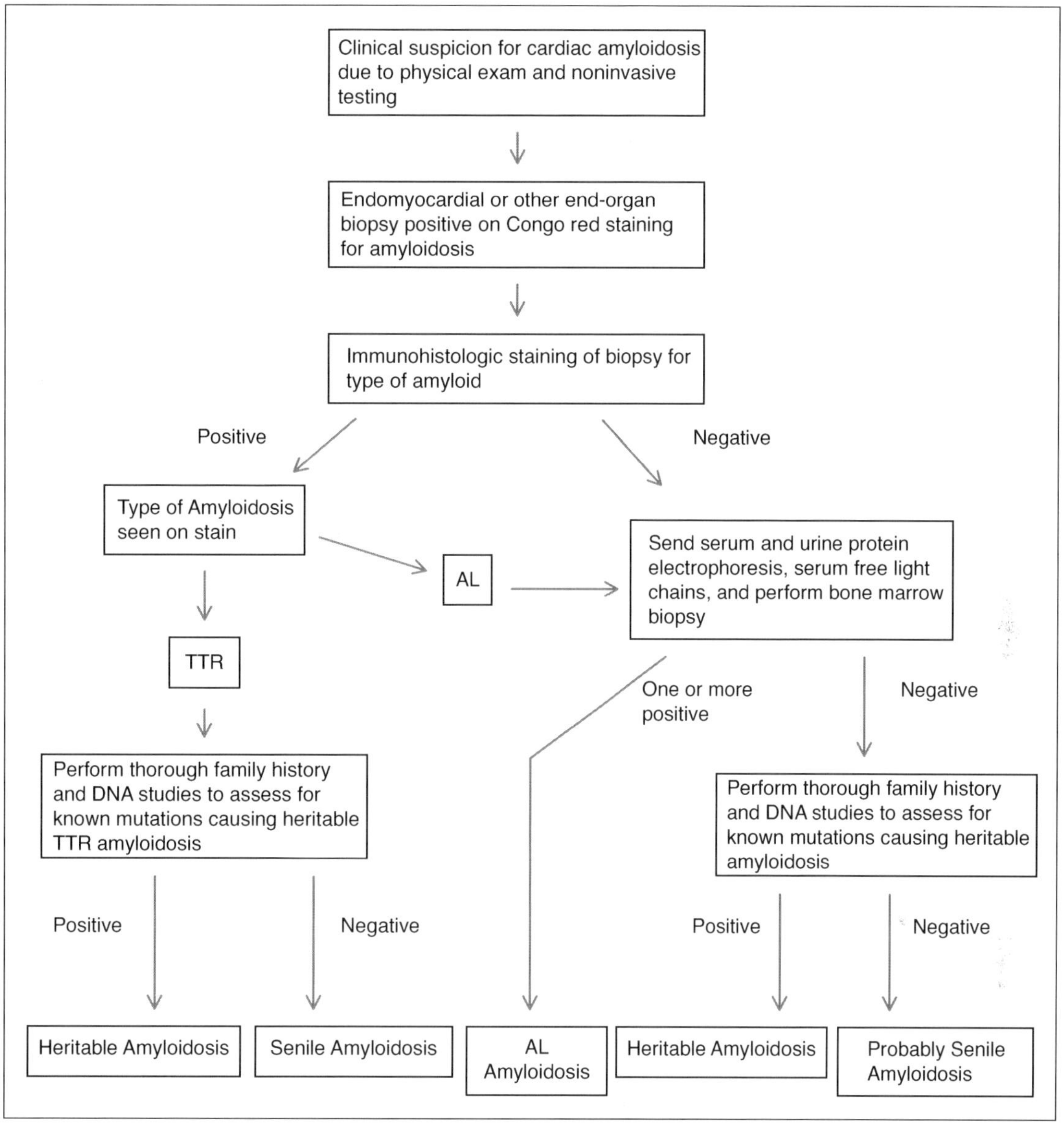

Figure 16-7
Work-up of newly diagnosed cardiac amyloidosis. In patients with previously diagnosed amyloidosis, the presence of a new restrictive cardiomyopathy indicates cardiac involvement and does not require endomyocardial biopsy.
Source: Adapted from reference 30.

Table 16-3
Survival in Cardiac Amyloidosis Following Peripheral Stem Cell Transplantation

STAGE	MEDIAN SURVIVAL (MONTHS)
I	27.2
II	11.1
III	4.1

Note: Stage I correlates with no elevation of either troponin I or NT-proBNP. Stage II correlates with elevation of either troponin I or NT-proBNP. Stage III correlates with elevation of both biomarkers (13).
NT-proBNP = N-terminal pro-brain natriuretic peptide.

DIAGNOSIS AND TREATMENT OF AL AMYLOIDOSIS

AL amyloidosis is the most common cause of cardiac amyloidosis, with cardiac infiltration affecting up to 50% of patients. The disease results when monoclonal light chains are over-produced due to inappropriate proliferation of plasma cells, resulting in systemic light chain deposition in β-pleated sheets and end-organ disruption.

The diagnosis of AL amyloidosis requires four criteria be met (14):

1. Presence of systemic amyloid deposit (within the kidney, liver, heart, gastrointestinal tract, peripheral nervous system, etc.)
2. Positive amyloid staining with Congo red in any tissue
3. Evidence that the amyloid is light chain-related (as opposed to another protein) by direct examination of the amyloid deposition (with immunohistochemical staining)
4. Evidence of monoclonal plasma cell proliferation via presence of a monoclonal protein band (M-band) in serum or urine, or clonal plasma cells on bone marrow biopsy

Cardiac deposition in AL amyloidosis occurs within the extracellular matrix of the heart, resulting in thickened myocardial wall and impaired relaxation. There is evidence that light chain deposition actually impairs myocardial systolic function, which may result in a slight reduction in ejection fraction (EF). This can improve with treatment. Deposition also disrupts the conduction system and contributes to the development of conduction delays and complete heart block. Amyloid deposits can also obstruct intramural coronary arteries and cause angina and myocardial infarction (MI). Epicardial artery involvement is rare. Valvular dysfunction rarely occurs from deposition on the valve leaflets, but thickening can be seen.

Treatment of patients with AL amyloidosis and CHF involves aggressive symptomatic treatment of the diastolic heart failure to allow definitive treatment of the amyloidosis. The severity of heart failure symptoms is often multifactorial, contributed to by increased right sided-filling pressures, low albumin from nephrotic syndrome and cardiac cachexia, and incomplete diuretic absorption due to intestinal edema. Maintaining an optimal fluid balance with fluid and salt restriction, coupled with high-dose diuretics, is the mainstay of heart failure therapy. Angiotensin-converting enzyme (ACE) inhibitor and beta-blockers should be used with extreme caution as they may result in severe hypotension. Due to autonomic nervous system dysfunction, amyloid patients are often reliant upon angiotensin for blood pressure maintenance. Blockage of ACE may therefore eliminate the patient's compensatory mechanism to maintain his or her blood pressure. Similarly, amyloid patients often rely on an increased pulse to maintain cardiac output as they develop reduced stroke volume. Use of beta-blockade may subsequently decrease cardiac output, resulting in hypotension. Digoxin and calcium-channel blockers should not be used due to preferential binding to amyloid fibers and increased myocardial concentrations (15,16).

If hypotension develops, it may be secondary to peripheral neuropathy and autonomic dysfunction, low cardiac output, or impaired peripheral vascular resistance. Similarly, auto correction of previous hypertension is frequently seen. If symptomatic autonomic dysfunction is present, treatment with midodrine (-agonist) can be effective.

Patients with amyloidosis are at risk for the development of thromboemboli as a result of atrial dysfunction and diminished atrial emptying from atrial amyloid infiltration, as well the thrombogenic nature of amyloid protein. Atrial stand-still demonstrated by a loss of a mitral inflow A-wave, loss of the mitral annular A-wave, and a sharply reduced or lost atrial reversal wave on pulmonary vein flow on echocardiography is therefore an indication for oral anticoagulation, even while maintaining an electrical sinus rhythm (17,18).

Treatment of AL amyloidosis requires chemotherapy directed at the plasma cell dyscrasia. Currently, treatment entails high-dose melphalan followed by autologous stem-cell transplant, with 10-year survival of 25%. Unfortunately, due to late presentation and advanced disease, only 20% to 25% of patients presenting with AL amyloidosis are eligible candidates for stem cell therapy (19). Response to stem cell transplant is particularly poor among patients with cardiac amyloidosis. An alternative regimen for patients not eligible for stem cell therapy includes use of melphalan with dexamethasone (19,20). Other agents currently under investigation include thalidomide, lenalidomide, or bortezomib (21).

CASE PRESENTATION

Six months after the initial diagnosis of cardiac amyloidosis and treatment initiation with melphalan and dexamethasone, the patient returns to clinic with a repeat echocardiogram. The left ventricular function has slightly improved to 55%, though the left and right ventricle walls remain thickened. A 12-lead ECG obtained at the time demonstrates progressive lengthening of the PR interval with widening of his QRS interval, a new right bundle branch block (RBBB), and occasional second-degree Type I atrioventricular (AV)-node block. The patient denies any syncopal episodes. Due to the rapidly progressive conduction dysfunction, a pacemaker is recommended without placement of an internal cardiac defibrillator.

TREATMENT OPTIONS

Patients with cardiac AL amyloidosis are at risk for sudden cardiac death, though it appears that a majority of those deaths are due to asystole and heart block from conduction system infiltration and electrical–mechanical dissociation rather than ventricular tachycardia or fibrillation (22). Therefore, prophylactic internal cardiac defibrillator placement is not recommended unless other indications, such as witnessed ventricular tachycardia, are present.

With evidence of rapidly progressive conduction system disease, the patient was at high risk for development of complete heart block.

CASE PRESENTATION

Despite placement of the pacemaker and chemotherapy, the patient's clinical condition continues to deteriorate with refractory right-sided heart failure symptoms and progressive neuropathy with autonomic dysfunction. He has rapidly reaccumulating, refractory pleural effusions due to amyloid infiltration into the pleural space requiring frequent drainage. Three months later, he enrolls in hospice and passes away several weeks later.

TREATMENT OF END-STAGE HEART FAILURE

Patients with cardiac involvement in AL amyloidosis have a poor prognosis, with a 4-year mortality of 80% (23). Patients who present with signs of heart failure have an even worse prognosis with a median survival of only 5 months (24), though these data were obtained from patients nearly two decades ago, before the introduction of modern chemotherapy. Predictors of sudden death include interventricular septum greater than 13 mm and the presence of couplets on Holter monitoring (25). More contemporary studies investigating the prognosis in patients with cardiac amyloidosis not eligible for stem cell therapy found a median survival of 10.5 months (26).

Mechanical support with left (27) or right (28) ventricular assist devices as destination therapy may offer palliation for patients suffering from debilitating restrictive cardiomyopathy and heart failure symptoms, though it is unclear whether this improves survival.

Cardiac transplantation for treatment of cardiac AL amyloidosis appears to offer improved survival compared with those who do not undergo cardiac transplant, though experience in this area is limited. At this time, patients considered for cardiac transplantation include those with amyloidosis limited to the heart without additional end-organ dysfunction or malnutrition (less than 5% of all patient presenting with AL amyloidosis; 10,11). Chemotherapy followed by autologous stem cell transplant should be performed within 6 months to 1 year of cardiac transplantation to avoid further amyloid deposition systematically or within the transplanted heart (29). Additional characterization of who may benefit from cardiac transplant, as well as the optimal protocol, is unclear due to the limited number of patients who have undergone this procedure.

REFERENCES

1. Rahman JE, Helou EF, Gelzer-Bell R, et al. Noninvasive diagnosis of biopsy-proven cardiac amyloidosis. *J Am Coll Cardiol.* 2004;43(3):410–415.
2. Maceira AM, Joshi J, Prasad SK, et al. Cardiovascular magnetic resonance in cardiac amyloidosis. *Circulation.* 2005;111(2):186–193.
3. Syed IS, Glockner JF, Feng D, et al. Role of cardiac magnetic resonance imaging in the detection of cardiac amyloidosis. *JACC Cardiovasc Imaging.* 2010;3(2):155–164.
4. Rapezzi C, Merlini G, Quarta CC, et al. Systemic cardiac amyloidoses: disease profiles and clinical courses of the 3 main types. *Circulation.* 2009;120(13):1203–1212.
5. Hurrell DG, Nishimura RA, Higano ST, et al. Value of dynamic respiratory changes in left and right ventricular pressures for the diagnosis of constrictive pericarditis. *Circulation.* 1996;93(11):2007–2013.
6. Talreja DR, Nishimura RA, Oh JK, Holmes DR. Constrictive pericarditis in the modern era: novel criteria for diagnosis in the cardiac catheterization laboratory. *J Am Coll Cardiol.* 2008;51(3):315–319.
7. Arbustini E, Merlini G, Gavazzi A, et al. Cardiac immunocyte-derived (AL) amyloidosis: an endomyocardial biopsy study in 11 patients. *Am Heart J.* 1995;130(3 Pt 1):528–536.
8. Pellikka PA, Holmes DR Jr, Edwards WD, Nishimura RA, Tajik AJ, Kyle RA. Endomyocardial biopsy in 30 patients with primary amyloidosis and suspected cardiac involvement. *Arch Intern Med.* 1988;148(3):662–666.
9. Shah KB, Inoue Y, Mehra MR. Amyloidosis and the heart: a comprehensive review. *Arch Intern Med.* 2006;166(17):1805–1813.
10. Dubrey SW, Cha K, Anderson J, et al. The clinical features of immunoglobulin light-chain (AL) amyloidosis with heart involvement. *QJM.* 1998;91(2):141–157.
11. Dubrey SW, Cha K, Simms RW, Skinner M, Falk RH. Electrocardiography and Doppler echocardiography in secondary (AA) amyloidosis. *Am J Cardiol.* 1996;77(4):313–315.
12. Palladini G, Campana C, Klersy C, et al. Serum N-terminal pro-brain natriuretic peptide is a sensitive marker of myocardial dysfunction in AL amyloidosis. *Circulation.* 2003;107(19):2440–2445.

13. Dispenzieri A, Gertz MA, Kyle RA, et al. Prognostication of survival using cardiac troponins and N-terminal pro-brain natriuretic peptide in patients with primary systemic amyloidosis undergoing peripheral blood stem cell transplantation. *Blood.* 2004;104(6):1881–1887.

14. Kyle RA, Rajkumar SV. Criteria for diagnosis, staging, risk stratification and response assessment of multiple myeloma. *Leukemia.* 2009;23(1):3–9.

15. Pollak A, Falk RH. Left ventricular systolic dysfunction precipitated by verapamil in cardiac amyloidosis. *Chest.* 1993;104(2):618–620.

16. Rubinow A, Skinner M, Cohen AS. Digoxin sensitivity in amyloid cardiomyopathy. *Circulation.* 1981;63(6):1285–1288.

17. Dubrey S, Pollak A, Skinner M, Falk RH. Atrial thrombi occurring during sinus rhythm in cardiac amyloidosis: evidence for atrial electromechanical dissociation. *Br Heart J.* 1995;74(5):541–544.

18. Feng D, Syed IS, Martinez M, et al. Intracardiac thrombosis and anticoagulation therapy in cardiac amyloidosis. *Circulation.* 2009;119(18):2490–2497.

19. Gertz MA. Immunoglobulin light chain amyloidosis: 2011 update on diagnosis, risk-stratification, and management. *Am J Hematol.* 2011;86(2):180–186.

20. Jaccard A, Moreau P, Leblond V, et al.; Myélome Autogreffe (MAG) and Intergroupe Francophone du Myélome (IFM) Intergroup. High-dose melphalan versus melphalan plus dexamethasone for AL amyloidosis. *N Engl J Med.* 2007;357(11):1083–1093.

21. Cohen AD, Comenzo RL. Systemic light-chain amyloidosis: advances in diagnosis, prognosis, and therapy. *Hematology Am Soc Hematol Educ Program.* 2010;2010:287–294.

22. Kristen AV, Dengler TJ, Hegenbart U, et al. Prophylactic implantation of cardioverter-defibrillator in patients with severe cardiac amyloidosis and high risk for sudden cardiac death. *Heart Rhythm.* 2008;5(2):235–240.

23. Felker GM, Thompson RE, Hare JM, et al. Underlying causes and long-term survival in patients with initially unexplained cardiomyopathy. *N Engl J Med.* 2000;342(15):1077–1084.

24. Kyle RA, Gertz MA, Greipp PR, et al. A trial of three regimens for primary amyloidosis: colchicine alone, melphalan and prednisone, and melphalan, prednisone, and colchicine. *N Engl J Med.* 1997;336(17):1202–1207.

25. Palladini G, Malamani G, Cò F, et al. Holter monitoring in AL amyloidosis: prognostic implications. *Pacing Clin Electrophysiol.* 2001;24(8 Pt 1):1228–1233.

26. Lebovic D, Hoffman J, Levine BM, et al. Predictors of survival in patients with systemic light-chain amyloidosis and cardiac involvement initially ineligible for stem cell transplantation and treated with oral melphalan and dexamethasone. *Br J Haematol.* 2008;143(3):369–373.

27. Siegenthaler MP, Westaby S, Frazier OH, et al. Advanced heart failure: feasibility study of long-term continuous axial flow pump support. *Eur Heart J.* 2005;26(10):1031–1038.

28. Krabatsch T, Potapov E, Stepanenko A, et al. Biventricular circulatory support with two miniaturized implantable assist devices. *Circulation.* 2011;124(11 Suppl):S179–S186.

29. Kristen AV, Sack FU, Schonland SO, et al. Staged heart transplantation and chemotherapy as a treatment option in patients with severe cardiac light-chain amyloidosis. *Eur J Heart Fail.* 2009;11(10):1014–1020.

30. Falk RH. Diagnosis and management of the cardiac amyloidoses. *Circulation.* 2005;112(13):2047–2060.

31. Ha JW, Ommen SR, Tajik AJ, et al. Differentiation of constrictive pericarditis from restrictive cardiomyopathy using mitral annular velocity by tissue Doppler echocardiography. *Am J Cardiol.* 2004;94(3):316–319.

32. Rajagopalan N, Garcia MJ, Rodriguez L, et al. Comparison of new Doppler echocardiographic methods to differentiate constrictive pericardial heart disease and restrictive cardiomyopathy. *Am J Cardiol.* 2001;87(1):86–94.

17

Left Ventricular Dysfunction and Associated Renal Failure: The Cardiorenal Syndrome

DAVID MURRAY

INTRODUCTION

The following case report illustrates the challenges of trying to facilitate volume removal in a congested patient with impaired renal function and diuretic refractoriness. The precise mechanisms responsible for the development of "cardiorenal" syndrome and worsening renal function are not known. Intrinsic renal disease, hemodynamic perturbations, increased central venous pressure (CVP), increased intra-abdominal pressure (IAP), and neurohormonal activation have been implicated (1–6).

The three most common causes for chronic kidney disease in our society are diabetic nephropathy, hypertension-induced nephrosclerosis, and atherosclerosis (4). Our patient did not have a history of diabetes or hypertension. Moreover, his urinalysis was bland without proteinuria, essentially ruling out glomerulonephritis and acute tubular necrosis. His renal ultrasound did not demonstrate hydronephrosis to suggest obstruction or cortical thinning to suggest repetitive ischemic insults and/or parenchymal kidney disease. Thus, our patient was felt to have a very good chance at achieving renal recovery with improvement in his hemodynamic profile.

CASE PRESENTATION

Mr. R is a 47-year-old male with severe ischemic dilated cardiomyopathy status post prior multivessel coronary artery bypass grafting (CABG) in 2000 and a repeat CABG in April 2004. His left ventricular systolic function was profoundly depressed (left ventricular ejection fraction [LVEF] less than 15%) despite reasonable beta-blockade (carvedilol 12.5 mg BID) and surgical revascularization. In addition, he had been troubled by paroxysmal atrial fibrillation; this had been treated with multiple direct current (DC) cardioversions and ultimately atrioventricular (AV) nodal ablation with implantation of a biventricular implantable cardioverter-defibrillator (ICD). He was able to maintain sinus rhythm with amiodarone. Despite aggressive treatment with loop (torsemide 100 mg daily), thiazide (metolazone 2.5 mg three times per week), and potassium sparing (spironolactone 25 mg daily) diuretics, Mr. R continued to have difficulty with volume overload. His diuretic refractoriness was felt to be related to both impaired absorption in the setting of gut edema and renal dysfunction (baseline creatinine [Cr] approximately 2.5 mg/dL). He was sent to our facility for management of his acute-on-chronic systolic heart failure and for consideration of advanced heart failure therapies.

At the time of admission on May 17, 2007, Mr. R was quite ill. He complained of daily paroxysmal nocturnal dyspnea, nonproductive cough, dyspnea with activities of daily living, and generalized fatigue. His sleep was disrupted by restlessness and anxiety. To be able to sleep, he had to sit upright in a chair. He could not walk more than 20 feet before needing to stop to rest. His appetite was poor and he was troubled by abdominal bloating and early satiety. He did not have nausea or vomiting.

On physical assessment, Mr. R was a cachectic, chronically ill appearing individual with a pale, grey complexion. He was short of breath at rest while sitting upright and he became dyspneic with conversation. His blood pressure was 117/82 mmHg with a heart rate of 70 beats/minute. Sclera were nonicteric and conjunctiva were pink. Lung exam was notable for diminished breath sounds and dullness to percussion at the bases with crackles approximately one third up the posterior thorax. He did not have any rhonchi or wheezes. On cardiac exam, he had a regular rate and rhythm with normal S1, loud P2, and a summation gallop. A grade 3/6 systolic murmur was heard at the left sternal border that increased with inspiration. He also had a Grade 3/6 holosystolic murmur at the apex. His jugular venous waveform had an accentuated "V" wave and right atrial pressure was estimated at greater than 20 mmHg. Kussmaul's sign was present and hepatojugular reflux was sustained. Mr. R's abdomen was protuberant with a fluid wave consistent with a large amount of ascites. His liver was enlarged and firm without nodularity. The abdominal wall and flanks were edematous. His lower extremities had marked, tense edema extending into the upper thighs. Capillary refill and pedal pulses were diminished.

Electrocardiogram (ECG) demonstrated an AV paced rhythm at 72 beats/minute. Chest x-ray was notable for cardiomegaly, hilar fullness, vascular redistribution, interstitial edema, and small bilateral effusions. Laboratory assessment revealed hyponatremia (Na^+ 121 mmol/L), hypokalemia (K^+ 3.6 mmol/L), metabolic alkalosis (bicarbonate 32 mmol/L), and renal insufficiency (blood urea nitrogen [BUN] 48 mg/dL, Cr 2.6 mg/dL). He had mild normocytic, normochromic anemia (hemoglobin 12.1 gm/dL), and thrombocytopenia (122K). Liver enzymes were normal and his bilirubin was mildly elevated at 1.3 mg/dL. Albumin was 4.3 g/dL, prealbumin 32.8 mg/dL. BNP was markedly elevated at 5,224 pg/mL. Urinalysis was bland. International normalized ratio (INR) was elevated at 5.1, reflective of warfarin-based anticoagulation for stroke prophylaxis coupled with impaired metabolism in the setting of hepatic congestion. Thyroid-stimulating hormone (TSH) was elevated at 12.59 mcIU/mL with free T4 1.1 ng/dL and free T3 56 ng/dL. His levothyroxine dose was increased from 25 mcg to 50 mcg daily.

Mr. R was perceived to have marked biventricular heart failure in the setting of profound left ventricular systolic dysfunction with superimposed severe mitral and tricuspid regurgitation. He had severe lower extremity edema, tense ascites, and interstitial pulmonary edema. His peripheral perfusion was felt to be impaired.

CASE PRESENTATION

Our initial treatment interventions were standard for the management of decompensated heart failure. As Mr. R was hyponatremic, his free water intake was limited to 500 mL daily (total fluid intake 1.5 L daily). Dietary sodium was restricted to 2 g/day as his total body sodium was deemed to be excessive. On the first day, he was given a bolus of IV furosemide 100 mg followed by a continuous infusion at a relatively low dose of 5 mg/hour.

DIURETIC THERAPY

IV loop diuretics are the mainstay of therapy for volume overload occurring in the setting of acute decompensated heart failure (ADHF; 7). Loop diuretics relieve dyspnea, reduce congestion, and decrease ventricular filling pressure. Diuresis may improve kidney function, possibly through alleviation of venous and/or abdominal congestion (see below; 1,3,7). Moreover, successful removal of excess fluid can enhance cardiac function and output via reductions in ventricular wall stress, improved subendocardial perfusion, and decreased AV valve regurgitation. Increases in cardiac output, in turn, may lead to increased glomerular filtration rate (GFR) via enhanced renal blood flow (RBF; **Figure 17-1**; 1,3,6–8).

That being said, diuretic therapy can worsen renal function in some patients. Unfortunately, we do not have any clinical or laboratory predictors to determine if a patient's renal function will improve or worsen with diuretic therapy. Overly aggressive diuresis can lead to intravascular volume depletion (arterial underfilling), resulting in hypotension, systemic vasoconstriction, reduced cardiac output, diminished GFR, and further impairment of renal function (2,3,7). In particular, these adverse effects may occur in a patient treated with conventional therapeutic agents used to treat heart failure such as angiotensin converting enzyme (ACE) inhibitors, angiotensin receptor blockers (ARBs), and vasodilators. Furthermore, diuretics promote neurohormonal activation (8,9). Volume contraction stimulates the secretion of renin from the juxtaglomerular apparatus and activates the sympathetic nervous system (SNS) via aortic arch and carotid sinus baroreceptors. Decreased atrial and ventricular stretch can suppress counterregulatory natriuretic peptide release. Also, loop diuretics augment renin secretion via two volume-independent mechanisms: (a) inhibition of sodium chloride uptake into the macula densa cells directly stimulates renin release (10), and (b) renal production of prostacyclin is enhanced, further promoting renin secretion (3). Clearly, diuretic management involves a delicate balance; the diuretic dose must be sufficient to effectively remove excess fluid without prompting adverse physiologic effects.

Diuretics (especially high-dose diuretics) have been associated with increased mortality in patients with heart failure. In the Studies of Left Ventricular Dysfunction (SOLVD) trial, the risk of hospitalization or death due to worsening heart failure was significantly increased in patients receiving non-potassium sparing diuretics compared with those not receiving

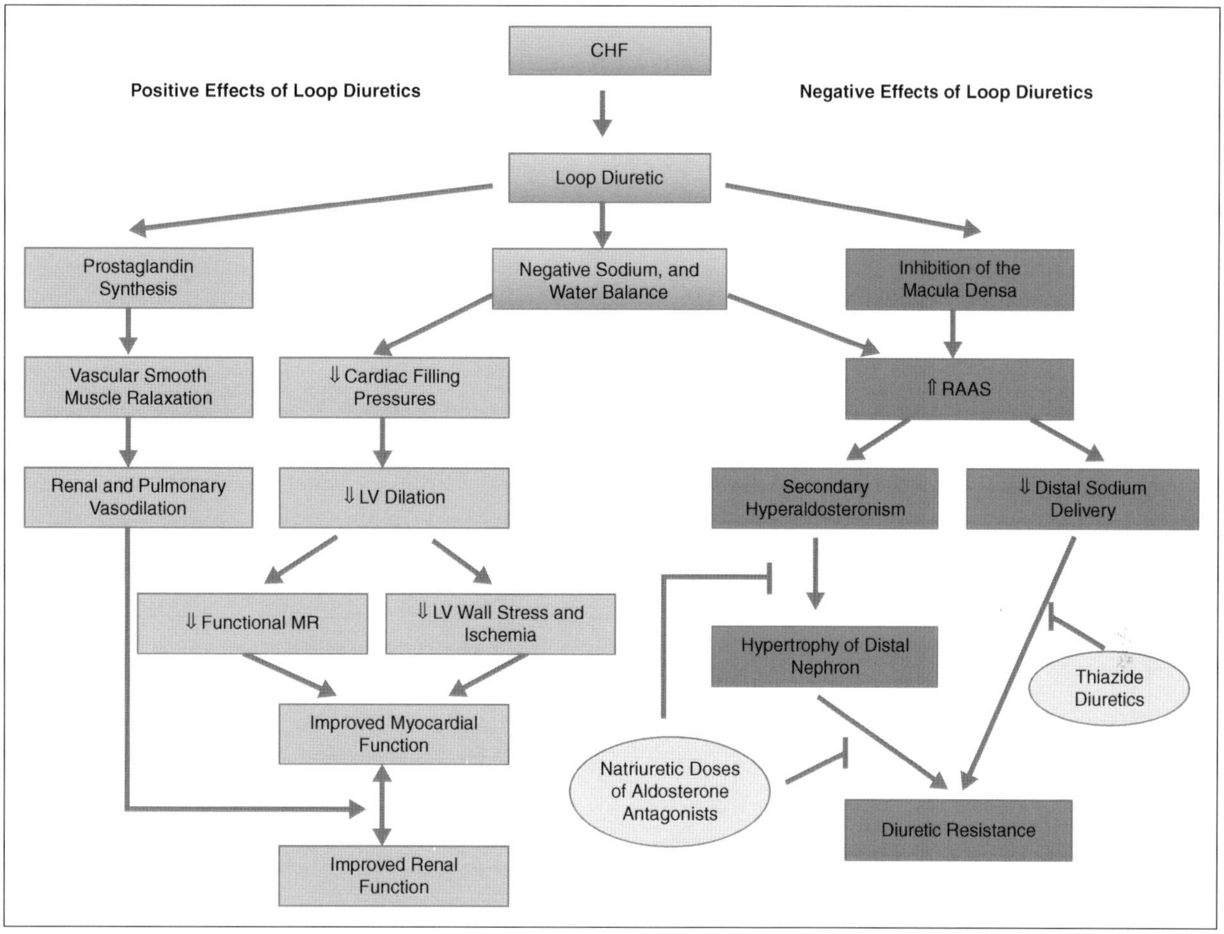

Figure 17-1
Mechanisms of diuretics. Positive and negative physiologic effects of loop diuretics as well as sites of action for thiazide diuretics and aldosterone antagonists.

Note: CHF = congestive heart failure; LV = left ventricular; MR = mitral regurgitation; RAAS = renin–angiotensin–aldosterone system.

Reprinted from Felker and Mentz (16) and adapted from Schrier (8) with permission from Elsevier.

diuretics (risk ratio, 1.31; 95% confidence interval [CI], 1.09–1.57; *P* = .0004; 11). In the Prospective Randomized Amlodipine Survival Evaluation (PRAISE) trial, use of high-dose diuretics was associated with increased total mortality (hazard ratio [HR], 1.37; *P* = .042), sudden death (HR, 1.39; *P* = .034), and pump failure death (HR, 1.51; *P* = .034; 12). Whether requiring higher doses of diuretics is merely a marker of more severe heart failure or whether higher doses of loop diuretics are contributing to adverse heart failure outcomes, perhaps via electrolyte imbalances (hyponatremia, hypokalemia, hypomagnesemia) and/or neurohormonal activation, is not known (13).

Loop diuretics, including furosemide, bumetanide, and torsemide, act by reversibly binding to and reversibly inhibiting the action of the Na^+-K^+-$2Cl^-$ cotransporter, thereby preventing salt transport out of the thick ascending loop of Henle (**Figure 17-2**). By inhibiting the concentration of solute within the medullary interstitium, loop diuretics reduce the driving force for water resorption in the collecting duct, even in the presence of antidiuretic hormone. The increase in delivery of Na^+ and water to the distal nephron markedly enhances potassium excretion, particularly in the presence of increased aldosterone. Loop diuretics are bound extensively to plasma proteins so delivery of these drugs to the tubule by filtration is limited. To gain access to the intraluminal-binding site on the Na^+-K^+-$2Cl^-$ cotransporter, these drugs are secreted by the organic acid transport system in the proximal tubule. Thus, the efficacy of loop diuretics is dependent on sufficient renal plasma blood flow and proximal tubular secretion to ensure delivery of these drugs to their site of action (14).

Although loop diuretics are commonly given by intermittent IV bolus, continuous infusion may have

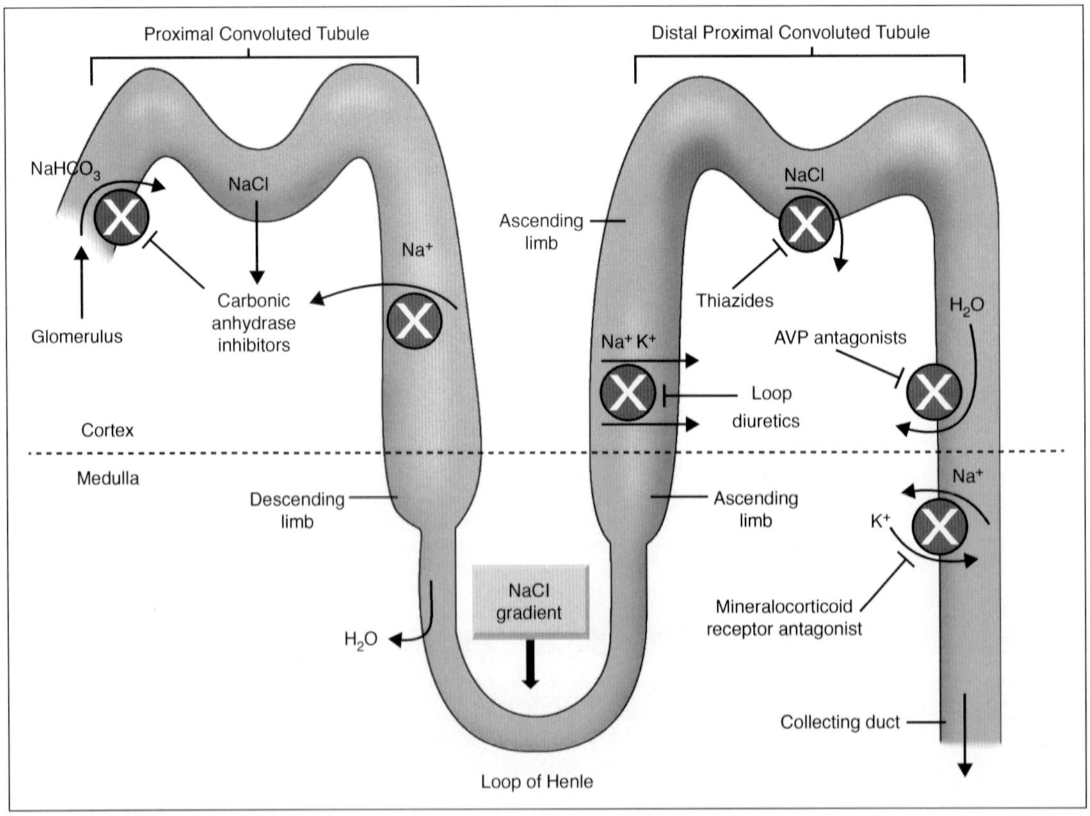

Figure 17-2
Sites of action of diuretics in the kidney.
Note: AVP = arginine vasopressin.
Source: Reprinted from Mann (14) with permission from Elsevier.

potential benefits. Theoretically, constant delivery of diuretic to the renal tubules could reduce postdiuretic "rebound" sodium retention and facilitate diuresis (7). Moreover, this strategy may reduce the rapidity of volume removal from the arterial space thereby preventing hypotension, sympathetic activation and worsening renal function. Indeed, a meta-analysis suggested greater urine output, shorter length of hospital stay, less renal impairment, and lower mortality rate in patients treated with a continuous loop diuretic infusion rather than an IV bolus-based approach (15). However, these findings were not confirmed in the recently published Diuretic Optimization Strategies Evaluation (DOSE) trial (16).

The DOSE trial was conceived to determine whether dose and method of loop diuretic administration influenced patient symptoms, volume removal, and renal function. Patients (n = 308) hospitalized with ADHF were randomly assigned to either a low-dose strategy (total IV furosemide dose equal to their daily oral loop diuretic dose in furosemide equivalents) or a high-dose strategy (total daily IV furosemide dose 2.5 times their total daily oral loop diuretic dose in furosemide equivalents). The "low-dose" and "high-dose" patients were then further randomized to receive their furosemide either by IV bolus every 12 hours or by continuous IV infusion. The study treatment was concealed and continued for up to 72 hours.

The strategy of continuous IV furosemide therapy did not confer additional benefit versus bolus-based IV therapy across a broad range of efficacy (dyspnea, freedom from congestion, change in weight, net fluid loss) and safety (worsening heart failure, increasing Cr greater than 0.03 mg/dL, death) endpoints. With respect to the comparison of the low-dose strategy versus the high-dose strategy, there was no significant difference in either of the coprimary endpoints of global assessment of symptoms or change in serum Cr over 72 hours. However, the high-dose strategy was associated with greater relief from dyspnea and more effective fluid and weight loss, albeit with a greater proportion of patients suffering from an increase in Cr greater than 0.3 mg/dL (23% of the patients in the high-dose group as compared with 14% in the low-dose group, $P = .04$). Although worsening of renal function occurred more frequently with the high-dose strategy in the short term, this did not lead to worsened clinical outcomes (death, rehospitalization, or emergency department visits) at 60 days. Thus, the method in which diuretics are administered (IV bolus vs. continuous IV) does not appear to influence efficacy of volume removal or renal function in patients with ADHF and moderate renal dysfunction. Conversely, administration of high-dose IV loop diuretics can more effectively alleviate dyspnea and remove volume, though with the potential cost of transient worsening of renal function (16).

Mr. R was severely hyponatremic. To treat his electrolyte abnormality, he was placed on a strict free water limitation and loop diuretics were used to eliminate excess water. Undoubtedly, our patient had marked increases in circulating arginine vasopressin (AVP). AVP is normally suppressed by hypo-osmolality. In heart failure, AVP secretion is markedly increased even in the setting of hyponatremia, secondary to nonosmotic baroreceptor-mediated release of the hormone (2). AVP stimulates the V1a receptors of vascular smooth muscle, resulting in arterial and venous vasoconstriction. In addition, AVP activates the V2 receptor on the basolateral surface of cells in the collecting ducts (**Figure 17-2**), resulting in expression and trafficking of the aquaporin 2 water channel to the apical surface (2). Consequently, water is reabsorbed. By virtue of increased plasma volume and venoconstriction, AVP increases cardiac preload, which can increase cardiac output and renal perfusion. Conversely, AVP-mediated arterial vasoconstriction increases afterload on the compromised heart, leading to a decrease in stroke volume. The influence of AVP on loading conditions of the heart can influence further remodeling of the myocardium.

Selective V1a antagonists block the vasoconstricting effects of AVP and V2 antagonists such as tolvaptan reduce the ability of the collecting duct to reabsorb water, preventing dilutional hyponatremia. Tolvaptan increases free water excretion and plasma osmolality, reduces body weight, improves symptoms of congestion, and modestly increases serum sodium concentrations. However, the results of the Efficacy of Vasopressin Antagonism in Heart Failure Outcome Study With Tolvaptan (EVEREST) trial demonstrated that adding oral tolvaptan (30 mg daily) to standard IV diuretic therapy in patients hospitalized with ADHF, followed by daily therapy after discharge, had no significant effect on the composite endpoint of cardiovascular death or hospitalization for heart failure (17). Conceivably, this drug may have increased our patient's serum sodium concentration but this treatment would not have influenced clinically important outcomes.

CASE PRESENTATION

To reduce the afterload stress on his compromised ventricles, nesiritide was infused at 0.01 mcg/kg/minute. His outpatient heart failure-related therapy (carvedilol 12.5 mg BID, amiodarone 150 mg daily, spironolactone 25 mg daily) was continued. He had not been on an ACE inhibitor or an ARB as an outpatient due to his kidney disease. As he did not make much clinical progress after the first day in the hospital, he was given another IV furosemide 100 mg bolus and his continuous drip was increased to 10 mg/hour. Nesiritide was increased to 0.02 mcg/kg/minute. After approximately 48 hours in the hospital, Mr. R's clinical status had not improved. While measures of his inputs and outputs suggested that 4 L had been removed, his weight had actually increased 0.8 kg. His symptoms and exam remained unchanged. Hyponatremia (Na^+ 121 mmol/L) and renal dysfunction (BUN/Cr 45/2.5) persisted. Nesiritide was discontinued.

NESIRITIDE THERAPY

The vasodilator nesiritide was used to reduce preload and afterload stress on his ventricles, with the intent of reducing AV valve regurgitation, augmenting cardiac output, and improving renal perfusion (18). Nesiritide is also a weak natriuretic and diuretic (18). In severe heart failure, characterized by extremely high renal vascular resistance (caused by neurohormonal activation) and markedly diminished RBF, GFR drops precipitously without further increase in filtration fraction (1). If Mr. R's renal dysfunction were to be secondary to poor cardiac output and excessive vasoconstriction, this approach should have led to improved renal function and diuretic responsiveness. In his case, this drug did not help, even at higher doses, so it was abandoned.

Nesiritide has Food and Drug Administration (FDA) approval for early relief of dyspnea in patients with acute heart failure. Yet, meta-analyses of small studies have suggested that this agent may worsen renal function and increase mortality (19,20). To address these concerns, Acute Study of Clinical Effectiveness of Nesiritide in Decompensated Heart Failure (ASCEND-HF) randomly assigned 7,141 patients with ADHF to receive either nesiritide or placebo for 24 to 168 hours in addition to standard care (21). Nesiritide did not lead to a significant reduction in self-reported dyspnea at 6 and 24 hours after treatment. The rate of rehospitalization for heart failure or death from any cause within 30 days was not statistically different. Nesiritide was not associated with worsening of renal function but it was associated with an increase in rates of hypotension (21). On the basis of these results (published 4 years after our patient's index hospitalization), nesiritide cannot be recommended for routine use in the broad population of patients with acute heart failure. The study did not address whether nesiritide is safe and effective in patients such as ours with impaired renal function (the median serum Cr in ASCEND-HF was 1.2 mg/dL).

Alternatively, we could have used other vasodilators in this clinical setting such as IV nitroglycerin, oral nitrates, hydralazine, ACE inhibitors, and ARBs. We elected not to use an oral vasodilator (nitrates, hydralazine) early in the course of his hospitalization due to concerns regarding effective absorption in a patient with visceral edema and the possibility of inducing sustained hypotension. IV vasodilators such as nesiritide and nitroglycerin are relatively short acting and can be titrated with less hemodynamic risk. Agents that block production (ACE inhibitors) and biologic effects (ARBs) of angiotensin II were avoided for fear of reducing GFR in a patient with diuretic refractoriness and pre-existing renal dysfunction.

CASE PRESENTATION

Mr. R was started on milrinone 0.25 mcg/kg/minute. IV chlorothiazide was added at 250 mg BID. Over the next day, his inputs and outputs were essentially matched and his weight increased another 0.4 kg.

MILRINONE THERAPY

Conceivably nesiritide failed as a consequence of Mr. R having inadequate cardiac reserve. In response to arterial vasodilation, his cardiac output may not have increased enough to meaningfully improve renal perfusion. Our next approach was to use inodilator therapy, initially with milrinone. Milrinone is a potent phosphodiesterase inhibitor. This drug increases myocyte intracellular cyclic adenosine monophosphate (c-AMP) levels by preventing its degradation. C-AMP is the secondary messenger responsible for activating protein kinase A, which in turn phosphoylates key calcium regulatory proteins responsible for enhancing inotropy and lusitropy. This drug is also a powerful pulmonary and systemic arterial dilator. Given that milrinone does not act via the beta-adrenergic receptor, this drug can circumvent the pharmacologic influences of beta-receptor blockade, in this case, carvedilol. If the myocardium has enough contractile reserve, milrinone increases cardiac output, reduces cardiac filling pressures, and decreases pulmonary and systemic arterial resistance.

From a pathophysiologic standpoint, milrinone should have been helpful. Traditionally, worsening renal function in the setting of decompensated heart failure has been attributed to impaired renal perfusion resulting from low cardiac output and arterial underfilling (2,22). Changes in cardiac output of approximately 25% lead to a reduction in RBF by 50% (22). Autoregulation of afferent and efferent glomerular arteriole vasomotor tone can preserve GFR via an increase in filtration fraction except at very low RBF values (22). We would have expected milrinone to improve RBF and GFR. As loop diuretic effectiveness is dependent upon GFR, an augmented response to furosemide was expected. In this case, milrinone was ineffective for 24 hours, even after the addition of low dose IV chlorothiazide (diuretic strategies are discussed below).

CASE PRESENTATION

In the hopes of promoting more vigorous diuresis, carvedilol was decreased to 6.25 mg BID and milrinone was replaced with IV dobutamine 5 mcg/kg/minute. IV furosemide was discontinued and instead he was given an IV bumetanide 3 mg bolus followed by a continuous drip at 2 mg/hour. IV chlorothiazide was changed to 1 g daily. With the aforementioned changes in his medical regimen, he began to effectively diurese. Over the next 24 hours, he lost 3.8 kg of fluid. Serum sodium improved a bit to 124 mmol/L, his BUN declined from 47 mg/dL to 41 mg/dL, and his Cr dropped from 2.6 mg/dL to 2.2 mg/dL. Given the profound drop in his serum potassium to 2.7 mmol/dL, IV chlorothiazide was discontinued and his bumetanide drip was decreased to 0.5 mg/hour. Potassium was aggressively supplemented. Dobutamine was maintained at 5 mcg/kg/minute. This regimen was quite effective over the next couple of days. Another 2.5 kg of fluid were removed. Serum sodium increased to 126 mmol/L and his BUN and Cr declined to 27 mg/dL and 1.6 mg/dL, respectively. His urine output began to taper so IV chlorothiazide was reinstated, initially at 250 mg daily, then increased to 500 mg twice daily. His weight dropped another 1.8 kg over 2 days but his serum sodium dropped to 124 mmol/L and his BUN and Cr increased to 30 mg/dL and 1.8 mg/dL, respectively.

DOBUTAMINE/DOPAMINE THERAPY

Like milrinone, dobutamine enhances myocardial contractility and relaxation. In addition, this drug has chronotropic properties and it is an arterial vasodilator. Dobutamine increases myocyte intracellular c-AMP via beta-adrenergic receptor occupancy, G-protein signaling, and activation of the effector enzyme adenyl cyclase. Mr. R seemingly responded to this drug better than milrinone. However, Mr. R's improved diuretic responsiveness and renal function was not necessarily attributable to the change in inotropic therapy. At the same time that he was started on dobutamine, he also received very high-dose IV bumetanide and adjunctive high-dose IV chlorothiazide. The change in diuretic strategy alone may have accounted for his improved diuretic responsiveness.

Although inodilators such as dobutamine and milrinone can significantly augment cardiac output, their effect on renal hemodynamics as well as on urine output in patients with ADHF has not been significantly investigated (23). Anecdotally, some but not all patients with very low cardiac output states have had improvements in diuretic responsiveness and renal function with inotropic support. That being said, the administration of these drugs in hospitalized patients with ADHF has been shown in a number of studies to be associated with increased risk of long-term morbidity and mortality (24) and their use has therefore been recommended only in selected patients with end-organ hypoperfusion (25).

Low-dose ("renal dose") dopamine has been suggested as a means of reducing diuretic refractoriness. At doses of 0.5 to 5 mcg/kg/minute, dopamine decreases renal vascular resistance, which leads to increased RBF and GFR. Dopamine also has direct natriuretic and diuretic effects mediated by the stimulation of the dopamine α-1 and dopamine α-2 receptors in the proximal tubule, the thick ascending loop of Henle, and the cortical collecting ducts (26). Moreover, the renal dopaminergic system collectively opposes the anti-natriuretic activity of the renin–angiotensin–aldosterone axis by downregulating the angiotensin-1 receptor (27). Low-dose dopamine can blunt the release of the vasoconstrictor norepinephrine from presynaptic nerve endings via activation of the dopamine α-2 receptor, thereby leading to modest systemic vasodilation and afterload reduction (28).

The effects of dopamine in patients with ADHF have not been extensively studied. The Dopamine in Acute Decompensated Heart Failure (DAD-HF) trial randomized ADHF patients (n = 60) to receive either a high-dose continuous infusion of furosemide at 20 mg/hour or a low-dose continuous infusion of furosemide at 5 mg/hour combined with dopamine 5 mcg/kg/minute (29). Per protocol, treatment was discontinued after 8 hours. No differences were seen between groups in terms of urine output and dyspnea relief (29). Worsening renal failure (greater than 0.3 mg/dL rise in Cr in 24 hours) occurred more frequently in the high-dose diuretic arm (30% vs. 9%; P = .04) but there was a similar length of stay and 60-day mortality/hospitalization (29). The lower rate of worsening renal function observed in the low-dose diuretic plus dopamine group could be ascribed to the lower furosemide dose, renoprotective effect of dopamine, or both. Ongoing trials are in process to determine the relative safety and efficacy of low dose dopamine in ADHF patients.

CASE PRESENTATION

Despite modest improvement in his condition, Mr. R remained profoundly volume overloaded with marked ascites. On the ninth day of his hospitalization, he underwent paracentesis with removal of 12.7 L of yellow ascitic fluid. Following this procedure, he had a profound diuresis of approximately 8 L over the next 16 hours. By the next morning, he had lost 20.4 kg. Not surprisingly, he was found to be hypokalemic (K^+ 2.7). Fortunately, his serum sodium actually improved (from 124 mmol/L to 128 mmol/L) as did his renal function (BUN 23 mg/dL, Cr 1.4 mg/dL). The ascitic fluid was not infected, cytology was negative for malignancy, and his serum-ascites albumin gradient was 0.7, consistent with right-sided heart failure (as opposed to primary liver disease) as the underlying cause. IV bumetanide (0.5 mg/hour) and IV chlorothiazide (500 mg every 12 hours) were discontinued to allow for mobilization of extravascular fluid to the vascular space and to facilitate correction of his hypokalemia. Twenty-four hours later, IV bumetanide was reinstated. He was given a 3 mg bolus followed by a continuous infusion at 0.5 mg/hour.

IMPORTANCE OF INCREASED IAP ON RENAL FUNCTION

The key to Mr. R's clinical improvement was his large volume paracentesis. Following removal of 12.7 L of ascitic fluid, he had marked diuretic responsiveness and improvement in renal function. Fortunately, he tolerated this massive loss of volume without hemodynamic insult. We did not intend to have him lose so much fluid in such a short period of time. Conceivably, he could have suffered from rapid volume and electrolyte shifts. In retrospect, his diuretics should have been held overnight.

Mr. R's improvement in renal function was likely a consequence of a reduction in IAP following paracentesis (1,30). The relatively compliant abdominal wall generally allows for increases in abdominal girth without meaningfully increasing IAP. However, once a critical volume is reached, the compliance of the abdominal wall decreases abruptly, leading to a rapid increase in IAP. Elevated IAP (defined as greater than 8 mmHg) can lead to renal compromise in the setting of abdominal compartment syndrome or other surgical interventions that lead to ascites or visceral edema. Elevated IAP may indirectly increase CVP and directly compress the renal parenchyma, leading to reduced renal perfusion and increased renal vein pressure (1). In turn, this leads to a reduced renal filtration gradient.

A substantial number of patients with ADHF present with intra-abdominal edema and sometimes with ascites. Until recently, the influence of IAP on renal function in patients with ADHF had not been evaluated. Mullens and colleagues prospectively enrolled 40 consecutive patients admitted to the ICU with ADHF (31). Each of the patients had depressed left ventricular systolic function (LVEF less than 30%) and elevated cardiac filling pressures (CVP greater than 8 mmHg, pulmonary capillary wedge pressure [PCWP] greater than 18 mmHg). IAP was measured with a standard Foley catheter connected to a pressure transducer. Elevated IAP was found in 60% of the patients. Patients with elevated baseline IAP had higher serum Cr levels at baseline (2.3 ± 1.0 mg/dL vs. 1.5 ± 0.8 mg/dL) compared with those with normal IAP (31). In patients with elevated baseline IAP, changes in IAP after intensive medical therapy correlated with changes in renal function; those who had a reduction in IAP had improved renal function and a subgroup with an increase in IAP had further deterioration in renal performance (31). These findings were independent of changes in cardiac filling pressures and output. Taken together, these data suggest that IAP mediated reductions in the renal filtration gradient leads to impairment of renal function.

CASE PRESENTATION

Over the next 3 days, Mr. R's serum sodium improved to 128, his BUN to 15 mg/dL, and Cr to 1.3 mg/dL. Three additional kilograms of fluid were removed. To help foster additional volume removal, he was given one dose of IV chlorothiazide 500 mg. As he had metabolic alkalosis, acetazolamide was started at 250 mg twice daily. With this regimen, he lost another 4.4 kg in 24 hours. Serum sodium and renal function remained stable. IV dobutamine was discontinued and he was successfully started on captopril 6.25 mg TID. Following these changes, his serum sodium dropped to 123 and his BUN increased to 21 mg/dL and Cr to 1.8 mg/dL.

During the course of his hospitalization, Mr. R lost 34 kg of fluid. He was evaluated for heart transplant and deemed an acceptable candidate. Mr. R ultimately underwent LVAD placement with a HeartMate XVE device for circulatory support and later underwent successful heart transplantation. Five years later, he continues to do exceedingly well.

ACE INHIBITORS, THIAZIDE DIURETICS, AND CARBONIC ANHYDRASE INHIBITORS

Mr. R was able to be weaned off IV dobutamine without deleterious effect on his renal function. He was started on low-dose captopril and subsequently had a modest decline in his GFR. His small bump in Cr was not surprising. Autoregulation of glomerular vasomotor tone is disrupted by the use of ACE inhibitors and ARBs. These agents effectively reduce angiotensin II-induced efferent arteriolar vasoconstriction, leading to reductions in intraglomerular pressure, filtration fraction, and GFR (3). These effects are magnified in the setting of hypotension and renal hypoperfusion. Persistent hypoperfusion may lead to renal parenchymal/cortical ischemia or infarction.

Thiazide-like diuretics block the Na^+-Cl^- transporter in the distal proximal convoluted tubule (**Figure 17-2**; 14). These diuretics decrease the kidney's ability to increase free water clearance and therefore may have contributed to hyponatremia in our patient. Thiazide-like diuretics enhance calcium resorption and diminish magnesium resorption. When loop diuretics are coadministered, the delivery of sodium to the distal proximal convoluted tubule is increased. Thiazide diuretics work synergistically with the loop diuretics by helping to prevent resorption of this excess sodium load, leading to enhanced natriuretic and diuretic effects.

Carbonic anhydrase plays an essential role in the $NaHCO_3$ resorption and acid secretion in the proximal tubule (**Figure 17-2**; 14). In our patient's case, the carbonic anhydrase inhibitor acetazolamide was used to correct metabolic alkalosis occurring as a result of loop and thiazide diuretic therapy. These agents are weak diuretics and when used repeatedly, they can lead to metabolic acidosis as well as severe hypokalemia.

IMPORTANCE OF CVP ON RENAL FUNCTION

With decline in his CVP, achieved via paracentesis and diuresis, Mr. R's renal indexes improved. The decrease in CVP in and of itself may have been responsible for his improved GFR. Growing evidence suggests that increased CVP is a major contributor to renal impairment (32,33). In a patient with volume overload and heart failure, the combination of increased CVP with low systemic arterial pressure (MAP) may lead to a severe compromise of the net renal filtration pressure (MAP – CVP) and GFR (32). In the presence of intrinsic renal disease related to diabetes, hypertension or atherosclerosis, glomerular filtration may be further reduced.

Support for this concept is evident from animal models. Using an isolated rodent kidney model, Winton demonstrated that increased renal venous pressure leads to reductions in RBF, urine flow, urinary sodium chloride excretion, and GFR. These abnormalities were reversed by lowering renal venous pressure (34). Experimentally induced hypervolemia in dogs directly decreased GFR, independent of cardiac index (35,36). Temporary renal vein compression reduces sodium excretion, increases renal interstitial pressure, and reduces GFR (37,38). Increased CVP may have adverse effects on renal structure and function independent of reductions in RBF. First, preclinical studies have shown that increased renal venous pressure is associated with increased renal interstitial pressure (37,38). Excessive renal interstitial pressure has detrimental consequences. When the renal interstitial pressure rises above the intraluminal tubular pressure, tubules will collapse (1,39). In addition, the pressure gradient across the glomerulus in Bowman's capsule will be negligible, impeding passive filtration. Secondly, increased CVP activates the renin-angiotensin-aldosterone system (RAAS) and the SNS, which eventually leads to a reduction in GFR via vasoconstriction and redistribution of blood flow (39). Lastly, increased interstitial pressure will induce tubule-interstitial inflammation and fibrosis, possibly as a consequence of a hypoxic state (40).

The importance of CVP in the development of the cardiorenal syndrome has been validated by clinical trials. Mullens et al evaluated 145 consecutive patients with ADHF treated with intensive medical therapy guided by invasive hemodynamics as assessed by pulmonary artery catheter (41). Increased CVP on admission as well as insufficient reduction of CVP during hospitalization were the strongest hemodynamic determinants of worsening renal function (41). In contrast, impaired cardiac index on admission and improvement in cardiac index with intensive medical therapy had a limited contribution to renal function (41). Systemic blood pressure, PCWP, and estimated renal perfusion pressure were similar between those with versus those without worsening renal function (41). Together, these data support the concept that the "congested kidney" resulting from increased renal venous pressure (increased renal afterload) and increased renal interstitial pressure (intrinsic renal compromise) might be a primary mechanism for the development of the cardiorenal syndrome.

ULTRAFILTRATION

As an alternative to diuretics, excess fluid can be removed directly via ultrafiltration (UF). This intervention was considered for our patient but not implemented as he responded to pharmacologic approaches and paracentesis. UF has theoretical advantages over loop diuretics (7). The ultrafiltrate is isotonic and isonatremic whereas loop diuretics lead to hypotonic urine (7). Thus, UF removes more sodium (and less potassium) than diuretics for an equivalent volume loss. In addition, if fluid removal does not exceed the interstitial fluid mobilization rate of 15 mL/minute, then intravascular volume can be preserved with UF, avoiding neurohormonal activation, and renal impairment that can be seen with diuretics (42).

The Ultrafiltration versus Intravenous Diuretics for Patients Hospitalized for Acute Decompensated Heart Failure (UNLOAD) trial was a prospective, randomized, multicenter trial of early UF versus IV diuretics in patients hospitalized with heart failure, hypervolemia, and moderate renal dysfunction (mean BUN 32 mg/dL, Cr 1.5 mg/dL; 43). Patients randomized to diuretic therapy received at least twice their outpatient furosemide-equivalent dose for each 24-hour period out to a minimum of 48 hours (43). For those assigned to UF, IV diuretics were prohibited for the first 48 hours (43). The duration and rate (up to 500 mL/hour) of fluid removal was left to the discretion of the treating physician (43). At 48 hours, weight loss was greater in the UF than in the standard-care group (5.0 ± 3.1 kg vs. 3.1 ± 3.5 kg; $P = .001$) though dyspnea scores were similarly improved (43). The percentage of patients with rises in serum Cr levels greater than 0.3 mg/dL was similar in the UF and standard-care group at 48 hours and at discharge (43). Lengths of index hospitalization stay were comparable (43). The New York Heart Association (NYHA) functional class, Living with Heart Failure scores, 6-minute walk distance, and Global Assessment scores were similarly improved in both groups (43). At 90 days, the UF group had fewer readmissions for heart failure. The reduction in 90-day hospitalization in the UF group was hypothesized to be due to more aggressive elimination of total body sodium (43). More effective removal of sodium results in greater reduction in extracellular volume. Furthermore, unlike diuretics, UF does not decrease sodium presentation to the macula densa and thus avoids a mechanism for renin secretion. Alternatively, patients undergoing UF had reduced diuretic exposure at the time of discharge, perhaps enhancing their diuretic responsiveness upon rechallenge. Critics of this study have argued that the results of the study were driven by the lack of aggressive diuretic use in the control arm.

The Cardiorenal Rescue Study in Acute Decompensated Heart Failure (CARRESS-HF) was designed to compare the effect of UF with that of stepped pharmacologic therapy (aggressive IV loop diuretic regimen ± thiazide diuretics and in some cases, IV vasodilators ± inotropic agents) in patients (n = 188) with ADHF (44,45). In the medical arm, investigators followed an algorithm to try to maintain a urine output between 3 and 5 L/day (44). All patients had worsening renal function (serum Cr increase of at least 0.3 mg/dL) within 12 weeks before or 10 days after the index hospitalization for heart failure (44). UF was inferior to pharmacologic therapy with respect to the bivariate end point of the change in the serum Cr level and body weight 96 hours after enrollment, driven primarily by an increase in the Cr level in the UF group (−0.04 mg/dL vs. 0.23 mg/dL; P = .003; 45). Weight loss was comparable between groups (45). Serious adverse events were more common in the UF group (45). Thus, CARRESS-HF suggests that UF is not justified for patients hospitalized for ADHF, worsened renal function, and persistent congestion.

CONCLUSION

The cardiorenal syndrome is a heterogeneous disorder characterized by renal dysfunction in the setting of impaired cardiac performance. Intrinsic renal disease may be a major contributing factor for diuretic refractoriness. Inspection of the urine for protein loss and/or active sediment is a simple but important test, which may indicate glomerular and/or tubular injury. A renal ultrasound can rule out hydronephrosis and long-standing injury (cortical thinning, decreased kidney size). Nephrotoxic agents such as nonsteroidal anti-inflammatory agents clearly can play a role and need to be eliminated. Impaired GFR and diuretic refractoriness may also be a consequence of poor renal perfusion, increased CVP, and/or increased IAP. Each patient needs to be assessed individually for the underlying cause(s) of their renal dysfunction. Therapy should be chosen accordingly, depending upon the patient's pre-existing kidney disease, perceived cardiac output, central venous pressure, and IAPs.

REFERENCES

1. Tang WH, Mullens W. Cardiorenal syndrome in decompensated heart failure. *Heart*. 2010;96(4):255–260.
2. Sarraf M, Schrier RW. Cardiorenal syndrome in acute heart failure syndromes. *Int J Nephrol*. 2011;2011:293938.
3. Rastogi A, Fonarow GC. The cardiorenal connection in heart failure. *Curr Cardiol Rep*. 2008;10(3):190–197.
4. Ronco C, Cruz DN, Ronco F. Cardiorenal syndromes. *Curr Opin Crit Care*. 2009;15(5):384–391.
5. Triposkiadis F, Starling RC, Boudoulas H, Giamouzis G, Butler J. The cardiorenal syndrome in heart failure: cardiac? Renal? Syndrome? *Heart Fail Rev*. 2012;17(3):355–366.
6. Martínez-Santos P, Vilacosta I. Cardiorenal syndrome: an unsolved clinical problem. *Int J Nephrol*. 2011;2011:913029.
7. Felker GM, Mentz RJ. Diuretics and ultrafiltration in acute decompensated heart failure. *J Am Coll Cardiol*. 2012;59(24):2145–2153.
8. Schrier RW. Role of diminished renal function in cardiovascular mortality: marker or pathogenetic factor? *J Am Coll Cardiol*. 2006;47(1):1–8.
9. Bayliss J, Norell M, Canepa-Anson R, Sutton G, Poole-Wilson P. Untreated heart failure: clinical and neuroendocrine effects of introducing diuretics. *Br Heart J*. 1987;57(1):17–22.
10. He XR, Greenberg SG, Briggs JP, Schnermann J. Effects of furosemide and verapamil on the NaCl dependency of macula densa-mediated renin secretion. *Hypertension*. 1995;26(1):137–142.
11. Domanski M, Norman J, Pitt B, Haigney M, Hanlon S, Peyster E; Studies of Left Ventricular Dysfunction. Diuretic use, progressive heart failure, and death in patients in the Studies Of Left Ventricular Dysfunction (SOLVD). *J Am Coll Cardiol*. 2003;42(4):705–708.
12. Neuberg GW, Miller AB, O'Connor CM, et al. Diuretic resistance predicts mortality in patients with advanced heart failure. *Am Heart J* 2002;144 (1):31–38.
13. Cooper HA, Dries DL, Davis CE, Shen YL, Domanski MJ. Diuretics and risk of arrhythmic death in patients with left ventricular dysfunction. *Circulation*. 1999;100(12):1311–1315.
14. Mann DL. Management of Heart Failure Patients with Reduced Ejection Fraction. In: Libby P, Bonow RO, Mann DL, Zipes DP, eds. *Braunwald's Heart Disease, a Textbook of Cardiovascular Medicine*, 8th edition. Philadelphia, PA: Elsevier; 2008:611–641.

15. Salvador DR, Rey NR, Ramos GC, Punzalan FE. Continuous infusion versus bolus injection of loop diuretics in congestive heart failure. *Cochrane Database Syst Rev*. 2005;(3):CD003178.
16. Felker GM, Lee KL, Bull DA, et al.; NHLBI Heart Failure Clinical Research Network. Diuretic strategies in patients with acute decompensated heart failure. *N Engl J Med*. 2011;364(9):797–805.
17. Konstam MA, Gheorghiade M, Burnett JC Jr, et al.; Efficacy of Vasopressin Antagonism in Heart Failure Outcome Study With Tolvaptan (EVEREST) Investigators. Effects of oral tolvaptan in patients hospitalized for worsening heart failure: the EVEREST Outcome Trial. *JAMA*. 2007;297(12):1319–1331.
18. Marcus LS, Hart D, Packer M, et al. Hemodynamic and renal excretory effects of human brain natriuretic peptide infusion in patients with congestive heart failure. A double-blind, placebo-controlled, randomized crossover trial. *Circulation*. 1996;94(12):3184–3189.
19. Aaronson KD, Sackner-Bernstein J. Risk of death associated with nesiritide in patients with acutely decompensated heart failure. *JAMA*. 2006;296(12):1465–1466.
20. Sackner-Bernstein JD, Skopicki HA, Aaronson KD. Risk of worsening renal function with nesiritide in patients with acutely decompensated heart failure. *Circulation*. 2005;111(12):1487–1491.
21. O'Connor CM, Starling RC, Hernandez AF, et al. Effect of nesiritide in patients with acute decompensated heart failure. *N Engl J Med*. 2011;365(1):32–43.
22. Damman K, Voors AA, Navis G, van Veldhuisen DJ, Hillege HL. The cardiorenal syndrome in heart failure. *Prog Cardiovasc Dis*. 2011;54(2):144–153.
23. Bayram M, De Luca L, Massie MB, Gheorghiade M. Reassessment of dobutamine, dopamine, and milrinone in the management of acute heart failure syndromes. *Am J Cardiol*. 2005;96(6A): 47G–58G.
24. Abraham WT, Adams KF, Fonarow GC, et al.; ADHERE Scientific Advisory Committee and Investigators; ADHERE Study Group. In-hospital mortality in patients with acute decompensated heart failure requiring intravenous vasoactive medications: an analysis from the Acute Decompensated Heart Failure National Registry (ADHERE). *J Am Coll Cardiol*. 2005;46(1):57–64.
25. Executive summary: HFSA 2006 Comprehensive Heart Failure Practice Guideline. *J Card Fail*. 2006; 12(1), 10–38.
25. Seri I, Kone BC, Gullans SR, Aperia A, Brenner BM, Ballermann BJ. Influence of Na+ intake on dopamine-induced inhibition of renal cortical Na(+)-K(+)-ATPase. *Am J Physiol*. 1990;258(1 Pt 2):F52–F60.
27. Gildea JJ. Dopamine and angiotensin as renal counterregulatory systems controlling sodium balance. *Curr Opin Nephrol Hypertens*. 2009;18(1):28–32.
28. Goldberg LI, Rajfer SI. Dopamine receptors: applications in clinical cardiology. *Circulation*. 1985;72(2):245–248.
29. Giamouzis G, Butler J, Starling RC, et al. Impact of dopamine infusion on renal function in hospitalized heart failure patients: results of the Dopamine in Acute Decompensated Heart Failure (DAD-HF) Trial. *J Card Fail*. 2010;16(12):922–930.
30. Mullens W, Abrahams Z, Francis GS, Taylor DO, Starling RC, Tang WH. Prompt reduction in intra-abdominal pressure following large-volume mechanical fluid removal improves renal insufficiency in refractory decompensated heart failure. *J Card Fail*. 2008;14(6):508–514.
31. Mullens W, Abrahams Z, Skouri HN, et al. Elevated intra-abdominal pressure in acute decompensated heart failure: a potential contributor to worsening renal function? *J Am Coll Cardiol*. 2008;51(3):300–306.
32. Ross EA. Congestive renal failure: the pathophysiology and treatment of renal venous hypertension. *J Card Fail*. 2012;18(12):930–938.
33. Damman K, van Deursen VM, Navis G, Voors AA, van Veldhuisen DJ, Hillege HL. Increased central venous pressure is associated with impaired renal function and mortality in a broad spectrum of patients with cardiovascular disease. *J Am Coll Cardiol*. 2009;53(7):582–588.
34. Winton FR. The influence of venous pressure on the isolated mammalian kidney. *J Physiol (Lond)*. 1931;72(1):49–61.
35. Abildgaard U, Amtorp O, Agerskov K, Sjøntoft E, Christensen NJ, Henriksen O. Renal vascular adjustments to partial renal venous obstruction in dog kidney. *Circ Res*. 1987;61(2):194–202.
36. Firth JD, Raine AE, Ledingham JG. Raised venous pressure: a direct cause of renal sodium retention in oedema? *Lancet*. 1988;1(8593):1033–1035.
37. Wathen RL, Selkurt EE. Intrarenal regulatory factors of salt excretion during renal venous pressure elevation. *Am J Physiol*. 1969;216(6):1517–1524.
38. Burnett JC Jr, Knox FG. Renal interstitial pressure and sodium excretion during renal vein constriction. *Am J Physiol*. 1980;238(4):F279–F282.
39. Jessup M, Costanzo MR. The cardiorenal syndrome: do we need a change of strategy or a change of tactics? *J Am Coll Cardiol*. 2009;53(7):597–599.
40. Gottschalk CW, Mylle M. Micropuncture study of pressures in proximal tubules and peritubular capillaries of the rat kidney and their relation to ureteral and renal venous pressures. *Am J Physiol*. 1956;185(2):430–439.
41. Mullens W, Abrahams Z, Francis GS, et al. Importance of venous congestion for worsening of renal function in advanced decompensated heart failure. *J Am Coll Cardiol*. 2009;53(7):589–596.
42. Marenzi G, Grazi S, Giraldi F, et al. Interrelation of humoral factors, hemodynamics, and fluid and salt metabolism in congestive heart failure: effects of extracorporeal ultrafiltration. *Am J Med*. 1993;94(1):49–56.
43. Costanzo MR, Guglin ME, Saltzberg MT, et al.; UNLOAD Trial Investigators. Ultrafiltration versus intravenous diuretics for patients hospitalized for acute decompensated heart failure. *J Am Coll Cardiol*. 2007;49(6):675–683.
44. Bart BA, Goldsmith SR, Lee KL, et al. Cardiorenal rescue study in acute decompensated heart failure: rationale and design of CARRESS-HF, for the Heart Failure Clinical Research Network. *J Card Fail*. 2012;18(3):176–182.
45. Bart BA, Goldsmith SR, Lee KL, et al.; Heart Failure Clinical Research Network. Ultrafiltration in decompensated heart failure with cardiorenal syndrome. *N Engl J Med*. 2012;367(24): 2296–2304.

V

Special Topics in Heart Failure

18

Evaluation and Workup of a Patient With Familial Dilated Cardiomyopathy

ANA MORALES AND RAY E. HERSHBERGER

INTRODUCTION

The following case illustrates the genetic evaluation process for a patient with familial dilated cardiomyopathy (FDC). Although at the time that our patient was seen, genetic testing was not routinely available, the role of research in the rapid evolution of cardiovascular genetic medicine can be appreciated as the timeline moves forward. Currently, clinical genetic testing is available to evaluate variants of strong clinical effects or, alternatively, for susceptibility variants of less effect that together can lead to disease. This case focuses on the role of genetic testing to assess for the presence of mutations of strong clinical effects while acknowledging that more subtle genome-wide variation and even environmental effects can play a role in any form of genetic disease. Universal clinical genetic principles such as those relevant to Mendelian disease and its complicating factors, as well as the role of gene-specific clinical presentation and presymptomatic counseling, among many others, will be applied in the analysis of this case.

CASE PRESENTATION

A 63-year-old female with a history of arrhythmia and heart failure is referred for heart transplant evaluation. She complains of fatigue and two to three pillow orthopnea. A year before, Holter evaluation revealed intermittent junctional heart beats (to 39 bpm), a PR interval of 300 ms, and paroxysmal atrial fibrillation, for which a dual chamber pacemaker was placed. At the time, coronary angiography was normal, but moderate mitral regurgitation was identified. Eventually her mitral regurgitation worsened, ejection fraction (EF) decreased to 50% to 55%, and a mitral valve replacement was performed. Postoperative evaluation showed decreased cardiac output and progressive global hypokinesis without evidence of myocardial infarction. By the time of visit, her condition had progressed to a late Class III New York Heart Association with maximal oxygen consumption (MVO_2, per treadmill exercise test) of 10 ml O_2/kg/min. Echocardiogram now shows a left ventricular end diastolic dimension (LVIDd) of 57 mm (> 99th percentile, as per Framingham Heart Study criteria (1) and EF of 20% with moderate pulmonary hypertension. She reported rare alcohol use; cigarette smoking and recreational drug use were denied. Previous medical history includes high cholesterol, hypothyroidism, gallbladder disease, cholecystectomy, and hysterectomy due to endometriosis. Her family history is remarkable for cardiovascular disease (**Figure 18-1**). Her father died suddenly at the age of 63 due to an unknown form of heart disease. Her mother also died at the age of 81 from an unknown form of heart disease. Her brother, 78, has a pacemaker/implantable cardiac defibrillator (ICD) and bradycardia. Another brother, 74, also has a pacemaker/ICD and a history of stroke. Her sister, 71, also with a pacemaker/ICD, has bradycardia and atrial fibrillation and is on anticoagulant therapy. The patient has two daughters, in their 30s, both reportedly unaffected. Given the medical and family history, a diagnosis of idiopathic dilated cardiomyopathy (IDC) with probable FDC was given. Cardiovascular screening

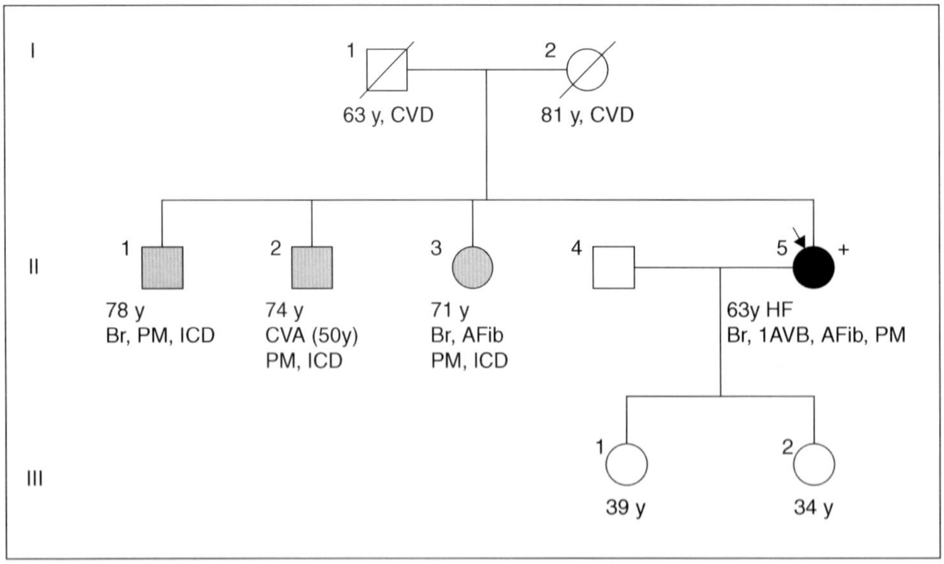

Figure 18-1
Pedigree of case study.

Note: AFib = atrial fibrillation; 1AVB = first-degree atrioventricular block; Br = bradycardia; CVA = cerebrovascular accident; CVD = cardiovascular disease; ICD = implantable cardiac defibrillator; PM = pacemaker; y = years of age.

Squares represent males; circles represent females, an arrow indicates the proband. The presence (+) of a *LMNA* mutation is indicated for the proband. The filled symbol indicates IDC. Gray symbols indicate another form of cardiovascular abnormality or diagnosis.

of her first-degree relatives was recommended. Clinical genetic testing for dilated cardiomyopathy (DCM) was not commonly available at the time. Instead, participation in genetic research was offered. She gave informed consent for a blood draw for research analysis of DCM gene mutations. The patient was accepted for transplant, and a year later, she was successfully transplanted. Five years after her heart transplant, research results revealed a novel *LMNA* 1114delG frameshift mutation (2), a likely disease causing variant. The genetic findings were confirmed by a certified clinical genetics laboratory. Genetic testing for the *LMNA* mutation identified in the patient was recommended for at-risk family members, who declined testing.

BACKGROUND

DCM, defined as left ventricular enlargement and systolic dysfunction (3), is a leading cause of heart failure (4). IDC is DCM of unknown cause, that is, when ischemia and other less common etiologies (except genetic) have been ruled out (**Table 18-1;** 5,6). IDC has an estimated prevalence of 36.5/100,000, however, recent estimates suggest a prevalence greater than 1/500 (53).

The phenotype (clinical features) of DCM include heart failure, arrhythmia, stroke, or thromboembolism representing advanced disease, as DCM can be clinically silent for years (8), with onset usually during the fourth to sixth decades (9); however, early (10) and late onset cases (11) have been reported.

Table 18-1
Causes of Dilated Cardiomyopathy[a]

Ischemic
Coronary artery disease
Structural heart disease
Congenital
Valvular
Toxic exposure
Anthracyclines
Imitanib
Alcohol
Cocaine
Endocrine
Hypothyroidism
Cushing's disease
Pheochromocytoma
Metabolic
Nutritional deficiencies
Electrolyte disturbances
Infectious disease
Human immunodeficiency virus
Parasitic, eg, Chagas disease
Infiltrative
Sarcoidosis
Amyloidosis
Other
Iron overload
Hypertension

Note: [a]This list is not exhaustive but provides those causes more likely to be encountered in North America.

Conduction system disease and cardiac arrhythmias can be the presenting feature in IDC (2), including sudden cardiac death (12). Onset of DCM during or soon after pregnancy is also thought to be part of the clinical spectrum (8,13–15).

Approximately 35% of IDC patients have FDC (two or more affected family members; 16). Most FDC is autosomal dominant (3,17,18), which means that the disease typically shows in every generation, with males and females affected in almost equal proportions (19). In autosomal dominant FDC, individuals with a disease causing mutation may show structural or hemodynamic changes with advancing age or may completely escape the disease (reduced, age dependent penetrance). Furthermore, age of onset, presentation, and disease course can be different among family members with the same disease-causing mutation (variable expression). Less frequent forms of FDC inheritance include autosomal recessive, X-linked, and mitochondrial patterns (8,20,21). Some DCM is associated with syndromic phenotypes (9,20,21). The clinical characteristics of individuals with usual nonsyndromic sporadic and familial disease DCM are indistinguishable from each other (22).

IDC exhibits locus heterogeneity, with mutations in >30 genes so far identified that account for approximately 40% of FDC (16,23). Represented across diverse functional cellular categories (from sarcomeric to RNA binding), the known DCM genes are expressed in the cardiomyocyte (16). Rare, truncating TTN mutations have been reported in 20% of cases, although truncating TTN mutations are also present in 3% of controls (54). Following TTN, mutations in *LMNA* are present in 5-8% of unselected IDC patients and in 15-30% with IDC and conduction system disease. Mutations in MYBPC3, MYH7, MYH6, TNNT2, and SCN5A are relatively frequent. DCM caused by these mutations is autosomal dominant.

Various pathogenesis mechanisms are thought to be involved (primarily depending on the gene mutation involved); however, myocardial injury is the end result (26). At the population level, a vast number of mutant alleles have been reported in each one of the known genes, all leading to essentially the same clinical picture (allelic heterogeneity). These mutations, frequently novel, elevate the complexity of adjudicating causality of genetic DCM variants to unprecedented levels (16,24).

Although early genetic studies demonstrated that FDC is a Mendelian disorder that follows defined patterns of inheritance resulting from single-gene mutations of large effects, evolving research suggests a more complex genetic model. Some families with *LMNA* mutations showing nonsegregation have been reported (2), in which functional studies show support causality of the identified variants (27), suggesting a possible second (likely genetic) factor leading to familial disease. The phenomenon of multiple mutations has been published in other cardiovascular genetic disorders (28–34). In fact, expanded multigene resequencing studies have identified a handful of IDC patients with more than one mutation (24,25,35). Whether these multiple variants modify penetrance and expression or are a requisite for the DCM phenotype is not well understood, but answers to these questions are essential for thorough patient care.

PATIENT EVALUATION

Following recognition that DCM has a genetic basis, guidelines for the genetic evaluation of cardiomyopathy (36,37) were developed, validating the concept that early detection can reduce morbidity and mortality (8,9,38,39). To achieve this goal, for every new diagnosis, a family history should be obtained; screening of asymptomatic first-degree relatives of affected individuals should be accomplished; and referral to centers specialized in genetic evaluation, molecular testing, and genetic counseling should be considered (36). **Figure 18-2** summarizes the genetic evaluation process.

FAMILY HISTORY

Family history information from at least three generations is essential in the genetic evaluation of cardiomyopathy (40,41). The pedigree, a graphic representation of family relationships and their medical histories, facilitates determination of inheritance patterns and, in turn, identification of at-risk family members for screening and molecular studies (36,40,41). Questionnaire formats, albeit useful in identifying other affected relatives in a time-efficient manner, are not as effective when assessing inheritance patterns. Family history questions should be open-ended and attentive to multisystem, syndromic disease, but the path of inquiry must strategically target cardiovascular disease (**Table 18-2**; 40,41). Ideally, medical records and relevant test results should be obtained to confirm any family history information (8).

In this case, a positive family history of heart disease and cardiomyopathy, as well as findings of pacemaker and ICD, supports FDC (**Figure 18-1**). The

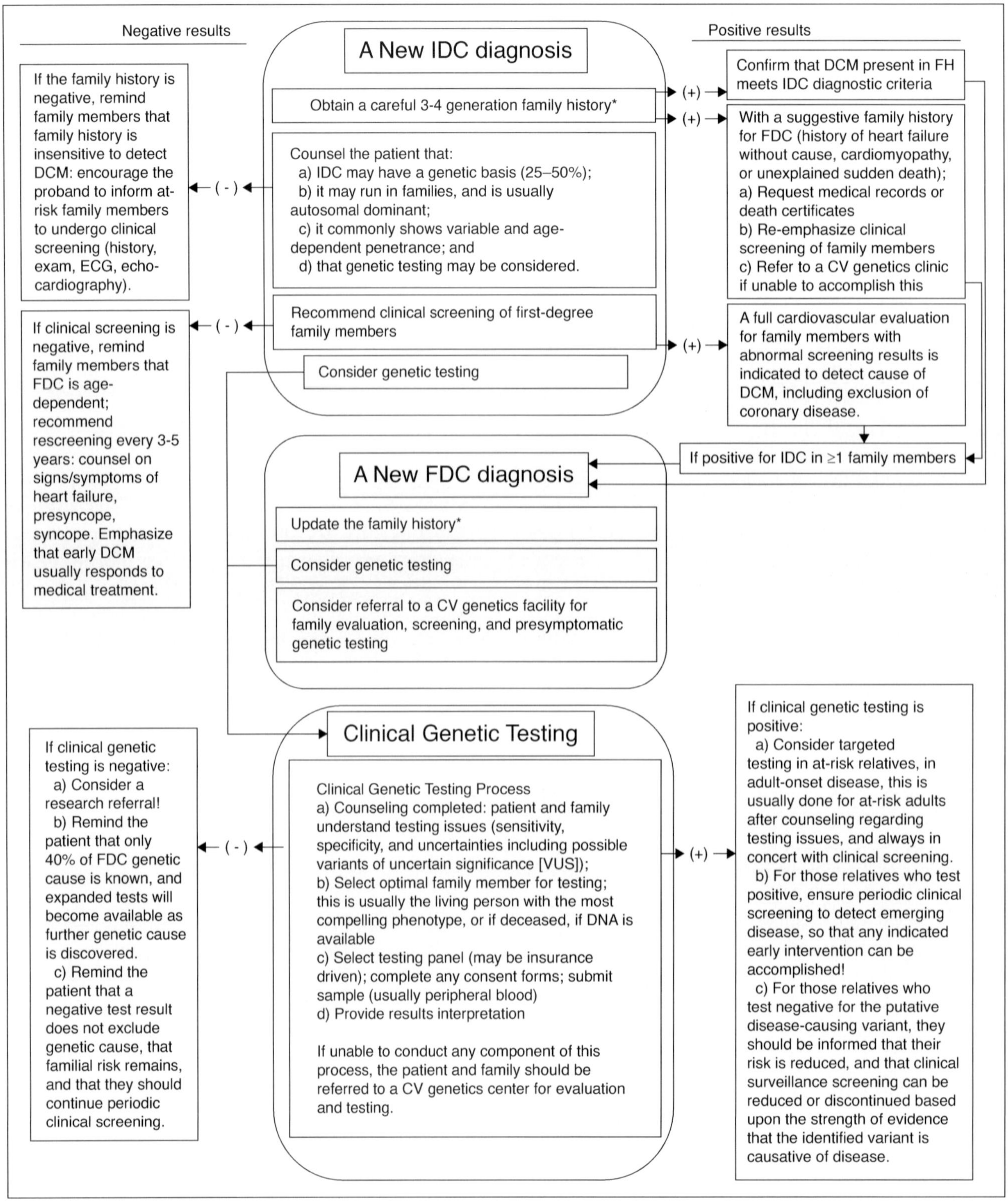

Figure 18-2
Flow diagram of genetic risk assessment for patients newly diagnosed with idiopathic dilated cardiomyopathy (IDC) or familial dilated cardiomyopathy (FDC).

Note: The left- and right-sided boxes provide guidance for negative or positive results, respectively, based on the results of history or testing recommended in the central boxes. *Always search for history or exam findings consistent with syndromic disease, particularly skeletal muscle symptoms. Figure used with permission from (16).

Table 18-2
Targeted Family History Information for Familial Dilated Cardiomyopathy[a]

HAS ANYONE IN YOUR FAMILY BEEN DIAGNOSED WITH DCM? IF SO, AT WHAT AGE? ARE ANY OF THE FOLLOWING SYMPTOMS, EVENTS, MEDICAL PROBLEMS PRESENT?
Arrhythmia (syncope, presyncope, palpitations, sudden cardiac death)
Heart failure (orthopnea, fatigue, dyspnea on exertion)
Stroke
Pregnancy associated cardiomyopathy
Extra-cardiac disease (hearing loss, myopathy)
HAS ANYONE IN YOUR FAMILY HAD ANY OF THE FOLLOWING TESTS OR PROCEDURES?
Echocardiogram
ECG
Heart catheterization
Chest x-ray
Genetic testing
ICD/pacemaker implant
Ventricular assist device implant
Heart transplantation

Note: [a]The above information should be sought regarding the affected individual and any first-, second- and third-degree family members. Consanguinity between the parents of an affected individual must be ruled out. Information regarding confounding factors (Table 18-1) should also be requested.

absence of dysmorphic features or multiorgan disease excludes syndromic disease. It is not uncommon for a patient to report a parent affected with DCM, heart failure, or an unknown form of heart disease. Although the father's sudden death at the age of 63 supports the possibility of paternal inheritance, this type of bias should be avoided, as a mutation could have been inherited from the mother or even from both parents (2,36).

Determining the pattern of inheritance is a process of elimination. X-linked recessive disease (19) is unlikely in this case due to the presence of three probably affected females (the proband, II.5, her sister II.3, and their mother, I.2). If X-linked recessive inheritance is present, DCM would have had to be inherited from the proband's mother (I.2, **Figure 18-1**), who would have a mutation in an X-linked, DCM-causing gene and a functional homologous copy. However, by definition, X-linked recessive disease would not usually be phenotypically apparent in females because the normal X chromosome allele, inherited from the father, would compensate for the nonfunctional allele, thereby preventing disease expression.

A mechanism by which females can show X-linked recessive disease is mediated by skewed X-inactivation (the preferential inactivation of the normal allele in a carrier female), a known phenomenon in X-linked recessive disease (19). Alternatively, a mechanism by which these three females could be affected with X-linked recessive disease would be if the father (Subject I.1, **Figure 18-1**) is affected with the same X-linked recessive disorder and the mother is either homozygous for or affected with the same disorder as the result of skewed X-inactivation. If the father is affected and the mother is homozygous for the same disorder, the father will pass his only X chromosome with the mutant allele to all of his daughters and by virtue of only having mutated alleles on both X chromosomes, the mother will only transmit the mutation, and all of her offspring would be affected If the mother is affected as a result of skewed X-inactivation, she would have one normal and one mutated X-linked gene. Following this scenario, as the father will only transmit the X chromosome harboring the mutation to his daughters, affected daughters could be possible if in all cases the mother's mutant X-linked allele was transmitted. While a couple formed by two affected individuals with the same X-linked disorder is not unheard of, it is rare, and thus very unlikely. Moreover, the actual proportion of X-linked DCM in all IDC is unknown, but appears to be relatively rare. Only two X-linked genes, *DMD* (Duchenne muscular dystrophy) and *TAZ* (Barth syndrome) have been identified, and these often include skeletal myopathy and infant onset disease, respectively (38).

Classic X-linked dominant inheritance, where only one copy of the mutant gene is needed to cause a phenotype in a female, is excluded, as X-linked dominant disorders in males are usually lethal (19), and it has not been reported in DCM (19). Autosomal recessive inheritance (19) is also rare in DCM (42,43), and in this case, only possible if both parents were carriers and both of their reported heart problems were unrelated to DCM. Furthermore, clues to autosomal recessive DCM, such as consanguinity and early onset disease (8) are absent. The observation of all four siblings being probably affected could be consistent with maternal mitochondrial inheritance (19), but it is unlikely that mitochondrial inheritance is present, as most mitochondrial DCM is associated with multisystem, syndromic disease (9,26).

CASE PRESENTATION

In this case, autosomal dominant inheritance provides the best fit. Not only is this pattern most common in FDC, but also supporting observations include two consecutive generations with affected individuals and both males and females affected in equal proportions. A complicating factor is the presence of two parents possibly affected with DCM, which poses the possibility of bilineal, multigenic inheritance (2). The patient was informed about the likely genetic basis of her condition and clinical implications. This included probable FDC and up to 50% DCM risk for the offspring of affected individuals.

It is important to note that the above assessment is principally based on Mendelian genetics principles and three key assumptions: (a) a correct conclusion usually follows the simplest explanation; (b) FDC follows a Mendelian pattern of inheritance; and (c) the information obtained is accurate (in the absence of medical records). In reality, a vast array of nuances can rule in every possible scenario. Also, as previously discussed, the genetics of DCM are increasingly recognized as going beyond classic Mendelian models. Last, because DCM can be silent for a number of years, family history, even if confirmed by medical records, cannot diagnose all FDC (38) especially when the history is noncontributory. Clinical cardiovascular screening, as described in the next section, is the gold standard to diagnose FDC.

Cardiovascular Screening

Cardiovascular screening should consist of a medical history (focused on heart failure symptoms, arrhythmias, presyncope, and syncope), physical examination (focused on cardiac and skeletal muscle systems), electrocardiogram, and echocardiogram. Creatine kinase (CK) levels have also been suggested only at initial evaluation to rule out combined cardiac and skeletal muscle disease, although care must be taken when drawing a CK to ensure that the individual has not recently undergone strenuous exercise (36). Given reduced, age dependent penetrance and variable expression in DCM, screening should be performed at intervals (**Table 18-3**; 36). Any abnormal screening results (regardless of genetic results) should be followed up in 1-year intervals (36). Cascade screening should be continued in the extended family for as long as IDC is identified. Thoughtfulness and flexibility should be applied in this process, as oftentimes, a key member is not willing or able to pursue screening. If so, screening should be performed on the next, immediate at-risk relative.

CASE PRESENTATION

In this case, the patient was informed that, regardless of genotype, cardiovascular screening is recommended as soon as possible in her two brothers and sister (who are all likely to be affected) as well as her daughters. If IDC is confirmed in any

Table 18-3
Recommended Time Intervals of Clinical Surveillance Screening for Family Members At-Risk for Dilated Cardiomyopathy[a]

	NEGATIVE GENETIC TESTING OR CARDIOVASCULAR SCREENING	KNOWN DISEASE CAUSING MUTATION
Children	Every 3–5 years	Yearly
Adults	Every 3–5 years	Every 1–3 years

Note: [a]History, exam, ECG, and echocardiogram are indicated at the above intervals, or at any time if symptoms occur. If a mutation is identified, screening should be more frequent. See reference (36).

of them, cardiovascular screening is recommended for their first-degree relatives. She was educated about the importance of communicating with her at-risk relatives about the importance of screening and the symptoms of heart failure, arrhythmia, and stroke. Emphasis was made on her understanding of seeking immediate medical care in the setting of potentially life-threatening symptoms such as syncope and presyncope.

Genetic Counseling and Molecular Evaluation

Although at the time when the guidelines were published in 2009 it was recommended that genetic testing begin with *LMNA, TNNT2*, and *MYH7* with reflex to additional genes if results are negative (9), single-gene testing has been replaced by more cost effective large gene panels (26,37). Currently, providers can choose from a variety of multiple gene panels or site-specific testing, depending on the case. While it has been estimated that up to 40% of genetic cause has been identified, a non trivial number of variants are of unknown significance. An analysis of clinical genetic results concluded that, among all positive results, likely pathogenic mutations were present in 17.4% (55).

In addition to collecting a family history, the genetic testing process involves providing clinical information, including genetic risk and reproductive options, discussing benefits and limitations of testing, and providing anticipatory guidance about possible results. For example, as some panels may include genes associated with syndromic disease, results may not only explain the cause of a patient's heart problem, but may also uncover risks for extra-cardiac disease (26). Moreover, to some individuals, knowledge of their results can generate feelings of confusion, anxiety, or for those escaping the family mutation, survivor guilt (39). Cost and potential issues of genetic discrimination should also be delineated. Contracting for the method for disclosing results (in person or by phone) should be agreed upon and an expected turnaround time for results should be given. For the above reasons, it is imperative that the provider has ensured that the patient understands the process and has voluntarily accepted to pursue genetic testing. Moreover, as mutation results are essential to risk stratification, the provider must also be extremely judicious when concluding that any identified variant is disease causing, an issue that will grow exponentially as more genes are discovered and larger panels become available. Unquestionably, the genetic evaluation process can be far from simple in some cases and therefore, referral to specialized centers should also be considered (36). These centers, many of which conduct genetic discovery studies, are usually staffed by cardiovascular genetics experts, genetic counselors, and medical geneticists.

When a genetic diagnosis has not been performed or is unavailable, it is recommended that testing begins with the individual with the strongest degree of supporting clinical diagnostic evidence (26) because this increases the probability of finding a mutation (9). Genetic testing for this individual should therefore include as many known DCM-causing genes as possible. If testing the most clearly affected family member is not possible, another relative may be offered testing. Preferably, this individual should be affected or should have potential early signs of DCM such as isolated left ventricular enlargement (26). However, this is not always possible, and, at times, the only candidate for genetic testing is the unaffected individual requesting risk assessment. Testing of such a less than ideal candidate requires careful consideration and frank discussion of the implications of any results (especially if negative). Offering testing from stored tissue (if the key family member is deceased) or DNA banking (for a key family member who, at the moment of inquiry, declines testing) are also recommended.

If a mutation that is known to cause IDC is identified in a patient (regardless of clinical status), at-risk relatives can be offered targeted or site-specific testing for the family mutation. Once the family mutation has been identified, targeted mutation testing, as opposed to a multigene panel, is indicated, as the genetic cause has been identified. First-degree relatives of individuals with the mutant allele are at 50% risk of inheriting the mutation, and if autosomal dominant, their DCM risk is significantly increased and ongoing screening is recommended (**Table 18-3**). Those testing negative for the family mutation can be discharged.

If, on the other hand, a patient with IDC undergoes genetic testing and results are negative, a genetic etiology cannot be ruled out as not all genetic causes have been identified. If pedigree analysis is consistent with autosomal dominant inheritance, risk to offspring of affected individuals remains at up to 50%. In this setting, first-degree relatives of affected individuals remain at high risk, but the clinical utility of their testing is null. There may be, however, a rationale to consider a multigene panel in another affected family member, preferably if the individual is a third-degree relative or greater. This is because in these cases, the possibility of a second, causative family mutation cannot be ruled out.

Excluding TTN, the vast majority of mutations identified in IDC are single-base exonic substitutions leading to amino acid changes (missense mutations). Missense mutations are hard to interpret clinically, as not all protein altering variants necessarily lead to an abnormal phenotype. Due to this, sequencing is the tool of choice in DCM, as it provides base-by-base reads of a DNA sample. A by-product of this degree of molecular thoroughness is the identification of variants of unknown significance (VUS). A VUS is a variant for which clinical causality cannot be established and therefore, is of little utility. Further complicating the landscape, in genetic DCM, a VUS finding is relatively more likely than in other genetic disorders. Additional research will only tell if this is a permanent fixture (reflecting the genetic nature of the disease) or temporary (reflecting a developing field). It is recommended that patients with VUS results recontact their medical genetics provider periodically, because with time, a VUS can be reclassified to pathogenic or benign.

Several methods are in place to classify a variant, including absence in control samples, functional studies, computer-based algorithms, and family-based segregation analyses (16). Segregation analyses, often the best way to prove the role of a variant in familial disease, require participation of multiple family members. Therefore, before ordering testing, the clinician should analyze the family history information and pay attention to the number of available affected and unaffected family members. The consenting process for genetic testing should, therefore, also include discussion of the possibility of a VUS finding, and how the patient's own family structure/availability can impact the interpretation of a possible inconclusive result.

CASE PRESENTATION

In addition to the positive family history in this case, the patient's presentation of conduction system disease should increase suspicion of a genetic etiology for her cardiomyopathy. In particular, the presence of conduction system disease increases the likelihood of a *LMNA* mutation (2,9,38). Personalized therapy for *LMNA*-cardiomyopathy, now under development, also supports genetic testing. However, at the time of her mitral valve replacement, genetic testing for DCM or *LMNA* testing, clearly indicated in this case, was not routinely available on a clinical basis.

Research participation proved valuable, as a genetic cause was eventually identified in her. Although research genetic testing opens the possibility of obtaining results, genetic research aims to further scientific understanding, with more clear benefits for society as a whole as opposed to for the individual. Moreover, in genetic research testing, which is free of cost, a turnaround time cannot be predicted and results cannot be guaranteed. The patient demonstrated understanding of these concepts and agreed to enroll in genetic research, not expecting to personally benefit from her participation.

Research genetic testing identified a novel deletion of a guanine base at position 1114 of the *LMNA* gene. Although segregation analysis of this variant was not possible in this case, various lines of evidence support its role in disease causation. First, *LMNA*, which codes for the lamin A/C protein (a component of the nuclear lamina expressed in many tissues; 44) is an established DCM gene (45–50). Second, the molecular nature of the observed defect is of the type expected to cause disease (51): the single-base deletion predicts a frameshift at amino acid position 372, resulting in the inclusion of 108 incorrect amino acids, followed by a premature stop codon, which truncates the protein 184 amino acids prematurely. Third, the personal and family history of conduction system disease is consistent with *LMNA*-DCM (12).

The researchers felt confident that the mutation was responsible for DCM in this case. In the United States, before these research results can be reported to the patient, they must be confirmed by a laboratory certified by the Clinical Laboratories Improvement Amendment of 1998 (CLIA). Confirmatory genetic testing usually involves a fee, which may or may not be covered by insurance. In this case, the patient was notified by the researchers that a genetic change was found that is thought to explain the heart problems in her family. Clinical genetic testing was offered to confirm and obtain specific results. Arrangements were made for a fresh blood sample to be drawn during a follow-up cardiology visit. The patient's sample was sent directly to a CLIA-certified clinical laboratory. The research laboratory provided the clinical laboratory with the necessary molecular information to confirm the *LMNA* mutation. Through her physician, the patient was informed of her specific results. Once results were confirmed by a CLIA-certified laboratory, and results were disclosed, genetic testing was recommended for her family members, including her daughters, who declined testing.

TREATMENT AND MANAGEMENT OF PATIENTS WITH GENETIC DCM

The guidelines state that treatment following usual guidelines for DCM (52) should also be undertaken for those with genetic DCM (36), including the early use of angiotensin converting enzyme (ACE)-inhibitors and/or beta blockers for those who have early DCM but are asymptomatic. Further, since some genetic DCM (such as that resulting from mutations in *LMNA*) may have an arrhythmic phenotype resulting in ventricular arrhythmia including sudden cardiac death (SCD), the use of implantable defibrillators is also indicated, even if the ejection fraction has not fallen to less than 35%, if there is evidence of a family history of SCD early in the course of DCM, or if the patient has had syncope or presyncope thought to be related to ventricular arrhythmias (36). In addition to ACE-inhibitors and beta blockers, heart failure is treated with diuretics as needed and cardiac transplantation as needed with advanced disease refractory to medical or device therapy.

This case raises an additional question: If genetic testing had revealed a *LMNA* mutation prior to the operation to replace this patient's mitral valve, would this information have affected the medical decision analysis? *LMNA* clinical genetic testing was not yet available when this operation was undertaken. However, her lack of responsiveness to the valve replacement surgery suggests that such operative or mechanical approaches to genetically based DCM may overall show reduced efficacy.

CURRENT STATE OF GENETIC TESTING FOR FDC

The last few decades have been witness to substantial progress. In only 6 years, the number of DCM genes grew from 19 to 34 (16). Once confined to research laboratories, subsequently limited to single-gene testing at the clinical level for a few genes, genetic testing for DCM has evolved into a variety of large, multigene panel options. To illustrate this, *LMNA* sequencing on a clinical basis has an 8% detection rate while a multigene panel with a much greater detection rate has a comparable cost. This dramatic improvement results from the maturation of DNA sequencing methods to the faster and more efficient Next Generation Sequencing (NGS), a group of technologies that employ high throughput methods. Currently used by some commercial laboratories offering genetic testing for DCM, NGS also made it possible to sequence an entire human exome (protein coding portion) or genome on a research basis (16).

While it is clear that FDC is genetic, and therefore, genetic testing should be offered, it is less clear if sporadic IDC is also genetic, and if as a result, whether genetic testing should be recommended for patients with a negative family history (24,25). Additional well-designed studies are needed to address this question. Regardless, it is reasonable to offer clinical genetic testing to individuals with IDC and a negative family history, as long as proper counseling is performed.

Other groups that may benefit from genetic testing include pregnant women with peripartum or pregnancy-associated cardiomyopathy (13–15) and pediatric populations (10). Unless the family history supports severe early onset, fetal DCM testing is not routinely indicated, as invasive procedures are rarely requested for late onset conditions. Syndromic disease involving DCM should always be ruled out before proceeding with testing, and if suspected (eg, if dysmorphic features, myopathy, hearing loss, immune deficiency, or other features are present), a referral to a medical geneticist is best (39). With the current detection rate of 40%, chances are high that a clinical genetic test will not identify a disease causing mutation. This is why it is reasonable to offer concurrent clinical and research testing.

Benefits of genetic testing include identifying at-risk family members, clarifying a diagnosis, and potentially informing clinical management (including conduction system disease risk). There are clear benefits associated with genetic testing for DCM, and as of 2013, insurance coverage of DCM genetic testing is steadily increasing. Nevertheless, letters of medical necessity and supporting medical records are often required to demonstrate how genetic information can guide medical treatment. If so, as in when genetic testing helps to clarify a diagnosis given a mixed cardiovascular phenotype (11), testing is often covered. Insurance companies are less likely to cover testing if the results are for the benefit of family members, unless these family members are also subscribers of the same policy. Some laboratories have customer service programs to assist patients with payment and insurance coverage issues. Knowing how to choose the right laboratory requires a consideration of the laboratory's reputation, their methodology, and detection rate, as well as the patient's financial situation. The GeneTests database, available online at www.genetests.org and periodically updated, provides a good starting point, with a directory of clinical and research laboratories offering genetic testing for DCM.

CONCLUSION

Mutations in a wide array of genes are present in some individuals with DCM. Although the DCM genetic landscape may not be completed until sometime in the future, a genetic evaluation is of significant clinical utility today. This evaluation includes a family history, cardiovascular screening, and genetic testing. In the coming decades, these recommendations will likely evolve as additional causation is identified and genetic information is integrated in treatments and therapies for DCM.

REFERENCES

1. Vasan R, Larson M, Levy D, et al. Distribution and categorization of echocardiographic measurements in relation to reference limits. The Framingham Heart Study: formulation of a height- and sex-specific classification and its prospective validation. *Circulation*. 1997;96(6):1863–1873.
2. Parks SB, Kushner JD, Nauman D, et al. Lamin A/C mutation analysis in a cohort of 324 unrelated patients with idiopathic or familial dilated cardiomyopathy. *Am Heart J*. 2008;156(1): 161–169.
3. Mestroni L, Maisch B, McKenna W, et al. Guidelines for the study of familial dilated cardiomyopathies. *Eur Heart J*. 1999;20(2):93–102.
4. Lloyd-Jones D, Adams RJ, Brown TM, et al. Heart disease and stroke statistics—2010 update: a report from the American Heart Association. *Circulation*. 2010;121(7):e46–e215.
5. Taylor MR, Carniel E, Mestroni L. Cardiomyopathy, familial dilated. *Orphanet J Rare Dis*. 2006;1(1):27.
6. Dec G, Fuster V. Idiopathic dilated cardiomyopathy. *N Engl J Med*. 1994;331:1564–1575.
7. Codd MB, Sugrue DD, Gersh BJ, et al. Epidemiology of idiopathic dilated and hypertrophic cardiomyopathy. A population-based study in Olmsted County, Minnesota, 1975–1984. *Circulation*. 1989;80(3):564–572.
8. Hanson E, Hershberger RE. Genetic counseling and screening issues in familial dilated cardiomyopathy. *J Genet Counseling*. 2001;10(5):397–415.
9. Hershberger RE, Cowan J, Morales A, et al. Progress with genetic cardiomyopathies: screening, counseling, and testing in dilated, hypertrophic, and arrhythmogenic right ventricular dysplasia/ cardiomyopathy. *Circ Heart Fail*. 2009;2(3):253–261.
10. Rampersaud E, Siegfried JD, Norton N, et al. Rare variant mutations identified in pediatric patients with dilated cardiomyopathy. *Prog Pediatr Cardiol*. 2011;31(1): 39–47.
11. Morales A, Pinto JR, Siegfried J, et al. Late onset sporadic dilated cardiomyopathy caused by a cardiac troponin T mutation. *Clin Trans Sci*. 2010;3(5):219–226.
12. Hershberger RE, Cowan J, Morales A. *LMNA-Related Dilated Cardiomyopathy*. Seattle, WA: GeneTests/GeneClinics; June 17, 2008. http://www.genetests.org.
13. Morales A, Painter T, Li R, et al. Rare variant mutations in pregnancy-associated or peripartum cardiomyopathy. *Circulation*. 2010;121(20):2176–2182.
14. van Spaendonck-Zwarts KY, van Tintelen JP, van Veldhuisen DJ, et al. Peripartum cardiomyopathy as a part of familial dilated cardiomyopathy. *Circulation*. 2010;121(20):2169–2175.
15. Anderson JL, Horne BD. Birthing the genetics of peripartum cardiomyopathy. *Circulation*. 2010;121(20):2157–2159.
16. Hershberger RE, Siegfried JD. State of the Art Review. Update 2011: clinical and genetic issues in familial dilated cardiomyopathy. *J Am Coll Cardiol*. 2011;57(16):1641–1649.
17. Baig MK, Goldman JH, Caforio AP, et al. Familial dilated cardiomyopathy: cardiac abnormalities are common in asymptomatic relatives and may represent early disease. *J Am Coll Cardiol*. 1998;31(1):195–201.
18. Grunig E, Tasman JA, Kucherer H, et al. Frequency and phenotypes of familial dilated cardiomyopathy [see comments]. *J Am Coll Cardiol*. 1998;31(1):186–194.
19. Nussbaum RL, McInnes, R. R., Willard, H. F., *Thompson & Thompson Genetics in Medicine*. 6th ed. Philadelpha, PA: Elsevier; 2004.
20. Judge DP, Johnson NM. Genetic evaluation of familial cardiomyopathy. *J Cardiovasc Trans Res*. 2008;1:144–154.
21. Dellefave L, McNally EM. The genetics of dilated cardiomyopathy. *Curr Opin Cardiol*. 2010;25(3):198–204.
22. Kushner JD, Nauman D, Burgess D, et al. Clinical characteristics of 304 kindreds evaluated for familial dilated cardiomyopathy. *J Cardiac Failure*. 2006;12(6):422–429.
23. Hershberger RE, Kushner JK, Parks SP. *Dilated Cardiomyopathy Overview*. In: GeneReviews at GeneTests: Medical Genetics Information Resource [database online]. Seattle, WA: GeneTests/ GeneClinics; July 27, 2007. http://www.genetests.org. Accessed July 10, 2008.
24. Hershberger RE, Norton N, Morales A, et al. Coding sequence rare variants identified in MYBPC3, MYH6, TPM1, TNNC1, and TNNI3 from 312 patients with familial or idiopathic dilated cardiomyopathy. *Circ Cardiovasc Genet*. 2010;3(2):155–161.
25. Hershberger RE, Parks SB, Kushner JD, et al. Coding sequence mutations identified in MYH7, TNNT2, SCN5A, CSRP3, LBD3, and TCAP from 313 patients with familial or idiopathic dilated cardiomyopathy. *Clin Translational Science*. 2008;1(1):21–26.
26. Hershberger RE, Morales A, Siegfried JD. Clinical and genetic issues in dilated cardiomyopathy: A review for genetics professionals. *Genetics in Medicine*. 2010;12(11): 655–667.
27. Cowan J, Li D, Gonzalez-Quintana J, et al. Morphological analysis of 13 LMNA variants identified in a cohort of 324 unrelated patients with idiopathic or familial dilated cardiomyopathy. *Circ Cardiovasc Genet*. 2010;3(1):6–14.
28. Hershberger RE. A glimpse into multigene rare variant genetics: triple mutations in hypertrophic cardiomyopathy. *J Am Coll Cardiol*. 2010;55(14):1454–1455.
29. Richard P, Charron P, Carrier L, et al. Hypertrophic cardiomyopathy: distribution of disease genes, spectrum of mutations, and implications for a molecular diagnosis strategy. *Circulation*. 2003;107(17):2227–2232.
30. Van Driest SL, Vasile VC, Ommen SR, et al. Myosin binding protein C mutations and compound heterozygosity in hypertrophic cardiomyopathy. *J Am Coll Cardiol*. 2004;44(9):1903–1910.
31. Sen-Chowdhry S, Syrris P, Ward D, et al. Clinical and genetic characterization of families with arrhythmogenic right ventricular dysplasia/cardiomyopathy provides novel insights into patterns of disease expression. *Circulation*. 2007;115(13):1710–1720.
32. Keating MT, Sanguinetti MC. Molecular and cellular mechanisms of cardiac arrhythmias. *Cell*. 2001;104(4):569–580.
33. Westenskow P, Splawski I, Timothy KW, et al. Compound mutations: a common cause of severe long-QT syndrome. *Circulation*. 2004;109(15):1834–1841.
34. Schwartz PJ, Priori SG, Napolitano C. How really rare are rare diseases? The intriguing case of independent compound mutations in the long QT syndrome. *J Cardiovasc Electrophysiol*. 2003;14(10):1120–1121.
35. Li D, Morales A, Gonzalez Quintana J, et al. Identification of novel mutations in RBM20 in patients with dilated cardiomyopathy. *Clin Trans Sci*. 2010;3(3):90–97.
36. Hershberger RE, Lindenfeld J, Mestroni L, et al. Genetic evaluation of cardiomyopathy--a Heart Failure Society of America practice guideline. *J Card Fail*. 2009;15(2):83–97.
37. Ackerman MJ, Priori SG, Willems S, et al. HRS/EHRA expert consensus statement on the state of genetic testing for the channelopathies and cardiomyopathies. This document was developed as a partnership between the Heart Rhythm Society (HRS) and the European Heart Rhythm Association (EHRA). *Heart Rhythm*. 2011;8(8):1308–1339.
38. Burkett EL, Hershberger RE. Clinical and genetic issues in familial dilated cardiomyopathy. *J Am Coll Cardiol*. 2005;45(7):969–981.

39. Cowan J, Morales A, Dagua J, et al. Genetic testing and genetic counseling in cardiovascular genetic medicine: overview and preliminary recommendations. *Congest Heart Fail.* 2008;14(2): 97–105.
40. Morales A, Cowan J, Dagua J, et al. Family history: an essential tool for cardiovascular genetic medicine. *Congest Heart Fail.* 2008;14(1):37–45.
41. Nauman D, Morales A, Cowan J, et al. The family history as a tool to identify patients at risk for dilated cardiomyopathy. *Prog Cardiovasc Nurs.* 2008;23(1):41–44.
42. Murphy RT, Mogensen J, Shaw A, et al. Novel mutation in cardiac troponin I in recessive idiopathic dilated cardiomyopathy. *Lancet.* 2004;363(9406):371–372.
43. Seliem MA, Mansara KB, Palileo M, et al. Evidence for autosomal recessive inheritance of infantile dilated cardiomyopathy: studies from the Eastern Province of Saudi Arabia. *Pediatr Res.* 2000;48(6):770–775.
44. Capell BC, Collins FS. Human laminopathies: nuclei gone genetically awry. *Nat Rev Genet.* 2006;7(12):940–952.
45. Fatkin D, MacRae C, Sasaki T, et al. Missense mutations in the rod domain of the lamin A/C gene as causes of dilated cardiomyopathy and conduction-system disease. *N Engl J Med.* 1999;341(23):1715–1724.
46. Brodsky GL, Muntoni F, Miocic S, et al. Lamin A/C gene mutation associated with dilated cardiomyopathy with variable skeletal muscle involvement. *Circulation.* 2000;101(5):473–476.
47. Becane HM, Bonne G, Varnous S, et al. High incidence of sudden death with conduction system and myocardial disease due to lamins A and C gene mutation. *Pacing Clin Electrophysiol.* 2000;23(11 Pt 1):1661–1666.
48. Jakobs PM, Hanson E, Crispell KA, et al. Novel lamin A/C mutations in two families with dilated cardiomyopathy and conduction system disease. *J Card Fail.* 2001;7(3):249–256.
49. Hershberger RE, Hanson E, Jakobs PM, et al. A novel lamin A/C mutation in a family with dilated cardiomyopathy, prominent conduction system disease, and need for permanent pacemaker implantation. *Am Heart J.* 2002;144(6):1081–1086.
50. Arbustini E, Pilotto A, Repetto A, et al. Autosomal dominant dilated cardiomyopathy with atrioventricular block: a lamin A/C defect-related disease. *J Am Coll Cardiol.* 2002;39(6):981–990.
51. Richards CS, Bale S, Bellissimo DB, et al. ACMG recommendations for standards for interpretation and reporting of sequence variations: revisions 2007. *Genet Med.* 2008;10(4):294–300.
52. Jessup M, Abraham WT, Casey DE, et al. 2009 focused update: ACCF/AHA Guidelines for the Diagnosis and Management of Heart Failure in Adults: a report of the American College of Cardiology Foundation/American Heart Association Task Force on Practice Guidelines: developed in collaboration with the International Society for Heart and Lung Transplantation. *Circulation.* 2009;119(14):1977–2016.
53. Hershberger RE, Hedges D, Morales, A. Dilated cardiomyopathy: the complexity of a diverse genetic architecture. *Nature Reviews.* 2013;10(9):531–547.
54. Herman DS, Lam L, Taylor MR, Wang L, Teekakirikul P, Christodoulou D, et al. Truncations of titin causing dilated cardiomyopathy. *N Engl J Med.* 2012;366:619–628.
55. Lakdawala NK, Funke BH, Baxter S, Cirino AL, Roberts AE, Judge DP, et al. Genetic testing for dilated cardiomyopathy in clinical practice. *J Card Fail.* 2012;18:296–303.

19

The Role of Risk Modeling in Heart Failure

ERIC S. KETCHUM AND WAYNE C. LEVY

CASE PRESENTATION

A 65-year-old male presents to his internal medicine clinic with lower extremity swelling and reduced functional capacity. He experiences heaviness in his chest with walking a mile at more than a moderate pace. He has had a long-standing history of poorly controlled hypertension and diabetes mellitus (DM). Workup leads to a new diagnosis of heart failure without evidence of ischemic contribution. His echocardiogram shows an ejection fraction (EF) of 40%. With the exception of a mild anemia (hemoglobin of 12) and a systolic blood pressure (SBP) of 150 despite being on 10 mg a day of amlodipine, his vital signs and laboratory studies are within normal limits. How does the diagnosis of heart failure affect this patient's expected survival? What aspects of his clinical picture are most reflective of his prognosis? How predictive are these features of his prognosis? What effect will initiating evidence-based heart failure therapies have on his survival?

PREDICTING SURVIVAL

The accuracy of patients and physicians in predicting survival in patients with heart failure has often been underwhelming, especially in patients with more advanced stages of heart failure. Physicians can be over-influenced by powerful anecdotes and memorable previous patient encounters in assessing patient prognosis (1). In a study of the use of pulmonary artery catheters in decompensated heart failure, both physicians and nurses assigned a probability of 1-year mortality of 60% to 70% to a cohort of patients whose actual 1-year mortality ended up 20% to 30% (2). Patients presenting to a heart failure clinic overestimated their expected life expectancy by an average of 40%, with the New York Heart Association (NYHA) I symptomology patients predicting the same life expectancy for themselves as the NYHA IV symptomology patients (3). This inaccuracy of prediction by holistic assessment alone is one argument for the use of objective, well-validated risk scores.

Many aspects of a patient's clinical presentation have at least some value in determination of expected morbidity and mortality. Examples of validated univariate predictors are listed in **Table 19-1**. These individual predictors can be combined via logistic regression or Cox proportional hazards modeling to generate multivariate models of risk. To assess prognosis in heart failure, models have used multiple variables that are associated with clinical history (age, gender, etiology of heart failure), vital signs, left ventricular function (left ventricular size, EF), exercise capacity (NYHA class, 6-minute walk distance, peak oxygen consumption, ventilatory efficiency), signs and symptoms of heart failure (rales, edema, elevated jugular venous pressure, or NYHA class), and laboratory values that may reflect dysregulation of the sympathetic nervous system, the renin–angiotensin–aldosterone system, cytokines, or other neurohormones.

Table 19-1
Predictors of Risk in Heart Failure

Patient History
Age
Gender
Comorbidities
Heart failure etiology
Physical Exam
Blood pressure
Heart rate and heart rate variability
Body mass index
Rales, elevated jugular venous pulsation, edema, S3 heart sound
Evaluation of Cardiac Structure and Function
Cardiomegaly on chest x-ray
Conduction delay and arrhythmias on EKG
Left ventricular ejection fraction
Right ventricular function
Chamber sizes
Valvular stenosis or regurgitation
Diastolic dysfunction (restrictive filling patterns)
Functional Capacity
NYHA class
Oxygen consumption with maximal exertion (peak VO_2)
Ventilatory efficiency (VE/VCO_2)
6-minute walk test
Serum Laboratory Markers
Cholesterol
Sodium
Hemoglobin
% Lymphocytes or % neutrophils
Uric acid
Creatinine, blood urea nitrogen, glomerular filtration rate
Albumin
Total bilirubin
Red cell distributaion width
Neurohormonal Dysregulation, Inflammation, and the Cardiac Stretch Response
BNP and NT-proBNP
Cardiac-specific troponin subtypes
C-reactive protein, tumor necrosis factor-α, interleukin-6
ST2, Galectin 3
Plasma metanephrines, renin, aldosterone
Metaiodobenzylguanidine cardiac imaging
Medical and Procedural Interventions
Evidence-based pharmacotherapy (ACE inhibitors, ARBs, beta-blockers, aldosterone blockers)
Dose of diuretic required to maintain euvolemia
Implantable cardiac defibrillator and cardiac resynchronization therapy
Ventricular assist devices and transplantation

Note: ARB = angiotensin receptor blocker; ACE = angiotensin-converting enzyme; BNP = B-type natriuretic peptide; NT-proBNP = N-terminal pro-brain natriuretic peptide; NYHA = New York Heart Association.

There is great variability in how predictive individual features are and to what extent they add information independently of other markers. Measuring the prognostic efficacy of an individual biomarker or lab parameter can be as simple as calculating a relative risk or odds ratio for patients above versus below a certain cut-point. The area under the receiver operator characteristic curve (AUC)—a measure of the sensitivity and specificity of a particular value for separating subjects into those who will live and those who will die during the period of observation—can be used to assess the efficacy of either individual predictors or of multivariate models. An AUC of 0.5 indicates no predictive power, while an AUC of 1 indicates perfect separation of survivors and nonsurvivors. Using the simple combination of age and gender, the Framingham Offspring Study was able to achieve an AUC of 0.75 for prediction of mortality in the general population (4). For a heart failure-specific population, age and gender are much less powerful predictors of outcome (5). As such, more sophisticated models are needed to accurately predict survival in the heart failure population. When looking at regression models or newer biomarkers, the integrated discrimination improvement or net reclassification improvement—how much adding a new risk marker to an existing schema changes a patient's pretest probability of adverse events during the observation period—can be used to aid in assessment (6).

THE SEATTLE HEART FAILURE MODEL

To return to the patient presented in the opening vignette, the Seattle Heart Failure Model (SHFM) is a well-validated tool for assessing his prognosis. The SHFM was derived in the Prospective Randomized Amlodipine Survival Evaluation (PRAISE 1) trial of amlodipine in patients with advanced heart failure (7). The model includes age, gender, EF, SBP, weight, and NYHA class. Proxies for neurohormonal activation and inflammation are included via the commonly collected laboratory biomarkers sodium, hemoglobin, percent lymphocytes, uric acid, and total cholesterol. Weight-adjusted diuretic daily dose required to maintain euvolemia is a powerful predictor of heart failure mortality, as shown in **Figure 19-1**, and is included in the SHFM. The SHFM was prospectively validated in 9,923 patients across several clinical trials, including Evaluation of Losartan in the Elderly (ELITE II), Valsartan Heart Failure Trial (Val-HeFT), Randomised Etanercept North AmerIcan Strategy to Study Antagonism of CytokinEs (RENAISSANCE), an Italian heart failure registry (real-world heart failure patients in Italian cardiology practices), and the University of Washington heart failure clinic (a younger patient population referred for transplant and left ventricular assist device [LVAD] evaluation). A subsequent validation in 4,077

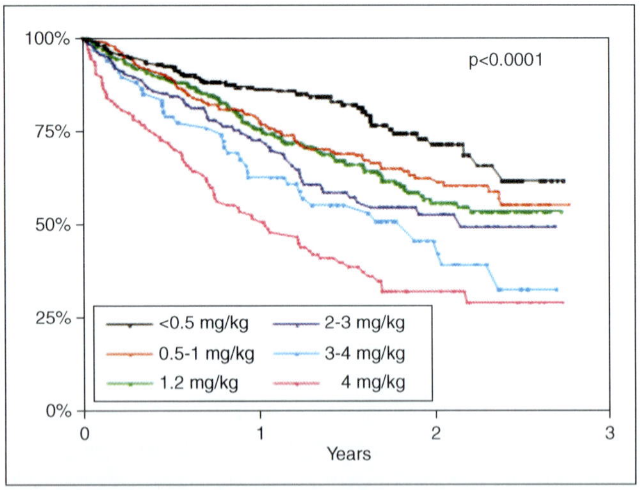

Figure 19-1
The impact of diuretic dosing on survival in heart failure is shown in this graphic depicting Kaplan–Meier survival curves for weight-adjusted daily doses of furosemide in NYHA IIIB/4 patients with EF ≤30%.

Note: EF = ejection fraction.

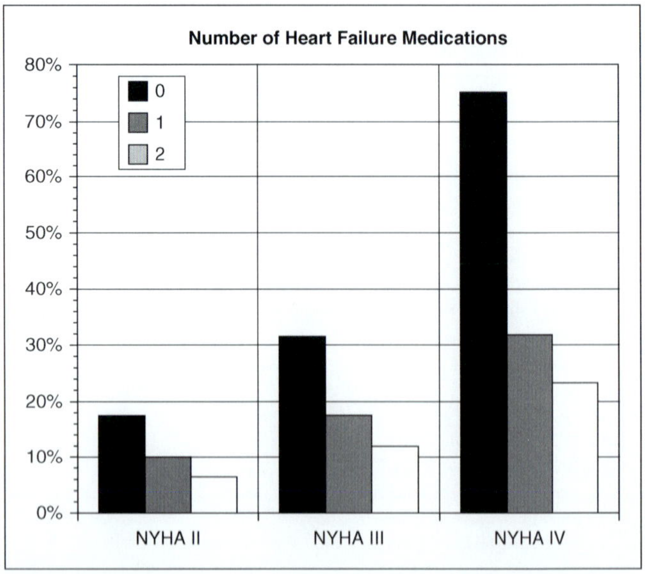

Figure 19-2
The impact of placing a patient on heart failure therapies is shown in this chart of survival by NYHA symptomology based on number of evidence-based medications tolerated.

community-based heart failure patients from 18 hospitals in Utah participating in the Intermountain Heart Collaborative Study Registry confirmed high correlation between SHFM predicted and actual survival (8). The validation receiver operating characteristic (ROC) varied from 0.68 to 0.81 in these diverse populations with the absolute estimate of mortality very close to the line of identity and an overall AUC of 0.73.

Use of evidence-based heart failure medications is associated with a marked reduction in mortality in patients with heart failure. **Figure 19-2** shows that the addition of one evidence-based heart failure therapy has about the same effect on mortality as having one category lower of NYHA symptomology. The SHFM includes the effects of angiotensin converting enzyme (ACE) inhibitors, angiotensin receptor blockers (ARBs), aldosterone blockers, beta-blockers, statins, and devices such as an implantable cardiac defibrillator (ICD) or cardiac resynchronization therapy with or without defibrillator (CRT or CRT-D; 7). An online calculator is available at http://seattleheartfailuremodel.org. A screenshot of the application with values plugged in for the patient presented in the opening vignette is depicted in **Figure 19-3**. For this patient with early-stage heart failure and not much evidence of laboratory or vital sign anomaly, we see that his life expectancy of 8.6 years is moderately reduced as compared to someone of the same age without heart failure. We also see that initiating evidence-based pharmacotherapy with an ACE inhibitor and a beta-blocker can provide him a life expectancy comparable to that based on his age of 12.5 years.

CASE PRESENTATION

Consider a more advanced heart failure patient. A 59-year-old female presenting with dyspnea on more than mild exertion is referred to a heart failure clinic. She has non-ischemic cardiomyopathy with an EF of 20%, blood pressure (BP) 86/58 mmHg, heart rate 95 beats/minute. She weighs 60 kg and is intolerant of beta-blocker therapy and aldosterone blockade. She has an ICD in place and evidence of intraventricular conduction delay on the electrocardiogram (ECG). Medications include torsemide 120 mg daily, enalapril 5 mg twice daily, allopurinol 300 mg daily, and digoxin 0.125 mg daily. Laboratory values include hemoglobin of 13 g/dL, a differential with 20% lymphocytes, uric acid of 8.0 mg/dL, total cholesterol of 160 mg/dL, and sodium of 134 mEq/L. Her inability to perform a cardiopulmonary exercise test suggests a peak exercise oxygen consumption (peak VO_2) less than 10 mL/kg/min. What is her risk of death? What advanced heart failure therapies should she be offered?

ADVANCED HEART FAILURE PROGNOSIS

Choosing to list for heart transplantation can be fairly straightforward in patients dependent on IV inotropic support or intra-aortic balloon pump for cardiogenic shock. However, there are many ambulatory patients with advanced symptoms in whom there is ambiguity as to appropriateness of listing for cardiac transplantation (9). A scoring system that was developed explicitly for this patient population

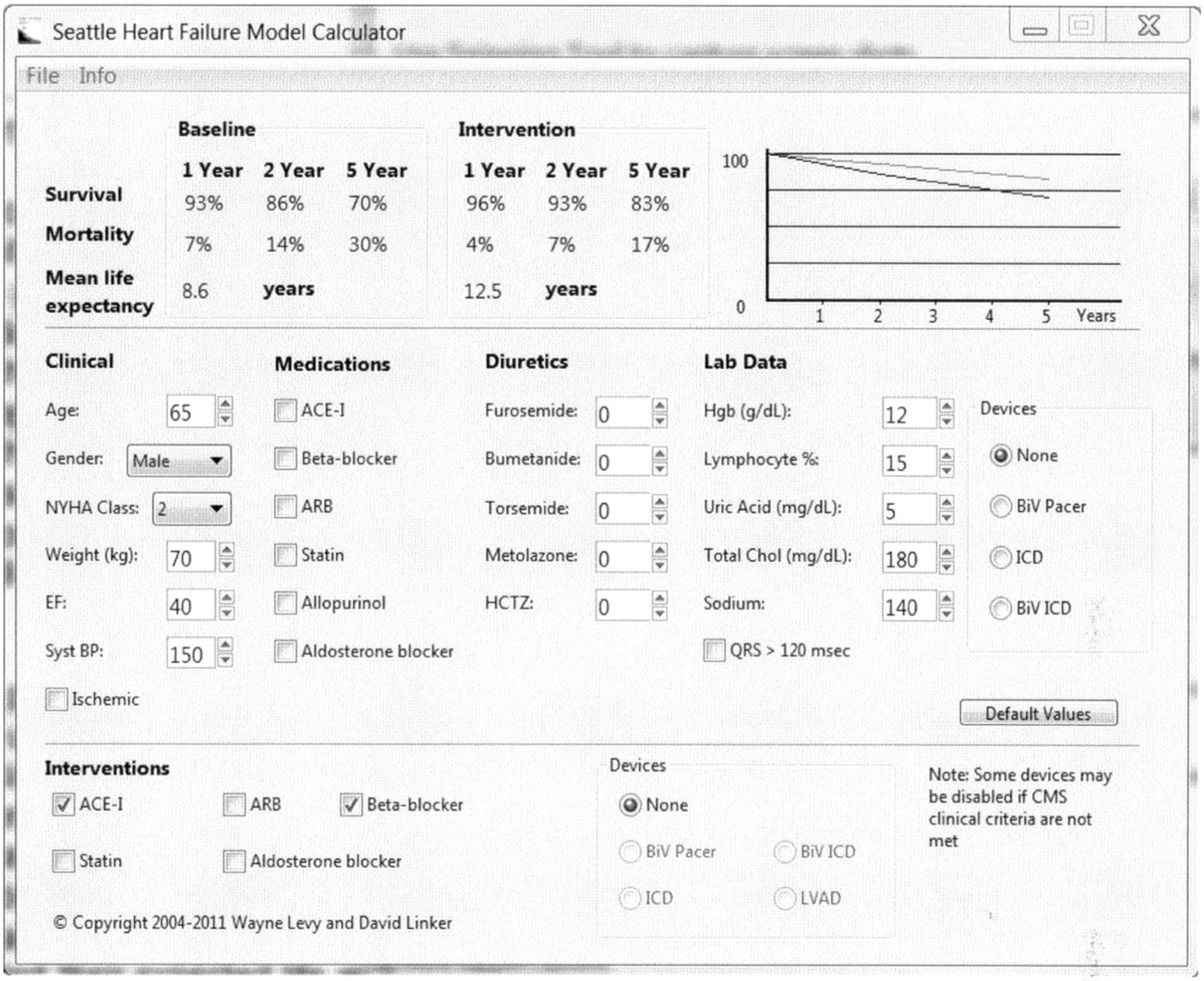

Figure 19-3
Clinical data for the patient presented in the opening clinical vignette is depicted in this screenshot of the windows application to calculate the Seattle Heart Failure Model risk score (available at http://seattleheartfailuremodel.org; 27).

is the Heart Failure Survival Score (HFSS). Its original description included an invasive version, requiring a mean pulmonary capillary wedge pressure (PCWP) for calculation, and a simpler, noninvasive version that did not (10). Given similar predictive power with either model, the noninvasive model entered uses as a more accurate tool than peak VO_2 alone in identifying candidates for cardiac transplantation. The HFSS is calculated as a sum of seven individual factors: -0.6931 if patient has ischemic cardiomyopathy; -0.6083 if patient has intraventricular conduction delay; -0.0216 × resting heart rate in beats/minute; + 0.0464 × left ventricular ejection fraction (LVEF) in percentage; + 0.0255 × mean blood pressure in millimeters of mercury; + 0.0546 × peak VO_2 in mL/kg/min; and + 0.0470 × serum sodium in mmol/L. Scores less than 7.2 are considered high risk, 8.1 or above are low risk, and values in between are of intermediate risk. One-year survival in the original validation cohort was 88%, 60%, and 35% in the low-risk, medium-risk, and high-risk groups. Survival for advanced heart failure patients has improved significantly since the original publication, with a recent validation suggesting 89%, 72%, and 60% 1-year survival for patients in the low-risk, medium-risk, and high-risk groups (11). Her HFSS of 7.2 places her just at the transition to the high-risk group.

The SHFM has been shown to be of value in advanced heart failure patients like this one, including in predicting mortality in patients presenting to a transplantation clinic (12) and in prediction of outcomes after placement of an LVAD (13,14). The SHFM suggests an annual mortality of 41% with a life expectancy of 1.9 years. With the most recent data demonstrating a median survival of over 10 years after cardiac transplantation (15), both the HFSS and the SHFM suggest this patient is high risk enough to benefit from listing for cardiac transplantation. One recent suggestion has been an SHFM 1-year mortality of greater than or equal to 20% as a clear indication for listing for heart transplantation, 10% to 20% as a borderline indication, and less than 10% as suggestive of deferral of listing (9). LVADs have seen rapidly increasing use in the last decade as either a bridge to transplantation or as destination therapy for patients with contraindications to or disinterest in transplantation (16). Her predicted mortality is high enough to benefit from evaluation for LVAD, with current Medicare criteria for LVAD implantation including a predicted 2-year mortality greater than 50% and current American College of Cardiology/American Heart Association (ACC/AHA) guidelines suggesting expected 1-year mortality greater than 50% (17). A trial is currently underway investigating the placement of LVADs in less ill patients meeting an overall annual mortality threshold in the 30% range, which will require a SHFM estimated survival of less than or equal to 16.5% for trial entry (18). This patient is right at the cusp of serious consideration for implantation of a LVAD, but certainly should be considered for listing for cardiac transplantation.

CASE PRESENTATION

A third patient with heart failure thought to be due to ischemic cardiomyopathy is admitted to the hospital. She is 63 years old and has been experiencing progressive fatigue, weight gain, and difficulty breathing over the few weeks prior to presentation. She has a history of moderate chronic obstructive pulmonary disease and a mild stroke 5 years prior to presentation. Her shortness of breath now occurs at rest. She is tachycardic at 105 beats/minute, tachypneic at 35 breaths/minute, hypotensive at 85/50, and weighs 70 kg. She ran out of her beta-blocker 3 weeks prior to presentation, but has been taking her ACE inhibitor and digoxin daily. She doubled her 100 mg of daily furosemide in an attempt to reduce the increased swelling in her legs. Her EF on echocardiogram conducted in the emergency department has declined to 15%. She has multiple lab abnormalities, including a creatinine of 1.8 mg/dL, blood urea nitrogen (BUN) of 53 mg/dL, sodium of 133 mEq/L, and B-type natriuretic peptide (BNP) of 1,100 pg/mmol. Other laboratory values include a differential showing 15% lymphocytes, hemoglobin of 11 g/dL, total cholesterol of 140 mg/dL, and uric acid of 9 mg/dL. Her ACE inhibitor is discontinued on the basis of her acute kidney injury and hypotension. She requires mechanical ventilation and IV inotropic support during her hospital stay, but ultimately shows enough improvement with medical therapy to be discharged from the hospital without IV pharmacologic support. At discharge, she is able to tolerate an ACE inhibitor and an aldosterone blocker with a blood pressure of 90/60. Her BNP has declined to 480 pg/mmol and her BUN to 25 mg/dL. She can complete a lap around the hospital floor in about 5 minutes. She requires 100 mg a day of furosemide to maintain euvolemia at a weight of 60 kg. Her differential now shows 25% lymphocytes.

She follows up in clinic 3 months later with symptoms not occurring until walking several blocks. She is able to tolerate a beta-blocker, an ACE inhibitor, and an aldosterone blocker. She is taking furosemide 80 mg daily and daily digoxin. Her BP is 100/70 mmHg, heart rate is 60 beats/minute, and her EF has improved to 25%. She has a left bundle branch block (LBBB) with a QRS of 160 ms. Notable changes to her laboratory values include hemoglobin of 12.9 g/dL, sodium of 139 mEq/L, and creatinine of 0.9 mg/dL. She has not performed a cardiopulmonary exercise test but you estimate that her peak VO_2 is greater than 14 mL/kg/min. What is her risk of mortality in the hospital, at discharge, and at her outpatient follow-up visit? What additional multivariate models are available that could aid in prognostication at different points in her presentation?

HEART FAILURE SCORING SYSTEMS

There have been dozens of heart failure scoring systems published in the literature over the last two decades (19), but only a few have achieved validation in external data sets and widespread use. Several validated models have been developed specifically for patients in the inpatient setting. **Table 19-2** compares the individual variables included in the models discussed in this chapter. The Enhanced Feedback for Effective Cardiac Treatment (EFFECT) score offers predictions of 30-day and 1-year mortality in hospital inpatients (20). Its calculation is depicted in **Table 19-3**. A notable inclusion in this model is the effect of comorbidities, such as cerebrovascular accident, cancer, and lung or liver disease, on survival. On presentation to the hospital, her EFFECT score of 151 for 30-day mortality and 161 for 1-year mortality places her into the very high-risk group, suggesting mortality in the range of 50% to 60% at 30 days and 75% to 80% at 1 year. The Acute Decompensated Heart Failure Registry (ADHERE) risk model includes both a logistic regression based formula and a recursive partitioning derived tree model to calculate risk of in-hospital mortality (21). Looking at the simplified tree model depicted in **Figure 19-4**, she falls into the intermediate risk group, suggesting a risk of in-hospital mortality of 12.5%. Although the tree model is easy to calculate, it is notable that the only way a patient can end up in the high-risk group is if he or she has

Table 19-2
A Comparison of the Individual Variables Required for Calculating Risk Scores Is Shown for the Various Models Presented in This Chapter

PREDICTIVE VARIABLE	HFSS	EFFECT	ADHERE LR	ADHERE TREE	ESCAPE	SHFM
Age		✓	✓		✓	✓
Gender						✓
Vital signs	SBP heart rate in beats/minute	SBP RR	SBP heart rate in beats/minute	SBP		Weight SBP
Diagnostic tests	LVEF					LVEF
	BBB					
	Peak VO_2					
Ischemic etiology	✓					✓
Comorbidities		✓				
CPR or ventilator					✓	
HF signs/symptoms					✓	✓
Labs	Sodium	Sodium	BUN	BUN	Sodium	Sodium Hemoglobin Lymphocytes
		BUN Hemoglobin		Creatinine	BUN BNP	Uric acid Cholesterol
HF medications					✓	✓
Devices (ICD, CRT)						✓
Output	Risk groups for 1-year event-free survival	Risk groups for 30-day and 1-year mortality	Risk groups for in-hospital mortality	Risk groups for in-hospital mortality	Risk groups for 6-month mortality after discharge	1- to 5-year survival and life expectancy

Note: BBB = bundle branch block; BNP = B-type natriuretic peptide; BUN = blood urea nitrogen; LVEF = left ventricular ejection fraction; Peak VO_2 = peak consumption of oxygen; RR = respiratory rate in breaths/minute; SBP = systolic blood pressure in mmHg.

Table 19-3
A Depiction of the Calculation of the Effect Model's 30-Day and 1-Year Mortality Risk for Inpatients (20)

PARAMETER	30-DAY SCORE	1-YEAR SCORE
Age	+1/year	+1/year
Respiratory rate (min 20; max 45)	+ # breaths/min	+# breaths/min
Systolic blood pressure		
< 90 mmHg	–30	–20
90–99 mmHg	–35	–25
100–119 mmHg	–40	–30
120–139 mmHg	–45	–35
140–159 mmHg	–50	–40
160–179 mmHg	–55	–45
> 179 mmHg	–60	–50

(Continued)

Table 19-3 *(Continued)*
A Depiction of the Calculation of the Effect Model's 30-Day and 1-Year Mortality Risk for Inpatients (20)

PARAMETER	30-DAY SCORE	1-YEAR SCORE
Blood urea nitrogen (up to 60)	+1/mg/dL	+1/mg/dL
Hemoglobin <10 g/dL	+0	+10
Serum sodium <136 mEq/L	+10	+10
Cerebrovascular disease	+10	+10
COPD	+10	+10
Cancer	+15	+15
Dementia	+20	+20
Hepatic cirrhosis	+25	+35

RISK SCORE	RISK STRATA	30-DAY MORTALITY	1-YEAR MORTALITY
< 61	Very low	0.4%–0.6%	2.7%–7.8%
61–90	Low	3.4%–4.2%	12.9%–14.4%
91–120	Intermediate	12.2%–13.7%	30.2%–32.5%
121–150	High	26%–32.7%	55.5%–59.3%
> 150	Very high	50%–59%	74.7%–78.8%

Note: The top portion shows the calculation of the score, while the bottom shows the division into five risk strata, with mortality ranges listed for the derivation and validation cohorts within each stratum. An online calculator is available at http://www.ccort.ca/CHFriskmodel.asp.

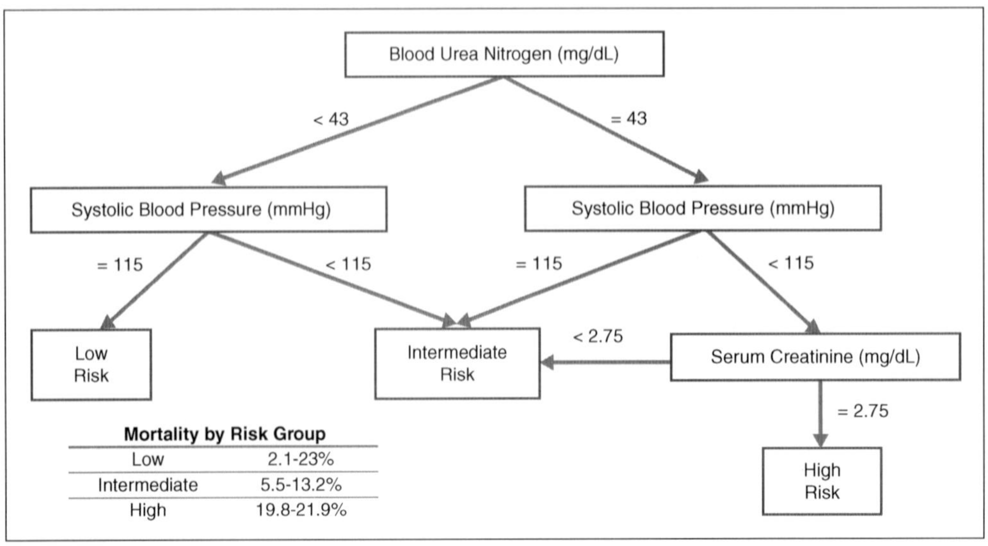

Figure 19-4
A depiction of the ADHERE tree model for calculation of in-hospital mortality (21). The range of risk predictions is based on the derivation and validation cohorts, with the original paper providing additional stratification within the intermediate risk group.

evidence of advanced renal dysfunction. Calculating her risk via the ADHERE logistic regression model, she does end up in a high-risk strata. The Evaluation Study of Congestive Heart Failure and Pulmonary Artery Catheterization Effectiveness (ESCAPE-HF) model was developed as a discharge model to predict 6-month mortality in patients receiving Swan-Ganz catheterization for management of acutely decompensated heart failure (22). A version with simplified risk categories is depicted in **Table 19-4**. Her clinical

Table 19-4
A Depiction of the Calculation of the ESCAPE-HF Discharge Score (22)

DISCHARGE PARAMETER	ADD IF TRUE
Age > 70 years	+1
BUN 40–90 mg/dL	+1
BUN > 90 mg/dL	+2
BNP 500–1,300 pg/mmol	+1
BNP >1,300 pg/mmol	+4
Serum sodium <130 mEq/L	+1
6-minute walk <300 feet	+1
Required CPR/ventilator	+2
Diuretic dose >240 mg	+1
No beta-blocker on discharge	+1
RISK SCORE	**6-MONTH MORTALITY**
0	7.7%
1–2	10.4%–16.7%
3–4	26.4%–44.8%
> 4	75%–100%

Note: The factors are summed together to divide patients into risk scores at the bottom, which have been pooled in this table into a smaller number of strata. Although the highest possible score is 13, only six of the 423 patients in the original study had a risk score > 5.

data at discharge gives her a score of 3, suggesting a 6-month mortality of 26.4%.

The SHFM has been shown to have value at multiple points in the patient evaluation process and has several applications to treatment planning. Although originally developed for outpatients, the SHFM has been shown to have predictive efficacy in the inpatient setting when compared against several other risk models (23). Its prediction of 79% 1-year mortality at the time of admission to the hospital suggests a very high-risk category comparable to that suggested by the EFFECT score. Her predicted 1-year mortality of 43% at time of discharge is comparable to that suggested by her ESCAPE-HF 6-month risk. A potential area of value of the SHFM in the discharge period is its ability to model the effects of devices and medications on outcomes. Intensification and optimization of medical therapy for heart failure was shown to occur in a pilot study of integration of risk modeling into patient–physician discussions (24). Selection of candidates for device therapy has been affected by several studies demonstrating a high-risk cohort of patients who do not benefit from placement of an ICD despite meeting current ACC/AHA criteria for implantation (25). Patients with a SHFM annual mortality of approximately 20% were shown in the Sudden Cardiac Death in Heart Failure (SCD-HeFT) trial to have no improvement in survival after placement of an ICD (26). Using the SHFM score, her annual mortality is 13% with a life expectancy of 5.7 years, while her HFSS of 8.46 would place her in the low-risk group. Thus, having survived her acute decompensation and further improved in the outpatient setting on appropriate heart failure medications, her mortality has markedly decreased. She is in the lower risk group of patients in SCD-HeFT and should benefit from a primary prevention ICD with CRT. The SHFM suggests that placement of a CRT-D would reduce her mortality further to 9% annually with an increase in her expected survival to 7.5 years.

In summary, there are many heart failure risk models with varying types of output for the specific clinical endpoint being prognosticated. The SHFM stands out for having been shown to be predictive and accurate in a variety of clinical settings and is probably the most useful, widely applicable single risk model.

REFERENCES

1. Hanratty B, Hibbert D, Mair F, et al. Doctors' perceptions of palliative care for heart failure: focus group study. *BMJ*. 2002;325(7364):581–585.
2. Yamokoski LM, Hasselblad V, Moser DK, et al. Prediction of rehospitalization and death in severe heart failure by physicians and nurses of the ESCAPE trial. *J Card Fail*. 2007;13(1):8–13.
3. Allen LA, Yager JE, Funk MJ, et al. Discordance between patient-predicted and model-predicted life expectancy among ambulatory patients with heart failure. *JAMA*. 2008;299(21):2533–2542.
4. Wang TJ, Gona P, Larson MG, et al. Multiple biomarkers for the prediction of first major cardiovascular events and death. *N Engl J Med*. 2006;355(25):2631–2639.
5. Rector TS, Ringwala SN, Ringwala SN, Anand IS. Validation of a risk score for dying within 1 year of an admission for heart failure. *J Card Fail*. 2006;12(4):276–280.
6. Pencina MJ, D'Agostino RB Sr, D'Agostino RB Jr, Vasan RS. Evaluating the added predictive ability of a new marker: from area under the ROC curve to reclassification and beyond. *Stat Med*. 2008;27(2):157–72; discussion 207.
7. Levy WC, Mozaffarian D, Linker DT, et al. The Seattle Heart Failure Model: prediction of survival in heart failure. *Circulation*. 2006;113(11):1424–1433.
8. May HT, Horne BD, Levy WC, et al. Validation of the Seattle Heart Failure Model in a community-based heart failure population and enhancement by adding B-type natriuretic peptide. *Am J Cardiol*. 2007;100(4):697–700.
9. Mancini D, Lietz K. Selection of cardiac transplantation candidates in 2010. *Circulation*. 2010;122(2):173–183.
10. Aaronson KD, Schwartz JS, Chen TM, Wong KL, Goin JE, Mancini DM. Development and prospective validation of a clinical index to predict survival in ambulatory patients referred for cardiac transplant evaluation. *Circulation*. 1997;95(12):2660–2667.
11. Goda A, Lund LH, Mancini D. The Heart Failure Survival Score outperforms the peak oxygen consumption for heart transplantation selection in the era of device therapy. *J Heart Lung Transplant*. 2011;30(3):315–325.
12. Kalogeropoulos AP, Georgiopoulou VV, Giamouzis G, et al. Utility of the Seattle Heart Failure Model in patients with advanced heart failure. *J Am Coll Cardiol*. 2009;53(4):334–342.
13. Ketchum ES, Moorman AJ, Fishbein DP, et al. Predictive value of the Seattle Heart Failure Model in patients undergoing left ventricular assist device placement. *J Heart Lung Transplant*. 2010;29(9):1021–1025.
14. Levy WC, Mozaffarian D, Linker DT, Farrar DJ, Miller LW; REMATCH Investigators. Can the Seattle heart failure model be used to risk-stratify heart failure patients for potential left ventricular assist device therapy? *J Heart Lung Transplant*. 2009;28(3):231–236.
15. Taylor DO, Stehlik J, Edwards LB, et al. Registry of the International Society for Heart and Lung Transplantation: Twenty-sixth Official Adult Heart Transplant Report-2009. *J Heart Lung Transplant*. 2009;28(10):1007–1022.
16. Kirklin JK, Naftel DC, Kormos RL, et al. Third INTERMACS Annual Report: the evolution of destination therapy in the United States. *J Heart Lung Transplant*. 2011;30(2):115–123.
17. Hunt SA, Abraham WT, Chin MH, et al. 2009 focused update incorporated into the ACC/AHA 2005 Guidelines for the Diagnosis and Management of Heart Failure in Adults: a report of the American College of Cardiology Foundation/American Heart Association Task Force on Practice Guidelines: developed in collaboration with the International Society for Heart and Lung Transplantation. *Circulation*. 2009;119(14):e391–e479.
18. Baldwin JT, Mann DL. NHLBI's program for VAD therapy for moderately advanced heart failure: the REVIVE-IT pilot trial. *J Card Fail*. 2010;16(11):855–858.
19. Bouvy ML, Heerdink ER, Leufkens HG, Hoes AW. Predicting mortality in patients with heart failure: a pragmatic approach. *Heart*. 2003;89(6):605–609.
20. Lee DS, Austin PC, Rouleau JL, Liu PP, Naimark D, Tu JV. Predicting mortality among patients hospitalized for heart failure: derivation and validation of a clinical model. *JAMA*. 2003;290(19):2581–2587.
21. Fonarow GC, Adams KF Jr, Abraham WT, Yancy CW, Boscardin WJ; ADHERE Scientific Advisory Committee, Study Group, and Investigators. Risk stratification for in-hospital mortality in acutely decompensated heart failure: classification and regression tree analysis. *JAMA*. 2005;293(5):572–580.
22. O'Connor CM, Hasselblad V, Mehta RH, et al. Triage after hospitalization with advanced heart failure: the ESCAPE (Evaluation Study of Congestive Heart Failure and Pulmonary Artery Catheterization Effectiveness) risk model and discharge score. *J Am Coll Cardiol*. 2010;55(9):872–878.
23. Nakayama M, Osaki S, Shimokawa H. Validation of mortality risk stratification models for cardiovascular disease. *Am J Cardiol*. 2011;108(3):391–396.
24. Prasad H, Sra J, Levy WC, Stapleton DD. Influence of predictive modeling in implementing optimal heart failure therapy. *Am J Med Sci*. 2011;341(3):185–190.
25. Goldenberg I, Vyas AK, Hall WJ, et al. MADIT-II Investigators. Risk stratification for primary implantation of a cardioverter-defibrillator in patients with ischemic left ventricular dysfunction. *J Am Coll Cardiol*. 2008;51(3):288–296.
26. Levy WC, Lee KL, Hellkamp AS, et al. Maximizing survival benefit with primary prevention implantable cardioverter-defibrillator therapy in a heart failure population. *Circulation*. 2009;120(10):835–842.
27. Mozaffarian D, Anker SD, Anand I, et al. Prediction of mode of death in heart failure: the Seattle Heart Failure Model. *Circulation*. 2007;116(4):392–398.

Index